Principles of Radiographic Imaging

An Art and a Science

4th Edition

Principles of Radiographic Imaging
An Art and a Science
4th Edition

Richard R. Carlton, M.S., R.T.(R)(CV), FAERS
Director of Radiologic and Imaging Sciences
Grand Valley State University
Grand Rapids, Michigan

Arlene M. Adler, M.Ed., R.T.(R), FAERS
Professor and Director, Radiologic Sciences Programs
Indiana University Northwest
Gary, Indiana

Contributors
Eugene D. Frank, Mary Ann Hovis, Bradley C. Johnson,
Robin Jones, Bernadette M. Kaufman, Barbara J. Smith

DELMAR
CENGAGE Learning™

Australia • Brazil • Japan • Korea • Mexico • Singapore • Spain • United Kingdom • United States

DELMAR
CENGAGE Learning

**Principles of Radiographic Imaging:
An Art and a Science, Fourth Edition**
by Richard R. Carlton and
Arlene M. Adler

Vice President,
Health Care Business Unit:
William Brottmiller

Director of Learning Solutions:
Matthew Kane

Acquisitions Editor: **Maureen
Rosener**

Product Manager: **Laurie Traver**

Senior Product Manager: **Darcy Scelsi**

Editorial Assistant: **Elizabeth Howe**

Marketing Director: **Jennifer McAvey**

Marketing Coordinator:
Christopher Manion

Marketing Director: **Jennifer McAvey**

Technology Director: **Laurie Davis**

Technology Project Manager:
Mary Colleen Liburdi

Production Director: **Carolyn Miller**

Production Manager:
Barbara A. Bullock

Art and Design Specialist:
Alexandros Vasilakos

Production Coordinator:
Kenneth McGrath

Project Editor: **Jennifer Luck**

For product information and technology assistance, contact us at
Professional & Career Group Customer Support, 1-800-648-7450
For permission to use material from this text or product, submit all requests
online at **www.cengage.com/permissions**
Further permissions questions can be emailed to
permissionrequest@cengage.com

ExamView® and ExamView Pro® are registered trademarks of FSCreations, Inc. Windows is a registered trademark of the Microsoft Corporation used herein under license. Macintosh and Power Macintosh are registered trademarks of Apple Computer, Inc. Used herein under license.

ISBN-13: 978-1-4018-7194-9

ISBN-10: 1-4018-7194-1

Delmar Cengage Learning
5 Maxwell Drive
Clifton Park, NY 12065-2919
USA

Cengage Learning products are represented in Canada by Nelson Education, Ltd.

For your lifelong learning solutions, visit **delmar.cengage.com**

Visit our corporate website at **www.cengage.com**

Notice to the Reader

Printed in Canada
6 7 8 9 13 12 11 10

DEDICATION

In memory of Richard Killar
Our art guy who always was willing
to do one more revision for us

In memory of Raymond P. Rossi
Our mentor, friend, teacher, and coauthor
We miss you, Ray

To Sidney Finkleman and Quentin Garlets
for teaching us to be radiographers,

to LaVerne Ramaeker, Kay Shriver, and our students
for teaching us to be teachers,

and most importantly,
to our families and friends
for sustaining us throughout.

CONTRIBUTORS

Mary Ann Hovis
Associate Professor
Engineering Technologies
Lima Technical College
Lima, Ohio

Bradley C. Johnson B.S., R.T.(R)
Lecturer
Radiologic Sciences Programs
Indiana University Northwest
Gary, Indiana

Robin Jones M.S., R.T.(R)
Clinical Coordinator
Radiologic Sciences Programs
Indiana University Northwest
Gary, Indiana

Eugene D. Frank, M.A., R.T.(R), FASRT, FAERS
Retired, Assistant Professor of Radiology
Mayo Clinic/Foundation
Rochester, Minnesota
Director, Radiography Program
Riverland Community College
Austin, Minnesota

Barbara J. Smith, M.S,. R.T.(R)(QM)
Portland Community College
Radiological Sciences
Portland, Oregon

Bernadette M. Kaufman, R.T.(R)(MR)
ISMRM SMRT Education Committee
Milwaukee, Wisconsin

The Founders of Radiography

Wilhelm Conrad Röntgen (1845–1923)

Wilhelm Conrad Röntgen became the first radiographer when he discovered x-rays on November 8, 1895, in his laboratory at the University of Würzburg in Germany. His original paper *On a New Kind of Rays* is printed in Appendix A. For his discovery he received the first Nobel prize in physics in 1901 and was decorated by Prussia, Bavaria, Great Britain, Austria, Mexico, Germany, France, the Netherlands, Sweden, Italy, Turkey, and the United States.

(Portrait courtesy of the American College of Radiology)

Eddy Clifford Jerman (1865–1936)

Ed. C. Jerman is known as "The Father of Radiography" in the United States because he was the first teacher of radiography. He began teaching x-ray techniques in 1897, he founded the American Association of Radiological Technicians (now known as the American Society of Radiologic Technologists), and personally examined the first 1,000 members of the American Registry of X-Ray Technicians. He brought order to the principles of radiographic exposure technique by naming the qualities of the radiographic image: density, contrast, detail, and distortion. In 1928 he published *Modern X-Ray Technic,* the first book on radiographic principles.

(Portrait courtesy of the American Society of Radiologic Technologists)

Arthur Wolfram Fuchs (1895–1962)

Arthur W. Fuchs is known as the inventor of the fixed kilovoltage technique of radiography. His father, Wolfram Fuchs, established the first x-ray laboratory in Chicago in 1896 but became one of the early martyrs to radiation, dying from excessive exposure. Arthur performed radiography for the United States Army in both World Wars I and II. During World War II he wrote the U.S. Army training manual, *Principles of Radiographic Exposure,* in which he outlined his success with the optimal fixed kVp technique system. In 1955 he first published his book, *Principles of Radiographic Exposure and Processing.*

(Portrait courtesy of the family of Arthur Fuchs)

Contents

UNIT II   Protecting
Patients and Personnel

UNIT III Creating the Image

CHAPTER 14
Vision and Perception

CHAPTER 15
Beam Restriction

CHAPTER 16
The Patient as a Beam Emitter

CHAPTER 17
The Pathology Problem

CHAPTER 18
The Grid

CHAPTER 19
Radiographic Film

CHAPTER 20
Film Processing

CHAPTER 21
Film Sensitometry

UNIT IV Analyzing the Image

CHAPTER 45
Magnetic Resonance Imaging

List of Tables

Foreword

It has been my pleasure to know Rick Carlton and Arlene Adler since early in my career as an educator. They became colleagues in the 1970s while they were at the University of Health Sciences of the Chicago Medical School, but it wasn't until they were both radiography program directors in the mid-1980s that they began to rely on one another for technical content and teaching ideas. They tell a story about how they were sitting in Arlene's kitchen in Crown Point, Indiana, in 1988, comparing notes on teaching principles of radiographic imaging. Their discussion began to focus on how they had organized the entire subject area so that it made sense to not only their students but to themselves as well. They decided to create a presentation to share their success with other educators when, suddenly, they looked at each other and realized they were talking about much more than another talk at a professional meeting. They changed their outline into a proposal for a complete textbook, and the rest has become part of the history of our profession.

Thirteen years and four editions later, that bit of radiologic epiphany has produced the most popular principles of radiographic imaging textbook in the United States. Their work has been widely adopted in Canada and is a respected authoritative reference for radiologic and imaging sciences professionals worldwide. Carlton and Adler have given hundreds of professional presentations and now stand with that small group of authors who have profoundly shaped the knowledge base of the entire profession.

This fourth edition of *Principles of Radiographic Imaging: An Art and a Science* is especially notable in that for the first time since the 1992 first edition, the text has been dramatically changed to reflect a digital imaging approach throughout. Chapter 24, Digital Image Processing, and Chapter 25, Digital Radiography, have been greatly expanded, and a new chapter, Chapter 26, Digital Image Management, addresses PACS management issues.

E. C. Jerman's classic image quality parameters of density, contrast, recorded detail, and distortion have remained intact but now fit into the scope of the five phases of image quality, which Carlton and Adler have identified as:

1. Image acquisition phase
2. Image processing phase
3. Image archiving phase
4. Image display phase
5. Image analysis phase

Finally, as you have come to expect, all updates have been completed of the critical foundation content in chapters such as X-Ray Tubes, Mammography, Computed Tomography, and Magnetic Resonance Imaging. Vascular Imaging has new authors and sports significant revision and updating as well. Overall, this fourth edition of *Principles of Radiographic Imaging: An Art and a Science* rises to a new standard for teaching and understanding the physics and instrumentation of the radiologic and imaging sciences.

Dr. Michael E. Madden, R.T.(R)(CT)(MR)
Director, Medical Diagnostic Imaging Programs
Fort Hays State University, Hayes, Kansas

Preface

 INTRODUCTION

As radiography educators, we designed this textbook with students and educators in mind: each chapter contains an outline, key terms, objectives, a summary, review questions, and a detailed bibliography. Although the order of the chapters is based on our experiences in reaching our students, most chapters stand alone and can be used in the order which is most appropriate within a given program.

We have made a special effort to represent our belief that professional development should be a prime objective of any radiography curriculum. This is best achieved through the demonstration of technical competence. This book is designed to assist students in developing this cornerstone of professionalism. Through technical competence and a professional demeanor students will be ready to assume their role as experts in the radiographic imaging process. In addition, we believe that true professionals take immense pride in their work to the extent that it becomes an art as well as a science.

There is a special focus on integrating digital imaging parameters into the mainstream of radiography practice. Special effort is made to emphasize both the technical information and the ethical importance of understanding the specifics of image receptor sensitivity in order to be able to reduce exposure to the patient.

References used extensively to assure both educator and students that we address all content expected for successful professional practice include the American Registry of Radiographic Technologists' *Content Specifications for the Examination in Radiography, the Radiography Curriculum* by the American Society of Radiologic Technologists, and various materials prepared by the Canadian Association of Medical Radiation Technologists.

 CONTENT

A special attempt was made to provide an introduction to physics and the imaging modalities, as well as exploring the details of the principles of radiographic exposure techniques. Well established image quality factors (density, contrast, recorded detail, and distortion) are incorporated into digital imaging while new considerations such as monitor brightness are added to the mix of understanding the image production and viewing chain. Five phases are introduced to digitized image production; Acquisition, Processing, Archiving, Displaying, and Analyzing. Each includes well known radiographic imaging parameters but each is also enhanced by the addition of digital factors that now impact on all imaging decisions. The overall design of the book separates the forty-five chapters into six units: Creating the Beam, Protecting Patients and Personnel, Creating the Image, Analyzing the Image, Comparing Exposure Systems, and Special Imaging Systems. This design helps organize the content for students by following a logical progression from introductory physics through the production and control of the beam to advanced modality systems.

We remain extremely pleased that our book remains one of the resources listed in the Radiography Curriculum of the American Society of Radiologic Technologists and we have long been pleased that this book continues to be recommended by the Canadian Association of Medical Radiation Technologists for preparation for their certification in Radiological Technology.

The rapid changes in technology present a challenge to textbook authors who are committed to providing current information for learners. The authors and contributors to the fourth edition carefully reviewed all content to identify areas requiring updating or new topics. As a result, numerous changes were made. The more significant changes are as follows:

- New section on digital radiography, including descriptions of current image receptor and detector systems, process of acquiring the digital radiography histogram and applying the display algorithm to the collected data, image quality issues, image acquisitions elements, DICOM-3 standard, and digital radiography artifacts
- Discussion of the latest research on subnuclear structures (M theory, including string theory)
- Daylight, laser, and dry film imaging systems
- "Darkroom disease" issues (including OSHA, ANSI, and ASHRAE ventilation recommendations)
- Vascular, mammography, CT, and MRI instrumentation chapters were updated by quality experts to reflect current technology

In addition to the updated and new content, this new edition continues to feature the following learning aids and critical content:

- Physical concepts are clearly explained and illustrated with many high-quality figures
- Effects of changing parameters on image quality are carefully described and illustrated with numerous images
- Criteria for image analysis are presented to help learners develop analytical skills
- High-quality radiographs are included throughout the text
- Radiation protection concepts and procedures are emphasized for both patients and radiographic personnel
- Chapter end summaries provide a quick reference to critical concepts and developments in the science of radiography
- Numerous troubleshooting tips are included to ensure quality radiographs
- Extensive references and recommended readings provide a historical perspective and provide learners a means to expand their understanding of concepts and systems
- Epigraphs and historical photos help trace the evolution of radiography to the present
- Unique emphasis on the art versus the science of radiography illustrates the broad applications of the technology

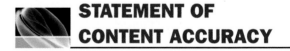 **STATEMENT OF CONTENT ACCURACY**

Although we assume full responsibility for any errors, including those which may be construed as arising from quoting other works out of context, we have made every effort to ensure the accuracy of the information. However, appropriate information sources should be consulted, especially for new or unfamiliar procedures. It is the responsibility of every practitioner to evaluate the appropriateness of a particular procedure in the context of actual clinical situations. Therefore, neither the authors nor the publisher take responsibility or accept any liability for the actions of persons applying the information contained herein in an unprofessional manner. This information is designed to supplement and enhance the instructional methodologies of educators in JRCERT [Joint Review Committee on Education in Radiologic Technologies (USA)] and CAMRT (Canada) approved radiography programs and should not be applied, especially to human subjects, without this background. In committing this book to print we fully realize that it is never finished, merely suspended for the time being.

Finally, as a reader your perceptions are important to us. We encourage you to communicate with us regarding facets of the book you appreciate or would like to see changed. We especially appreciate constructive comments and notice of errors. Our intention is to present the principles of radiography in an interesting format that provides a base from which true professionalism can develop. Any commentary readers care to make towards this end will be valued and welcomed.

Richard R. Carlton
Grand Valley State University
Radiologic and Imaging Sciences
Center for Health Sciences
Suite 200
301 Michigan St. NE
Grand Rapids, MI 49503
616-331-5953
carltonr@gvsu.edu

Arlene M. Adler
Indiana University Northwest
3400 Broadway
Gary, Indiana 46408
1-219-980-6540
aadler@iun.edu

Acknowledgments

We wish to acknowledge the support and inspiration provided by Dean Jane Toot, Bonita Pawloski, and Gunter Tusch at Grand Valley State University in Grand Rapids, Michigan; Dean Linda Rooda and the wonderful radiologic sciences faculty at Indiana University Northwest including Robin Jones, Sandy Piehl, Rachel Davids, Brad Johnson, Sharon Lakia, Sue Woods, Theresa Kempfer, Becky Bilyak, Jan Borden, Helen Campbell, Carol Collins, Martha Foreman, Char Gilpin, Pat Lewis, Becky Wantland, Sue Wilson, Jane Wuchenich and Laura Zlamal.

The fourth edition has been produced by our most dedicated team at Delmar Cengage Learning. It includes Maureen Rosener, our publishing mentor, and our editors Darcy Scelsi, Alex Vasilakos, and Laurie Traver.

We are especially grateful to Joe Chovan, the most spectacular artist we have ever worked with. Joe's artistic skills are on exhibit throughout the Delmar radiologic catalog and in our fourth edition we have been able to bring new insight into complex content through his sparkling and insightful illustrations.

We are indebted to the unstinting contributions from Barbara Smith of Portland Community College. A significant portion of the accuracy of the book derives from the constant inspection and contributions made by Barry Burns at the University of North Carolina who routinely went far beyond our wildest hopes in critiquing our text, producing films to illustrate his points, disproving old wives tales in his laboratory, and generously sharing his results (and venison) with us. Much more than a friend, Barry has become a backbone of the technical aspects of this book. Eugene Frank at Riverland Community College in Minnesota. continued his persistent and knowledgeable critique of our efforts. We are grateful for Gene's unique contributions, especially his ability to never let nearly two decades of friendship come between us and a more accurate reworking of verbiage or the details of an illustration. Gene revised his chapter on mammography instrumentation, which adds immeasurably to the depth of this work.

We acknowledge detailed contributions for this edition from John Skinner at Mid Michigan Community College, Jeff Lloyd at Spectrum Butterworth in Grand Rapids, Michigan, John Godisak at Grand Rapids Community College, Michigan and Jennifer Lockhart from Saint Anthony Medical Center in Crown Point, Indiana.

The students, faculty, and staff at Arkansas State University played a major role in the third edition. Special thanks is due Dean Susan Hanrahan, Ray Winters, Jeannean Rollins, Lyn Hubbard, Tracey White, and Deanna Harris for unremitting support and constant enthusiasm for what we are trying to accomplish in the radiologic sciences.

We thank the faculty and students who have found our work valuable in the process of radiography education and practice since the first edition was published. The success of this book and the invitation to produce a new edition are a direct result of the acceptance of our work by the radiography profession, which we gratefully acknowledge.

Our families once again deserve our thanks for their understanding. Don Adler and Lynn Carlton have both given countless hours that were rightfully theirs, for which we extend a peace offering of love. Arlene's family has grown by two, and appreciation goes to her daughters Meri and Katie (who now come first) as well as to Edyta for all her help. Rick's extended family now includes grandson Nathan and Michael, who gets their time, book or not.

Once again, we have been assisted in our work by a wide spectrum of colleagues in the radiologic sciences and related fields. In addition to those who assisted us during the first edition, we wish to add Irven Rule of the Siemens Training and Development Center in Cary, North Carolina; Alfred Hufnagl of the Northern Alberta Institute of Technology, Canada; Penelope Roberts of the Department of Medical Physics and Medical Engineering at Southampton University Hospitals, UK; Kathheryn Root of Holyoke Community College, Massachusetts; Dr. Appel and Kevin Sisak at DuPont; Garry Harris at Agfa; and Gregory Wheeler of Wheeler and Associates, San Francisco, California.

Our ability to devote the countless hours necessary to make this book what it has become is in great part due to the support we have received from our bosses, Robert Moon at Indiana University Northwest and Sam Bassitt at Lima Technical College. Our faculties have also made significant contributions through their consistent willingness to comment on the countless details we have explored with them over the years. Thank you Jody Ellis, Sandy Piehl, Laura Richards, Marie Ross, Debra Sobota, Andy Shappell, and Deb Scroggins. Special thanks goes to Barb Hanna and Wil Reddinger who provided us with their expertise in verifying laboratory results, producing new images, and refining our clumsy attempts to illustrate many concepts. Allen Lindmark from the Department of Chemistry at Indiana University Northwest also needs our thanks for his review of our basic explanations of chemistry concepts.

And finally, we thank those fellow educators who have taken the time to sit down with us at meetings, write letters, make phone calls, compose email, and fax their comments and suggestions to us. Although we are certain we have not remembered all of you (for which we apologize), these include John Clouse of Owensboro Community College, Kentucky; Marianne Tortorici and Mike Mixdorf at the University of Nevada, Las Vegas; Bob Misiak, Orange County Community College, New York; Jack Thomas at Lakeland Community College, Ohio; Lisa Iacovelli at Crozer-Chester Medical Center, Pennsylvania; Max Grady at Kettering College of Medical Arts, Ohio; Donna Mitchell at John Peter Smith Hospital, Texas; Anita Slechta of California State University at Northridge; Elwin Tilson of Armstrong State College, Georgia; Shay Mercer at New Mexico State University; Judy Williams of Grady Memorial Hospital, Georgia; Marilyn Sinderbrand of Northern Virginia Community College; Bill Sykes of Shawnee State University, Ohio; Bart Schraa of Daniel Denhoed University, Rotterdam, Netherlands; Frank Porter at St. Vincent Infirmary Medical Center, Arkansas; Mitchell Bieber, University of Virginia Medical Center; Donna Foster at Northern New Mexico Community College; Bill May of Iatwamba Community College, Mississippi; Lorraine Henry of Orange Coast Community College, California; and Steve Dowd of the University of Alabama at Birmingham.

Appreciation is also expressed to the colleagues who reviewed the manuscripts for this edition. Their critical reviews helped to guide us in the preparation of the final manuscript.

Reviewers

Abbey Freeman, MSA, RT(R)
Sanford Brown College
Fenton, Missouri

Jeff L. Berry, MS, RT(R)(CT)
Fort Hays State University
Hays, Kansas

Donna Lyke, MS, RT(R)(M)(QM)
University of Saint Francis
Fort Wayne, Indiana

Gary Morrison, Med, RT (R)
Midwestern State University
Wichita Falls, Texas

Denise Orth, BS, RT (R)(M)
Fort Hays State University
Hays, Kansas

Robert Slothus, RT(R), MS
The Pennsylvania College of Technology
Williamsport, Pennsylvania

Barbara Smith, BS, RT(R)(QM)
Portland Community College
Portland, Oregon

Edwin Viglia, RT(R)
Kankakee Community College
Kankakee, Illinois

The production of this book would not have been possible without the support of our spouses, Don and Lynn. In addition, we gratefully acknowledge the role played by Delmar Cengage Learning; Indiana University Northwest; Lima Technical College; and St. Rita's Medical Center of Lima, Ohio. Special thanks are due Dr. LaVerne Ramaeker, Sam Bassitt, Marlene Ledbetter, and Dennis Spragg for their continued support. A major contribution to the accuracy of the information and illustrations was made by the consistent presence of Eugene Frank, of the Mayo Clinic Foundation, throughout.

We are in the professional debt of many who inspired us, taught us, and collaborated with us throughout the years. Much of what is contained in this work is a direct result of these efforts. Those to whom we are especially indebted are Tracy Ahdel, Janice Akin, Judy Baron, Karen Brinkman, John Cortez, Marion Frank, Mick Jagger, Karen Jefferies, Robin Jones, Dr. George Koptik, Judy Koptik, Jon Lilly, Dr. Marzuto, Kathy Miller, Joe Mosqueda, Traci O'Donnell, LaVerne Ramaeker, Karen Schmidl, Kay Shriver, Tracy Thegze, Jean Widger, Rob Wilcoxen, and Sue Wilson. And of course our students at Indiana University Northwest, Lima Technical College, Wilbur Wright College, Malcolm X College, and Michael Reese Hospital and Medical Center.

Like our colleagues and students, we owe much to the institutions that contributed to our professional expertise. We wish to thank Indiana University Northwest, Lima Technical College, Michael Reese Hospital and Medical Center, Lutheran General Hospital, Mercy Hospital and Medical Center (Chicago), Northwestern Memorial Hospital (Chicago), Wilbur Wright College, Illinois Central College, Carl Sandburg College, Evanston Hospital, Methodist Medical Center (Peoria), and Community Memorial Hospital (Monmouth).

We owe special thanks to many people for sharing their personal expertise and material collections. One of the highest forms of professionalism, the willingness of radiologic technologists to freely give of their time and knowledge, was demonstrated again and again by everyone from whom we requested assistance in our compilation of the multitude of photographs, drawings, radiographs, and other illustrative materials in the text and those who assisted in the numerous reviews of our writing. Among these deserving special thanks are Gene Frank and Norlin Winkler of the Mayo Clinic Foundation and Ray Rossi of the University of Colorado for their commentary and technical assistance above and beyond the normal bonds of friendship; Philip W. Ballinger of the Ohio State University; Terry West of Toronto, Secretary-General of the International Society of Radiographers and Radiological Technicians; Stewart Bushong of Baylor College of Medicine; Terry Eastman of Dallas; Joe Fodor of the University of Cincinnati Medical Center; Nina Kowalczyk of Riverside Methodist Hospital, Columbus, Ohio; Denise Moore of Sinclair Community College, Dayton, Ohio; Bruce Long of Indiana University Medical Center; Marilyn Holland of the University of Iowa Hospitals and Clinics; Charles R. Griffith of FGHB Certified Radiation Physicists; Loren Garlets of Hays State University, Kansas; Pat Sharp of Gannon University, Erie, Pennsylvania; Tim Penning of Athens Regional Medical Center, Georgia; Seymour Sterling, FASRT, of Yardley, Pennsylvania; Jerome Taubel of the Mayo Clinic Foundation, Rochester, Minnesota; Bob Kobistek in Cleveland and Martin Ratner and Steve Szeglin in Carle Place, New York, both of Victoreen, Inc./Nuclear Associates; Terry Hanby of DuPont; Robert Trinkle, formerly of DuPont; Mike Wilsey of Agfa Matrix; Robert Lockery and Walter Weigl of Siemens Corporation; Robert Busic of General Electric Medical Systems; William Conklin of Orangeburg, SC; Rene Abgrall of Thoard, France; Toshinori Komba of Komazawa University, Tokyo, Japan; Angela Pickwick of Montgomery County Community College, Maryland; Jerry Conlogue of Gulf

Coast Community College, Florida; Barb Imber of St. Rita's Medical Center, Lima, Ohio; Rick Halker of Lima Memorial Hospital, Ohio; The Radiology Department of Van Wert County Hospital, Van Wert, Ohio, John Stone of Emory University Medical School, Atlanta; Tom Beery and Will Wells of Lima Technical College; Judy Shaw of Lima Technical College; Doug Raver and Chris Innskeep of Lima Technical College for video and software graphics; and Jan Krietemeyer of Lima, Ohio for bibliographic research.

How to Use StudyWARE™ to Accompany Principles of Radiographic Imaging: An Art and a Science

The StudyWARE™ software helps you learn terms and concepts in *Principles of Radiographic Imaging: An Art and a Science.* As you study each chapter in the text, be sure to explore the activities in the corresponding chapter in the software. Use StudyWARE™ as your own private tutor to help you learn the material in your *Principles of Radiographic Imaging: An Art and a Science* textbook.

Getting started is easy. Install the software by inserting the CD-ROM into your computer's CD-ROM drive and following the on-screen instructions. When you open the software, enter your first and last name so the software can store your quiz results. Then choose a chapter from the menu to take a quiz or explore one of the activities.

Menus

You can access the menus from wherever you are in the program. The menus include Quizzes, Activities, and Scores.

Quizzes

Quizzes include multiple choice, true/false, fill-in-the-blank, and matching questions. You can take the quizzes in both Practice Mode and Quiz Mode. Use Practice Mode to improve your mastery of the material. You have multiple tries to get the answers correct. Instant feedback tells you whether you're right or wrong—and helps you learn quickly by explaining why an answer was correct or incorrect. Use Quiz

Mode when you are ready to test yourself and keep a record of your scores. In Quiz Mode, you have one try to get the answers right, but you can take each quiz as many times as you want.

Activities

Activities include flashcards, concentration, hangman, crossword puzzles, and case studies. Have fun while increasing your knowledge!

Scores

You can view your last scores for each quiz and print your results to hand in to your instructor.

UNIT 1   # Creating the Beam

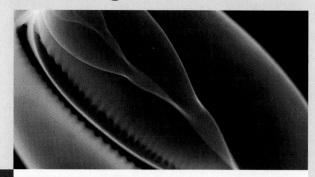

An inherent quality of a professional is the possession of expertise regarding the technical aspects of a field far above that of a nonprofessional. Knowledge of the principles of radiographic image production is part of the technical expertise of the professional radiographer. Radiography programs provide students with classroom instruction, laboratory experience, and clinical practice in this subject. No other medical professional experiences as intensive or comprehensive a study of radiographic imaging. This unit is designed to provide the basics necessary for this knowledge by building a framework of information regarding the creation of the diagnostic X-ray beam.

The framework begins with an elementary review of **basic mathematics** and **radiation concepts,** including atomic theory, X-ray properties, and necessary units of measurement. Although this may be a review of previous science course work for many readers, it is important to make sure everyone is on the same wavelength before using the information in the remainder of the book. **Electricity** and **electromagnetism** are large chapters that lay the foundation for understanding how to control the beam. **X-ray equipment,** the **X-ray tube,** and **X-ray production** provide an understanding of exactly how basic physics is used to create the X-ray beam.

CHAPTER 1

Basic Mathematics

Mary Ann Hovis

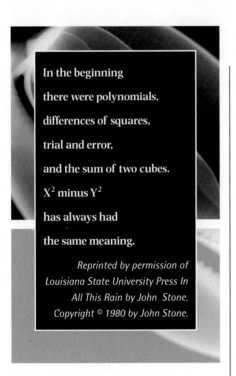

In the beginning
there were polynomials,
differences of squares,
trial and error,
and the sum of two cubes.
X^2 minus Y^2
has always had
the same meaning.

Reprinted by permission of Louisiana State University Press In All This Rain by John Stone. Copyright © 1980 by John Stone.

KEY TERMS

absolute value	equation	kilogram
algebraic expression	equivalent equation	like term
coulomb per kilogram	gray	meter
direct variation	identity	open equation
	inverse variation	second
		sievert

OBJECTIVES

Upon completion of this chapter, the student should be able to:

- Perform functions with fractions and decimals.
- Determine significant digits in a number.
- Perform calculations in scientific notation with signed numbers and exponents.
- Simplify algebraic expressions.
- Convert units within the SI system.

Mathematics is the language of science. Radiographers need to be able to speak this language. This math review is intended to refresh essential skills in this area.

 ARITHMETIC

Fractions

Addition and Subtraction. To add or subtract two fractions with **like** denominators, add or subtract the numerators and keep the like denominator.

EXAMPLES:

$$\frac{3}{8} + \frac{2}{8} = \frac{5}{8}$$

$$\frac{7}{8} - \frac{4}{8} = \frac{3}{8}$$

$$\frac{a}{b} + \frac{c}{b} = \frac{a + c}{b}$$

$$\frac{a}{b} - \frac{c}{b} = \frac{a - c}{b}$$

To add or subtract two fractions with **unlike** denominators, rewrite each fraction with a like or common denominator. Then add or subtract the numerators and keep the like or common denominator.

EXAMPLES:

$$\frac{1}{4} + \frac{5}{6} = \frac{3}{12} + \frac{10}{12} = \frac{13}{12}$$

$$\frac{7}{5} - \frac{1}{3} = \frac{21}{15} - \frac{5}{15} = \frac{16}{15}$$

$$\frac{a}{b} + \frac{c}{d} = \frac{ad}{bd} + \frac{bc}{bd} = \frac{ad + bc}{bd}$$

$$\frac{a}{d} - \frac{c}{d} = \frac{ad}{bd} - \frac{bc}{bd} = \frac{ad - bc}{bd}$$

Multiplication. Multiplication can be written in several ways (Table 1-1). To multiply two frac-

TABLE 1-1. **Multiplication Notation**

Throughout this review the algebraic notation for multiplication will be used.

Example: 3 × 4 will be written as 3 · 4.

A · (dot) is used as a symbol for multiplication.

Example: a × b will be written as a · b or as ab.

When two letters are used the dot is usually omitted.

Example: 3 × a will be written as 3a or as 3 · a.

Parentheses can also be used to represent multiplication.

Example: 3 × 4 can be written as (3)(4).

tions, multiply the numerators and multiply the denominators.

EXAMPLES:

$$\frac{2}{5} \times \frac{3}{7} = \frac{2 \times 3}{5 \times 7} = \frac{6}{35}$$

$$\frac{a}{b} \times \frac{c}{d} = \frac{a \times c}{b \times d}$$

Division.   To divide two fractions, rewrite the division problem as a multiplication problem by multiplying the first fraction by the second fraction inverted.

EXAMPLES:

$$\frac{2}{5} \div \frac{3}{7} = \frac{2}{5} \times \frac{7}{3} = \frac{2 \times 7}{5 \times 3} = \frac{14}{15}$$

$$\frac{a}{b} \div \frac{c}{d} = \frac{a}{b} \times \frac{d}{c} = \frac{a \times d}{b \times c}$$

Decimals

Decimal number place value (columns) is determined as shown in Figure 1-1.

Addition and Subtraction. To add or subtract two decimal numbers, line up the decimal points in each number, adding or subtracting as with whole numbers. Remember to add in zeros to fill out the decimal positions if necessary. The decimal point must remain in the same position.

Decimal number place value (columns)

FIGURE 1-1 Decimal number place values.

EXAMPLES:

Add:	Subtract:	Rewrite as:
76.81	76.1	76.10
+ 384.1	− 2.96	− 2.96
460.91		73.14

Multiplication. To multiply two decimal numbers, multiply the numbers as if they were whole numbers. Place the decimal point in the product so the number of places in the product equals the sum of the number of decimal places in each number.

EXAMPLE:

Multiply:

```
    2.31        2 decimal positions
  × 6.8         1 decimal position
   1848
   1386
  15.708        3 decimal positions
```

Division. To divide two decimal numbers, set up as if doing whole number division. Move the decimal point in the divisor to the right to make the divisor a whole number. Move the decimal point in the dividend the same number of places to the right (as was done for the divisor). Add zeros if necessary to maintain the position of the decimal. Divide the numbers as if they were whole numbers. Place the decimal point in the quotient directly above the decimal point in the dividend. Add zeros if necessary to maintain the position of the decimal.

EXAMPLES:

```
.25)1250

     5000.
.25)125000.

1.3)733.2

     564.
13.)7332.
    65
    83
    78
    52
    52
     0
```

Convert a Fraction into a Decimal Number.
To convert a fraction into a decimal, divide the denominator into the numerator.

EXAMPLE: Convert 7/8 into a decimal:

```
     .875
  8)7.000
    64
    60
    56
    40
    40
```

Convert a Percent to a Decimal. To convert a percent to a decimal, move the decimal point two places to the left.

> *EXAMPLE:* Convert 78.5% to a decimal:
>
> 78.5% = .785

Convert a Decimal to a Percent. To convert a decimal to a percent, move the decimal point two places to the right.

> *EXAMPLE:* Change .452 to a %:
>
> .452 = 45.2%

Computation with Values (Numbers)

Exact. Some numbers are exact values, like the counting numbers (1, 2, 3, . . .). For example, there are exactly four legs on a chair. Exact numbers in computations are as accurate or as precise as needed.

Significant Digits. Some values are obtained by measurement and are only as accurate as the measuring device. The last digit in the reading is usually estimated. **When dealing with these values in computations, the results will only be as accurate as the least accurate value.** This is the concept of significant digits.

To determine the number of significant digits in a value (number):

1. Count all nonzero digits.
2. Count all zeros between nonzero digits.
3. Count all zeros at the end of a decimal value.

The number of significant digits in a value is the sum of the numbers obtained in steps 1, 2, and 3.

> *EXAMPLES:* The following are measured values from a radiation dose meter (dosimeter).
>
> 7.14 mR has three significant digits.
> 90.104 mR has five significant digits.
> 0.048 mR has two significant digits.
> 7300 mR has two significant digits.
> 6.900 mR has four significant digits.

Precision. The precision of a value refers to the decimal position of the last significant digit.

> *EXAMPLE:*
>
> .0218 is precise to the ten-thousandths.

Rounding Off. To round a number the last digit to be retained is:

1. Left unchanged if the digit to the right of the last digit to be retained is less than 5.
2. Is increased by one if the digit to the right of the last digit to be retained is 5 or greater.

> *EXAMPLES:*
>
> 75.2581 rounded to 4 significant digits is 75.26.
> 6836.66 rounded to 2 significant digits is 6800.
> 0.0381 rounded to 2 significant digits is 0.038.
> 0.0299 rounded to 2 significant digits is 0.030.

Multiplication and Division of Approximate Values. When multiplying or dividing two or more approximate values, the number of significant digits in the final answer is no greater than the number of significant digits in the value with the least number of significant digits.

> *EXAMPLE:* Using the calculator, (103.81) · (1.34) = 139.1054. However, since 1.34 has only three significant digits, the answer should have only three significant digits. Therefore, 139.1054 needs to be rounded to three significant digits, making it 139.

Addition and Subtraction of Approximate Values. When adding or subtracting two or more approximate values, the final answer should be no more precise than the **least** precise of the values.

> *EXAMPLE:* Add the following:
>
> 123.1
> 89.123
> <u>103.3456</u>
> 315.5686

Since the least precise number is 123.1, the answer should be rounded to 315.6.

Powers of 10

The decimal system is based on powers of 10, as is the metric system. These are very important systems to the radiographer. When a^n is written, a is called the base and n is the exponent. Integers are defined as the numbers $\ldots -3, -2, -1, 0, 1, 2, 3, \ldots$.

Positive Integer Exponents. Definition:

$$a^n = \underbrace{a \cdot a \cdot a \cdots a}_{n \text{ times}} \text{ (multiply n times)}$$

EXAMPLES:

$10^1 = 10$
$10^2 = 10 \cdot 10 = 100$
$10^3 = 10 \cdot 10 \cdot 10 = 1000$
$10^n = 10 \cdot 10 \cdot 10 \cdots 10 = 100 \ldots 0$ (n zeros)

Negative Integer Exponents. Definition:

$$a^{-n} = \frac{1}{a^n} \text{ (for a} \neq 0)$$

$$10^{-1} = \frac{1}{10} = .1$$

$$10^{-2} = \frac{1}{10^2} = .01$$

$$10^{-3} = \frac{1}{10^3} = .001$$

$$10^{-n} = \frac{1}{10^n} = .00 \ldots 001 \text{ (n} - 1) \text{ zeros}$$

Zero Exponents. Definition: $a^0 = 1$ (for a $\neq 0$)

EXAMPLE:

$10^0 = 1$

Scientific Notation

A number written in scientific notation is written as the product of a number between 1 (including 1) and 10 times a power of 10. In other words, $N \times 10^p$ where $1 \leq N < 10$ and p is an integer.

EXAMPLES:

7.15×10^4 is a number in scientific notation.
1.598×10^{-5} is a number in scientific notation.
7.58×10^0 is a number in scientific notation.

Converting Numbers from Ordinary to Scientific Notation. To write a number in scientific notation, the decimal point must be moved to the position following the first nonzero digit.

EXAMPLES:

$70.57 = 7.057 \times 10^1$ (p = 1)
$.00815 = 8.15 \times 10^{-3}$ (p = −3)
$7.58 = 7.58 \times 10^0$ (p = 0)

In the first example, the decimal point is moved one digit to the left, making the power of 10 (p), 1. In the second example, the decimal point is moved three digits to the right, making the power of 10, −3. In the third example, the decimal point is not moved and the power of 10 is 0.

In general, when moving the decimal point to the left the power of 10 will be the number of positions moved. When moving the decimal point to the right the power of 10 will be negative the number of positions moved. When the decimal point is not moved, the power of 10 will be zero.

Converting Numbers from Scientific to Ordinary Notation. To convert a number in scientific notation to ordinary notation, the decimal position is moved according to the following:

1. If the power of 10 is positive, move the decimal point to the right the number of positions in the exponent.

2. If the power of 10 is negative, move the decimal point to the left the number of positions in the exponent.

3. If the power of 10 is zero, the decimal remains in the same position.

In all of the above, once the decimal point has been moved, the 10 and its power are dropped. Zeros are added if necessary.

EXAMPLES:

$3.7 \times 10^4 = 37,000$
$5.56 \times 10^{-5} = .0000556$
$1.34 \times 10^0 = 1.34$

Dimensional Analysis

The concept of dimensional analysis is very useful when converting from one set of units to another. The principle is based on fractions whose quotients are 1.

EXAMPLE:

$$\frac{12 \text{ in}}{1 \text{ ft}} = 1 \text{ or } \frac{1 \text{ ft}}{12 \text{ in}} = 1$$

Recall that multiplying a quantity by 1 does not change the value of the quantity. In order to convert from one set of units to another, algebraic operations are performed with units in the same way they are with algebraic symbols.

EXAMPLE: Convert 7.0 ft to inches.

$$7.0 \text{ ft} = 7.0 \text{ ft} \cdot \frac{12 \text{ in}}{1 \text{ ft}} = 7 \cdot 12 \text{ in} = 84 \text{ in}$$

Note that it is possible to "cancel" the feet unit, leaving the inches unit.

Convert 70.0 km/hr to m/s.

$$70.0 \frac{\text{km}}{\text{hr}} =$$

$$70.0 \frac{\text{km}}{\text{hr}} \cdot \frac{1000 \text{ m}}{1 \text{ km}} \cdot \frac{1 \text{ hr}}{60 \text{ min}} \cdot \frac{1 \text{ min}}{60 \text{ s}} =$$

$$70.0 \cdot 1000 \cdot \frac{1}{60} \cdot \frac{1 \text{ m}}{60 \text{ s}} = 19.4 \frac{\text{m}}{\text{s}}$$

Recall that 1 km = 1000 m, 1 hr = 60 min, and 1 min = 60 s. Note that it is possible to "cancel" the km unit, the hr unit, and the min unit.

When converting cubic units or square units, extra attention needs to be given to the conversion factors. Study the following example carefully.

EXAMPLE: Convert 3.8000 ft³ (cubic feet) to cubic inches (in³).

$$3.8000 \text{ ft}^3 = 3.8000 \text{ ft}^3 \cdot \frac{12 \text{ in}}{1 \text{ ft}} \cdot \frac{12 \text{ in}}{1 \text{ ft}} \cdot \frac{12 \text{ in}}{1 \text{ ft}}$$

$$= 6566.4 \text{ in}^3$$

or

$$3.8000 \text{ ft}^3 = 3.8000 \text{ ft}^3 \cdot \left(\frac{12 \text{ in}}{1 \text{ ft}}\right)^3 = 6566.4 \text{ in}^3$$

EXAMPLE: Convert 10 roentgens per hour to roentgens per minute.

$$10.0 \frac{\text{roentgens}}{\text{hour}} = 10.0 \frac{\text{roentgens}}{\text{hour}} \cdot \frac{1 \text{ hour}}{60 \text{ minutes}}$$

$$= .167 \frac{\text{roentgens}}{\text{minute}}$$

ALGEBRA

Signed Numbers

Numbers are not always positive. For example, the thermometer indicates that it is very cold at −20°F. Negative numbers can be illustrated by using a number line (Figure 1-2). Positive numbers are assigned to the right of the zero point and negative numbers to the left of the zero point. A statement that 7 is less than 10 (written as $7 < 10$) indicates that 7 is to the left of 10 on the number line. A statement that −5 is greater than −9 (written as $-5 > -9$) indicates that −5 is to the right of −9 on the number line.

Absolute Value. The **absolute value** of a number is the distance from 0 to that number on the number line. Since distance is a non-negative quantity, that means that the absolute value of a number is always positive or zero. The notation used for absolute value is two vertical bars ($|\ |$).

EXAMPLES:

$$|-2| = 2 \qquad |4| = 4 \qquad |0| = 0$$

Since −2 is two units from zero on the number line, the absolute value is 2. Since 4 is four units from zero on the number line, the absolute value is 4. Since 0 is zero units from zero on the number line, the absolute value is 0.

Addition. To add two positive numbers, add their absolute values and attach a positive sign to the result. The positive sign is usually omitted.

EXAMPLE:

$$(+7) + (+8) = +15 \qquad 7 + 8 = 15$$

To add two negative numbers, add their absolute values and attach a negative sign to the result.

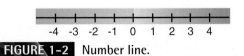

FIGURE 1-2   Number line.

EXAMPLE:

$$(-7) + (-8) = -15 \qquad -7 + (-8) = -15$$

To add two numbers with unlike signs, subtract the smaller in absolute value from the larger in absolute value and attach the sign of the larger in absolute value to the result.

EXAMPLES:

$$(-10) + (3) = -7 \qquad 4 + (-9) = -5$$
$$(8) + (-5) = 3 \qquad -3 + (7) = 4$$

Negative of a Number. The negative of a number is the opposite of the number in sign.

> **EXAMPLES:** The negative of 7 is -7; the negative of -7 is 7.
>
> If $b = 7$, then $-b = -7$.
> If $b = -7$, then $-b = -(-7) = 7$.

Subtraction. Subtraction is rewritten as addition, as in $a - b = a + (-b)$.

EXAMPLES:

$$8 - 10 = 8 + (-10) = -2$$
$$8 - (-10) = 8 + 10 = 18$$
$$-8 - 10 = -8 + (-10) = -18$$
$$-8 - (-10) = -8 + 10 = 2$$

All of the above subtraction problems are rewritten as addition and then the rules for addition of signed numbers are used.

Multiplication. To multiply two numbers, multiply their absolute values. If both numbers are positive or both numbers are negative, attach a positive sign to the result. If the numbers are opposite in sign, attach a negative sign to the result.

EXAMPLES:

$$(2)(3) = 6$$
$$(-2)(-3) = 6$$
$$(2)(-3) = -6$$
$$(-2)(3) = -6$$

Division. To divide two numbers, divide their absolute values. If both numbers are positive or both numbers are negative, attach a positive sign to the

result. If the numbers are opposite in sign, attach a negative sign to the result.

EXAMPLES:

$$8 \div 2 = 4$$
$$-8 \div -2 = 4$$
$$8 \div (-2) = -4$$
$$-8 \div 2 = -4$$

Order of Operation

Order-of-operation problems may occur when parentheses are not indicated. For example, evaluate $2 + 3 \cdot 4$. Depending on whether addition or multiplication is performed first the answer might be 20 or 14. The answer actually depends on the order of operation. Rules have been established that make the correct result 14.

The difference between the unary minus sign $(-)$ and the subtraction sign $(-)$ and the difference between the unary plus sign $(+)$ and the addition sign $(+)$ must be understood before order-of-operation rules can be learned.

A subtraction sign $(-)$ is used between two numbers:

EXAMPLE:

$7 - 8$ (subtraction sign)

A unary minus sign $(-)$ is used before one number.

EXAMPLE:

-7 (unary minus sign)

An expression can have both a subtraction sign and a unary minus sign.

EXAMPLE:

$-7 - 8$ (the first is a unary minus, the second a subtraction sign)

An addition sign $(+)$ is used between two numbers:

EXAMPLE:

$8 + 10$ (addition sign)

A unary plus sign $(+)$ is used before one number.

EXAMPLE:

$+8$

Rules for Order of Operation

1. Perform all operations inside grouping symbols (parentheses, radical symbols, fraction bar, brackets, etc.)
2. Exponentiation (raising to a power or roots)
3. Unary minus $(-)$ or unary plus $(+)$
4. Multiplication and division
5. Addition and subtraction

Operations are performed from the lowest level (#1) to the largest level (#5). Operations on the same level are evaluated left to right.

EXAMPLES:

$2 + \fbox{$3 \cdot 4$}$ (multiplication first)

$= 2 + 12$ (addition)

$= 14$

$\fbox{$8 \cdot 6$} - \fbox{$12 \div 2$}$ (multiplication and division first)

$= \fbox{$48 - 6$}$ (subtraction)

$= 42$

$\dfrac{8 + 7}{2 + 3}$ (bar acts as grouping symbol)

$= \dfrac{15}{5}$ (add numerator and add denominator first)

$= 3$ (divide)

$(-2)^3$ (exponentiation first)

$= -8$

$-(2)^4$ (exponentiation first)

$= -(16)$ (unary minus sign)

$= -16$

$3(\fbox{$7 + 4$})$ (add inside parenthesis first)

$= \fbox{$3 \cdot 11$}$ (multiply)

$= 33$

$2(\fbox{$6 + 1$})^2$ (add inside parenthesis first)

$= 2\fbox{$(7)^2$}$ (exponentiation next)

$= 2 \cdot 49$ (multiply)

$= 98$

Algebraic Expressions

Algebraic expressions are letters and/or numbers that are multiplied, divided, added, subtracted, or raised to a power.

EXAMPLES:

$3x^3 + 5x^2 - 7x + 8$

$x + 5$

$$\dfrac{}{y - 7}$$

There are several rules for combining algebraic expressions.

Distributive Law. The statement of the distributive law is:

$a(b + c) = a \cdot b + a \cdot c$

EXAMPLES:

$7(x + y) = 7x + 7y$
$7(3 + 5) = 7 \cdot 3 + 7 \cdot 5 = 21 + 35 = 56$
$p(x + 4) = px + 4p$ (The numeral is normally written in front of the letter.)

If the addition sign were a subtraction sign, then:

$a(b - c) = a \cdot b - a \cdot c$

EXAMPLES:

$7(x - 7) = 7x - 7y$
$7(3 - 5) = 7 \cdot 3 - 7 \cdot 5$
         $= 21 - 35 = 21 + (-35) = -14$
$p(x - 4) = px - 4p$

Care needs to be taken when one or two negative signs are involved.

EXAMPLES:

$-7(x + y) = -7x + (-7y)$ (distributive law)
         $= -7x - 7y$ (the reverse definition of subtraction)
$-7(x - y) = -7x - (-7y)$ (distributive law)
         $= -7x + 7y$ (definition of subtraction)
$-7(-3 - 8) = (-7)(-3) - (-7)(8)$
                (distributive law)
        $= 21 - (-56)$ (multiply)
        $= 21 + 56$ (definition of subtraction)

        $= 77$

Addition and Subtraction of Like Terms.

Like terms are terms with identical literal factors. A literal factor is a factor denoted by a letter. Like terms may be added or subtracted.

EXAMPLE:

$7x + 3x = 10x$ (like terms)

EXAMPLE:

$7x + 3y = 7x + 3y$ (unlike terms may not be added)

EXAMPLE:

$7x - 3x = 4x$

EXAMPLE:

$-7x - 3x = -7x + (-3x)$ (definition of subtraction)

$= -10x$ (combine like terms)

EXAMPLE:

$-7x - (-3x) = -7x + 3x$ (definition of subtraction)

$= -4x$ (combine like terms)

Parentheses.

When an algebraic expression involves parentheses, the parentheses need to be removed in order to simplify the expression.

EXAMPLE:

$7(x + y) + 4(x + y)$

$= 7x + 7y + 4x + 4y$ (distributive law)

$= 11x + 11y$ (combine like terms)

EXAMPLE:

$7(x + y) - 4(x + y)$

$= 7(x + y) + (-4)(x + y)$ (definition of subtraction)

$= 7x + 7y + (-4x) + (-4y)$ (distributive law)

$= 3x + 3y$ (combine like terms)

EXAMPLE:

$7(x - y) - 4(x - y)$

$= 7(x - y) + (-4)(x - y)$ (definition of subtraction)

$= 7x - 7y + (-4x) - (-4y)$ (distributive law)

$= 7x + (-7y) + (-4x) + (4y)$ (definition of subtraction)

$= 3x + (-3y)$ (combine like terms)

$= 3x - 3y$ (reverse of definition of subtraction)

EXAMPLE:

$x - (y - x) = x + (-1)(y - x)$

$= x + (-y) - (-x)$

$= x + (-y) + x$

$2x - y$

If an expression involves parentheses within parentheses, then it is simplified from the innermost parentheses out.

EXAMPLE:

$7 - [6x - (x - 4)]$

$= 7 - [6x - x + 4]$ (remove innermost parentheses)

$= 7 - [5x + 4]$ (simplify within parentheses)

$= 7 - 5x - 4$ (remove parentheses [square bracket])

$= 3 - 5x$ (combine like terms)

Exponents. Definition:

$$a^n = \underbrace{a \cdot a \cdot a \cdots a}_{n \text{ times}}$$

where a is the base and n is the exponent

EXAMPLE:

$3^4 = 3 \cdot 3 \cdot 3 \cdot 3 = 81$

Laws of Exponents

Law 1: $a^m \cdot a^n = a^{m+n}$

EXAMPLES:

$a^4 \cdot a^3 = a^{4+3} = a^7$

$a \cdot a^5 = a^{1+5} = a^6$

Law 2: $\dfrac{a^m}{a^n} = \begin{cases} a^{m-n} & \text{if } m \geq n \\ \dfrac{1}{a^{n-m}} & \text{if } n > m \end{cases} \quad a \neq 0$

EXAMPLES:

$$\frac{x^5}{x^2} = x^{5-2} = x^3$$

$$\frac{x^7}{x^{10}} = \frac{1}{x^{10-7}} = \frac{1}{x^3}$$

Law 3: $(ab)^m = a^m b^m$

EXAMPLE:

$$(ab)^4 = a^4 b^4$$

Law 4: $\left(\dfrac{a}{b}\right)^m = \dfrac{a^m}{b^m}, b \neq 0$

EXAMPLE:

$$\left(\frac{a}{b}\right)^5 = \frac{a^5}{b^5}$$

Law 5: $(a^m)^n = a^{m \cdot n}$

EXAMPLE:

$$(a^4)^5 = a^{4 \cdot 5} = a^{20}$$

Definition: $a^0 = 1$ for $a \neq 0$

EXAMPLES:

$$5^0 = 1$$
$$x^0 = 1$$
$$(5x)^0 = 1$$
$$5x^0 = 5 \cdot 1 = 5$$

Definition: $a^{-n} = \dfrac{1}{a^n}$ for $a \neq 0$

EXAMPLES:

$$x^{-7} = \frac{1}{x^7}$$

$$2^{-3} = \frac{1}{2^3} = \frac{1}{8}$$

It can also be shown that:

$$\frac{1}{a^{-n}} = a^n \text{ for } a \neq 0.$$

EXAMPLES:

$$\frac{1}{5^{-2}} = 5^2 = 25$$

$$\frac{1}{x^{-5}} = x^5$$

Multiplying Numbers in Scientific Notation.

When multiplying two numbers in scientific notation, the Ns are multiplied and the powers of ten are added. This is simply using the rule of exponents when the bases are the same.

EXAMPLE:

$$(2.4 \times 10^3)(3.8 \times 10^{11})$$
$$= (2.4 \cdot 3.8) \times 10^{3+11}$$
$$= 9.1 \times 10^{14}$$

Dividing Numbers in Scientific Notation.

When dividing two numbers in scientific notation, the Ns are divided and the exponents are subtracted. This is another example of using the rules of exponents.

EXAMPLE:

$$(8.3 \times 10^4) \div (2.7 \times 10^{11})$$
$$= 8.3 \div 2.7 \times 10^{4-11}$$
$$= 3.1 \times 10^{-7}$$

Evaluating Algebraic Expressions

To evaluate an algebraic expression, replace each unknown with the given value and then perform the indicated operations.

EXAMPLE: Evaluate $2a^2 + 5b$ for $a = 3$ and $b = 4$.

$$2a^2 + 5b = 2(3)^2 + 5(4)$$
$$= 2 \cdot 9 + 20$$
$$= 18 + 20$$
$$= 38$$

Formulae are examples of equations where algebraic expressions are evaluated.

Convert 60.0°F to C.
The formula involved is C = 5/9(F − 32°).
Determine C when F = 60.0°.

C = 5/9(F − 32°)
C = 5/9(60.0° − 32°)   (substitute 60.0° for F)
C = 5/9(28°)
C = 15.6°C

Convert 20.0°C to F.
The formula to use is F = 9/5C + 32°.
Determine F when C = 20.0°.

F = 9/5(20°) + 32°
F = 36° + 32°
F = 68°

Equations

An **equation** is a statement that contains an equal sign. For example, A = B is an equation. An equation can be either a true or a false statement.

5 + 3 = 7   (false statement)
5 + 3 = 8   (true statement)

Both of these statements are equations but only one is true.

An equation that contains at least one unknown (variable) is an **open equation**.

x + 5 = 7
3x + 5 = 7 − 2x

An open statement becomes either true or false when the unknown (variable) is replaced (substituted) with a numeric value.

In x + 5 = 7, replace x with 3.
   3 + 5 = 7 is a false statement.
In x + 5 = 7, replace x with 2.
   2 + 5 = 7 is a true statement.

The solution of an equation is that numeric value which, when substituted in the equation, gives a true statement. In the earlier example, 2 is the solution to the equation.

There may be many solutions to an equation. For example, in the equation x + 5 = x + 5, all numeric values for x will give a true statement. **This type of equation is called an identity.**

There may be no solutions to an equation. For example, in the equation x + 5 = x + 6, there are no numbers that, when substituted in the equation, give a true statement. Therefore, there are no solutions to the equation.

Equivalence Principles. The principles of equivalence are needed to solve equations. **Equivalent equations are equations that have the same solutions.**

Addition and Subtraction Principle. If the same number is added to each side or subtracted from each side of an equation, the equation remains equivalent.

x − 5 = 7   (add 5 to both sides)
x − 5 + 5 = 7 + 5   (equivalent equation to
x = 12   x − 5 = 7)

      x + 3 = 12   (subtract 3 from both sides)
x + 3 − 3 = 12 − 3   (equivalent equation to
        x = 9   x + 3 = 12)

Multiplication and Division Principle. If the same nonzero number is multiplied or divided by each side of the equation, the equation remains equivalent.

$\dfrac{x}{5} = 6$ (multiply each side by 5)

$5 \cdot \dfrac{x}{5} = 5 \cdot 6$ (equivalent equation)

x = 30

EXAMPLE:

$$3x = 12 \qquad \text{(divide each side by 3)}$$
$$\frac{3x}{3} = \frac{12}{3} \qquad \text{(equivalent equation)}$$
$$x = 4$$

To find a solution to an equation, the unknown (variable) must be isolated on one side of the equation.

EXAMPLE:

Solve: $x + 7 = 12$ for x

$$x + 7 = 12$$
$$x + 7 - 7 = 12 - 7 \quad \text{(subtract 7 from each side)}$$
$$x = 5$$

Check:

$$x + 7 = 12$$
$$5 + 7 = 12 \qquad \text{(substitute value for x)}$$
$$12 = 12 \qquad \text{(statement is true; therefore,}$$
$$\text{5 is solution to equation)}$$

EXAMPLE:

Solve: $\dfrac{x}{6} = 18$ for x

$$\frac{x}{6} = 18$$
$$6 \cdot \frac{x}{6} = 6 \cdot 18 \qquad \text{(multiply both sides by 6)}$$
$$x = 108$$

Check:

$$\frac{x}{6} = 18$$
$$\frac{108}{6} = 18 \qquad \text{(substitute 108 for x)}$$
$$18 = 18 \qquad \text{(statement is true)}$$

EXAMPLE:

Solve: $5a = 30$ for a

$$5a = 30$$
$$\frac{5a}{5} = \frac{30}{5} \qquad \text{(divide both sides by 5)}$$
$$a = 6$$

Check:

$$5a = 30$$
$$5(6) = 30 \qquad \text{(substitute 6 for a)}$$
$$30 = 30 \qquad \text{(statement is true)}$$

EXAMPLE:

Solve: $7x - 5 = 3x + 7$ for x

$$7x - 5 = 3x + 7$$
$$7x - 5 + 5 = 3x + 7 + 5 \quad \text{(add 5 to both sides)}$$
$$7x = 3x + 12$$
$$7x - 3x = 3x + 12 - 3x \quad \text{(subtract 3x from both sides)}$$
$$4x = 12$$
$$\frac{4x}{4} = \frac{12}{4} \qquad \text{(divide both sides by 4)}$$
$$x = 3$$

Check:

$$7x - 5 = 3x + 7$$
$$7(3) - 5 = 3(3) + 7 \qquad \text{(substitute 3 for x)}$$
$$21 - 5 = 9 + 7$$
$$16 = 16 \qquad \text{(statement is true)}$$

To solve an equation with parentheses, the parentheses need to be eliminated using some correct procedure, usually the distributive law.

EXAMPLE:

Solve: $7(x + 6) = 21$ for x

$$7(x + 6) = 21 \qquad \text{(distributive law)}$$
$$7x + 42 = 21 \qquad \text{(subtract 42 from each side)}$$
$$7x = -21 \qquad \text{(divide each side by 7)}$$
$$x = -3$$

Check:

$$7(x + 6) = 21 \qquad \text{(substitute } -3 \text{ for x)}$$
$$7(-3 + 6) = 21$$
$$7(3) = 21$$
$$21 = 21 \qquad \text{(statement is true)}$$

Sometimes a formula needs to be rearranged. This is just like solving an equation for an unknown (variable).

EXAMPLE:

Solve for t when a = bt + c

$$a = bt + c$$
$$a - c = bt + c - c \quad \text{(subtract c from each side)}$$
$$a - c = bt \qquad\qquad\qquad \text{(divide by b)}$$
$$\frac{a - c}{b} = \frac{bt}{b}$$
$$\frac{a - c}{b} = t$$

Check:

$$a = bt + c$$
$$a = b \cdot \frac{a - c}{b} + c \quad \left(\text{substitute } \frac{a - c}{b} \text{ for t}\right)$$
$$a = a - c + c$$
$$a = a \qquad\qquad\qquad \text{(statement is true)}$$

Variation

There are two types of variation that will be discussed here—direct and inverse.

Direct Variation. Direct variation means that one quantity is a multiple of a second quantity. An example of direct variation is y = kx where k is the constant of proportionality. Here y is a multiple of x, making y directly proportional to x.

Another example is $y = kx^2$ where k is the constant of proportionality, making y directly proportional to the square of x. Another way to think of direct variation is that the quotient of the two quantities is always a constant. It is possible, knowing the values for the quantities, to find the constant.

Inverse Variation. Inverse variation means that when two quantities are multiplied their product is a constant.

An example of inverse variation is y = k/x where k is the constant of proportionality. Here the product of x and y is a constant, namely k. This is usually read as y is inversely proportional to x.

Another example is $y = k/x^2$ where k is the constant of proportionality. Here the product of x^2 and y is a constant. This is usually read as y is inversely proportional to the square of x (or x^2).

It is also possible to combine the two variations. As an example, consider $y = kx/z^2$. Here y is directly proportional to x and inversely proportional to the square of z.

UNITS OF MEASUREMENT

In order to quantify scientific phenomena, standard units of measurement have been established. These units allow scientists to describe quantities. In physics, the primary or fundamental units of measurement are **mass, length,** and **time.** These units, although they have the same meaning and have been standardized by international organizations, are measured by the use of two widely different systems. These are the British (foot-pound-second) system, also called the United States customary system, and the metric [MKS (meter-kilogram-second) or CGS (centimeter-gram-second)] system. Although most countries utilize the metric system of measurement, attempts to switch to this system in the United States have not been very successful. In the United States, length is measured in inches and feet rather than meters and kilometers. By combining one or more of the fundamental units, scientists arrive at secondary or derived units. For example, the area of an object is derived from the fundamental unit of length. The area of a rectangle is determined by multiplying the lengths of the two sides of the object.

SI Units

In 1960, at the Eleventh General Conference of Weights and Measures, the Système Internationale d'Unites (SI) was defined and officially adopted. This system of units, used to measure various quantities, is now accepted as the metric system. In the SI system, there are seven base units (Table 1-2). All other units are derived from these units, although some derived units are given special names. It is important to become familiar with SI units since they have been internationally adopted.

In addition, although the United States does not use SI/metric units for the public, all scientific in-

TABLE 1-2.   SI Units of Measurement

Base Units		
Quantity	Unit Name	Symbol
Mass	kilogram	kg
Length	meter	m
Time	second	s
Electric current	ampere	A
Temperature	kelvin	K
Amount of substance	mole	mol
Luminous intensity	candela	cd

Derived Units			
Quantity	Unit Name	Symbol	British Units
Absorbed dose	gray	Gy	rad
Charge	coulomb	C	esu
Electric potential	volt	v	
Dose equivalent	sievert	Sv	rem
Energy	joule	J	erg
Exposure	coulomb/ kilogram	C/kg	roentgen
Frequency	hertz	Hz	cycles per second
Force	newton	N	
Magnetic flux	weber	Wb	
Magnetic flux density	tesla	T	gauss
Power	watt	W	
Radioactivity	bequerel	Bq	curie

TABLE 1-3.   SI Unit Values

Factors	Prefixes	Symbols
10^{12}	tera	T
10^{9}	giga	G
10^{6}	mega	M
10^{3}	kilo	k
10^{2}	hecto	h
10^{1}	deka	da
10^{-1}	deci	d
10^{-2}	centi	c
10^{-3}	milli	m
10^{-6}	micro	μ
10^{-9}	nano	n
10^{-12}	pico	p
10^{-15}	femto	f
10^{-18}	atto	a

Fundamental Units

Mass. Mass is the amount or quantity of matter. The standard unit of mass is the **kilogram** (kg). It is represented by a cylinder of platinum-iridium, which is kept in a vault at the International Bureau of Weights and Measures in Paris, France.

Length. The unit of length is the **meter** (m). The meter was defined in 1983 as the distance that light travels in a vacuum in 1/299,792,485 second.

Time. The unit of time is the **second** (s). The second was originally defined in terms of the rotation of the earth on its axis (the mean solar day) but, like the meter, the need for greater accuracy resulted in redefining the unit. Time is now measured by the vibrations of cesium—133 atoms. This method is sometimes called the atomic clock.

Prefixes

The metric system uses prefixes to units to denote different orders of magnitude, as shown in Table 1-3.

quiries utilize the SI system. The seven base SI units are mass, length, time, electric current, temperature, amount of substance, and luminous intensity. Radiologically important derived units are the **coulomb per kilogram** (C/kg), formerly the roentgen (R); the **gray** (Gy), formerly the rad (radiation absorbed dose); and the **sievert** (Sv), formerly the rem (radiation equivalent man). These radiologic units are described in greater detail in Chapter 8.

To convert from grams to kilograms or micrograms, or to grams with any other prefix, the decimal point is moved. If the prefix moves up the table, the decimal point is moved to the left the number of exponent positions moved. If the prefix moves down the table, the decimal point is moved to the right the number of exponent positions moved. Dimensional analysis can also be used.

EXAMPLES:

23.4 g = 0.0234 kg	Move the decimal point 3 positions left.
23.4 g = 23,400 mg	Move the decimal point 3 positions right.
23.4 mg = 0.0000234 kg	Move the decimal point 6 positions left.
23.4 kg = 2,340,000 cg	Move the decimal point 5 positions right.

Using dimensional analysis:

$$23.4 \text{ g} = 23.4 \text{ g} \frac{\text{g}}{1000\text{g}} = 0.0234 \text{ kg}$$

TABLE 1-4. Commonly Used SI Prefixes

Unit	Symbol	Meaning
kilovolt	kV	10^3 volts
centimeter	cm	10^{-2} meter
milliampere	mA	10^{-3} amp
milligray	mGy	10^{-3} Gy
nanosecond	ns	10^{-9} second

Some commonly used prefixes are shown in Table 1-4.

Conversion from one system to another is needed from time to time. For example, 1 inch = 2.54 cm is the conversion fact for changing inches to centimeters. See the section on dimensional analysis under the math review for the procedure to convert from one set of units to another.

SUMMARY

A basic review of arithmetic, algebra, and units of measurement has been presented. The arithmetic review includes fractions, decimals, computation with values, powers of ten, scientific notation and dimensional analysis. The algebra review includes signed numbers, order of operation, algebraic expressions, exponents, evaluating algebraic expressions, equations, and variation. Both SI and British (U.S. customary) units of measurement are introduced.

In order to quantify science, standard units of measurement were established. The fundamental units of measurement are mass, length, and time. Units of measurement were officially defined on an international level through the adoption of the SI units. The seven base SI units are mass, length, time, electric current, temperature, amount of substance, and luminous intensity. Radiologically important derived units are the coulomb per kilogram (C/kg), formerly the roentgen (R); the gray (Gy), formerly the rad (radiation absorbed dose); and the sievert (Sv), formerly the rem (radiation equivalent man).

REVIEW QUESTIONS

1. $\dfrac{4}{7} + \dfrac{1}{2} =$

2. $\dfrac{2}{9} \cdot \dfrac{3}{8} =$

3. $571.1 - 182.572 =$

4. $725 \div 0.25 =$

5. Change .325 to a percent.

6. What are the significant digits of each of the following:

   a. 20.10

   b. 192

   c. 38.04

   d. 2,700

   e. 1,800.004

7. Add the following numbers, leaving the results with the correct number of significant digits if each number is assumed to be approximate.

   a. $2.1 + 2.824$

   b. $3.2 + 4.19$

8. Change the following numbers to scientific notation:

   a. .0081

   b. 7,811.2

   c. .00024

   d. 78,432

9. Change the following numbers to ordinary notation:

   a. 3.614×10^2

   b. 1.876×10^{-4}

   c. 1.823×10^3

   d. 5.67×10^6

10. Convert 1,500 seconds to hours.

11. Convert 10 meters^2 to centimeters^2.

12. Simplify the following algebraic expressions:

    a. $-3(x + y) + 7(2x + 1)$

    b. $-4(x + 2y) - 8(2x - y)$

13. Simplify the following expressions, leaving the answer with only positive exponents:

    a. $a^2 \cdot b^3 \cdot a^4 \cdot b^2$

    b. $(a^4)^3 \cdot (a^2)^{-3}$

14. Evaluate the expression for a = 5 and b = 3.

    $\dfrac{3}{8}(a^2 - b^2)$

15. Evaluate the expression for a = 2, b = −4, and c = 6.

    $3(a + b) - c$

16. Solve for x: $2x - 8 = 4$

17. Solve for x: $2(3x - 8) = 3(4 - x) + 6x$

18. Solve for a: $\dfrac{2}{3} = \dfrac{a}{15}$

REFERENCES AND RECOMMENDED READING

Aufmann, R. N., & Barker, V. C. (2003). *Basic college mathematics* (7th ed.). Boston: Houghton Mifflin.

Burns, J. E. (1979). The new SI units: Problems with conversion. *The Canadian Journal of Radiography, Radiotherapy, and Nuclear Medicine, 10*(2), 60–70.

Dunworth, J. V. (1976). SI units for ionizing radiations. The use of the "Gray." *Radiography, 42*(496), 84.

Martin-Gay, K. E. (2004). Pre-algebra (4th ed.). Upper Saddle River, NJ: Prentice Hall.

The SI for the health profession. (1979). *The Canadian Journal of Medical Radiation Technology, 10*(4), 138.

Washington, A. J. (1999). *Basic technical mathematics* (7th ed.). Upper Saddle River, NJ: Pearson Addison Wesley.

Wyckoff, H. O. (1978). The international system of units (SI). *Radiology, 128*, 833–835.

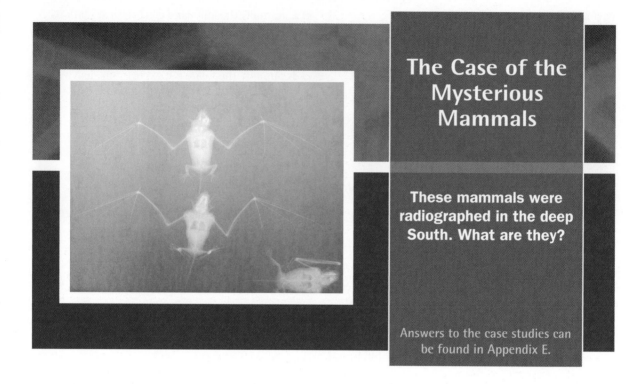

The Case of the Mysterious Mammals

These mammals were radiographed in the deep South. What are they?

Answers to the case studies can be found in Appendix E.

CHAPTER 2

Radiation Concepts

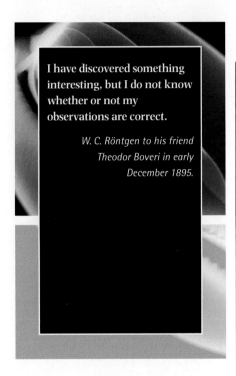

I have discovered something interesting, but I do not know whether or not my observations are correct.

W. C. Röntgen to his friend Theodor Boveri in early December 1895.

KEY TERMS

amplitude
atom
atomic mass number (A)
atomic mass unit (amu)
atomic number
chemical energy
compound
electrical energy
electricity
electromagnetic energy
electromagnetic radiation (EM)
electromagnetic spectrum
electron (e⁻)
electron binding energy (E_b)

electron volt (eV)
element
excitation
frequency
heat
ion
ionization
isotope
kinetic energy
K-shell
lambda
M theory
mass
mechanical energy
mixture
molecule
neutron (n⁰)
nu
nuclear energy
nucleon

nucleus
octet rule
period
photon
potential energy
proton (p⁺)
quantum
quark
radiation
shell
string theory
substance
temperature
thermal energy
valence
wavelength
weight
Z number

OBJECTIVES

Upon completion of this chapter, the student should be able to:

- Describe the branches of science.

- Differentiate between matter and energy.

- Describe the basic structure of matter.

- Identify the various types of energy.

- Explain the basic concepts of atomic theory.

- Differentiate between the radiations along the electromagnetic spectrum.

- Describe the wave and particle theories for electromagnetic radiation.

- Identify the properties of x-rays.

- Explain the standard units of measurement.

MATTER AND ENERGY

Radiography is the recording of images created by the use of x-ray energy. It is both an art and a science. In order to perform the duties of a radiographer, it is necessary to understand the art of the profession as well as the science.

Science is the use of knowledge in an organized and classified manner. The scientific method has been used by men and women to understand the world in which we live. This method systematically involves collecting facts, studying their relationships, and arriving at conclusions based on analysis. Natural science is the study of the universe and its contents. It can be divided into two categories: (1) the study of nonliving matter, known as physical science, and (2) the study of living matter, known as biological science. Radiographers learn about biological science through a study of human anatomy and physiology and about physical science through a study of x-ray production and imaging processes.

Physics is a branch of physical science that studies matter and energy and their interrelationships. Matter is defined as anything that has mass and occupies space. Energy is the ability to do work.

Matter

Matter is a very general term used to describe the substance that comprises all physical objects. It has shape, form, and it occupies space. A principle characteristic of matter is **mass.** Mass is the quantity of matter contained in an object. It is best described by its energy equivalence, although the term weight is generally used to mean the same thing. **Weight** is the force that an object exerts under the influence of gravity. An object may be weightless in a zero gravity environment, such as in space, but the mass of that object would remain unchanged.

The unit of mass is the kilogram, which equals 1,000 grams. The kilogram represents the weight of a standard piece of platinum-iridium kept at the International Bureau of Weights and Measures in Paris, France. It is equal to the mass of 1,000 cm^3 of water at 0° Celsius (C) or Centigrade.

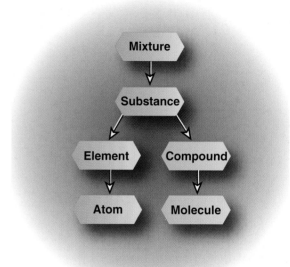

FIGURE 2-1 Structure of matter.

The structure of matter has been studied throughout history. In nature, matter is most commonly found as a mixture of substances (Figure 2-1). A **substance** is defined as a material that has a definite and constant composition. When two or more substances are combined, they form a **mixture.** For example, air is a mixture of oxygen, hydrogen, nitrogen, and a variety of other substances.

Substances may be either simple or complex. Simple substances are known as **elements** and complex substances are known as **compounds.** An element is a substance that cannot be broken down into any simpler substances by ordinary means. There are 92 naturally occurring elements identified on the periodic table of elements (Figure 2-2). Elements include such substances as hydrogen, oxygen, carbon, calcium, copper, silver, gold, lead, and barium. When two or more elements are chemically united in definite proportion, compounds are formed. Water and salt are both examples of compounds. Water is formed by the chemical union of two hydrogen atoms and one oxygen atom and is referred to as H_2O (Figure 2-3). Each element has an abbreviated letter or letters to identify it. These

IUPAC
Periodic Table of the Elements

Key:

| atomic number |
| symbol |
| name |
| standard atomic weight |

	1	2		3	4	5	6	7	8	9	10	11	12	13	14	15	16	17	18
K or 1	1 H hydrogen 1.007 94(7)																		2 He helium 4.002 602(2)
L or 2	3 Li lithium 6.941(2)	4 Be beryllium 9.012 182(3)												5 B boron 10.811(7)	6 C carbon 12.0107(8)	7 N nitrogen 14.0067(2)	8 O oxygen 15.9994(3)	9 F fluorine 18.998 4032(5)	10 Ne neon 20.1797(6)
M or 3	11 Na sodium 22.989 770(2)	12 Mg magnesium 24.3050(6)												13 Al aluminium 26.981 538(2)	14 Si silicon 28.0855(3)	15 P phosphorus 30.973 761(2)	16 S sulfur 32.065(5)	17 Cl chlorine 35.453(2)	18 Ar argon 39.948(1)
N or 4	19 K potassium 39.0983(1)	20 Ca calcium 40.078(4)	21 Sc scandium 44.955 910(8)	22 Ti titanium 47.867(1)	23 V vanadium 50.9415(1)	24 Cr chromium 51.9961(6)	25 Mn manganese 54.938 049(9)	26 Fe iron 55.845(2)	27 Co cobalt 58.933 200(9)	28 Ni nickel 58.6934(2)	29 Cu copper 63.546(3)	30 Zn zinc 65.409(4)	31 Ga gallium 69.723(1)	32 Ge germanium 72.64(1)	33 As arsenic 74.921 60(2)	34 Se selenium 78.96(3)	35 Br bromine 79.904(1)	36 Kr krypton 83.798(2)
O or 5	37 Rb rubidium 85.4678(3)	38 Sr strontium 87.62(1)	39 Y yttrium 88.905 85(2)	40 Zr zirconium 91.224(2)	41 Nb niobium 92.906 38(2)	42 Mo molybdenum 95.94(2)	43 Tc technetium [97.9072]	44 Ru ruthenium 101.07(2)	45 Rh rhodium 102.905 50(2)	46 Pd palladium 106.42(1)	47 Ag silver 107.8682(2)	48 Cd cadmium 112.411(8)	49 In indium 114.818(3)	50 Sn tin 118.710(7)	51 Sb antimony 121.760(1)	52 Te tellurium 127.60(3)	53 I iodine 126.904 47(3)	54 Xe xenon 131.293(6)
P or 6	55 Cs caesium 132.905 45(2)	56 Ba barium 137.327(7)	57-71 lanthanoids	72 Hf hafnium 178.49(2)	73 Ta tantalum 180.9479(1)	74 W tungsten 183.84(1)	75 Re rhenium 186.207(1)	76 Os osmium 190.23(3)	77 Ir iridium 192.217(3)	78 Pt platinum 195.078(2)	79 Au gold 196.966 55(2)	80 Hg mercury 200.59(2)	81 Tl thallium 204.3833(2)	82 Pb lead 207.2(1)	83 Bi bismuth 208.980 38(2)	84 Po polonium [208.9824]	85 At astatine [209.9871]	86 Rn radon [222.0176]
Q or 7	87 Fr francium [223.0197]	88 Ra radium [226.0254]	89-103 actinoids	104 Rf rutherfordium [261.1088]	105 Db dubnium [262.1141]	106 Sg seaborgium [266.1219]	107 Bh bohrium [264.12]	108 Hs hassium [277]	109 Mt meitnerium [268.1366]	110 Ds darmstadtium [271]	111 Uuu unununium [272]							

57 La lanthanum 138.9055(2)	58 Ce cerium 140.116(1)	59 Pr praseodymium 140.907 65(2)	60 Nd neodymium 144.24(3)	61 Pm promethium [144.9127]	62 Sm samarium 150.36(3)	63 Eu europium 151.964(1)	64 Gd gadolinium 157.25(3)	65 Tb terbium 158.925 34(2)	66 Dy dysprosium 162.500(1)	67 Ho holmium 164.930 32(2)	68 Er erbium 167.259(3)	69 Tm thulium 168.934 21(2)	70 Yb ytterbium 173.04(3)	71 Lu lutetium 174.967(1)
89 Ac actinium [227.0277]	90 Th thorium 232.0381(1)	91 Pa protactinium 231.035 88(2)	92 U uranium 238.028 91(3)	93 Np neptunium [237.0482]	94 Pu plutonium [244.0642]	95 Am americium [243.0614]	96 Cm curium [247.0704]	97 Bk berkelium [247.0703]	98 Cf californium [251.0796]	99 Es einsteinium [252.0830]	100 Fm fermium [257.0951]	101 Md mendelevium [258.0984]	102 No nobelium [259.1010]	103 Lr lawrencium [262.1097]

FIGURE 2-2   **Periodic Table of Elements.** *Copyright © 2003 IUPAC, the International Union of Pure and Applied Chemistry.*

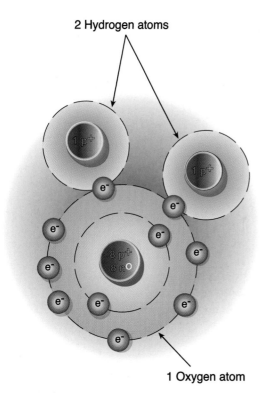

2 Hydrogen atoms

1 Oxygen atom

FIGURE 2-3 A water molecule is formed when two atoms of hydrogen combine with one atom of oxygen.

abbreviations for the elements are outlined on the periodic table. For example, in the compound salt, the element sodium (Na) is chemically combined with the element chlorine (Cl), in equal proportions, to form sodium chloride (NaCl).

When broken down and examined in its purest form, matter is actually comprised of very small invisible particles known as atoms. An **atom** is the smallest particle of an element that still possesses the chemical properties of that element. When two or more atoms are chemically united, they form a **molecule,** which is the smallest particle of a compound that still possesses the characteristics of the compound. For example, in the compound water, two hydrogen (H) atoms combine with one oxygen (O) atom to form one water (H_2O) molecule. With salt, one sodium (Na) atom combines with one chlorine (Cl) atom to form one sodium chloride (NaCl) molecule.

Atoms are tightly bonded to one another when a molecule is formed. These bonds cannot be broken by ordinary physical means, such as crushing. Atoms and molecules are, however, bound to one another by varying degrees of attraction. The degree of attraction between atoms or molecules will determine if the substance is a solid, a liquid, or a gas. The attraction is weakest with a gas and strongest with a solid. For example, depending on the degree of molecular attraction, water can exist in its usual state as a liquid, or it can exist as a gas (steam) or a solid (ice). The state is determined by the heat or thermal energy that the substance possesses.

Energy

Energy is defined as the ability to do work. The unit of energy is the joule (J). When energy is emitted and transferred through matter, it is called **radiation.** Radiation is a term applied to many forms of energy, such as heat and light. When the burner on a stove is lit, it can be described as radiating heat. A light bulb is capable of radiating light. When any form of matter is struck by a form of radiant energy, it is described as being exposed or radiated.

There is a unique relationship between matter and energy. They are interchangeable. This relationship was described in 1905 by the German American physicist, Albert Einstein (1879–1955), in his well-known theory of relativity. Einstein mathematically described the relationship between matter and energy in the equation:

$$E = mc^2$$

where: E = energy
m = mass
c = constant (the speed of light in a vacuum)

At the basis of Einstein's work is the Law of Conservation. This law states that the sum total of all matter and energy in the universe is a constant: matter and energy cannot be created or destroyed but can be converted from one form to another. Although recent research has demonstrated certain circumstances when Einstein's theory has been disproved, for practical purposes it is essentially true.

ATOMIC THEORY

Matter is comprised of very small particles known as atoms. To understand how small atoms really are, it has been estimated that one teaspoon of water (about 1 cm^3) contains about three times as many atoms as the Atlantic Ocean contains teaspoons of water.

Atoms can be subdivided into three basic subatomic particles: **protons (p^+), neutrons (n^0),** and **electrons (e^-).**

Historical Overview

The composition of the atom has been a topic of scientific investigation for thousands of years. The Greeks theorized that matter has four basic components: air, water, earth, and fire. They named the smallest division of these components the atom. This theory was accepted until the early 1800s, when an English schoolteacher named John Dalton (1766–1844) published his work on atomic theory. Dalton concluded that all elements could be differentiated from one another based on the characteristic of mass. He further concluded that each of the elements was composed of atoms that behaved in an identical fashion during a chemical reaction. During the mid-1800s, a Russian scientist, Dmitri Mendeleev (1834–1907), developed the first periodic table of the elements. This table arranges the elements in order of ascending atomic mass and on the basis of the repetition of similar chemical properties (Figure 2-2). More detailed information on a specific element on the periodic table, including specific characteristics, electron configurations, and electron binding energies, can be found at www.webelements.com.

Investigation of the structure of matter continued and, in 1911, English physicist Ernest Rutherford (1871–1937) developed a model for the atom that contained a central, small, dense nucleus, which possessed a positive charge and was surrounded by a negative cloud of randomly placed electrons, which had a negative charge. In 1913, Niels Bohr (1885–1962), a Danish physicist, expanded on Rutherford's work and proposed a model for the atom that is considered the most representa-tive of the structure of matter. Bohr's atom is likened to a miniature solar system where electrons orbit around a central nucleus just as the planets revolve around the sun.

Although the atom is far more complex than Bohr's simple model suggests, this model is still the most widely used in explaining the composition of matter. One key distinction between Bohr's model and an actual atom is that electrons orbit the nucleus in many planes, while the planets orbit the sun in essentially the same plane.

Bohr's simple model was difficult to apply to high atomic number elements. Both Niels Bohr and the Austrian physicist, Erwin Schrödinger, working with their associates, developed a theoretical approach to understanding atomic behavior. Both Bohr and Schrödinger were successful, but physicists primarily use Schrödinger's concept because it has been found to be more convenient. This approach is the foundation of modern physics and is known as quantum or wave mechanics.

According to the principles of quantum mechanics, orbital electrons are assigned probabilities for occupying any location within the atom. The greatest probabilities are associated with Bohr's original model.

Basic Atomic Particles

The atom is best described as having a small, dense center known as the **nucleus,** which is surrounded by electrons that orbit it at various levels (Figure 2-4). The nucleus contains two of the three basic particles of the atom, protons and neutrons, which are responsible for almost all of the mass of an atom. Protons and neutrons together are referred to as **nucleons.** The third basic particle, the electron, is located outside the nucleus and has a relatively insignificant mass, 1/1,826 that of a proton.

Electrons cannot be divided into smaller parts, but protons and neutrons are both composed of even smaller subnuclear structures called **quarks.** There are new theories that may explain them as well as find a way for quantum physics and relativity theory to work together. The overall concept is being referred to as **M theory.** It postulates that electrons and quarks may not be particles, but instead

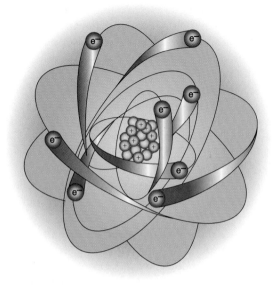

FIGURE 2-4 A three-dimensional diagram of an atom of oxygen, which contains eight protons, eight neutrons located within the center nucleus, and eight electrons within orbital shells moving around the nucleus.

may be extremely small loops of rapidly vibrating string-like matter. One idea is that matter behaves differently depending on the vibrations of the string (like a guitar string playing many different sounds depending on the position of the fingers on the frets, force applied via finger or pick, and the shape and size of the body of the guitar or the electronics in the pickup). In fact, this concept is now being called **string theory.** There are actually five different string theories and they require the addition of several new dimensions in addition to the four we know (as well as the need to invent new forms of mathematics to figure out how they function). Although this begins to sound like a science fiction story, many physicists are beginning to agree that these new theories may be the next frontier for research and hold hope for better explanations about how matter behaves. It is likely that our knowledge of radiation will expand along with these theories throughout your career in the radiologic sciences.

The subatomic particles possess electrical charges. There are two types of electrical charges: positive and negative. The proton is a positively charged particle and the electron is a negatively charged particle. The neutron contains no charge and is said to be electrically neutral. When the number of positively charged protons equals the number of negatively charged electrons, the atom is neutral or stable. Because of its electrical nature, the atom is dynamic and ever moving. It is in a constant, vibrating motion because of the strong positive nuclear force field, which is surrounded by the negatively charged spinning and orbiting electrons.

Each of the elements has its own specific number of nuclear protons. This is the key characteristic that distinguishes one element from another. The number of nuclear protons in an atom is known as the **atomic number** or **Z number.** The simplest element, hydrogen, possesses only one proton and therefore has an atomic number of 1. Helium comes next on the periodic table and has two protons, giving it an atomic number of 2. Lead has an atomic number of 82, indicating that within the nucleus of an atom of lead there are 82 protons. The periodic table lists the elements in ascending order according to the element's atomic number (Figure 2-2). In a neutral atom the number of protons is equal to the number of electrons. For example, in a stable, neutral atom of hydrogen there is one proton and one electron. In a stable atom of lead there are 82 protons and 82 electrons.

Although not a common occurrence in nature, when an atom of a given element loses or gains a proton, that atom becomes a different element. For example, if an atom of carbon with atomic number 6 gains a proton, the atom then becomes an atom of nitrogen with atomic number 7. Atoms of one element do change to atoms of another element during the natural process of radioactive decay. Radium, with an atomic number of 88, decays over a very long period of time to form the element radon, which has atomic number 86. Radon is a naturally occurring gas that is also radioactive. Recent studies have found increased radon levels in homes around the country. Radon testing kits are now commercially available to measure radon levels in the home.

Changes in the number of protons change the identity of the element completely, but this is not the case with changes in the number of neutrons or electrons. If an atom gains or loses neutrons, the result is an atom called an **isotope.** Isotopes are atoms that have the same number of protons in the nucleus but

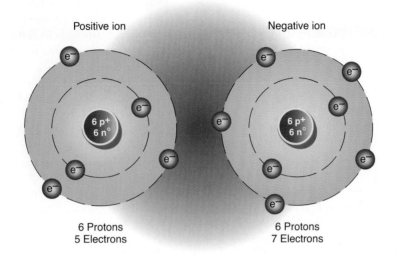

Positive ion   Negative ion

6 Protons   6 Protons
5 Electrons   7 Electrons

FIGURE 2-5   The ionization process. When an electron is either added to or removed from an atom, the atom is ionized. A neutral carbon atom contains six protons and six electrons; a positive ion of carbon would contain more protons than electrons, and a negative ion of carbon would contain more electrons than protons.

differ in the number of neutrons. Deuterium is an isotope of hydrogen. It contains the same number of protons as hydrogen but also contains one neutron.

If an atom gains or loses an electron, it is called an **ion** and the atom is said to be ionized. **Ionization** is the process of adding or removing an electron from an atom. When an electron is removed from an atom, the atom becomes a positive ion; that is, the atom possesses an extra positive charge. When an electron is added to an atom, the atom becomes a negative ion; that is, it possesses an extra negative charge (Figure 2-5).

Atomic Mass

The mass of an atom is extremely small; however, it is important to understand the differences in the mass of each of the basic particles of an atom. Each individual particle has its own unique mass. As stated earlier, the mass of an atom is almost entirely concentrated in the nucleus. The mass of a proton is approximately 1.673×10^{-27} kilograms and the mass of a neutron is almost identical, at 1.675×10^{-27} kilograms. While these numbers seem remarkably small, they are still significantly greater than the mass of an electron, at 9.109×10^{-31} kilograms. Protons have approximately 1,836 times the mass of

TABLE 2-1.   Atomic Particles

Particle	Mass Number	Mass (Kilograms)	amu	Charge
Proton	1	1.673×10^{-27}	1.00728	Positive
Neutron	1	1.675×10^{-27}	1.00867	Neutral
Electron	0	9.109×10^{-31}	0.000548	Negative

electrons, and neutrons have approximately 1,838 times more. The mass of the particles of an atom is sometimes described in **atomic mass units (amu).**

In order for science to be as exact as possible, scientists defined an atomic mass unit as equal to one twelfth of a carbon 12 atom. The amu of a proton is approximately 1.00728, a neutron has an amu of approximately 1.00867, and an electron has an amu of approximately 0.000548. When precision is not necessary, the mass of an atom is described by an **atomic mass number** symbolized by the letter **A.** The atomic mass number is equal to the number of protons and neutrons in the nucleus. For our purposes, each proton and neutron can be considered to have a mass number of one and an electron to have a mass number of zero (Table 2-1).

Orbital Electrons

Each of the electrons around the nucleus is in continuous motion. According to quantum mechanics, each of these electrons resides in an orbit that may be described as a "probability density." The orbital describes the region over which the electron is most likely to be at any given time.

The distance from the nucleus determines the energy level or **shell** the electron occupies. Each energy level has a certain **electron binding energy (E_b).** The binding energy of an electron is defined as that amount of energy needed to remove the electron from the atom. If a free electron at rest is assumed to have an energy of zero, then the total energy of an orbital electron would be zero minus the binding energy or the negative of the binding energy. The closer an electron is to the nucleus, the more tightly it is bound to its orbit or shell. The charge felt by any electron at various distances from the nucleus is termed the shielded nuclear charge.

Certain forces are responsible for maintaining the electron's position and motion in its orbit. The stability of this orbit is contributed to by two opposing forces: the centrifugal force and the attractive electrostatic force. The centrifugal force tends to cause the electron to fly out in space. The attractive electrostatic force between the positively charged nucleus and the negatively charged electron tends to cause the two to fly together. These forces are exactly equal and opposite in a stable orbital. The end result is an electron that is in motion in a specific orbit around the nucleus. The closer an electron is to the nucleus, the higher the electron binding energy is and the more difficult it is to remove the electron from the atom.

The orbital shell closest to the nucleus is called the **K-shell;** the next shell is called the L-shell, then M-, N-, O-, P-, and, finally, the Q-shell. These letters for the shells are actually no longer used by chemists and physicists. They identify the shells by the principal quantum number (n). The first shell (K) is designated as n = 1. The second shell (L) is n = 2; the third shell (M) is n = 3, etc. Two additional quantum numbers, the angular momentum quantum number and the magnetic quantum number, are further used by chemists and physicists to describe more precisely the location of an electron within an atom.

In a neutral atom, the number of protons and electrons is equal. This means that each element has a different number of orbital electrons. The element hydrogen has only one proton and one electron. The electron of a hydrogen atom orbits in the K-shell. There is a maximum number of electrons that can occupy a given shell. The maximum number is determined by the formula $2n^2$, where n equals the shell or principal quantum number, starting with K as the first shell. According to this formula, the maximum number of electrons in each of the shells would be:

$$K = 2(1)^2 = 2$$
$$L = 2(2)^2 = 8$$
$$M = 2(3)^2 = 18$$
$$N = 2(4)^2 = 32$$
$$O = 2(5)^2 = 50$$
$$P = 2(6)^2 = 72$$
$$Q = 2(7)^2 = 98$$

Electrons may begin to appear in the next shell before a shell contains its maximum number of electrons. For example, electrons may appear in the N-shell before the M-shell has 18 electrons in it. This is because the number of electrons in the outermost shell never exceeds eight electrons. This is commonly referred to as the **octet rule.** Atoms that contain exactly eight electrons in their outermost shell are considered inert and chemically stable. The specific electron configuration will determine an element's position within the groups of the periodic table.

As the number of electrons and protons increases, so does the binding energy of a given electron. This is due to the increase in the positive charge in the nucleus. This means that the electrons in atoms of high atomic number elements are bound more tightly than the electrons in atoms of lower atomic number elements. The binding energy of electrons in the K-shell of lead is much higher than the binding energy of the K-shell electrons in hydrogen or oxygen. In addition, the binding energy of an electron decreases as the distance from the nucleus is increased (Figure 2-6). It takes more energy to remove a K-shell electron from its path than it would to remove an electron from a shell at a greater distance from the nucleus, such

74 p+ 110 n⁰

2 e⁻	8 e⁻	18 e⁻	32 e⁻	12 e⁻	2 e⁻
K	**L**	**M**	**N**	**O**	**P**
n = 1	n = 2	n = 3	n = 4	n = 5	n = 6
~ 69.5 keV	~ 12 keV	~ 3 keV	~ 0.6 keV	~ 0.08 keV	~ 0.02 keV

FIGURE 2-6   The closer an electron is to the nucleus, the greater will be the binding energy of the electron.

as the L-, M-, or N-shell. This will become important to remember when studying the effect of x-rays on atoms.

The binding energy of an electron is measured in a unit called the **electron volt (eV).** This is the same unit used to describe x-ray energies. The electron volt is the energy one electron will have when it is accelerated by an electrical potential of one volt. Because x-ray and binding energies are great, the usual unit used to express these energies is the kilo-electron volt (keV). One keV equals 1,000 electron volts.

The atomic configuration and the approximate binding energies of certain elements are important because of their significance in radiology. These elements include hydrogen (H), carbon (C), and oxygen (O) because they are the principal elements that comprise the human body; iodine (I) and barium (Ba), because these elements are used as contrast media for a variety of radiologic examinations; tungsten (W) and molybdenum (Mo), because they are x-ray tube target materials; and lead (Pb), because it is the element used for radiation protection devices. A diagram of these elements shows that as the atomic number of an element increases, the K-shell binding energy of the element increases (Figure 2-7). This means that a K-shell electron of lead (Pb) is more tightly bound and more difficult to remove from the atom than a K-shell electron of smaller atomic number elements, such as hydrogen (H) or oxygen (O).

To remove the K-shell electron from an atom of tungsten or lead requires much more energy than would be necessary to remove a K-shell electron from an atom of hydrogen, carbon, or oxygen. When an electron is removed from an atom, the atom is said to be ionized. X-rays are capable of ionizing atoms. The x-ray energy must be greater than the binding energy of the electron in order for ionization to occur (Figure 2-8).

The Periodic Table

The present-day periodic table lists the 92 naturally occurring elements and an additional 18 elements that have been created in the laboratory through scientific investigation (Figure 2-2). The elements are listed in ascending order based on the atomic number located above the element's symbol. The relative atomic mass of the element is identified below the symbol. Each of the elements is also arranged into one of seven horizontal periods and one of eight vertical groups. The periods represent elements with the same principal quantum number or number of electron shells and the groups represent elements with the same number of electrons in the outermost shell. For example, each element in the last group has eight electrons in its outermost shell. These elements are chemically very stable atoms.

The number of electrons in the outermost shell of an atom determines the chemical combining characteristic or **valence** of the element. An element that has only one electron in the outermost shell is described as having a valence of $+1$ and would be located in Group 1 on the periodic table. This element will freely give up this electron to bind with another element to form a compound. An element that has seven electrons in its outermost shell has a valence of -1 and would be located in Group 7. This element will freely accept an electron to form a chemical bond because atoms prefer the stable octet configuration. An example of this bond,

known as an ionic bond, is the salt molecule. Sodium (Na), having a valence of $+1$, can easily combine with chlorine (Cl), with a valence of -1, to form sodium chloride (NaCl), salt (Figure 2-9). The valence of an element determines the way the atoms will combine in definite proportions. Because of the element's valence number, **two** hydrogen atoms combine with **one** oxygen atom to form water. Hydrogen has a valence of $+1$, while oxygen has a valence of -2. Oxygen has room for two hydrogen atoms and will share electrons, a type of bond known as a covalent bond (Figure 2-10).

 TYPES OF ENERGY

Energy is the ability to do work. It exists in many different forms. Regardless of form, all types of energy possess an actual or potential ability to do work. Work is the result of a force acting upon an object over a distance. It is expressed in the equation **work = force × distance.** When a force acts upon an object over a distance, energy is expended. For example, when a book is lifted 1 foot above a table, work is done and energy is expended. If the same book is lifted 2 feet above the table, twice as much work and energy are expended.

Mechanical

Mechanical energy is the result of the action of machines or physical movement. There are two types of mechanical energy: potential and kinetic. **Potential energy** is the energy that an object has because of its position. It is stored, by virtue of its position, in the object until it is converted to another form of energy. A car located at the top of a hill possesses more potential energy than the same car located at the bottom of a hill. If the car's brakes are released, the potential energy is then converted to kinetic energy as the car moves to the bottom of the hill (and a lower energy state). **Kinetic energy** is the energy of motion. An object in motion is able to perform work because it is moving. For example, the energy of water as it moves in a river can be used to perform work. When a dam is built across a river, the kinetic energy of the moving water can be used to produce electric energy. No electricity will be produced if the water is not moving.

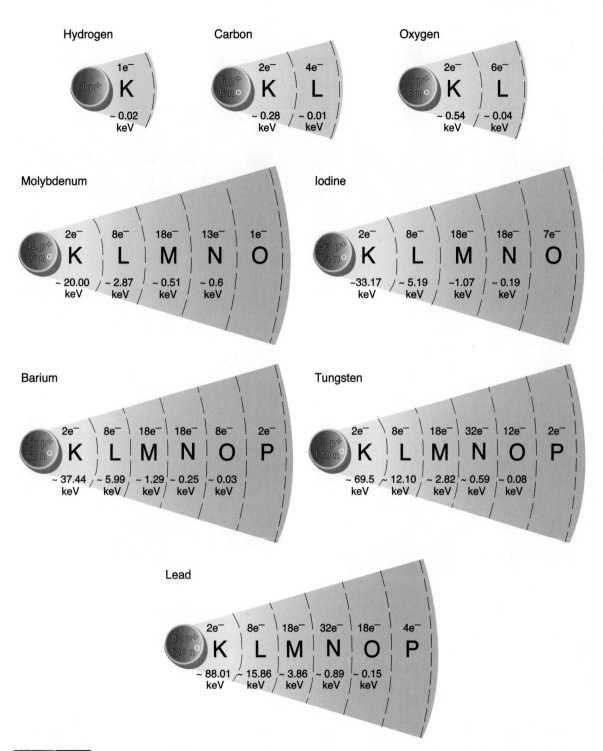

FIGURE 2-7 The atomic configurations and binding energies of elements that have significance in radiology.

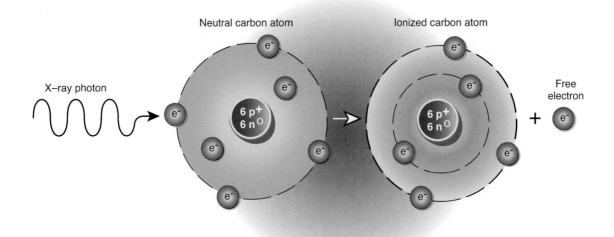

FIGURE 2-8 An x-ray photon can interact with an electron and eject it from an atom. This removal of an electron results in the ionization of the atom.

FIGURE 2-9 An ionic bond is formed between sodium (Na) and chlorine (Cl) to form table salt, sodium chloride (NaCl).

Chemical

Chemical energy is the form of energy released during a chemical reaction. A battery operates using chemical energy. The purpose of a battery is to convert chemical energy into electrical energy.

Heat

Heat, also called **thermal energy,** is the result of the motion of atoms and molecules. The faster the atoms and molecules within a substance are moving or vibrating, the greater the thermal energy of the sub-

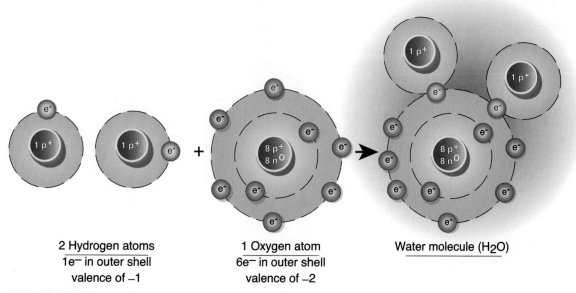

2 Hydrogen atoms
$1e^-$ in outer shell
valence of -1

1 Oxygen atom
$6e^-$ in outer shell
valence of -2

Water molecule (H_2O)

FIGURE 2-10   A covalent bond is formed between two hydrogen atoms and one oxygen atom to form water, H_2O.

stance. **Temperature** is a measure of thermal energy. As the temperature of a substance increases, the motion of the atoms in the substance increases. When a pan of water is placed on an electric burner, the electrical energy is converted to heat energy, which raises the temperature of the water and increases the motion of its atoms and molecules.

Electrical

Electrical energy, or **electricity,** is the result of the movement of electrons (electrical charges). Electricity is the study of resting or moving electrical charges. There are numerous appliances that operate by the use of electrical energy. When a lamp is turned on, a flow of electrons passes along a wire in a light bulb. The light bulb is a device that converts electrical energy to light, which is a form of electromagnetic energy. In a toaster, electrical energy is converted to heat, or thermal energy.

Nuclear

Nuclear energy is stored in the nucleus of each atom and holds the nuclear particles in a tight bond. A tremendous amount of energy is stored in the nucleus of an atom. In the 1940s scientists working at the University of Chicago learned how to control the release of this energy and, as a result of this knowledge, developed the atomic bomb. Today, nuclear power plants convert nuclear energy, within a very controlled environment, to electricity.

Electromagnetic

Electromagnetic energy is a form of energy that is the result of electric and magnetic disturbances in space (Figure 2-11). This type of energy travels through space as a combination of electric and magnetic fields and is produced by the acceleration of a charge. There are many very familiar forms of electromagnetic energy, including radio waves, microwaves, infrared light, visible light, and cosmic rays. X-rays are a form of man-made electromagnetic energy that is created in an x-ray tube when high-speed electrons are suddenly stopped. Physically they are identical to gamma rays, differing only in origin. Gamma rays originate from the nucleus of radioactive materials, while x-rays originate in an x-ray tube.

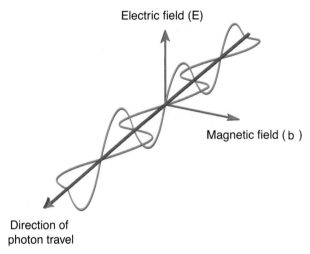

Electric field (E)

Magnetic field (b)

Direction of
photon travel

 Overlapping sine waves, one representing an electric field and the other a magnetic field,
illustrate electromagnetic radiation.

ELECTROMAGNETIC SPECTRUM

Electromagnetic radiation (EM) is a natural part of the environment in which we live. Although the term may not be a common one, we are all familiar with many forms of this energy. The nature of electromagnetic radiation was discovered in scientific experiments using visible light. Visible light was shown to have both electric and magnetic properties and was therefore described as being electromagnetic. Shortly after these investigations, other forms of electromagnetic radiation, invisible to man, were studied and a theory to explain this form of energy was proposed.

Electromagnetic radiation spans a continuum of wide ranges of magnitudes of energy. This continuum is termed the **electromagnetic spectrum** (Figure 2-12). The electromagnetic spectrum details all of the various forms of EM radiation. One of the common properties of all forms of EM radiation is velocity. The velocity of EM energy is equal to the speed of light (c), which is 3×10^8 meters/second (186,400 miles per second) in a vacuum.

Electromagnetic radiation with energies of approximately 10 eV and higher are capable of ionizing an atom or molecule. Ultraviolet, x-ray, and gamma radiations are all capable of ionization. When they interact with matter, they can remove an electron from an orbital shell. Electromagnetic radiation is also capable of transferring energy to an atom by a process known as **excitation.** In the excitation process, electrons in an atom are moved to a higher energy state without actually being removed from the atom.

In studying EM radiation, scientists found that under certain circumstances it behaved as a wave and at other times it behaved as a particle. **This dual nature is known as the wave-particle duality of radiation. To best understand x-rays, it is necessary to consider them as both waves and particles of energy.**

Wave Theory

Electromagnetic energy travels through space in the form of waves. Waves are disturbances in a medium. Ocean waves and sound waves are examples of disturbances of the mediums of water and air. When a rock is dropped into water, waves result. During speech, sound waves are created as disturbances in the air. **Electromagnetic waves are unique in that no medium is required.** They can travel in a vacuum.

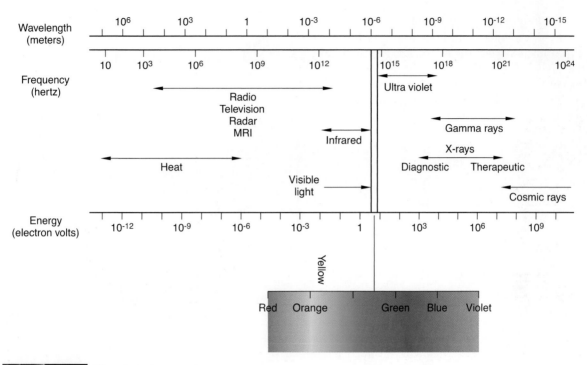

FIGURE 2-12   The electromagnetic spectrum.

All types of waves have an associated wavelength, frequency, amplitude, and period. To illustrate the wave concept, a sine wave is used because electromagnetic waves travel in the form of a sine wave (Figure 2-13). Sine waves can be mathematically described, but these definitions are beyond the scope of this book. Instead, we will use the primary descriptions of electromagnetic waves: wavelength and frequency. The **wavelength** is the distance between any two successive points on a wave. Wavelength is usually measured from crest to crest or trough to trough. It is represented by the Greek letter **lambda** (λ), the character for length. Wavelengths vary from kilometers to Angstroms. The Angstrom (represented by the symbol Å) is equal to 10^{-10} meters, which is one ten-billionth of a meter. The Angstrom is of special interest because the wavelength of diagnostic x-rays is 0.1–0.5 Å. **Amplitude** is the intensity of the wave defined by its maximal height.

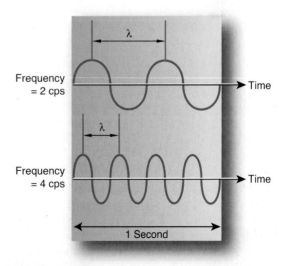

FIGURE 2-13   Two sine waves. With electromagnetic waves, if wavelength decreases, frequency will increase.

The **frequency** is the number of waves that passes a particular point in a given time frame, or the number of cycles per second. It is represented by the Greek letter **nu** (ν), the initial for number. The unit of frequency is the hertz (Hz) or cycles per second (cps). **Period** is the time required to complete one cycle of the wave.

A relationship exists between the frequency, wavelength, and velocity of a wave. This relationship is expressed by the formula:

velocity = frequency $\times$ wavelength,
   or c = $\nu\lambda$

where: c = constant (the speed of light)
     ν = the frequency
     λ = the wavelength

This is known as the wave equation. Recall that with electromagnetic waves, velocity was a constant equal to the speed of light. Because velocity is a constant, an increase in frequency would result in an associated decrease in wavelength and vice versa. Therefore, **frequency and wavelength are inversely proportional.**

Radiation along the electromagnetic spectrum will vary according to the associated frequency and wavelength. Low frequencies and long wavelengths are at the bottom end of the spectrum with radio waves and microwaves, visible light is in the center of the spectrum, and at the top of the spectrum are gamma and x-rays, with associated high frequencies and short wavelengths.

Particle Theory

When high-frequency electromagnetic radiation interacts with matter, it behaves more like a particle than a wave. With this model, electromagnetic radiation acts like a small bundle of energy, known as a **photon** or **quantum.** The photon carries a specific amount of energy that is dependent on frequency. **Photon energy and frequency are directly proportional.** If the frequency of an x-ray is doubled, the energy is doubled. This relationship was first described by the German physicist Max Planck (1858–1947). The relationship between photon energy and frequency is mathematically described in the formula:

$$E = h\nu$$

where: E = photon energy (eV)
     h = Planck's constant
        (4.15×10^{-15} eV-sec)
     ν = photon frequency (Hz)

From this formula, it is possible to calculate the frequency of an x-ray when given the x-ray photon's energy.

EXAMPLE: What is the frequency of a 72 keV x-ray photon?

Answer:

$$E = h\nu$$

$$\nu = \frac{E}{h}$$

$$\nu = \frac{72 \text{ keV}}{4.15 \times 10^{-15} \text{ eV-sec}}$$

$$\nu = \frac{7.2 \times 10^4 \text{ eV}}{4.15 \times 10^{-15} \text{ eV-sec}}$$

$$\nu = 1.73 \times 10^{19} \text{ Hz}$$

THE DISCOVERY OF X-RAYS

On November 8, 1895, the German physicist Wilhelm Conrad Röntgen discovered an unusual phenomenon while working in his laboratory at the University of Würzburg. Röntgen had been repeating various experiments with cathode rays, notably those of his colleagues Hertz, Hittorf, Crookes, and Lenard. These investigators had developed equipment for exploring the effects of high tension discharges in evacuated glass tubes. By late 1895, this small group of physicists was beginning to explore the properties of cathode rays outside the tubes. Early in November of 1895, Röntgen was repeating an experiment with one of Lenard's tubes in which a thin aluminum window had been added to permit the cathode rays to exit the tube. Lenard had supplied the tube with a tightly fitting cardboard covering to protect the aluminum window from damage by the strong electrostatic field necessary to produce the cathode rays. This covering also prevented any visible light from escaping. Röntgen had successfully repeated the experiment and had observed that the invisible cathode rays caused a fluorescent effect on a small cardboard screen painted with barium platinocyanide when it was placed very close to the aluminum window.

It occurred to Röntgen that the Hittorf-Crookes tube, which had a much thicker glass wall than the Lenard tube, might also cause this fluorescent effect. In the late afternoon of November 8, he determined to test his idea. He carefully constructed a black cardboard covering similar to the one he had used on the Lenard tube. He covered the Hittorf-Crookes tube with the covering and attached electrodes to the Ruhmkorff coil to generate an electrostatic charge. Before setting up the barium platinocyanide screen to test his idea, Röntgen darkened the room to test the opacity of his cardboard cover. As he passed the Ruhmkorff coil charge through the tube, he determined that the cover was light-tight and turned to prepare the next step of the experiment. It was at this point that he noticed a faint shimmering from a bench a meter away from the tube. To be sure, he tried several more discharges and saw the same shimmering effect each time. Striking a match, Röntgen discovered the shimmering had come from the location of the barium platinocyanide screen he had been intending to use next.

Röntgen spent the next few hours repeating the experiment again and again. He quickly determined that the screen would fluoresce at a distance from the tube much greater than in his previous tests. He speculated that a new kind of ray might be responsible. November 8 was a Friday, and Röntgen took advantage of the weekend to repeat his experiments and make his first notes. In the following weeks, he investigated nearly all the known properties of the rays, even eating and sleeping in his laboratory.

Röntgen's discovery of x-rays was no accident, and he was not working alone. With the investigations he and his colleagues in various countries were pursuing, the discovery was imminent. The idea that he just happened to notice the barium platinocyanide screen totally misrepresents his investigative powers. He had planned to use the screen in the next step of the experiment.

At one point while he was investigating the ability of various materials to stop the rays, he brought a small piece of lead into position while a discharge was occurring. Imagine Röntgen's astonishment as

he saw the first radiographic image, his own flickering ghostly skeleton on the barium platinocyanide screen. He later reported that it was at this point that he determined to continue his experiments in secrecy, because he feared for his professional reputation if his observations were in error.

Röntgen became the first radiographer when he produced a series of four photographs to accompany the first draft of his paper: the hand of his wife (Figure 2-14), a set of weights, a compass, and a piece of metal. Röntgen's original paper, "On a New Kind of Rays," was published 50 days later on December 28. It is translated in Appendix A. Röntgen assigned the mathematical term for an unknown, X, to the rays he discovered. In later years they were officially given his name to honor his work. Today, either term, x-rays or Röntgen rays, is acceptable. Röntgen published a total of three papers on x-rays between 1895 and 1897. His investigative powers

FIGURE 2-14 The first x-ray image of the human hand. The radiograph was taken by Röntgen of his wife's hand. *(Courtesy of American College of Radiology, Chantilly, VA)*

were so phenomenal that none of his conclusions have yet been proven false. Röntgen received many honors for his discovery, including, in 1901, the first Nobel Prize for physics. He died of carcinoma of the bowel in 1923.

X-RAY PROPERTIES

When Röntgen began his study of the invisible x-rays, it was unlikely that he would be able to identify all of the properties of this new discovery. Röntgen's investigation was so thorough, however, that no scientist since has been able to add to the list of properties Röntgen identified.

Through his use of the scientific method, Röntgen found that x-rays:

1. Are highly penetrating, invisible rays which are a form of electromagnetic radiation.

2. Are electrically neutral and therefore not affected by either electric or magnetic fields.

3. Can be produced over a wide variety of energies and wavelengths (polyenergetic and heterogeneous).

4. Release very small amounts of heat upon passing through matter.

5. Travel in straight lines.

6. Travel at the speed of light, 3×10^8 meters per second in a vacuum.

7. Can ionize matter.

8. Cause fluorescence (the emission of light) of certain crystals.

9. Cannot be focused by a lens.

10. Affect photographic film.

11. Produce chemical and biological changes in matter through ionization and excitation.

12. Produce secondary and scatter radiation.

SUMMARY

The physical universe can best be understood through physics—the study of matter and energy and their interrelationships. Matter is the substance which comprises all physical objects. The smallest subdivision of matter is the atom, which is comprised of three basic subatomic particles: the proton, the neutron, and the electron. Energy is the ability to do work. There are many forms of energy, including x-rays, which are a form of electromagnetic radiation. Matter and energy cannot be created or destroyed but are interchangeable, as described in Einstein's theory of relativity ($E = mc^2$).

The atom is best described as having a small, dense center, known as the nucleus, that is surrounded by electrons located within orbital shells. Protons and neutrons are located within the nucleus and are responsible for almost all of the mass of an atom. The electron is located outside the nucleus and has a relatively insignificant mass. Protons possess a positive charge, electrons possess a negative charge, and neutrons are electrically neutral.

Each of the elements has its own specific number of nuclear protons. This is the key characteristic that distinguishes one element from another. The number of nuclear protons in an atom is known as the atomic number or Z number. The periodic table lists the elements in ascending order according to the element's atomic number.

Electromagnetic radiation behaves as both a wave and a particle. As a wave, EM radiation has an associated frequency and wavelength. As a particle, it behaves as a bundle of energy, called a photon. X-rays are a man-made form of electromagnetic radiation that is created when high-speed electrons are suddenly stopped. X-rays were discovered by Wilhelm Conrad Röntgen on November 8, 1895, in Germany. From his thorough investigation, 12 properties of x-rays were identified.

REVIEW QUESTIONS

1. What are the two major branches of natural science?

2. How do matter and energy differ?

3. Define an atom and a molecule.

4. What are the three basic subatomic particles?

5. What is ionization?

6. What is the formula used to determine the maximum number of electrons that can be contained in a given shell? How many electrons can be contained in the N-shell?

7. The periodic table of elements arranges the elements into periods and groups. How are the elements similar within each period? Within each group?

8. How do radiations differ along the electromagnetic spectrum?

9. List five types of energy.

10. For electromagnetic radiation, what is the relationship between frequency and wavelength? Between frequency and photon energy?

11. List five properties of x-rays.

REFERENCES AND RECOMMENDED READING

Ball, J. L., & Moore, A. D. (1997). *Essential physics for radiographers* (3rd ed.). Oxford: Blackwell Scientific.

Bushberg, J. T., Seibert, J. A., Leidholdt, E. M., & Boone, J. M. (2002). *The essential physics of medical imaging* (2nd ed.). Philadelphia: Lippincott Williams & Wilkins.

Bushong, S. C. (2004). *Radiologic science for technologists: Physics, biology, and protection* (8th ed.). St. Louis, MO: Elsevier C. V. Mosby.

Curry, T. S., Dowdey, J. E., & Murry, R. C. (1990). *Christensen's introduction to the physics of diagnostic radiology* (4th ed.). Philadelphia: Lea and Febiger.

Eisenberg, R. L. (1992). *Radiology: An illustrated history.* St. Louis, MO: Elsevier C. V. Mosby.

Fuchs, A. W. (1960). Radiography of 1896. *Image, 9,* 4–17.

Glasser, O. (1958). *Dr. W. C. Röntgen* (2nd ed.). Springfield, IL: Charles C Thomas.

Handbook of chemistry and physics (78th ed.). (1998). Boca Raton, FL: CRC Press.

Hennig, U. (1989). *Deutsches Röntgen-Museum Remscheid-Lennep.* Remscheid, Germany: Westermann.

Meredith, W. J., & Massey, J. B. (1977). *Fundamental physics of radiology* (3rd ed.). Chicago: Yearbook Medical.

Röntgen, W. C. (1896). On a new kind of rays, *Science, 3*(59), 227–231.

Röntgen, W. C. (1896). On a new kind of rays. *Nature, 53*(1369), 274–276.

Selman, J. C. (2000). *The fundamentals of imaging physics and radiobiology: For the radiologic technologists* (9th ed.). Springfield, IL: Charles C Thomas.

CHAPTER 3

Electricity

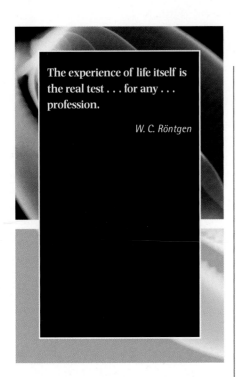

The experience of life itself is the real test . . . for any . . . profession.

W. C. Röntgen

KEY TERMS

admittance
alternating current (AC)
amp (A)
ampere (A)
atomic reactor
battery
circuit breaker
concentration
conductance
conduction band
conductor
contact
current
direct current (DC)
distribution
electrical circuit
electric current

electric field
electrification
electromotive force (emf)
electrostatic
friction
fuse
gasses
generator
induction
insulator
inverse square law
ionic solution
laws of electrostatics
metallic conductor
milliamperage (mA)
movement
ohm Ω

parallel circuit
potential difference
potentiometer
power loss formula
repulsion–attraction
resistance
rheostat
semiconductor
series circuit
solar converter
static discharge
superconductor
vacuum
valence energy band
volt
voltage (V)
zero or ground potential

OBJECTIVES

Upon completion of this chapter, the student should be able to:

- Explain the atomic nature of electricity.
- State the elementary laws of electrostatics.
- Describe the methods of electrification.
- Interpret the results of various electrostatic interactions.
- Differentiate conductors from insulators.

- Describe the basic factors of electrodynamics.
- Calculate the effect of changes in voltage, amperage, and resistance according to Ohm's law.
- Calculate voltage, amperage, and resistance in simple series and parallel circuits.

To control x-rays it is necessary to understand how they are produced. X-rays are produced when extremely high-energy electricity produces high-speed electrons that interact with matter. Electricity must be understood at the subatomic level for this process to become clear. The distribution and movement of electrons, along with their associated charges, make up electricity. Understanding atomic structure, including how electrons interact both in and outside of atoms, becomes the key to understanding electricity. It is the distribution and movement of atomic charges that can cause forces to interact.

Atoms contain both kinds of electrical charges, the **positive charge** of the proton, which is locked within the nucleus by very strong forces, and the **negative charge** of the electron, which is located outside the nucleus, bound by relatively weak forces. Electrons may not be associated with a nucleus at all, in which case they are called "free" electrons. In either case, **the positive charge of the proton and the negative charge of the electron are equal in strength.** Because electrons, with their negative charges, are free to move between atomic orbital shells and even between atoms, electricity concerns the distribution and movement of electrons and has little to do with the positively charged protons locked within the atomic nucleus.

ELECTROSTATICS

Electrostatics is the study of the distribution of fixed charges, or electrons that are at rest. Just as all atoms are charged (neutral, positive, negative), objects become charged by their composite individual atomic charges. Some atoms include electrons in their outer shells, or beyond the outer shell but within the atom's sphere of influence, that are very easily removed. There are instances, as when walking across a heavy rug in winter, when electrons are easily transferred (literally scooped up) onto another object. It is this type of distribution and redistribution of charged electrons that makes up electrostatics.

The term **electrification** is used to describe the process of electron charges being added to or sub-

tracted from an object. When one object has more electrons than another, it also has more negative charges. Therefore, it can be considered to be negatively electrified, or to have a negative charge. The concept of positive electrification, a positive charge, is more complicated because protons, which carry true positive charges, are not easily distributed. Therefore, a positive charge usually refers to something with a weaker negative charge, or fewer electrons. The so-called positively electrified, charged, object has a negative charge; it is just a weaker negative charge than the object with which it is being compared. It is less negative, and therefore termed positive, by comparison. It is important to remember that electrification is a relative term and that nearly all objects have negative charges. **When discussing electricity, the terms negative and positive refer to the relationship between two objects, not to their true atomic charges.**

In conjunction with the idea that negative and positive charges are relative to each other, another concept is required in order to establish a neutral reference point. This is done by defining the earth as **zero or ground potential.** Because the earth contains what is essentially an infinite number of charges, both positive and negative, in equal distribution, it is considered to be neutral and is the reference point for discussing charges. It has zero potential because the equally balanced charges have no potential to perform work and release energy. The symbol for ground is ⏚.

Laws of Electrostatics

Before attempting to understand how objects are electrified, it is helpful to learn five fundamental **laws of electrostatics.** These important laws have many corollaries in physics and will be used again and again throughout this book. The five laws are:

1. **Repulsion-attraction** (Figure 3-1). Like charges repel; unlike charges attract.

2. The **inverse square law** (Figure 3-2). The force between two charges is directly proportional to the product of their magnitudes and inversely proportional to the square of the distance between them. As a charged object gets further away, the influencing charge decreases because

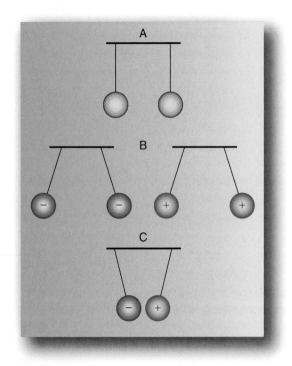

FIGURE 3-1 Repulsion-attraction law:
(A) neutral charge; (B) repulsion of like charges;
and (C) attraction of unlike charges.

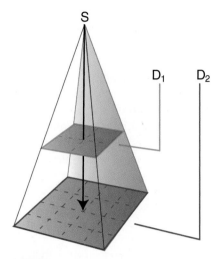

FIGURE 3-2 The inverse square law: If S is the source and D_2 is twice the distance of D_1, the area covered by the diverging field at D_2 is four times the area covered at D_1.

of the increased area it affects. The law is expressed as:

$$\frac{I_1}{I_2} = \frac{D_2^2}{D_1^2}$$

where: I_1 = old intensity

   I_2 = new intensity

   D_1^2 = old distance squared

   D_2^2 = new distance squared

EXAMPLE: If an object has a charge of 4 coulombs at 4 mm, what will the charge be at 8 mm?

Answer:

$$\frac{I_1}{I_2} = \frac{D_2^2}{D_1^2}$$

$$\frac{4 \text{ coulombs}}{x} = \frac{(8 \text{ mm})^2}{(4 \text{ mm})^2}$$

$$\frac{4}{x} = \frac{64}{16}$$

$$64x = 64$$

$$x = 1 \text{ coulomb}$$

In this example, as the distance doubled, the charge was reduced to 25 percent of its original value. Although this inverse square formula is usually sufficient for radiographic needs, it is important to understand that the true relationship of the force between two charges is accurately expressed in Coulomb's law:

$$F = \frac{kq_1q_2}{R^2}$$

where: F = electrostatic force in newtons

   k = constant of proportionality
   (9×10^9 for coulombs and meters)

q_1 and q_2 = charges in coulombs

   R = distance in meters

This formula takes into account the true definition: the force between two charges (q_1 and q_2) is directly proportional to the product of their magnitudes ($q_1 \times q_2$), and inversely proportional to the square of the distance between

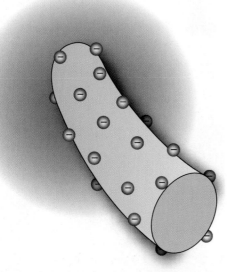

FIGURE 3-3   The law of distribution of charge: As individual electrons are repelled from one another, they distribute at the outer limits of a conductor.

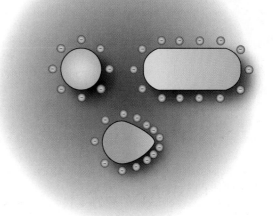

FIGURE 3-4   The law of concentration of charge: Because each negative charge is repelled by all other negative charges, they tend to concentrate at points of greatest curvature.

them (($q^1 \times q^2)/R^2$). Ironically, although the French physicist Coulomb (1736–1806) received the credit for development of this law, the original inquiry was initiated by the American scientist Benjamin Franklin (1706–1790).

3. **Distribution** (Figure 3-3). Charges reside on the external surfaces of conductors and equally throughout nonconductors. This law is a result of the effect of the repulsion-attraction law as electrons, all with negative charges, attempt to repel each other as much as possible. In a solid conductor this results in equal distribution on the surface, which is the point where electrons can obtain maximum distance from each other. In a nonconductor, such as a cloud, charge movement is not facilitated and equal distribution throughout the object results.

4. **Concentration** (Figure 3-4). The greatest concentration of charge will be on the surface where the curvature is sharpest. If enough electrons congregate they can induce ionization of the surrounding air and even discharge to the nearest point of lower concentration.

Therefore, x-ray tubes, which are subjected to extremely high charges, must not have sharp or rough edges where concentrations of electrons could occur and discharge at the wrong moment or in an undesirable direction. Consequently, the interior components of x-ray tubes are rounded and highly polished to eliminate sharply curved surfaces.

5. **Movement.** Only negative charges move along solid conductors. Because the positive charges, the protons, are tightly bound inside the atomic nuclear field, only the electrons, which exist outside the nucleus, are easily moved along conductors.

Electrification

Objects can be electrified by three methods: **friction, contact,** and **induction.**

Friction. Electrification by friction occurs when one object is rubbed against another and, due to differences in the number of electrons available on each, electrons travel from one to the other. Ideal conditions for electron transfer occur during cold weather when low humidity removes stabilizing electrons from the air, decreasing the resistance to electron movement between objects. An example is a common trick that delights children—rubbing a balloon against a wool sweater will permit the balloon to stick to a wall. In low humidity, electrons will transfer from the wool to the balloon, giving it a negative charge, which can cause it to stick to a smooth wall with a relatively positive charge. This is an example of opposites attracting one another. A common example of like charges repelling one another occurs when hair is electrified by friction during combing in low humidity conditions. The comb removes electrons from the strands of hair, often accompanied by crackling sounds, leaving each more positively charged. The strands are then repelled by those adjoining, which now also have stronger positive charges. The result is wild strands of hair standing straight out from your head. The solution to the problem is to increase the humidity, or the amount of water in the air, causing a slight condensation on all surfaces. This thin film of moisture becomes a pathway for the distribution of electrons. The use of a humidifier in a radiographic darkroom during cold weather thus helps eliminate electrostatic discharges that can cause artifacts on film.

Contact. Electrification by contact occurs when two objects touch, permitting electrons to move from one to the other. This process is a simple equalization of charges, with both objects having similar charges after the contact. Walking across a woolen carpet in a room with low humidity may cause shoes to scoop electrons from the carpet fibers that are then distributed over the entire body. This is an example of electrification by friction. However, when a positively charged object with fewer electrons is touched, the contact will cause electrons to move to the less negatively charged object in an attempt to equally distribute the charges. A metal doorknob or another person are examples of positively charged objects that would attract electrons from a person who had just walked across a rug. After the contact, both objects would have a more equal distribution of electrons. This is caused by the individual force fields of the electrons satisfying the repulsion-attraction law over

FIGURE 3-5 A typical tree-branch static discharge artifact on a radiograph.

the entire surface of the conductors. In many instances, actual physical contact does not occur before the electrons equalize. As soon as the oppositely charged objects are in close proximity, the electrons often jump the gap in the form of a **static discharge.** This occurs as soon as the difference in charges becomes sufficiently great and the intervening distance sufficiently small. In most cases the static discharge releases excess energy in the form of light photons. When this occurs between a piece of radiographic film and a cassette, darkroom bench, or the body of the person handling the film, the light forms an image on the film. Figure 3-5 illustrates one of the common types of static discharge that appears as a radiographic film artifact.

An electroscope is a simple device that illustrates the laws of electrostatics. It consists of a rod connected to a pair of thin, easily charged metallic leaves, which are protected from air currents by a glass flask

Metal Knob
and Rod

Foil Leaves

A   B

FIGURE 3-6 Charging an electroscope by contact: Electrons distribute equally when they are permitted to move from one object (the rod) to another (the electroscope) by contact.

(Figure 3-6A). When a charged object (such as the metallic rod shown in Figure 3-6B) is brought into contact with the rod, the excess electrons obey the third law of electrostatics and distribute equally throughout the rod and leaves. The resultant increase in the number of electrons present on both leaves causes the two leaves to obey the first law of electrostatics and, because they possess like charges, repel each other. Consequently, it is possible to see the two leaves move further apart.

If an electroscope is subjected to an intense beam of ionizing x-ray photons, the air becomes ionized. The ionized atoms draw excess electrons from the leaves, thus causing the charge on the leaves to be reduced. Consequently, the electroscope leaves relax and move closer together.

Induction. Electrification by induction is the most important method because it is the one used in the operation of electronic devices. **Induction is the process of electrical fields acting on one another without contact.** Every charged body is surrounded by a force field, much like the fields that surround individual atoms. Like atoms, force fields are a result of the composite forces of the charges residing within the object. These force fields are called **electric fields** and they can cause induction. When a strongly and a weakly charged object come close to one another, the electrical fields will begin to act on one another before contact occurs (Figure 3-7A). As can be seen in Figure 3-7B, charges will migrate to one end of an object in anticipation of contact. However, as seen in Figure 3-7C, when the stronger object is removed before contact, the charges in the weaker object will redistribute themselves as they were before the induction occurred. This temporarily induced movement of charges is useful in many electronic devices, such as motors, transformers, and solenoids.

With an understanding of friction and induction electrification, it becomes possible to understand one of the greatest of natural phenomena—lightning. Lightning discharges occur as the masses of atoms making up the water vapor in clouds move rapidly through the atmosphere. Under conditions where many electrons are available, such as when there are numerous storm clouds, the movement of the water vapor atoms tends to cause electrons to be picked up or lost. As an individual cloud becomes predominantly positively or negatively charged, it becomes a candidate for a huge electrostatic discharge. Clouds often pick up electrons on their upper edges and lose them on their lower edges and vice versa. In these instances the difference in charges makes the cloud a candidate for a cloud-to-cloud discharge as soon as the insulating effect of the vapor between the two surfaces has been overcome. But the most interesting part of lightning is cloud-to-ground discharges. The ground often develops a temporary opposite charge from the underside of the cloud because of the induction effect of the cloud on the ground. This causes the electrons to spread out, which in turn tends to rapidly increase the difference in charges between cloud and ground and can quickly overcome the insulating effect of the air between the cloud and the ground. The result is lightning discharges occurring much more rapidly than if induction had not taken place. Lightning discharges do not occur as a single transfer of electrons from one area to another. Instead, vast numbers of electrons may be transferred from

A B C

FIGURE 3-7 Charging an electroscope by induction: Electrons are induced to move away from the heavily charged rod (B) but return to their normal distribution when the rod is removed (A and C).

cloud to ground, overloading the ground, which in turn transfers electrons back to the cloud, which again transfers them to the ground, over and over until the charges are somewhat equally distributed. A short lightning discharge often transfers electrons back and forth between cloud and ground many times within a microsecond.

ELECTRODYNAMICS

Electrons that are moving in predominantly the same direction are often referred to as an **electric current.** A number of conditions encourage electron movement, thus permitting the flow of electric current. A **vacuum** is a space from which air has been removed. Since it has few atoms to oppose electron flow, it is especially useful in permitting electrons to reach the speed necessary to produce x-rays. Some **gasses** (such as neon) will promote the drift of electrons from a negative electrode (cathode) to a positive electrode (anode). These

gasses also promote the drift of positive ions toward the negative cathode while negative ions move toward the positive anode. **Ionic solutions** can cause electrons to migrate to positive or negative poles during electrolysis, when they are subjected to an electric current.

Electrolysis becomes possible when two neutral atoms with complementary valences (e.g., −1 and +1) are brought together in a solution. They become ions in the solution when the positive valence atom gives up an outer-shell electron to the negative valence atom. The atom missing an electron becomes a positive ion (because a negative charge has been removed), while the one receiving the electron becomes a negative ion (because a negative charge has been added). When metallic rods are connected to a battery and immersed in the solution, the negative pole will attract the positive ions while the positive pole will attract the negative ions. This migration of electrons during the electrolytic process comprises an electrical current. **Metallic conductors,** such as copper wire, are the most common pathways provided for the movement of elec-

FIGURE 3-8 Electron drift along a conductor.

Ball   Tube filled with balls

Ball

FIGURE 3-9 As when balls are pushed into a tube, each electron needs to move only a short distance for the effect of current movement to be achieved at the other end.

trical current. The atoms of metallic conductors permit valence electrons to drift. In common household wiring the actual physical movement is about 2 mm per second (Figure 3-8). The electrical current, as a whole, is similar to a tube filled with balls, as in Figure 3-9. If the tube is full and a new ball is pushed into one end, a ball will drop instantly from the far end, although each ball moved or drifted only a short distance. Electrons move along a conductor with a similar domino effect, resulting in movement of electrons at the far end. This movement occurs extremely rapidly, nearly at the speed of light (3×10^8 meters/second).

The movement of electrons is facilitated by materials that easily permit electrons to flow. These materials are called **conductors** and **superconductors.** Examples of conductors are metals such as copper and aluminum. Conversely, electron movement is inhibited by materials that resist the flow of electrons. These nonconducting materials

are called **insulators.** Examples of insulators are plastic, rubber, and glass. The third classification of materials is **semiconductors.** They have the ability to conduct under certain conditions and insulate under others. The actual conditions causing these changes in conductivity are complex and are addressed later in this chapter. They result primarily from changes in the energy states of atoms, causing outer-shell electrons to move in a particular direction (Table 3-1).

An **electrical circuit** is a pathway (commonly copper wire) that permits electrons to move in a complete circle from their source, through resisting electrical devices and back to the source. As in electrostatics, an electrical circuit must have an excess charge at one end and a comparative deficiency at the other to allow electrons to flow. There are several sources of the excess electrons necessary to cause current flow. Examples include **batteries,** which convert chemical energy to electrical; **generators,** which convert mechanical energy to electrical; **solar converters,** which convert solar photons to electrical energy; and **atomic reactors,** which convert nuclear energy to electrical. Only batteries and generators are efficient devices at present. Solar converters and atomic reactors have yet to be developed to directly convert energy for widespread commercial use. Solar converters remain expensive, while nuclear reactors, although efficient on a large scale, continue to meet significant public opposition. They operate by using the massive energy of the atom to produce steam, which is then used to run turbine generators.

TABLE 3-1.	Properties of Conducting Materials	
State	**Material**	**Characteristics**
Insulator	Plastic, Rubber, Glass	Large energy difference between conduction and valence bands; resists electron flow.
Semiconductor	Silicon, Germanium	Small energy difference between conduction and valence bands; conducts OR resists, depending on temperature and other conditions.
Conductor	Copper, Aluminum	Overlapping conduction and valence bands; conducts with minor resistance, varying depending on temperature and other conditions.
Superconductor	Titanium	Greatly overlapping conduction and valence bands; conducts with little or no electrical potential; most current systems require extreme cold to function although research indicates room temperature superconductors may be developed soon.

Describing Current Flow

Electrons move from the highest concentration to the lowest. There is much confusion regarding how to describe their movement because early pioneers in electrical phenomena assumed that the moving charges were positive when actually they were negatively charged electrons. The negative pole is the source of electrons that move toward the positive receiving pole. Consequently, **conventional electric current is described as going from positive to negative poles while electron flow is actually from negative to positive poles.**

It is important to specify whether descriptions are of electrical current or electron flow, as they are exact opposites. It may be useful to think of negative charges moving in one direction as being equivalent to a positive charge effect in the opposite direction. The importance of these definitions will become apparent later in this text, especially when discussing the interactions of both electrical and magnetic forces.

The nature of the flow of electrons that make up an electric current can be described in many different ways. The most common factors used as descriptors are the **quantity** of electrons flowing, the **force** with which they travel, the amount of **opposition** to the current flow in the circuit and the **direction** of travel.

The direction of travel of the electrons is defined as either **direct current (DC)**, when all electrons move in the same direction, or **alternating current (AC)**, when electrons move first in one direction and then reverse and move in the opposite direction. Through the use of various electrical devices, which we will investigate later, it is possible to change the current from DC to AC and back, as necessary.

Current

The quantity, or number, of electrons flowing is sometimes referred to as the **current.** It is useful to think of the measurement of current as the number of electrons flowing past a given point per unit of time (usually per second). The French scientist André Ampère (1775–1836) did much original work in defining electricity and magnetism. Consequently, the unit of current bears his name. The **ampere** is sometimes called the **amp** for short and is represented by the symbol **A.** It consists of the movement of 6.24×10^{18} **electrons per second** past a given point; therefore, the technical definition is **one coulomb of electrical charge flowing per second (1 ampere = 1 coulomb/ 1 second).** Earlier, the drift of electrons was given as less than 1 mm per second. The fact that 1 ampere flowing in a household wire causes 6,240,000,000,000,000,000 electrons to move less than 1 mm per second should help in understanding the small size of electrons. Diagnostic radiographic equipment utilizes milliamperage units to regulate the number of electrons available to produce x-ray photons. The **milliamperage (mA)** is found on nearly all x-ray machines and adjustment by the radiographer operating the equipment will cause the number of electrons and the number of x-ray photons produced to vary. The adjustment of an x-ray machine to add an additional 100 mA (a common increment) causes 6.24×10^{17} more electrons per second to pass through the x-ray tube.

> **EXAMPLE:** If an x-ray machine is operating at 0.01 second and the amperage is 100 mA, how many electrons would move through the tube?
>
> **Answer:**
>
> $(6.24 \times 10^{17}$ electrons/second$) \times 0.01$ seconds $= 6.24 \times 10^{15}$ (6.24 million billion or 6,240,000,000,000,000)

The word current is used to describe the presence of electron flow as well as to describe exactly how much current is flowing. It is important to distinguish which use of the word is intended.

Potential Difference

The force with which the electrons travel is a function of the difference between the number of electrons in excess at one end of the circuit and the deficiency at the other end. The attempt of the unequal forces to balance is the cause of the force of electron movement. Because the difference is present while the source is connected into the circuit, **there does not have to be an actual flow of current for the difference to exist.** Therefore, the simple potential for a difference is used to describe the force, or strength of movement, behind electrons.

Potential difference is the best term to describe the force or **strength** of electron flow. It should be remembered that potential difference continues to exist even when a switch is opened in a circuit, breaking the actual flow of electrons (current). Because potential difference is the prime force causing electrical devices to convert electrical energy to mechanical, the term **electromotive force (emf)** has also been used. Electromotive force is actually the total maximum difference of potential between the positive and negative ends of the electron source,

but it is not incorrect to use the term in place of potential difference.

The unit of potential difference is the **volt,** represented by the symbol **V** (named for the Italian physicist Alessandro Volta [1745–1827]). The term *voltage* is also used to describe potential difference. The technical definition of a volt is **1 joule (J) of work done on 1 coulomb of charge (1 volt = 1 joule/1 coulomb).** A joule is the SI unit for both mechanical energy and work.

Thus, for the reasons previously stated, the force with which electrons travel can be described by the terms potential difference, electromotive force (emf), and **voltage (V).**

As the current flows along the circuit, the potential difference is reduced because the closer the electrons come to the deficient end of the circuit, the farther they are from the excess end (the driving source) and the closer they are to becoming part of the deficiency themselves. With this understanding of potential difference, the concept of grounding electrical circuits for safety should become clear. When equipment is properly grounded and the radiographer, who is also grounded, comes in contact, there is no potential difference. However, when equipment is not properly grounded, the radiographer may become a better path to ground. The passage of electrons (voltage) through the radiographer may be shocking, to say the least.

High voltage is extremely dangerous because there does not have to be an actual flow of current for the potential difference to exist. This means high potential difference or voltage remains a hazard at all times (and explains why warnings must be posted in these areas). All that is required for a high difference in voltage to achieve equalization is for a conductor to present itself. If this happens to be a patient who inadvertently uses a wet hand to grasp a cracked high-voltage cable or a radiographer who touches two connection points inside a control console, the shocking result is the same.

Resistance

The amount of opposition to the current in the circuit is called the **resistance.** Research into the interrelationships of current, potential difference, and resistance was done by the German physicist Georg Ohm

(1787–1854). As a result, the unit of resistance is called the **ohm.** It is represented by the symbol Ω (omega). The technical definition of an ohm is the resistance to a flow of current provided by a column of mercury 106.3 cm long with a diameter of 1 mm^2 at 0° C. A practical definition of an ohm will be provided later, based on the interaction of several characteristics of a conductor. Resistance and impedance are the terms used to describe current opposition. There are numerous factors that impede the flow of electrons, thus increasing resistance. The primary factors for electrical circuits are the ability to conduct electrons, the length of the conductor, the cross-sectional diameter, and temperature.

When the expression 1/R is used, the resistance of a DC circuit is measured as **conductance,** while that of an AC circuit is measured as **admittance.** The SI unit for conductance and admittance is the siemens, which is represented by the symbol S and is named after the English electrical engineer Sir William Siemens (1823–1883), brother of Werner von Siemens, founder of the German electrical and x-ray equipment corporation.

The ability to conduct electrons has already been discussed enough to define a conductor as a material that permits electrons to flow easily, and an insulator as one that inhibits their movement. The tendency of an atom to permit electrons nearby or within one of the orbital shells is the prime factor in determining conductivity, semiconductivity and insulation properties. The **valence energy band** (the outermost and sometimes next-to-outermost orbital shell) not only determines the chemical properties of the atom, as discussed previously, but has much to do with conductivity as well. Orbital shells lower or closer to the nucleus (and of less energy) than the valence band are normally completely full (Figure 3-10). Valence has much to do with the ability of a material to conduct electrons. Any element with one valence electron is a good conductor (e.g., copper, silver, and gold). In addition, the further the valence electron is from the nucleus, the better a conductor it is. For example, gold is a better conductor than silver because its valence electron is in the sixth shell, while silver's is in the fifth. Silver is a better conductor than copper because copper's valence electron is in the fourth shell. Since copper has a higher melting point and is much cheaper, it is more commonly used than silver or gold.

There is also an area beyond the valence band that is referred to as the **conduction band.** The conduction band is not an orbital shell but is within the force field (area of influence) of the atom (see Figure 3-10). Conductors have conduction bands that are populated by free electrons and, in solid materials, they are able to move freely from one atom's conduction band to another's, as in Figure 3-10C. This is why many of the best conductors are solids. Conversely, insulators

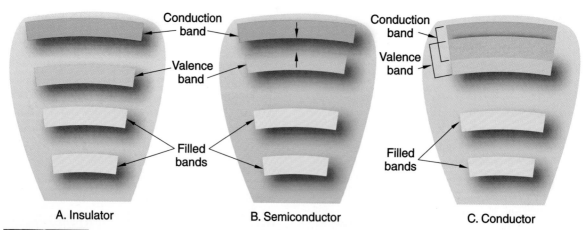

A. Insulator   B. Semiconductor   C. Conductor

FIGURE 3-10 The arrows demonstrate the difference between the energy levels of conduction and valence bands in an (A) insulator; (B) semiconductor; and (C) conductor. Note that the conduction and valence bands overlap in a good conductor.

have very poor or nonexistent conduction bands. The number of electrons in the conduction band is determined by the energy difference between the valence band and the conduction band. Although the conduction band is always at a higher energy level than the valence band, the energy required of an individual electron to place it in the conduction band will determine how many electrons can possibly exist there. In fact, the difference between the energy levels required of conduction band electrons as compared to valence band electrons is the factor that differentiates conductors from semiconductors from insulators. In Figure 3-10, the differences are shown as (C) a good conductor with overlapping valence and conduction bands; (B) a semiconductor with closely related bands; and (A) a good insulator with a wide gap between the bands. Metals often have overlapping bands with conduction bands, including portions of the valence bands, thus placing large numbers of electrons into the conduction bands. Therefore, metals, especially silver and copper, make the best conductors. The best insulators are materials with complex molecular structures, such as wood, plastic, glass, and rubber.

The length of the conductor has a directly proportional relationship to resistance. In other words, as the length of the conductor doubles, the resistance will also double. Just as a short garden hose will spray water with greater force than a long hose, so a short conductor will permit a greater force of electrons while a longer conductor offers greater resistance.

The cross-sectional diameter of the conductor has an inversely proportional relationship to resistance. In other words, as the cross-sectional diameter doubles, the resistance will be halved. A garden hose with a small diameter will impede water flow more than a large-diameter hose, just as a small-diameter conductor will resist electron flow more than a conductor with a large diameter.

Finally, the temperature of the conductor can also influence the resistance. Heat is simply a measurement of the amount of atomic and molecular energy, often seen as vibration. As temperature increases, atomic collisions provide enough energy to some electrons to permit them to jump into the atom's conduction band. In conductors, increased temperature increases free electron collisions, and this in turn lessens electrical current flow. In insula-

tors the increased number of collisions because of increased temperature causes some electrons to lose energy and fall back into the valence band, thus decreasing the energy difference between the bands and consequently decreasing the insulating ability of the material. Semiconductors become more conductive as temperature increases, for the same reason, with a resultant narrowing of the gap between their already close bands.

An approximation of these relationships is shown in Figure 3-11. A close examination of this figure illustrates that increased resistance from heat is significant. In fact, it becomes a major problem with the large heat-producing transformers used in x-ray equipment, and unique methods have been adopted to overcome its effect. In addition, extrapolation of the conductor curve to the left illustrates that if conductors can be supercooled, as they are in modern magnetic resonance imaging equipment, a significant increase in conductivity can be achieved.

In recent years, superconductivity has been achieved to reduce resistance to the point where current is apparently flowing without potential difference. Table 3-1 provides information on the conductive properties of materials important in electronics.

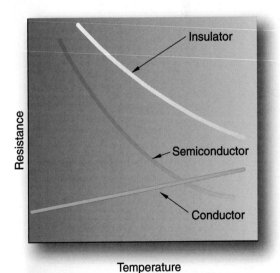

FIGURE 3-11   The effect of temperature on conductors, semiconductors, and insulators.

The total resistance is calculated as:

$$R = \frac{\rho L}{A}$$

where: R = resistance in ohms
  ρ = resistivity (a function of atomic
    structure and temperature)
    (ρ is the Greek letter rho)
  L = length in meters
  A = area in square meters

This total resistance formula is the true technical definition of an ohm as a unit.

Ohm's Law

Georg Ohm discovered a mathematical relationship between the factors of current, potential difference, and resistance that applies to all resistance circuits and is known as Ohm's law. The law describes the relationship between current and potential difference as **the current along a conductor is proportional to the potential difference.** It is easier to remember this relationship as a formula:

$$\frac{V}{I}$$

V = potential difference in volts
 I = current in amperes

This expression does not include the resistance factor, which is a critical element. Therefore, Ohm's law is usually expressed as the algebraic derivation with resistance times current equal to potential difference, or:

$$V = IR$$

where: V = potential difference in volts
  I = current in amperage
  R = resistance in ohms

This version solves for voltage when the current and resistance are known. Of course, Ohm's law can also be stated in its other forms to solve for unknown currents and resistances:

$$I = \frac{V}{R}$$

and

$$R = \frac{V}{I}$$

EXAMPLE: What is the amperage in a circuit of 20 volts and 10 ohms?

Answer:

I = V/R
I = 20 volts/10 ohms
I = 2 amperes

EXAMPLE: What is the voltage in a circuit of 100 amperes and 5 ohms?

Answer:

V = IR
V = 100 amperes $\times$ 5 ohms
V = 500 volts

EXAMPLE: What is the resistance in a circuit of 80 kilovolts and 200 milliamperes?

Answer:

R = V/I
R = 80 kV/200 mA
R = 80,000 volts/0.2 ampere
R = 400,000 ohms

A memory device used by many students is known as an Ohm's law triangle (Figure 3-12A). To determine the correct formula for one of the variables in the Ohm's law equation, V = IR, simply write the variables as shown (V over I and R), and then cover the variable to be solved with a finger. For example, Figure 3-12B is to solve for R. The correct relationship is given of V/I equals the covered R. Moving a finger around the triangle produces V/R = I and I • R = V as well.

It is useful to be able to calculate the total amount of power used in an electric circuit. **The unit of**

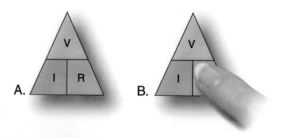

FIGURE 3-12 Ohm's law triangle.

power is the watt. Because the total amount of energy available in a circuit is determined by the current (amperage) and potential difference (voltage), **the watt is defined as 1 ampere flowing through 1 volt.** Power is calculated with the following formula:

$$P = IV$$

where: P = power in watts
I = current in amperes
V = potential difference in volts

Common household appliances tend to operate between 500 and 2,000 watts (most have labels indicating their wattage ratings), and all circuits in buildings have wattage safety limitations. The use of equipment whose total wattage ratings exceed the safety limit of the circuit will cause the circuit to overload and shut down because of excessive heat generation. Radiographic equipment capabilities can be measured by the power rating, usually by calculating the greatest possible energy output.

EXAMPLE: What is the power rating, in kilowatts, of an x-ray generator capable of 800 milliamperes at 100 kilovolts?

Answer:

P = IV
P = 800 mA × 100 kV
P = 0.8 A × 100,000 V
P = 80,000 watts
P = 80 kilowatts

EXAMPLE: If a mobile x-ray machine operates from a 110 V wall receptacle and is rated at a total resistance of 12 Ω, how much current does it draw during exposure?

Answer:

$I = \dfrac{V}{R}$

$I = \dfrac{110 \text{ V}}{12 \text{ Ω}}$

I = 9.2 A

EXAMPLE: How much power does it use?

Answer:

P = IV
P = 9.2 A × 110 V
P = 1,012 W

With this information it is also possible to calculate the expense of the power for a radiographic examination.

EXAMPLE: If the power company charges 5¢ per kWhr, what is the cost of the power for 10 minutes of fluoroscopy at 5 mA and 100 kV?

Answer:

The power is calculated as:

P = IV
P = 5 mA × 100 kV
P = 0.005 A × 100,000 V
P = 500 W

The total energy consumed is calculated as:

total energy = power × seconds
total energy = 500 W × 10 minutes
total energy = 500 W × 600 seconds
total energy = 300,000 Ws
total energy = 300 kWs

The total cost is calculated as:

total cost = total energy used × $0.05/kWhr
total cost = 300 kW/second × $0.05/kWhr
total cost = 0.08 kW/hr × $0.05/kWhr
total cost = $0.004, or
total cost = 0.4¢

The heat that is produced during the operation of electrical equipment becomes of great concern as power use increases. The importance of changes in resistance to heat output can best be understood if the power formula, P = IV, is converted to what is sometimes called the **power loss formula, P = I²R.** This is calculated from:

the power formula, P = IV
substituting IR for V
(because Ohm's law states that V = IR)
resulting in P = I × IR
or P = I²R (watts).

This equation clarifies that power loss from current heat is proportional to the resistance, and heat power loss increases very rapidly with current increase. As illustrated in the formula, heat power loss is proportional to the square of the amperage. In other words, doubling the amperage increases power loss by a factor of 4, etc.

SERIES AND PARALLEL CIRCUITS

An electric circuit can be designed to send electrons through various resistance devices by linking them one after the other in a **series circuit** (Figure 3-13A) or by giving each component an individual branch in a **parallel circuit** (Figure 3-13B). The effect of each type of circuit on current, potential difference, and resistance is summarized in Table 3-2. The best way to understand the effects of both series and parallel circuitry is to work through a series of problems that demonstrate these differences.

EXAMPLE: What is the total current in a series circuit with three resistances, each supplied with 10 amperes?

Answer:

$I_t = I_1 = I_2 = I_3$
$I_t = 10 \text{ A} = 10 \text{ A} = 10 \text{ A}$
$I_t = 10$ amperes

EXAMPLE: What is the total current in a parallel circuit with three resistances, each supplied with 10 amperes?

Answer:

$I_t = I_1 + I_2 + I_3$
$I_t = 10 \text{ A} + 10 \text{ A} + 10 \text{ A}$
$I_t = 30$ amperes

Note that the series circuit supplies a current of 10 amperes, while the parallel circuit supplies 30 amperes. Parallel circuits supply a greater total current

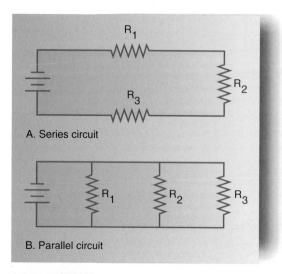

A. Series circuit

B. Parallel circuit

FIGURE 3-13 (A) Series and (B) parallel circuits.

TABLE 3-2. Effect of Circuit Type on Current, Potential Difference, and Resistance (with an example circuit of three resistances)

	Series	Parallel
Current	Same in each element, each element same as total circuit, $I_t = I_1 = I_2 = I_3$	Sum of all elements equals total circuit, $I_t = I_1 + I_2 + I_3$
Voltage	Sum of all elements equals total circuit, $V_t = V_1 + V_2 + V_3$	Same in each element, each element same as total circuit, $V_t = V_1 = V_2 = V_3$
Resistance	Sum of all elements equals total circuit, $R_t = R_1 + R_2 + R_3$	Sum of reciprocal of each element is inversely proportional to the total, $\dfrac{1}{R_t} = \dfrac{1}{R_1} + \dfrac{1}{R_2} + \dfrac{1}{R_3}$

Note: A reciprocal ohm, as in 1/R, is known as a siemens (S).

than series circuits when all other factors are the same. An interesting phenomenon occurs when the effect on voltage is compared, instead of current, using resistances.

EXAMPLE: What is the total voltage in a series circuit with three resistances, each supplied with 10 volts?

Answer:

$V_t = V_1 + V_2 + V_3$
$V_t = 10\text{ V} + 10\text{ V} + 10\text{ V}$
$V_t = 30\text{ volts}$

EXAMPLE: What is the total voltage in a parallel circuit with three resistances, each supplied with 10 volts?

Answer:

$V_t = V_1 = V_2 = V_3$
$V_t = 10\text{ V} = 10\text{ V} = 10\text{ V}$
$V_t = 10\text{ volts}$

Note that the series circuit supplies 30 volts, while the parallel circuit supplies 10 volts. Series circuits supply greater total potential difference than parallel circuits when all other factors are the same. The difference between series and parallel circuits when the same resistances are used is also notable.

EXAMPLE: What is the total resistance of a series circuit with resistances of 2.5 Ω, 4.2 Ω, and 6.8 Ω?

Answer:

$R_t = R_1 + R_2 + R_3$
$R_t = 2.5\ \Omega + 4.2\ \Omega + 6.8\ \Omega$
$R_t = 13.5\ \Omega$

EXAMPLE: What is the total resistance of a parallel circuit with resistances of 2.5 Ω, 4.2 Ω, and 6.8 Ω?

Answer:

$$\frac{1}{R_t} = \frac{1}{R_1} + \frac{1}{R_2} + \frac{1}{R_3}$$
$$\frac{1}{R_t} = \frac{1}{2.5\ \Omega} + \frac{1}{4.2\ \Omega} + \frac{1}{6.8\ \Omega}$$

$$\frac{1}{R_t} = 0.4\text{ S} + 0.24\text{ S} + 0.15\text{ S}$$
$$\frac{1}{R_t} = 0.785\text{ S}$$
$$R_t = \frac{1}{0.785\text{ S}}$$
$$R_t = 1.274\ \Omega$$

Note that the series circuit provides 13.5 Ω of resistance, while the parallel circuit has only 1.274 Ω. Parallel circuits offer less total resistance to electrical current when all other factors are the same. In addition, parallel circuits are not broken when a single resistance is interrupted (as when a light bulb burns out). Series circuits require all resistances to be operable, otherwise there is no pathway for the current to take. The classic example of the difference is illustrated by comparing strings of Christmas lights in series versus parallel circuits. When a single series-wired light burns out, it breaks the circuit and all the lights go out. When a single parallel-wired light burns out, it breaks the circuit in its parallel branch only and the other lights continue to operate. Electrical devices use a wide variety of both types of circuits, including complicated combinations of both. It is also interesting to calculate the effect of both circuit types on amperage by figuring resistance and then applying Ohm's law.

EXAMPLE: What is the total amperage in a series circuit with resistances of 2.5 Ω, 4.2 Ω, and 6.8 Ω with a potential difference of 10 volts?

Answer:

The total resistance is calculated as:

$R_t = R_1 + R_2 + R_3$
$R_t = 2.5\ \Omega + 4.2\ \Omega + 6.8\ \Omega$
$R_t = 13.5\ \Omega$

The total amperage is calculated with Ohm's law:

$$I = \frac{V}{R}$$
$$I = \frac{10\text{ V}}{13.5\ \Omega}$$
$I = 0.74\text{ amperes}$

EXAMPLE: What is the total amperage in a parallel circuit with resistances of 2.5 Ω, 4.2 Ω, and 6.8 Ω and a potential difference of 10 volts?

Answer:

The total resistance is calculated as:

$$\frac{1}{R_t} = \frac{1}{R_1} + \frac{1}{R_2} + \frac{1}{R_3}$$

$$\frac{1}{R_t} = \frac{1}{2.5\ \Omega} = \frac{1}{4.2\ \Omega} + \frac{1}{6.8\ \Omega}$$

$$\frac{1}{R_t} = 0.4\ S + 0.24\ S + 0.15\ S$$

$$\frac{1}{R_t} = 0.785\ S$$

$$R_t = \frac{1}{0.785\ S}$$

$$R_t = 1.274\ \Omega$$

The total amperage is calculated with Ohm's law:

$$I = \frac{V}{R}$$

$$I = \frac{10V}{1.274\ \Omega}$$

$$I = 7.85\ \text{amperes}$$

Note that the series circuit operates with a current of 0.74 ampere, while the parallel circuit operates with a current of 7.1 amperes. Parallel circuits operate with greater current when all other factors are the same. It is also interesting to study the effect of both circuit types on voltage by calculating resistance and then applying Ohm's law.

EXAMPLE: What is the total voltage of a series circuit with resistances of 2.5 Ω, 4.2 Ω, and 6.8 Ω with a current of 50 amperes?

Answer:

The total resistance is calculated as:

$$R_t = R_1 + R_2 + R_3$$

$$R_t = 2.5\ \Omega + 4.2\ \Omega + 6.8\ \Omega$$

$$R_t = 13.5\ \Omega$$

The total voltage is calculated with Ohm's law:

$$V = IR$$

$$V = 50\ A \times 13.5\ \Omega$$

$$V = 675\ \text{volts}$$

EXAMPLE: What is the total voltage of a parallel circuit with resistances of 2.5 Ω, 4.2 Ω, and 6.8 Ω and a current of 50 amperes?

Answer:

The total resistance is calculated as:

$$\frac{1}{R_t} = \frac{1}{R_1} + \frac{1}{R_2} + \frac{1}{R_3}$$

$$\frac{1}{R_t} = \frac{1}{2.5\ \Omega} + \frac{1}{4.2\ \Omega} + \frac{1}{6.8\ \Omega}$$

$$\frac{1}{R_t} = 0.4\ S + 0.24\ S + 0.15\ S$$

$$\frac{1}{R_t} = 0.785\ S$$

$$R_t = \frac{1}{0.785\ S}$$

$$R_t = 1.274\ \Omega$$

The total voltage is calculated with Ohm's law:

$$V = IR$$

$$V = 50\ A \times 1.274\ \Omega$$

$$V = 63.68\ \text{volts}$$

Note that the series circuit operates at 675 volts, while the parallel circuit operates at 64 volts. Parallel circuits operate at lower voltage than series circuits when all other factors are the same.

Parallel circuits are used for the electrical wiring of buildings because the failure of a single device does not break the electrical supply to other devices. As can be seen from these problems, the addition of current-using devices to a series circuit causes the voltage to drop, thus reducing the potential difference to the other devices in the circuit. In a series circuit of lights, for example, the addition of more bulbs will cause all the bulbs to burn dimmer. **As more resistances are added to a parallel circuit, total resistance drops, total amperage increases and total voltage remains unchanged.** The total resistance of a parallel circuit is always less than the amount of the lowest resistor (usually about half of the lowest resistor).

A disadvantage to parallel circuits is that with the addition of resistances, the increasing amperage can short circuit the entire system. This creates the possibility of wires becoming hot enough to start a fire. To prevent this from occurring, either a **circuit breaker** or a **fuse** is placed in the line. These devices are constructed to permit the breaking of the circuit before a dangerous temperature is reached. Circuit breakers simply pop open and can be reset once the cause of the problem has been located and removed from the circuit. Fuses are constructed with a metal tab that will melt when dangerously heated, thus breaking the circuit. Fuses are not reusable and must be replaced.

A variable resistor called a **potentiometer** or **rheostat** permits a variable contact to slide along a series circuit of resistance coils. When resistors are connected in a series circuit, Ohm's law dictates that an increase in resistance will result in a decrease in

voltage and vice versa if the amperage remains unchanged. When a knob is connected to the variable slide contact (as in a radio volume control), a simple twist permits voltage and amperage regulation (with a corresponding increase or decrease in speaker volume). Unfortunately, rheostats cause significant energy waste in heat, and the direct application of Ohm's law results in voltage changing when only an amperage change is desired and vice versa. For these reasons, rheostats are not practical in high-voltage situations. Their prime use is to control current but they have never been adaptable to high-voltage transformers.

SUMMARY

The distribution and movement of electrons, along with their associated charges, make up electricity. Electrostatics is the study of the distribution of fixed charges that are at rest. When one object has more electrons than another, it also has more negative charges and is considered to have an overall negative charge. A positive charge refers to something with a weaker negative charge, or fewer electrons. The terms negative and positive refer to the relationship between two objects, not to their true atomic charges. Because the earth contains what is essentially an infinite number of charges, it is considered to be neutral, or at zero ground potential. The five laws of electrostatics are: (1) repulsion–attraction; (2) the inverse square law; (3) distribution; (4) concentration; and (5) movement. Objects can be electrified by friction, contact, and induction.

The movement of electrons is facilitated by materials that permit electrons to flow easily. These materials are called conductors or superconductors. Nonconducting materials are called insulators, while materials that conduct under certain conditions and insulate under others are known as semiconductors.

An electrical circuit is a pathway that permits electrons to move in a complete circle from their source, through resisting electrical devices, and back to the source. Electrons move from the high-

est concentration to the lowest. Conventional electric current is described as going from positive to negative poles, while electron flow is actually from negative to positive poles. It is important to specify whether descriptions are of electrical current or electron flow, as they are exact opposites.

The quantity of electrons flowing is referred to as the current and is measured in amperes. The force with which the electrons travel is referred to as the potential difference, electromotive force, or voltage and is measured in volts. There does not have to be current flow for voltage to exist. The opposition to the current flow is referred to as resistance and is measured in ohms. The relationship between these factors is expressed in Ohm's law: $V = IR$. The resistance of metallic conductors is affected by length, diameter, and temperature. When $1/R$ is used to express resistance in an AC circuit, it is measured in siemens.

The valence energy band of an atom has much to do with the ability of a material to conduct electrons. There is also an area beyond the valence band that is referred to as the conduction band. Conductors have conduction bands that are populated by electrons that are able to move freely from one atom's conduction band to another's. Insulators have widely separated valence and conduction bands, while semiconductors have intermediate properties.

Circuits are known by several parameters. These include the direction the electrons travel, which is defined as either direct current (DC) or alternating current (AC). It is possible to change the current from DC to AC and back, as necessary. The total amount of energy in a circuit is described as the power of the circuit and is measured in watts so that $P = IV$. Circuits can be described as series or parallel, depending on how the components are connected. The total resistance of a series circuit is measured in ohms, as $R_t = R_1 + R_2 + R_3$. The total resistance of a parallel circuit is measured in siemens, as

$$\frac{1}{R_t} = \frac{1}{R_1} + \frac{1}{R_2} + \frac{1}{R_3}$$

Parallel circuits operate with greater current through resistances, and they supply a greater total current from the power supply than series circuits when all other factors are the same. Parallel circuits are often used because the failure of a single device does not break the electrical supply to other devices. Circuit breakers and fuses prevent damage to electrical components by permitting the breaking of an overloaded circuit before a dangerous temperature is reached. A potentiometer or rheostat is a variable resistor.

REVIEW QUESTIONS

1. State the five elementary laws of electrostatics.
2. Describe the three methods of electrification.
3. How are conductors different from insulators?
4. Explain the difference between conventional electrical current and actual electron flow.
5. State the four basic factors that are used to describe the nature of the flow of electrons in electrodynamics.
6. What are the units used to describe potential difference, current flow, and opposition to current flow?
7. State Ohm's law.
8. What is the potential difference in a circuit of 20 amperes and 10 ohms? 30 amperes and 6 ohms? 100 mA and 5 ohms?
9. What is the power rating of an x-ray generator capable of 1,000 mA at 110 kV?
10. What is the voltage in a parallel circuit of 20 amperes with resistances of 6, 10, and 15 ohms?
11. What is the amperage in a series circuit of 110 volts with resistances of 5, 10, and 20 ohms?

REFERENCES AND RECOMMENDED READING

Ball, J. L., & Moore, A. D. (1997). *Essential physics for radiographers* (3rd ed.). Oxford: Blackwell Scientific.

Bushberg, J. T., Seibert, J. A., Leidholdt, E. M., & Boone, J. M. (2003). *The essential physics of medical imaging* (2nd ed.). Philadelphia: Lippincott, Williams & Wilkins.

Bushong, S. C. (2004). *Radiologic science for technologists: Physics, biology, and protection* (8th ed.). St. Louis, MO: Elsevier Mosby.

Carroll, Q. B. (1993). *Fuchs's radiographic exposure, processing and quality control* (5th ed.). Springfield, IL: Charles C Thomas.

Dendy, P. P., & Heaton, B. (1999). *Physics for diagnostic radiology* (2nd ed.) Institute of Physics. Bristol, England.

Hay, G. A., & Hughes, D. (1972). *First-year physics for radiographers.* London: Bailliere Tindall.

Johns, H. E., & Cunningham, J. R. (1983). *The physics of radiology* (4th ed.). Springfield, IL: Charles C Thomas.

Meredith, W. J., & Massey, J. B. (1977). *Fundamental physics of radiology* (3rd ed.). Chicago: Yearbook Medical.

Selman, J. (2000). *The fundamentals of imaging physics and radiobiology for the radiologic technologist* (9th ed.). Springfield, IL: Charles C Thomas.

van der Plaats, G. J. (1980). *Medical x-ray techniques in diagnostic radiology* (4th ed.). The Hague: Martinus Nijhoff.

Wilks, R. J. (2003). *Principles of radiological physics.* (4th ed.) Edinburgh: Churchill Livingstone.

Wolbarst, A. B. (1993). *Physics of radiology.* Norwalk, CT: Appleton & Lange.

CHAPTER 4

Electromagnetism

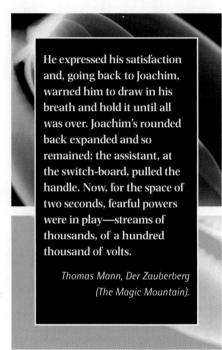

He expressed his satisfaction and, going back to Joachim, warned him to draw in his breath and hold it until all was over. Joachim's rounded back expanded and so remained; the assistant, at the switch-board, pulled the handle. Now, for the space of two seconds, fearful powers were in play—streams of thousands, of a hundred thousand of volts.

Thomas Mann, Der Zauberberg
(The Magic Mountain).

KEY TERMS

air core transformer	galvanometer	rectification
ammeter	gauss (g)	retentivity
armature	generator	rotor
artificial permanent magnet	half-wave rectification	secondary coil
autotransformer	hysteresis loss	self-induction
brush	I^2R loss	self-rectification
capacitor	inductive reactance	shell-type transformer
closed–core transformer	lines of flux	silicon-controlled rectifier (SCR)
coercivity	lines of force	sine wave
commutator ring	magnet	slip ring
diamagnetic	magnetic dipole	solenoid
dielectric	magnetic domain	space charge cloud
diode	magnetic field	spin magnetic moment
dynamometer	motor	stator
eddy current loss	mutual induction	step-down transformer
electromagnetic relay	natural magnet	step-up transformer
electromagnet	nonmagnetic	tesla (T)
farad (f)	open–core transformer	thermionic emission
ferromagnetic	orbital magnetic moment	thyristor
Fleming's hand rules	paramagnetic	transformer
flux density	permeability	voltmeter
full–wave rectification	primary coil	Weber (Wb)

OBJECTIVES

Upon completion of this chapter, the student should be able to:

- Explain the atomic nature of magnetism.
- Classify materials according to their magnetic properties.
- State Fleming's hand rules of electromagnetics.
- Explain how a solenoid and an electromagnet function.
- Describe magnetic and electromagnetic induction.

- List the types of movement that will produce electromagnetism.
- State the factors that regulate the strength of electromagnetic induction.
- Explain self-induction.
- Illustrate the generator and motor principles.
- Explain the waveform produced by direct- and alternating-current generators and motors.
- Describe the function of a transformer.

- Calculate voltage and amperage according to the transformer law.

- Discuss various factors affecting transformer efficiency and construction.

- Explain the function of an autotransformer and a capacitor.

- Describe the function of a silicon-controlled rectifier at the atomic level.

- Describe the process of thermionic emission.

- Explain the waveforms that are produced by half-wave and full-wave rectification.

MAGNETISM

Magnetism is one of the fundamental forces. Materials that have the ability to attract iron are classified as having a strong magnetic force. To understand magnetism it is important to return to atomic structure for a detailed examination of the effects of particle movement around the nucleus. **When a charged particle is in motion, a magnetic force field perpendicular to the motion will be created** (Figure 4-1). In the case of the negatively charged electrons orbiting the nucleus of an atom, the closed loop of the orbit cancels all but the field that is perpendicular to the plane of the motion (Figure 4-2). This perpendicular magnetic force is called **orbital magnetic moment.**

A magnetic effect is also established by electrons spinning on their axes. The effect created by the movement of these electrons is called **spin magnetic moment.** The disruption of this axial spinning and the energy released as it reorients itself are the physical basis that permits magnetic resonance imaging (see Chapter 45).

Atoms having a significant number of electrons with their magnetic moments in the same direction, especially when the outer shells are involved, will exhibit a net magnetic field in a distinct direction (see Figure 4-2A). Groups of atoms with this net magnetic field are known as **magnetic dipoles** or **magnetic domains.** This is the basis of the domain theory of magnetism. It has been theorized that 10^{15} (1,000,000,000,000,000 or 1 million billion) atoms make up a single dipole. This is not a standard number, as it has been shown that dipoles vary in size and actually grow or shrink, depending on local conditions. In nonmagnetic objects the magnetic dipoles are randomly arranged, essentially can-

Magnetic field lines

FIGURE 4-1 Magnetic field created by a charged particle in motion. The movement of a charged particle creates a magnetic field perpendicular to the motion of the particle.

celling out each other. If an external force field has the time or strength to orient enough of the dipoles in the same direction and/or cause those dipoles to grow in size, the object exhibits a uniformly strong magnetic field and is referred to as a **magnet** (see Figure 4-2B).

The force fields that are created when magnetic dipoles orient to create a magnet are called **lines of force, lines of flux,** or the **magnetic field.** These lines of force flow not only through the magnet itself but outside the magnetic material, forming a three-dimensional field surrounding the magnet (see Figure 4-2B). The stronger the magnetic field, the more lines of flux. Placing small iron filings on a surface under which a strong magnet is placed will map out the magnetic lines of flux. Figure 4-3 illustrates the lines of flux emanating from the poles of a bar and

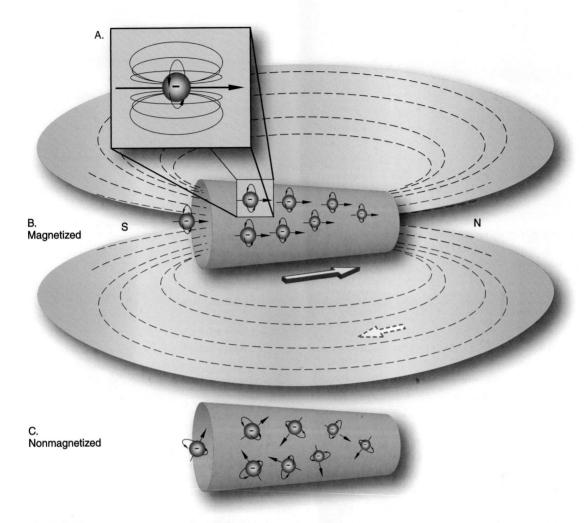

FIGURE 4-2 The concept of magnetism: (A) The spinning of an individual electron is the spin magnetic moment, and the magnetic field created by the spin is the orbital magnetic moment (heavy arrows). Groups of atoms with most of the magnetic moment force in a single direction form a magnetic dipole or domain. (B) When the magnetic dipoles or domains are in a predominant direction, a magnet is formed with an external magnetic field. (C) When the magnetic dipoles or domains are not in a predominant direction, the object is not magnetized.

a horseshoe magnet. The ends of a magnet are defined as the north and south poles; **lines of force always flow from north to south outside a magnet and from south to north within a magnet** (see Figure 4-2B). It is important to remember that **lines of force** never intersect. In some cases they are described as being parallel. However, many circumstances may cause the magnetic field to contract or expand. Under these conditions the lines of

force bend closer or further from one another, no longer making them truly parallel.

The stronger the magnetic field, the greater the number of lines of flux or the greater the **flux density.** Flux density is determined both by field strength and by the area in which the lines of flux are located.

$$\text{magnetic flux} = \frac{\text{field strength}}{\text{area}}$$

FIGURE 4-3 Strong permanent magnets placed under a surface containing loose iron filings will demonstrate magnetic lines of flux as the filings orient to the magnetic field (forming the initials of Indiana University Northwest).

There are two primary units used to measure the strength of magnetic fields. The **SI unit for magnetic flux is the Weber,** represented by the symbol Wb, (for the German physicist Wilhelm **Weber** [1804–1891], who proposed the basic theory of magnetism discussed above). 1 Wb $= 10^8$ lines of flux. **The units for magnetic flux density are the tesla,** represented by the symbol T (for the American physicist Nikola **Tesla** [1857–1943]), and the **gauss,** represented by the symbol G (for the German mathematician Johann **Gauss [1777–1855]). 1 tesla = 10,000 gauss.** 1 T = 1 Wb/m², or 1 Wb per square meter. The earth's magnetic field averages about 0.0001 T (1 G or 100,000 lines of flux per square meter), while an ordinary household magnet (used, for example, to keep papers on a refrigerator) might have a strength of 0.1 T (1,000 G or 10,000,000 lines of flux per square meter). Modern magnetic resonance imaging (MRI) equipment often operates in the range of 0.3–2.0 T (3,000 to 20,000 G or 30,000,000 to 200,000,000 lines of flux per square meter).

Because the earth itself is a magnet, with a north and a south pole, lines of force, although relatively weak, are present everywhere. This fact is used in the design of a magnetic compass. The pointer is simply a small piece of permanent magnet which will align itself with the earth's magnetic lines of force and indicate direction. Because of this, a compass is a use-

ful tool in detecting magnetic lines of force, including those induced by electrons moving in electrical circuits and devices. Worth noting is the fact that the earth's true magnetic poles are not located in Antarctica and the Arctic Ocean. Instead, the true magnetic north pole is located in Canada's far north, while the true magnetic south pole is near Australia. Both poles tend to drift to new locations as geological conditions beneath the earth's crust change.

Magnets can be classified by type of production as **natural, artificial permanent,** and **electromagnets. Natural magnets** are created when iron oxide (magnetite) remains in the earth's magnetic field for ages, slowly orienting the magnetic dipoles in the same direction. These natural magnets are called lodestones. They were recognized by primitive man and investigated by Greek academics. In some regions entire mountains of iron ore that have remained undisturbed for eons have magnetic properties. Natives of Thunder Bay, Ontario, delight in watching tourists follow signpost instructions to place their cars in neutral gear at the bottom of a magnetic mountain's gentle grade in hopes that the magnetic field will pull their cars up the hill.

Artificial permanent magnets are manufactured from a steel alloy called alnico, composed of aluminum, nickel, and cobalt. While it is hot, alnico is subjected to the field of a strong commercial magnet to permit easier orientation of the magnetic dipoles. Upon cooling, the magnetic field becomes relatively permanent.

Electromagnets are temporary magnets produced by moving electric current. Because the electrons comprising the flow of current create magnetic fields in exactly the same manner as do the orbiting and spinning atomic electrons, any flow of current produces a magnetic field. When the current ceases flowing, the magnetic field collapses, making these electrical magnets temporary.

It is possible to create a fourth type of magnet by vibration. Prior to the 20th century, experienced blacksmiths were easy to spot because the tongs they used to handle heated metals had become magnetized. After many years of standing in the same position (in orientation to the earth's magnetic lines of force), heating the tongs in the forge, and then pounding the hot metal into shape on the anvil, the tongs had become well magnetized. A request to see

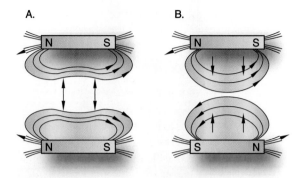

FIGURE 4-4 Repulsion-attraction of magnetic lines of force: (A) Lines of force in the same direction will repel each other. (B) Lines of force in opposite directions will attract each other.

a horseshoe hanging from a rafter would prove a smith's experience when he used the magnetized tongs to easily lift it down.

The laws governing magnetism are similar to the laws of electrostatics. However, only three are of importance for this text:

1. **Repulsion-attraction.** Like poles repel; unlike poles attract. In addition, like lines of force repel and unlike lines of force attract, when placed within each other's force fields (Figure 4-4).

2. **The inverse square law.** The force between two magnetic fields is directly proportional to the product of their magnitudes and inversely proportional to the square of the distance between them. Exactly as with electrostatics, as an object gets further away, the influencing field decreases because of the increased area it affects.

3. **Magnetic poles.** Every magnet has two poles, a north and a south, as discussed earlier. No matter how much a magnet is divided, even into individual moving electrons, both poles continue to exist.

Because the laws of electrostatics, magnetism, and gravity have so many similarities, physicists have long searched for a mathematical theory to relate the three forces into a unified field theory. Albert Einstein worked unsuccessfully toward this goal until he died and the search continues to the present time, in the work of Stephen Hawking.

Magnetic Induction

When a nonmagnetized iron bar is brought within the lines of force of a strong magnet, the dipoles will temporarily align themselves with the lines of force passing through the iron bar. If the bar is removed from the field after a short time, the dipoles will return to their random orientation, thus leaving the bar unmagnetized. This process is termed magnetic induction and operates like electromagnetic induction. Instead of temporary repulsion of electrons, magnetic poles are induced through the temporary orientation of the dipoles.

The ease with which sensitive devices can be magnetized or demagnetized by stray electrical fields makes magnetic shielding desirable in many situations. Because there is no magnetic insulator, shielding is accomplished by providing a highly permeable ferromagnetic material, such as iron, through which stray magnetic fields can be directed, thus protecting sensitive devices from exposure to the stray field. This technique is used to shield some magnetic resonance imaging (MRI) units, although they require radio frequency (RF) shielding as well.

Magnetic Classification of Materials

Permeability is the ease with which a material can be magnetized, while **retentivity** is the ability of a material to stay magnetized. These two factors are inversely proportional because, if it is difficult to orient the dipoles (low permeability), it is also difficult to disorient them (high retentivity). The major classifications of the magnetic properties of materials according to their relative permeabilities are:

1. **Ferromagnetic** (or simply magnetic) materials such as iron, cobalt, and nickel are highly permeable and greatly susceptible to induction. These materials have a majority of their dipoles lying in the same direction, thus setting up a natural magnetic field. In addition, the material must permit the atoms to be oriented, thus permitting the growth of magnetic dipoles in predominantly the same direction. Specialized alloys such as alnico, permalloy, or mumetal (some alloys, strangely enough, contain no

ferromagnetic elements) are designed to enhance permeability and exhibit dramatically increased magnetic field strength.

2. **Paramagnetic** materials, such as platinum and aluminum, have low permeability and weak attraction to magnetic fields. These materials have only a slight majority of dipoles in the same direction and there is little tendency for the size of the dipoles to grow. MRI contrast media are usually paramagnetic.

3. **Diamagnetic** materials, such as beryllium, bismuth, and lead, are actually weakly repelled by all magnetic fields, including both north and south poles. Strangely, water is slightly diamagnetic. This property is so weak that it is easily obscured by other types of magnetic induction.

4. **Nonmagnetic** materials, such as wood, glass, rubber, and plastic, are not affected by magnetic fields and cannot be magnetized. Nonmagnetic materials are most often composed of atoms locked into crystalline or molecular patterns, thus forming ionic and covalent bonds and eliminating the ability of electrons to freely orient themselves to external magnetic lines of force. This classification includes most materials.

ELECTROMAGNETISM

Electricity and magnetism are actually different aspects of the same force, electromagnetism. Although the study of magnetism dates to ancient times, and the study of electricity to Queen Elizabeth I's physician, William Gilbert (1540–1603), it was not until 1820, when the Danish physicist Hans Oersted (1777–1851) observed the deflection of a compass during a classroom demonstration of electrical phenomena, that the relationships between the two began to be established. Oersted's discovery, and subsequent investigations by many others, permitted the generation, control, and practical use of electricity and initiated the electronic revolution that continues today.

Oersted's experiment proves that when there is no current flowing in the wire, the compass needle aligns itself with the earth's magnetic field (Figure 4-5). However, when current is flowing, the needle is de-

A. Without current flow

B. With current flow

FIGURE 4-5 Oersted's experiment: A compass placed near a wire conductor will indicate the direction of the earth's magnetic field (A) when no current is flowing in the wire. Because flowing current creates a magnetic field around the wire conductor that is stronger than the earth's field, the compass will indicate the direction of the current-induced field while the switch is closed (B).

flected toward the wire and when the current stops, the needle returns to alignment with the earth's field. This led to the conclusion that **any moving charge produces a magnetic field.** As was stated earlier in the section on magnetism, this applies to even a single electron's negative charge in orbit around an atom. A slightly different arrangement of Oersted's experiment (Figure 4-6) permits the mapping of the magnetic field surrounding the flow of current.

The English scientist John Fleming (1849–1945) developed a series of easily remembered aids to help with the relationship between electricity and mag-

Current Flow

Compass

FIGURE 4-6 Relationship of induced magnetic field to direction of current flow: A variation of Oersted's experiment maps out the magnetic field induced by flowing current.

netism. They are known as **Fleming's hand rules.** There are several "hand" rules that are quite useful for remembering various electromagnetic relationships. The rules are divided into four groups: (1) **hand thumb rules along a conductor;** (2) **hand thumb rules for solenoid and electromagnet poles;** (3) **hand generator effect rules; and** (4) **hand motor principle rules.** These are summarized in Table 4-1. Before learning any of the rules, it is critical to remember that **hand rules which are based on current flow (conventional current direction) and hand rules which are based on electron flow (actual direction of electron movement) will be exact opposites.** For example, the right-hand thumb rule applies to conventional current flow. This is identical to the left-hand thumb rule applied to actual electron flow.

The hand thumb rule, the first of the hand rules, applies to remembering the relationship between the direction of current along a conductor and the direction of the resulting magnetic lines of force field. **Fleming's right-hand thumb rule states that if the right hand is used to grasp a conducting**

TABLE 4-1.   Fleming's Hand Rules for Electromagnetic Relationships

		Conventional Current Flow	Electron Flow
Along a Conductor			
thumb	= conventional current or electron flow	right-hand thumb rule (see Figure 4-7)	left-hand thumb rule (left-hand version)
fingers	= magnetic field		
Solenoid and Electromagnet Poles			
thumb	= direction of north pole	right-hand thumb rule (see Figure 4-9)	left-hand thumb rule (left-hand version)
fingers	= conventional current or electron flow		
Generator Effect			
thumb	= movement of conductor on armature	right-hand generator rule (see Figure 4-12)	left-hand generator rule (left-hand version)
index finger	= magnetic lines of force field		
middle finger	= current or electron flow		
Motor Principle			
thumb	= movement of conductor on rotor	left-hand motor rule (see Figure 4-18)	right-hand motor rule (right-hand version)
index finger	= magnetic lines of force field		
middle finger	= current or electron flow		

Direction of magnetic field lines

Current

Wire

FIGURE 4-7 Fleming's right-hand thumb rule: When the right hand is positioned so the thumb points in the direction of conventional current flow, the fingers indicate the direction of the induced magnetic field. Fleming's left-hand thumb rule does the same for actual electron flow.

wire with the thumb in the direction of the current flow, the fingers will indicate the direction of the magnetic field lines of force surrounding the conductor (Figure 4-7). (If the thumb points in the direction of actual electron flow, then a left-hand thumb rule must be used to show the direction of the magnetic field lines of force surrounding the conductor.) Table 4-1 compares this rule with the other "hand" rules.

SOLENOIDS AND ELECTROMAGNETS

An interesting phenomenon occurs when conducting wire is looped (Figure 4-8A). Using the right-hand thumb rule to determine the direction of the magnetic lines of flux, it is apparent that inside the loop the magnetic fields from both sides join to double the magnetic flux density. If a series of loops are made, creating a coil (Figure 4-8B), the flux density is greatly increased. When current is flowing through this type of coil it is called a **solenoid.** The flux density can be increased further still by adding a ferro-

magnetic core. This configuration is called an *electromagnet.* **The strength of solenoids and electromagnets is determined by the number of loops (or turns) of wire, the current strength and the permeability of the core.** The right-hand thumb rule can also be applied to a solenoid or an electromagnet to determine the location of the magnetic poles. **If the fingers point in the direction of the current, the thumb will point toward the north pole** (Figure 4-9). (If the fingers point in the direction of actual electron flow, then a left-hand thumb rule must be used for the thumb to point toward the north pole.) Table 4-1 compares this rule with the other "hand" rules.

Both the solenoid and the electromagnet demonstrate magnetic properties only while electric current is flowing. If the current stops flowing, the magnetic properties vanish, and if the current is adjusted up or down, the magnetic strength changes accordingly. The factors that govern the effectiveness of solenoids and electromagnets are the **diameter** of the coil, its **length,** and the **current** passing along the coil. Electromagnets are used as remote control devices in circuit breakers and in the temporary locks, sometimes called detents, on radiographic equipment. In a typical circuit breaker configuration, a wire from the circuit to be protected is incorporated into an electromagnet, which, when the current becomes dangerously high, has been calculated to attract a movable contact, which breaks the circuit.

Solenoids are often used as detent locks on the overhead crane of x-ray tubes. The detent can be activated by a switch at the x-ray tube controls. The switch activates the magnetic properties of the solenoid, which in turn attracts a metal latch or bolt. This temporarily locks the tube to the center of the x-ray table or at the proper distance from a film holder. **Electromagnetic relays** are similar to circuit breakers. They are used to protect radiographers from electrical shock by isolating control buttons on the x-ray console from the actual circuit in which high voltage is flowing.

Electromagnetic Induction

Once it became known that electrical current could generate a magnetic field, the obvious question was whether the reverse was true. In fact it

A. Loop of conductor

B. A solenoid

FIGURE 4-8   A solenoid: (A) When a conductor is looped to form a coil, the magnetic fields from both sides join to double the magnetic field strength inside the loop. (B) A solenoid is a helix coil through which current is flowing; it uses the coil loops to produce a greatly strengthened magnetic field.

was demonstrated by the English physicist Michael Faraday (1791–1867) the year after Oersted's discovery. The simple presence of a magnetic field is not sufficient to cause electrons to move along a wire. Faraday discovered that the magnetic lines of force and the wire must have a motion relative to each other to induce an electrical current (Figure 4-10). There are three ways to create the motion between lines of force and a conductor:

1. **Move the conductor** through a stationary, unchanging strength magnetic field.
2. **Move magnetic lines of force** through a stationary conductor with an unchanging strength magnetic field.
3. **Vary the magnetic flux** strength from a stationary magnet through a stationary conductor. As the flux strength varies, the lines of force will expand and contract, in effect causing the relative motion necessary to induce current.

FIGURE 4-9 Fleming's right-hand thumb rule applied to determining the pole of a solenoid or electromagnet. When the fingers point in the direction of the current, the thumb will point toward the north pole.

The exact definitions of "magnetic flux strength" and "lines of force" are critical to understanding these differences.

There are two primary laws that govern the induction of current by magnetic fields. Faraday's law (sometimes called The First Law of Electromagnetics) states that four factors regulate the strength of induced current when magnetic lines of force and a conductor are in motion relative to one another:

1. the **strength** of the magnetic field,
2. the **speed** of the motion between lines of force and the conductor,
3. the **angle** between the magnetic lines of force and the conductor and
4. the **number of turns** in the conducting coil.

This law makes it possible to determine the direction in which the induced current will flow. This application of the law was established by the Russian scientist Heinrich Lenz (1804–1865). Lenz's law (sometimes called The Second Law of Electromag-

A. Without relative motion

B. With relative motion

FIGURE 4-10 Faraday's experiment: A meter will not indicate current flow (A) until the magnetic lines of force from the magnet and wire have a motion relative to one another (B).

netics) states that induced current flow sets up a magnetic field opposing the action that produced the original current, or, simply, that induced current opposes any flux change.

These two laws apply to both forms of induction: mutual induction and self-induction. **Mutual**

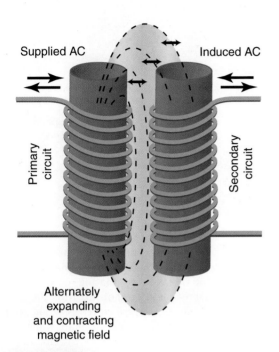

Supplied AC

Induced AC

Primary circuit

Secondary circuit

Alternately
expanding
and contracting
magnetic field

FIGURE 4-11 Mutual induction: A varying current supplied to the primary coil induces a similar flow in the second coil. The constantly expanding and contracting magnetic lines of force induced in the primary coil provide the relative motion with the secondary coil necessary to induce current flow in the secondary coil.

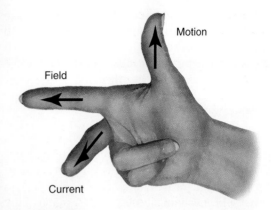

Motion

Field

Current

FIGURE 4-12 Fleming's right-hand generator rule: When the thumb points in the direction the conductor (or armature) is moving and the index finger points in the direction of the magnetic lines of force field, the middle finger indicates the direction of conventional current flow. Fleming's left-hand generator rule does the same for actual electron flow.

induction occurs when two coils are placed in proximity and a varying current supplied to the first coil (as an electromagnet) induces a similar flow in the second coil (Figure 4-11). The coil supplied with current is called the **primary coil,** while the coil in which the current is inducted is called the **secondary coil.** The flow occurs in the secondary coil because the primary current alternates. This follows the rule that moving lines of force from a varying intensity current will induce electron flow in the wire through which it passes. In this case the secondary coil is cut by the varying (and therefore moving) lines of force from the current in the primary coil.

Self-induction is much more complicated but is more understandable when comparing a coil supplied with direct current, where there is self-induction only at the turn-on moment, with a coil supplied with alternating current, where self-induction occurs regularly. Alternating current is present when the electrons constantly change direction. A coil supplied with alternating current permits a steady flow of electrons and establishes an electromagnetic effect for half the cycle. However, at the instant the current supply reverses, the previously established electromagnetic north and south poles will induce an opposing potential difference, thus attempting to induce against the incoming supply of electrons. This tendency of an alternating current is called **inductive reactance** and is measured in ohms of resistance. Self-induction is useful when it is desirable to permit direct current to flow while at the same time hindering alternating current.

An important relationship exists between the direction of movement of a wire coil (the armature), the direction of the magnetic lines of force field, and the direction in which the induced current will flow. This relationship is best remembered by the use of another "hand" rule (Figure 4-12). **Fleming's right-hand generator rule states that if the thumb points in the direction the conductor (or armature) is moving and the index finger points in the direction of the magnetic lines of**

force field, then the middle finger will indicate the direction of the conventional current. (If the direction of actual electron flow is desired, then a left-hand generator rule must be used.) Table 4-1 compares this rule with the other "hand" rules.

Generators

A **generator,** or dynamo, is a device that converts mechanical energy to electrical energy using Faraday's discovery of moving lines of flux in relationship to a conductor to induce current. This process converts the mechanical energy of the motion (any of the three ways) to electrical energy. A simple generator is composed of a conductor and magnets arranged as shown in Figure 4-13. The conductor is a coil of wire, called an **armature,** set between opposing magnetic poles so that it encounters the strongest lines of force. If the armature is rotated by a strong source of mechanical energy (such as a steam or water turbine), the generator can produce massive amounts of electrical energy. It is important to note the method that is used to convey the electrical current from the armature to the circuit. A set of **slip rings** and **brushes** permits the circuit to remain stationary while the armature rotates without breaking the electrical contact between them. This allows the electrons to flow without interruption. **Each slip ring connects to one end of the armature wire** (see Figure 4-13).

To understand exactly how the current is produced, it is necessary to follow the production step by step (Figure 4-14). Notice that the armature coil wire is shown in cross-section at the top, three-dimensionally in the middle, and that the graph at the bottom represents the voltage produced. It is important to understand the relationship of the angle between this wire's motion and the lines of force between the stationary magnets. In Figure 4-14A the wire's motion is parallel to the lines of force. This produces no emf, as shown on the graph. In Figure 4-14B the rotation of the armature has changed the wire's motion until it is at a 45° angle to the lines of force. Fleming's right-hand generator rule demonstrates that the conventional electrical current is moving into the page (electron flow would be out of the page). Because of the 45° angle, the magnitude of the emf, although rising, has

Rotating shaft
(attached to turbine or
other source of mechanical
energy)

Brush

N

S

Armature

Slip ring

FIGURE 4-13 An AC generator: Mechanical energy rotates the shaft to which the armature is attached. As the wires of the armature rotate, they cut through the magnetic lines of flux from the magnets and produce electrical current. The slip rings and brushes permit the armature to rotate while maintaining contact with the wires of the circuit.

not yet reached its peak. In Figure 4-14C, the motion of the wire is 90° to the lines of force (the maximum angle), resulting in the peak emf. As the wire begins to turn back to parallel in Figure 4-14D, the emf begins to drop back toward zero. When the wire reaches a parallel position, as in Figure 4-14E, the emf has returned to zero. As the wire begins to move into a 270° position (which is a 90° position in the opposite direction), notice that the relationship between the wire's motion and the lines of force has changed. Using Fleming's right-hand generator rule again, it is simple to see that the conventional electrical current has now reversed and is moving out of the page (while the electron flow has reversed to move into the page). **It is at this point that alternating current is produced.** This has occurred because **alternating current is produced when the wire's motion relative to the lines of force is reversed.** In Figures 4-14F, G, H, and I, the rise to peak and drop back to zero emf is repeated but in the opposite direction. This explains not only why generator-produced current must be alternating but also accounts for its pulsating nature.

The type of curve produced by an AC generator will always appear as in Figure 4-14. It is called a

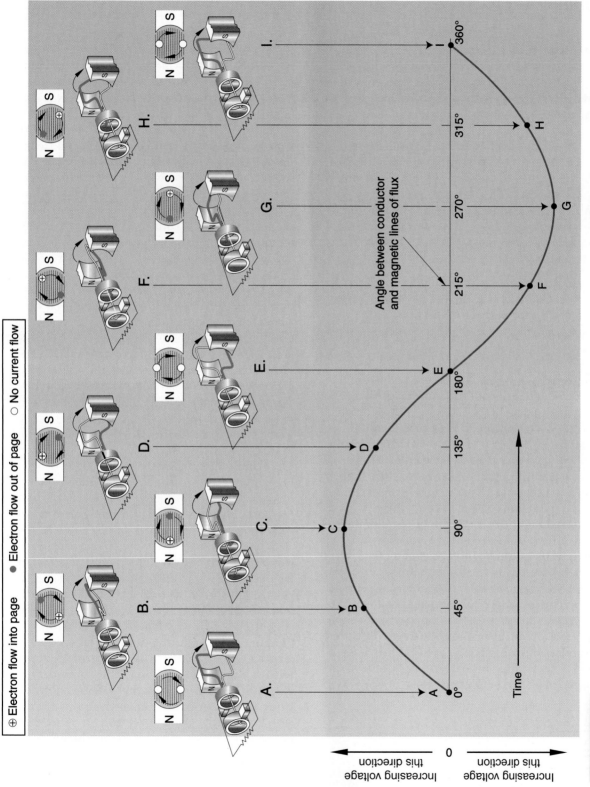

⊕ Electron flow into page   ● Electron flow out of page   ○ No current flow

Angle between conductor and magnetic lines of flux

Time

Increasing voltage this direction

0

Increasing voltage this direction

FIGURE 4–14 The production of alternating current: Armature coil wire is shown in cross section (top). Three-dimensional view of generator (middle). Graph of the voltage produced (bottom). See text for step-by-step description.

sine wave because it depends on the mathematical sine between the plane of the armature and a plane perpendicular to the lines of force. **One complete turn of the generator armature represents one cycle.** The sine wave illustrates one complete turn of the armature as the distance between two corresponding points. Note that this would be represented by the distance between *a* and *i* in Figure 4-14. **The frequency of the sine wave is determined by the number of cycles per second (cps). The unit of frequency is the hertz, represented by the symbol Hz. 1 cps = 1 Hz.** American and Canadian generators operate at 60 Hz. Most of the rest of the world operates at 50 Hz.

> *EXAMPLE:* How many times per second do the electrons in a 60 Hz alternating current change their direction of movement?
>
> *Answer:*
>
> 60 Hz × 2 directions = 120 changes per second

From Figure 4-14, it also becomes apparent that the **peak voltage is not the same as the average voltage** throughout the entire sine wave. The same is true of amperage and resistance (Ohm's law). This makes the measurement of all factors very difficult in pulsating alternating current because of the constant fluctuation of the sine wave. This is solved by using the root mean square (rms) values of the amperage and voltage. **Root mean square (rms) values of the total voltage and amperage in an alternating current are equivalent to the effect that would be produced in a direct current resistance by the same factors.** Resistance in alternating currents is calculated from a complicated series of factors, resulting in measurement of the apparent total resistance. **Apparent total resistance of an alternating current is called impedance, which is represented by the symbol Z.** This permits a revised version of Ohm's law to be applied for alternating current as:

$$I = \frac{V}{Z}$$

where: I = rms amperage
V = rms voltage
Z = impedance

When using an x-ray machine, it is worth remembering that the **kilovoltage settings represent peak kilovoltage, not average or rms values.**

A direct-current generator is made by exchanging the slip rings for a **commutator ring,** as shown in Figure 4-15. **A commutator is a single ring that is divided in half, with each half connected to one end of the armature wire.** The single commutator's two halves replace the pair of slip rings. Instead of each end of the armature wire being connected to its own slip ring, each end of the armature wire is connected to half of the commutator ring. When a generator has its armature connected to a commutator, the sine wave of the output is dramatically different from that produced by a pair of slip rings. Although the armature turns exactly as in an alternating current generator, the commutator routes the current very differently. This current produces a sine wave exactly as in an alternating current generator (Figures 4-15A–C). The use of Fleming's right-hand generator rule demonstrates that the conventional electrical current is moving into the page (electron flow would be out of the page). In Figure 4-15D the wire has begun to move toward the second phase of the cycle. As in the alternating-current generator, the relationship between the wire's motion and the lines of force has changed. Using Fleming's right-hand generator rule again, it is simple to see that the conventional electrical current has now reversed and is moving out of the page (while the electron flow has reversed to move into the page). However, it is extremely important to note that in Figure 4-15D, the commutator ring has also changed the brush with which it was in contact. This has the same effect as switching the exiting connections on the armature wires. **Although Fleming's right-hand generator rule demonstrates the change in direction of current within the armature wire, the commutator ring has also reversed the exiting connections, thus keeping the current in the circuit flowing in the same direction. It is at this point that direct current is produced.** Note that the direct current is not as steady as would be expected with a battery source. Instead a pulsating direct current has been produced.

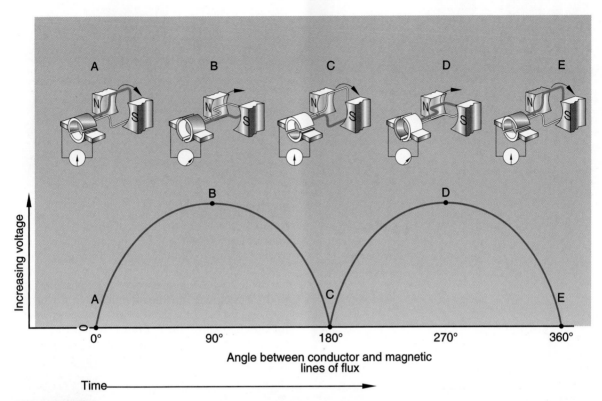

FIGURE 4-15 A DC generator: The slip rings have been exchanged for a commutator ring, with each half connecting to one end of the armature wire. Although the armature turns exactly as in an AC generator, the commutator routes the current as shown on the graph. See text for step-by-step description.

Multiple-coil direct-current generators are used in place of the simple single-coil generators diagrammed in Figures 4-14 and 4-15. These DC generators utilize numerous coils and a commutator divided into a corresponding number of segments, as shown in Figure 4-16A. This type of generator produces a sine wave, as shown in Figure 4-16B. The combined current generated never drops to zero and has the advantage of a much steadier flow, although the pulsations have not been completely eliminated.

Motors

A device that is supplied with electrical current to produce mechanical motion is called a **motor.** Motors have essentially the same parts as generators and operate on the same principles but in reverse. In addition, some of the parts have been slightly redesigned and carry names different from those in a generator.

The motor principle is a result of the interaction of magnetic fields when an electric current is sent along a conductor that is residing in a magnetic field. As current flows through the conducting coil, a magnetic field is established, according to Fleming's right-hand thumb rule (Figure 4-17). Because the conducting coil lies within the lines of force from the stationary magnets, the induced lines of force will be attracted in one direction (downward for the left wire and upward for the right wire) while at the same time being repelled in the other direction (upward for the left wire and downward for the right wire). The net result is that the conductor begins to move in the direction of the arrows.

A.

B.

Increasing Voltage

Time

FIGURE 4-16   Multiple coil, split commutator, DC generator: More than one coil, or armature, with a split commutator (A) will produce DC current as shown in the graph (B).

FIGURE 4-17   The motor principle: Because the conducting wires of the armature lie within the lines of force from the stationary magnets, when current begins to flow through the armature, the induced lines of force will be attracted downward for the left wire and upward for the right wire while at the same time being repelled in the other direction (upward for the left wire and downward for the right wire). The net result is that the conductor begins to move in the direction of the arrows.

Fleming's left-hand motor rule states that if the index finger points in the direction of the magnetic lines of force field and the middle finger points in the direction of the conventional current, the thumb will indicate the direction the conductor will move (Figure 4-18). (This would be a right-hand motor rule if the direction of electron flow is being considered.) Table 4-1 compares this rule with the other "hand" rules.

Different motor configurations are required depending on whether alternating or direct current is supplied. **Direct-current motors use commutator rings.** As with a DC generator, the commutator is required in order to switch the flow of current when the conducting coil begins to reach a 180° position, where the induced and stationary lines of

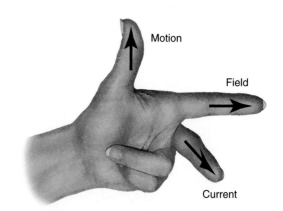

Motion

Field

Current

FIGURE 4-18   Fleming's left-hand motor rule: If the index finger points in the direction of the magnetic lines of force and the middle finger points in the direction of the conventional current flow, the thumb will indicate the direction the conductor will move. (This would be a right-hand motor rule if the direction of actual electron flow is being considered.)

Stator electromagnets

N   N

N

3   1

2

Rotor

3   2

N

2   3

S   S

1

Rotor wire
windings

S   S

FIGURE 4-19 Alternating-current induction
motor: The rotor windings obey the motor
principle as they move perpendicular to the
magnetic lines of flux, in the direction of the
arrows. The stator electromagnets are supplied
with multiphase current to activate them in
sequential pairs to maintain maximum
perpendicular motor principle force.

force no longer attract or repel one another. When
the current flow is switched by the commutator
ring, the magnetic lines of force also reverse. Continuing this switching of current flow results in the
conductor continually being simultaneously repelled and attracted in a circle, thus turning a shaft
and supplying the mechanical motion as a conversion of the applied electrical energy.

These direct-current motors use many turns of
wire in the conductor coil to increase the strength of
the field. This requires numerous pairs of stationary
magnets to force the conductor coil to cut the stationary lines of force as near to 90° (the maximum
inducing angle) as often as possible (Figure 4-19).

Alternating-current motors use slip rings.
Unlike direct-current motors, the incoming current
switches direction, making the commutator unnecessary. There are two major types of alternating
current motors.

**Synchronous alternating-current motors
have conducting coils that turn at the same
speed as the generator armature supplying the
current (or a multiple of the armature's
speed).** Synchronous motors are useful when a
steady speed is necessary, as in a timing device. They
tend to be relatively weak because insufficient motor
principle force is established at the conducting coil.

**Alternating-current induction motors uti-
lize a rotor coil with the exterior magnetic
field supplied by several pairs of electromagnets, thus producing a strong magnetic field,
increasing the power of the motor and permitting it to run at any desired speed.** Instead of
supplying current to the coil in the magnetic field,
an induction motor uses a device called a **rotor. A
rotor consists of bars of copper around an
iron core** (see Figure 4-19). No commutator or slip
rings are required. Instead, a device called a **stator**
is used. **A stator consists of pairs of stationary
magnets (or, more commonly, electromagnets)
arranged around the rotor. The stator must be
supplied with multiphase current.** The stator
electromagnets are energized in sequence. As the
copper bars of the rotor reach a point where the motor principle forces are equalized, the multiphase
current activates the next pair of electromagnets
and the motor principle forces pull the rotor around
to the next position. This continuing sequential en-
ergization causes the motor principle forces to continually turn the rotor. Extremely powerful
induction motors are made by increasing the
strength and number of pairs of electromagnets;
these motors are popular for industrial and consumer uses.

Induction motors are used in rotating anode
x-ray tubes where the target anode is attached to
the induction motor rotor inside the glass vacuum
tube. Because magnetic lines of force will pass
through glass and a vacuum, the electromagnets
can be positioned outside the vacuum tube, thus
avoiding interference with the high voltages required to produce x-rays.

The motor principle is also used in meters: **gal-
vanometers for direct current**, when permanent
magnets are used, to indicate current, and **dy-
namometers for alternating current**, when electromagnets are used (Figure 4-20A). To a great

A. A galvanometer   B. Ammeter in circuit   C. Voltmeter in circuit

FIGURE 4–20   (A) A simple galvanometer uses an electromagnet to attract a coil of wire to which a needle is attached. When a scale is calibrated, amperage or voltage can be measured. (B) Ammeter connection. (C) Voltmeter connection.

extent they are being replaced by digital meters that provide numerical indications of current. **When a meter is connected in series,** it measures current in amperes and is called an **ammeter** (see Figure 4-20B). **When connected in parallel, it measures potential difference in volts and is called a voltmeter** (see Figure 4-20C).

CONTROLLING ELECTRICAL CURRENT

Transformers

Alternating current, because of its changing direction, constantly establishes, collapses, reestablishes, and re-collapses its surrounding magnetic field. This aspect can be used to change electricity by combining electromagnetic mutual induction with an application of Ohm's law to form a device called a **transformer.** Transformers are composed of two coils placed near one another (but without electrical connection). If current is supplied to one coil, the lines of force that are induced will pass through the other coil and induce a flow of electrons (see Figure 4-11). The coil that is supplied with current is the **primary,** while the coil in which current is induced is the **secondary.**

The number of turns of wire in the primary coil is designed to be different from the number of turns of wire in the secondary. This causes the induced current to be different in the secondary coil. For example, the lines of force induced by a single primary coil loop may cut two loops of the secondary. In this case the voltage in the primary would be induced in **both** secondary loops, thus doubling the secondary voltage. When the voltage is increased from primary to secondary it is called a **step-up transformer.** When the voltage is decreased from primary to secondary it is called a **step-down transformer.** The **transformer law** expresses this phenomenon:

$$\frac{V_s}{V_p} = \frac{N_s}{N_p}$$

where: V = potential difference in volts
N = number of turns of wire in the coil
p = primary coil
s = secondary coil

EXAMPLE: If a transformer is supplied with 400 volts to the primary coil, has 100 turns of wire on the primary coil and 20,000 turns of wire on the secondary coil, what will the voltage be in the secondary coil?

Answer:

$$\frac{V_s}{V_p} = \frac{N_s}{N_p}$$

$$\frac{V_s}{400V} = \frac{20,000 \text{ turns}}{100 \text{ turns}}$$

$$100 \, V_s = 400V \times 20,000 \text{ turns}$$

$$V_s = \frac{8,000,000}{100}$$

$$V_s = 80,000 \text{ volts or } 80 \text{ kilovolts}$$

EXAMPLE: If a transformer has 120 turns of wire on the primary coil, 80 volts in the primary coil, and 20 volts in the secondary coil, how many turns of wire must there be in the second-ary coil?

Answer:

$$\frac{V_s}{V_p} = \frac{N_s}{N_p}$$

$$\frac{20V}{80V} = \frac{N_s}{120 \text{ turns}}$$

$$\frac{2,400 \text{ turns}}{80} = N_s$$

$$N_s = 30 \text{ turns}$$

Transformers are used to change voltage. However, Ohm's law is in effect and the effect of the transformer on amperage, voltage and number of turns in the coils can be calculated by combining the transformer law with Ohm's law:

$$\frac{I_s}{I_p} = \frac{V_p}{V_s}$$

and:

$$\frac{I_s}{I_p} = \frac{N_p}{N_s}$$

It is helpful to remember that voltage and number of turns are directly proportional, while voltage and amperage are inversely proportional. Therefore, the number of turns and amperage must also

be inversely proportional. It is also important to note that a step-up transformer increases voltage from primary to secondary while decreasing amperage. Conversely, a step-down transformer decreases voltage from primary to secondary while increasing amperage. Because transformers are designed to change voltages, the descriptive terms step-up and step-down refer to the voltage change, not the amperage change. You should remember that Ohm's law requires the consideration of resistance and this is indeed an important factor. However, this book will not address that aspect. **All transformers must operate on alternating current to provide the establishing and collapsing magnetic fields that induce the voltage changes in the secondary coil.**

Although transformer efficiency, the ability of a transformer to avoid power loss, is usually above 95 percent, a number of factors influence how much energy is lost. Because the high-voltage transformer used in x-ray equipment must step up voltage into the kilovolt range, it uses large amounts of secondary coil windings. This massive amount of wire and the high induced voltage cause several problems that greatly affect the efficiency of the transformer.

1. **I^2R loss,** sometimes called copper loss, is caused by the inherent resistance to current flow that is found in all conductors. The power lost due to this resistance is proportional to the square of the current. It is minimized by using low-resistance wire, such as large-diameter copper, and by using high voltage and low amperage. Lost power is given off as heat. This is the reason why power transmitted long distances between cities is carried on high-voltage power lines. The high voltage permits low amperage and greatly reduced I^2R loss. Because high voltages are extremely dangerous, they are carried on high towers. Step-down transformers are used at receiving stations to lower the voltage (and increase the amperage) to make the power safe for use in buildings.

2. **Hysteresis loss** (lagging loss) in the core occurs because energy is expended as the continually changing AC current magnetizes, demagnetizes, and remagnetizes the core material. Demagnetization leaves some dipoles in the

original orientation, and this residual magnetism causes the remagnetic effort to lag, thus producing more heat loss. The characteristic that requires energy to carry out this constant reorientation of the magnetic dipoles is called **coercivity.** Coercivity can be minimized by using a core material such as silicon iron.

3. **Eddy current loss** in the core is a result of currents opposing the cause which produced them, according to Lenz's law, as discussed earlier. They are produced in any conducting material subjected to changing magnetic fields. Laminating the transformer core reduces the eddy current loss by dividing the core into thin layers. This reduces the strength of the eddy currents (Figure 4-21).

These factors result in a great amount of heat build-up which can be felt by placing your hand on the exterior of the transformer cabinet in a diagnostic x-ray room. Although the transformer is highly insulated and immersed in insulating dielectric oil, there is a definite warmth to the cabinet after the machine has been in use for a few hours. The size of the x-ray transformer makes its efficiency an important factor.

There are numerous types of transformer configurations. The simple arrangement of two coils of wire in proximity to facilitate induction, that has been used so far to explain transformer function, is called an **air core transformer.** If the primary and secondary coils are filled with an iron core, the strength of the magnetic field is greatly increased, forming an **open-core transformer.** Various types of cores have been designed to enhance the lines of force and thereby increase the magnetic field strength (Figure 4-22). The field from an open core tends to diverge as it forms the external lines of force. Closing the core to form a **closed-core transformer** (by placing a top and bottom to the cores) will direct the lines of force from primary and secondary cores toward each other and result in a significant system net increase in field strength. The **shell-type transformer** goes one step further by converging both the inside and outside lines of force through an iron core. In addition, a great efficiency is obtained by insulating the wiring and wrapping the primary and secondary coils atop one another,

Primary

Secondary

A. Closed core transformer

B. Nonlaminated core

C. Eddy currents

D. Laminated core

E. Eddy currents

FIGURE 4-21 (A) Closed-core transformer; (B) nonlaminated core; (C) nonlaminated core eddy currents; (D) laminated core; and (E) laminated core eddy currents.

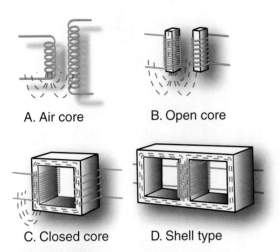

A. Air core   B. Open core

C. Closed core   D. Shell type

FIGURE 4-22   Various types of transformer core configurations; (A) air core; (B) open core; (C) closed core; and (D) shell type.

FIGURE 4-23   An autotransformer.

thus minimizing the distance between coils and maximizing the coupling effectiveness of the induction. X-ray generators use laminated core, shell-type transformers, which are the most common type in use today.

Autotransformers

It is possible to construct a variable transformer, called an **autotransformer,** by connecting both primary and secondary coils in series instead of insulating them. This also permits a single coil on a central core. Connections are made along a single coil at different points for primary and secondary. The primary side has a selection of taps available to permit a variable number of turns in the primary coil (Figure 4-23). When the connections to the taps are attached to control buttons, an effective means of changing voltage is available.

Autotransformers are not suitable for use in the high-voltage transformers in x-ray machines. However, they are suitable for controlling voltage on the low-voltage side of the x-ray circuit before it has been increased by the main step-up transformer, thereby varying the voltage on the high-voltage side as well.

There are three important transformers in the x-ray circuit (Figure 4-24). The autotransformer is used to vary the incoming-line voltage to an appropriate level for the high-voltage step-up transformer. The high-voltage step-up transformer is used to raise the incoming-line voltage to the kilovoltage range necessary for x-ray production. The filament step-down transformer is used to decrease the incoming-line voltage to the 5–15 volt and 3–5 ampere range used to heat the x-ray tube filament.

Capacitors

A **capacitor** is a device capable of accumulating and storing an electrical charge. A simple capacitor consists of two insulated metal plates with opposite charges (Figure 4-25). The repulsion between the charges on the two plates permits a greater number of electrons to be stored on each. The insulation between the plates is called the **dielectric,** and its value is determined by the insulating ability as well as the plate size, distance between the plates, and charge. The unit of capacitance is named for Faraday but has been shortened to **farad.** It is represented by the symbol **f** and is expressed as:

$$C = \frac{q}{V}$$

where: c = capacitance in farads
q = charge on either plate in coulombs
V = potential difference between plates in volts

FIGURE 4-24 Three critical transformer locations in the diagnostic x-ray circuit. The autotransformer permits selection of the voltage (by controls labeled kV on the console). The high-voltage transformer steps the incoming-line voltage up to the kV range before sending it to the x-ray tube. The filament transformer steps the incoming-line voltage down to heat the x-ray tube filament.

FIGURE 4-25 A simple parallel plate capacitor.

Because of the immense size of the coulomb, the farad is very large, making the microfarad (µf) the more common unit.

Capacitors must be charged to be operable; this is done by applying a direct-current voltage. The capacitor will accept a charge until it equals the DC voltage. When discharged, the capacitor has the ability to deliver the stored charge in short and easily controlled intervals. This uniform direct current is especially useful in mobile x-ray units where it is convenient to have a battery charge a capacitor and then initiate a burst of high voltage for the x-ray exposure. Capacitors are also used to supply a more constant voltage to the x-ray tube in some stationary units.

RECTIFICATION

X-ray tubes operate best when receiving direct current. In fact, there is a danger in supplying alternating current because if a flow of electrons occurs in the wrong direction the tube may be damaged beyond repair. **Rectification is the process by which alternating current is changed to pulsating direct current,** and requires the use of one-way electrical devices called rectifiers. Although solid-state semiconductor diodes are most commonly used, it is easier to understand the operation of a vacuum-tube rectifier. Both of these devices create electrical "one-way streets" by permitting electrons to flow easily in one direction while offering a high resistance to movement in the other direction.

The operation of semiconductors was mentioned earlier, in Chapter 3, during the discussion of conductor valence bands. There are numerous types of semiconductors but they all operate in the same manner. The simplest to explain is the p-n junction semiconductor, which is composed of solid materials of two predominant categories, n-type and p-type. N-type materials have loosely bound electrons that move freely between an atom's conduction bands. P-type materials have electron traps made up of positively charged holes that tend to attract and hold electrons instead of permitting them to move freely to another atom. Both types of materials are affected by slight amounts of impurities which are intentionally added to change the conduction properties. For example, arsenic has a valence that permits it to form covalent bonds with silicon crystals, but it makes an extra electron available for conduction, thus forming an n-type material. Conversely, gallium also has a valence permitting covalent bonding with silicon, but it leaves a need for an additional electron, thus forming an electron "hole" and a p-type material.

A rectifying semiconductor called a **diode** is made by sandwiching a p-type crystal with an n-type to form a p-n junction (Figure 4-26). When a potential difference is established with the positive charge at the p side of the junction and the negative charge at the n side, the positive holes from the p side are attracted to the junction, as are the available electrons

from the n side. This permits easy movement of electrons into the p holes. **In a diode, electrons flow from the n to the p side of the p-n junction and conventional electrical current moves from the p to the n side.** When alternating current reverses and the positive charge is at the n side of the junction and the negative charge is at the p side, the positive holes from the p side are repelled from the junction, as are the available electrons from the n side. This makes movement of electrons from the n side of the junction to the p side very unlikely, as both the repulsion-attraction of the charges and the distance between p holes and electrons are working against the electron movement. The result is that no electrons move across the junction, thus creating a one-way street for electrons. The electronic symbol for a diode reflects this movement for conventional electrical current (see Figure 4-26D). Remember that electron flow will be opposite the direction of the arrow.

A thyristor, or silicon-controlled rectifier (SCR), is a more complex semiconductor that has proven useful for high-speed switching of the primary high-voltage x-ray circuit. SCRs are composed of two p-type and two n-type layers, making three p-n junctions (Figure 4-27). Both n-p-n-p and p-n-p-n sequences are possible. In either case, the third section serves as a gate. This gate can change the polarity of the entire SCR by receiving a given charge. Rapid pulses of current to the gate permit it to hold or release large amounts of current. The SCR functions extremely rapidly and has replaced mechanical switchers and thyratrons (gas-filled predecessors to thyristors) in high kilowattage x-ray generators.

A valve tube was a vacuum tube that operated in the same manner as a diode but was constructed like an x-ray tube. Although they are no longer used in x-ray circuitry, they are a useful example in learning how a modern diode circuit functions. The difference between a valve tube and an x-ray tube is that a valve tube operated at energies below the range necessary to produce x-ray photons. The cathode and anode were arranged to permit electrons to jump without requiring the energy necessary to produce x-rays (Figure 4-28). Current could flow from cathode to anode because the jump to the

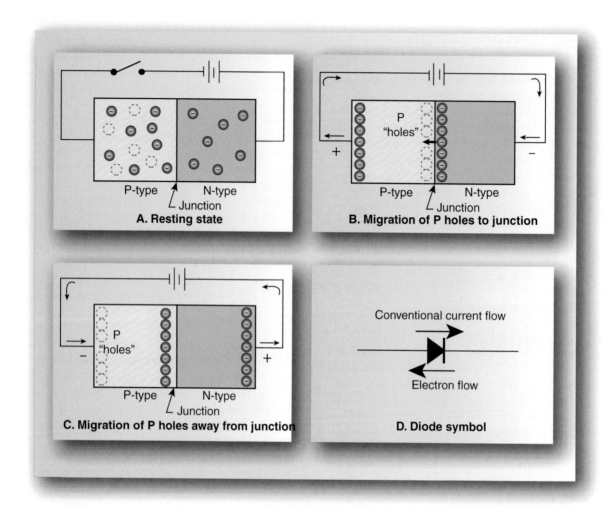

A. Resting state

B. Migration of P holes to junction

C. Migration of P holes away from junction

D. Diode symbol

Conventional current flow

Electron flow

FIGURE 4-26 The functioning of a p–n junction of a solid–state semiconductor diode.

massive anode was easy. However, as electrons repelled one another, they spread out over the entire surface of the anode and could not develop sufficient repulsive force to jump to the cathode. This made the tube a one-way street for electrons to move from cathode to anode.

The cathode included a coil of small-diameter tungsten wire, called the filament, through which current was passed. Of course the small diameter of the wire caused a greatly increased resistance to the flow of electrons. This resulted in

heat increase to the extent that electron movement actually ejected individual electrons from the surface of the wire. Sometimes this phenomenon is described as a boiling of electrons from the surface. The result was the formation of an electron cloud (see Figure 4-28B). This process is called **thermionic emission** because the heat (therm) has caused ionization (ionic), resulting in electrons being expelled (emission) from the surface of the wire. This effect is sometimes called a **space charge cloud.** It is important to note that the small diame-

FIGURE 4-27 Silicon-controlled rectifier (SCR) n-p-n-p and p-n-p-n junctions.

A. Valve tube anode and cathode

B. Filament enlargement

FIGURE 4-28 Anode and cathode of a valve tube.

ter of the cathode's thin filament wire makes it extremely fragile. At the high kilovoltages supplied to x-ray tubes, a single electron striking the heated filament would cause it to break, thus rendering the tube useless. All modern x-ray machines use safety devices to prevent the anode side of the tube from

receiving electrons, even during the opposing flow of alternating current.

The anode is a relatively large metallic surface, usually a cup, disk, or flat plate, depending on the desired function of the tube. The shape of the anode varies between a valve tube and an x-ray tube and this accounts for the fact that x-ray tubes emit primarily x-ray range photons while valve tubes do not. Diagnostic x-ray tubes utilize angled disks, while dental x-ray tubes and other types of relatively low-voltage tubes use flat-plate anodes. A valve-tube anode consists of a cold metallic cup that surrounds the coiled filament (see Figure 4-28).

Valve tubes permit electrons to flow from cathode to anode when a large enough potential difference exists to cause the electrons of the thermionically emitted cloud to be simultaneously repelled from the cathode and attracted to the anode. This is done by creating a **negative charge at the cathode and a positive charge at the anode** (Figure 4-29). **Remember that electron flow will always be from cathode to anode and this means conventional electrical current will always be from anode to cathode.** It is important to note that electrons cannot move from anode to cathode due to the charges and to the shapes of the anode and cathode. The anode is shaped much larger than the cathode filament and this causes the electrons to distribute themselves over the entire surface as they follow the law of repulsion in regard to one another (see Figure 4-29). With such a large distribution surface, the electrons should not build up enough repulsion or heat to make movement from anode to cathode possible. When direct current causes the anode to remain positive at all times, there is a force of attraction working to keep the electrons on the anode. On the other hand, the cathode is relatively small and carries a negative charge at all times. The small size not only causes heating, it also restricts the flow of electrons so much that thermionic emission is enhanced. The negative charge works to encourage thermionic emission by actively repelling the electrons from the filament surface. Together these forces make the anode very attractive to electrons, while making the cathode undesirable. Consequently, as electron movement from cathode to

Electron flow

FIGURE 4-29 Electron flow through an x-ray tube.

anode is made easy, movement from anode to cathode is made extremely difficult. This creates a one-way street for electron flow, just as in a diode.

Half-Wave Rectification

In both solid-state diodes and valve tubes the forces create an electronic one-way street and effectively suppress the opposing half of the incoming current flow. A supply of alternating current to either type of rectifier will result in a pulsating direct current due to the suppression of half of the incoming wave (Figure 4-30). This type of suppression rectification is called **half-wave rectification** because only half of the incoming alternating current is being converted to pulsating direct current. The opposing half of the flow is simply ignored and not utilized. In early radiography this type of circuit was called **self-rectification** (Figure 4-31). The danger was that overheating of the anode might cause thermionic emission. This condition could result in electrons moving to the cathode filament during the half of the alternating-current cycle when the anode was negatively charged. This of

Diode

Oscilloscope

FIGURE 4-30 Half-wave rectification with one diode rectifier on the anode side of the x-ray tube circuit. Note the waveforms that would result if an oscilloscope was connected to the circuit.

FIGURE 4-31 Half-wave rectification without a diode rectifier (self-rectification).

course would break the filament and destroy the x-ray tube. In even the simplest of modern x-ray equipment the x-ray tube is protected from this occurrence by the addition of a single rectifier on the anode side of the circuit (see Figure 4-30). This protects the x-ray tube anode from receiving a negative charge. In addition, if overheating should occur, the protecting rectifier would be destroyed and could be replaced, costing much less than it would to replace the x-ray tube.

Full-Wave Rectification

It is possible to convert the opposing half of the incoming electron flow so that electrons are always moving in the same direction, instead of discarding half the cycle by suppression. This is done through an ingenious arrangement of four rectifiers in a bridge circuit called a **full-wave rectification** circuit (Figure 4-32). A full understanding of the circuit requires following the electron flow completely from the secondary coil of the high-voltage step-up transformer to the x-ray tube during both halves of the AC cycle. Figure 4-32A illustrates the electron flow by the sequence of numbered arrows.

1. Electron flow is induced from the secondary coil of the high-voltage step-up transformer.

2. Electron flow reaches the first circuit junction and flows both ways.

3. Electron flow on this path reaches the anode of valve tube II and distributes over the large, unheated surface, attempting to build up enough charge to jump to the cathode.

4. Electron flow on this path reaches the heated cathode of valve tube I and easily jumps to the anode (thus never permitting enough charge to accumulate for the electron flow at arrow 3 to jump across valve tube II).

5. Electron flow reaches the second junction and flows both ways.

6. Electron flow on this path reaches the anode of valve tube III and distributes over the large, unheated surface, attempting to build up enough charge to jump to the cathode.

7. Electron flow on this path moves without resistance toward the x-ray tube.

8. Electron flow reaches the x-ray tube heated cathode and jumps to the anode.

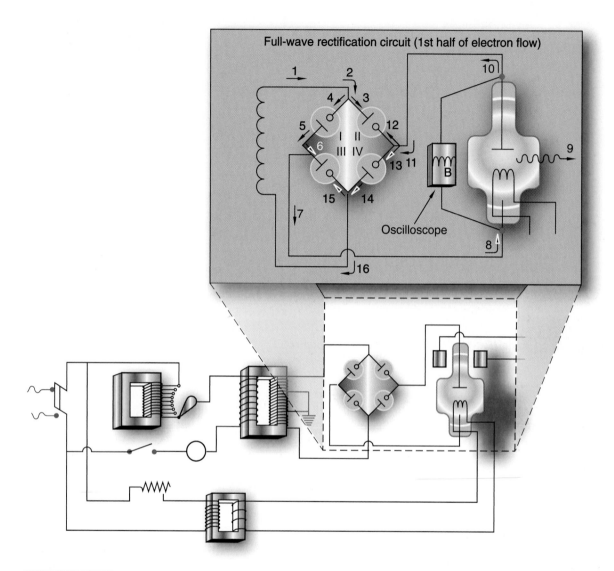

Full-wave rectification circuit (1st half of electron flow)

Oscilloscope

9. X-rays are produced as a result of the electrons striking the anode.

10. Electron flow from the anode moves without resistance back toward the rectification circuit.

11. Electron flow reaches the third junction and flows both ways.

12. Electron flow on this path reaches the heated cathode of valve tube II but cannot jump to the

anode because the anode is still loaded with the charge moving at arrow 3. Because these are like charges, they repel one another.

13. Electron flow on this path reaches the heated cathode of valve tube IV and easily jumps to the anode.

14. Electron flow reaches the fourth junction and flows both ways.

15. Electron flow on this path reaches the heated cathode of valve tube III but cannot jump to the anode because the anode is still loaded with the charge moving at arrow 6. Because these are like charges, they repel one another.

16. From this point on, electron flow on this path moves without resistance toward the secondary coil of the high-voltage step-up transformer. This completes the circuit.

Following the same logic, to trace the current path for the opposite half of the alternating current cycle

in Figure 4-32 results in reorientation of the direction of electron flow. This is full-wave rectification and it produces the sine wave shown in Figure 4-14.

Note that **the x-ray tube will emit x-ray photons during both halves of the full-wave rectified AC cycle.** The double efficiency of full-wave rectification permits a significant increase in the power output capability of radiographic equipment. This results in an ability to use higher mA and kVp settings. Consequently, nearly all modern x-ray equipment is full-wave rectified.

SUMMARY

A magnetic force field surrounds all charged particles when they are in motion. These force fields are magnetic lines of force. Electromagnets are temporary magnets produced by moving electric current. The laws governing magnetism are similar to the laws of electrostatics. Electromagnetic induction is an important phenomenon basic to nearly all electrical devices. It is produced by movement between magnetic lines of force and a conductor.

A generator is a device that converts mechanical energy to electrical energy. Either AC or DC current can be produced through the use of either slip rings or a commutator ring. One complete turn of the generator armature represents one cycle (1 Hz). A device that is supplied with electrical current to produce mechanical motion

is called a motor. Motors have essentially the same parts as generators and operate on the same principles, but in reverse. A meter may be connected in parallel to measure current or in series to measure voltage.

A transformer is used to change voltage through the use of Ohm's law. A capacitor is a device capable of accumulating and storing electrical charge. Rectification is the process by which alternating current is changed to pulsating direct current. Silicon-controlled rectifiers are solid-state semiconductors that are used for high-speed switching of the primary high-voltage x-ray circuit. Both self-wave and half-wave rectification are infrequently used in modern x-ray equipment. Diodes replaced valve tubes as one-way circuits that permit full-wave rectification.

REVIEW QUESTIONS

1. What is magnetism?

2. What is an electromagnet?

3. Explain the difference between electron flow and conventional current flow.

4. What is indicated by the direction of the thumb, index, and middle finger in one of Fleming's hand rules?

5. What are the three ways to induce electromagnetic current flow in a conductor?

6. Name the four factors controlling the strength of electromagnetically induced current.

7. What is the difference between a generator and a motor?

8. Describe the functions of slip rings and of a commutator ring.

9. How is an ammeter different from a voltmeter?

10. What is the function of a transformer?

11. State the transformer law.

12. What is the function of an autotransformer?

13. What is a diode?

14. What is rectification?

15. What components are necessary to produce a full-wave rectified circuit?

REFERENCES AND RECOMMENDED READING

Ball, J. L., & Moore, A. D. (1997). *Essential physics for radiographers* (3rd ed.). Oxford: Blackwell Scientific.

Bushberg, J. T., Seibert, J. A., Leidholdt, E. M., & Boone, J. M. (2003). *The essential physics of medical imaging.* (2nd ed.) Philadelphia: Williams & Wilkins.

Bushong, S. C. (2004). *Radiologic science for technologists: Physics, biology, and protection* (8th ed.). St. Louis, MO: Elsevier Mosby.

Carroll, Q. B. (1993). *Fuchs's radiographic exposure, processing and quality control* (5th ed.). Springfield, IL: Charles C Thomas.

Del Toro, V. (1993). *Principles of electrical engineering* (4th ed.). Englewood Cliffs, NJ: Prentice-Hall.

Dendy, P. P., & Heaton, B. (1999). *Physics for diagnostic radiology.* (2nd ed.) Institute for Physics. Bristol, England.

Gates, E. D. (1987). *Introduction to electronics: A practical approach.* Clifton Park, NY: Thomson Delmar Learning.

Glasser, O., Quimby, E. H., Taylor, L. S., Weatherwax, J. L., & Morgan, R. H. (1961). *Physical foundations of radiology* (3rd ed.). New York: Paul B. Hoeber Division of Harper & Brothers.

Graham, B. J., & Thomas, W. N. (1975). *An introduction to physics for radiologic technologists.* Philadelphia: W. B. Saunders.

Hay, G. A., & Hughes, D. (1972). *First-year physics for radiographers.* London: Bailliere Tindall.

Hendee, W. R., & Ritenour, R. (1993). *Medical imaging physics* (3rd ed.) St. Louis, MO: Elsevier Mosby.

Johns, H. E., & Cunningham, J. R. (1983). *The physics of radiology* (4th ed.). Springfield, IL: Charles C Thomas.

Nadon, J. M., Gelmine, B. J., & McLaughlin, E. D. (1989). *Industrial electricity* (4th ed.). Albany: Delmar Publishers.

Roderick, J. F., & Sutherland, B. (1952, March). A study of the static electricity problems in the x-ray darkroom. *The X-Ray Technician, 23.* 23:5, 343–348, 365.

Roller, D., & Roller, H. D. (1967). The development of the concept of electric charge: Electricity from the Greeks to Coulomb, case 8. *Harvard Case Histories in Experimental Science.* Cambridge, MA: Harvard University Press.

Wilks, R. J. (2003). *Principles of radiological physics.* (4th ed.) Edinburgh: Churchill Livingstone.

Wolbarst, A. B. (1993). *Physics of radiology.* Norwalk, CT: Appleton & Lange.

CHAPTER 5

X-Ray Equipment

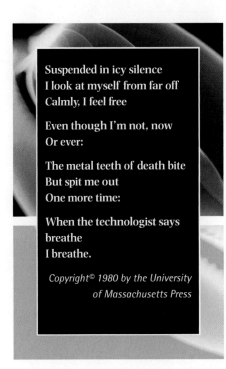

Suspended in icy silence
I look at myself from far off
Calmly, I feel free

Even though I'm not, now
Or ever:

The metal teeth of death bite
But spit me out
One more time:

When the technologist says
breathe
I breathe.

*Copyright© 1980 by the University
of Massachusetts Press*

KEY TERMS

automatic exposure
  control
automatic exposure
  device
C-arm tube
  suspension system
compression band
computed
  tomography unit
diagnostic
exposure switch
filament circuit
fixed
floor suspension
  system
floor-to-ceiling
  suspension system

footboard
handgrip
head unit
incoming-line
  current
ionization chamber
  device
main circuit
main switch
mains
mammography
  unit
milliampere-second
  timer
minimum reaction
  (or response) time
mobile system

overhead suspension
  system
panoramic dental and
  facial unit
phototimers
shoulder supports
simulator unit
single-phase power
therapeutic
three-phase 12-pulse
three-phase power
three-phase six-pulse
tilting
timer
tomography unit
urologic unit
voltage ripple

OBJECTIVES

Upon completion of this chapter, the student should be able to:

- Describe various diagnostic equipment, table, tube-support, and ancillary equipment configurations.

- State incoming line current characteristics.

- Describe the differences between single-phase and three-phase power.

- Explain the functions of the basic components of the main and filament x-ray circuits.

- Discuss the differences between single-phase, three-phase six- and twelve-pulse, and high-frequency waveforms on generator output.

- Describe the function of capacitor discharge and battery-operated mobile units.

- Explain the function of a falling load generator.

- Differentiate phototimers from ionization chamber automatic exposure controls.

- Describe the placement and function of a phototimer and an ionization chamber automatic exposure control.

- Describe potential problems that could be caused by minimum reaction times.

- Justify the use of backup time when using automatic exposure controls.

TYPES OF X-RAY EQUIPMENT

A vast number of uses for x-rays have been found in medicine and this has led to the development of a wide variety of categories and types of equipment (Figure 5-1). Medical x-ray units can be classified as **diagnostic** or **therapeutic.** Most diagnostic units are designed for specific procedures, such as general procedures, cardiac catheterization, head procedures, fluoroscopy, etc. All of these units operate within the diagnostic x-ray range. This range is approximately $10-1,200$ milliamperes (mA), $0.001-10$ seconds, at a peak kilovoltage (kVp) of approximately 25 to 150.

Tables

The radiographic table is designed to support the patient in a position that will enhance radiographic examination. As any patient can attest, comfort is not the primary purpose of the table, although some institutions permit foam pads for lengthy examinations.

The tabletop must be uniformly radiolucent to easily permit x-rays to pass through. A Bakelite or similar surface is most common, although specialized applications, such as angiography, may use a carbon graphite fiber to reduce absorption of photons. Although flat tops are most common, curved tops are available. Curved (or dished) tops are usually used for fluoroscopic examinations. They are usually more comfortable for the patient and permit the body part to be placed slightly closer to the image receptor for a more accurate image. Curved tops have two serious disadvantages. It is difficult for the radiographer to maintain a patient accurately in an oblique or lateral position on a curved top, and the top is entirely useless as a level support surface for a film cassette during tabletop radiography.

FIGURE 5-1 A typical diagnostic radiographic and fluoroscope room. *(Courtesy of Philips Medical Systems)*

The tabletop must be **easily cleaned, hard to scratch, and without crevices where radiographic contrast media can accumulate.** It is sometimes necessary to remove body fluids after an examination, and this must be possible to achieve in a quick and sanitary manner.

The table must **include space for a tray to hold cassettes and a radiographic grid.** The tray is often called a "Bucky tray" in honor of Dr. Gustav

Bucky (1880–1963), the inventor of the radiographic grid that is installed over the cassette tray. The grid installation usually consists of a mechanism that will automatically move the grid during exposure. Many units include automatic exposure control sensors in the tray. Some tables use a stationary tray with a movable tabletop. Others use a tray that is movable along rails extending the length of the table with a stationary tabletop. Still others use a tray and top that are both partially movable. Some tabletops are motor driven and movable along their length. Others are floating tops which can be moved along their length and width simultaneously when an electromagnetic brake is released. The brake may be controlled by hand, knee, or foot. Floating tops save radiographers significant amounts of time and effort, especially when positioning large patients.

Tables are available in **fixed** and **tilting** models. Fixed tables do not permit tilting the patient's head or feet down. They are designed for diagnostic radiographic work only. Tilting tables are sometimes described by their tilting capability (for example, 90–15 would indicate a table capable of tilting 90° in one direction and 15° in the other). Rooms designed to perform both diagnostic radiographic and fluoroscopic (R&F) examinations are equipped with tilting tables, although some rooms designed only for radiographic examinations may also use them.

The table is usually at a height that reduces physical strain on the radiographer, who must stretch and bend over and around the table as the patient, ancillary equipment, cassette, and x-ray tube are positioned. This is usually 30–40 inches or 75–100 cm from the floor. This is not a safe or convenient height for patients and it causes problems for ambulatory patients who are not in good physical condition. A primary concern for all radiographers must be proper assistance to these patients when they are getting onto and down from the table. Fixed tables are available in adjustable models that can be lowered while a patient is assisted onto the table and then raised to a working height.

Ancillary equipment for tilting tables includes a **footboard** for patients to stand on when the table is upright. The footboard is often used for gastrointestinal studies when the patient begins the examination in an erect position and is then brought horizontal during the procedure, or vice versa. In these instances it is critical to ascertain that the footboard is securely in place and will support the full weight of the patient. This is best done when the table is horizontal by pulling hard on the footboard. Procedures requiring tilting the patient's head down, such as myelography, may require the use of **shoulder supports** to keep patients from sliding off the table. In these instances, **handgrips** give the patient an added feeling of security.

Compression bands serve two functions: they restrain patients who are unable to cooperate, and they compress abdominal tissue for a more uniform subject density. Both functions improve radiographic image quality. A compression band should never be used as the sole restraint device.

Tube Supports

The tube support system is designed to permit the x-ray tube to be manipulated to the various locations necessary to obtain examination procedure projections and to hold the tube immobile during the exposure. Tube suspension systems are available in numerous configurations such as: *overhead, floor-to-ceiling, floor, mobile,* and *C-arm.* Both flexibility and cost are reflected in this order, with overhead supports being the most flexible and costly.

The **overhead suspension system,** sometimes called ceiling suspension, allows controls of longitudinal and transverse positioning as well as vertical distance.

Each of these complex motions is locked into place by a solenoid with a control placed where it can be easily reached by the radiographer. Also included in the control mechanisms are "detents," or centering locks, to verify common tube positions (for example, centered to the cassette in the Bucky tray or at a routine distance from the table or upright Bucky unit). Unfortunately, each manufacturer uses a different placement and labeling for these controls. For this reason, it is helpful to practice manipulating the controls prior to using the equipment to perform radiographic procedures.

The **floor-to-ceiling suspension system** uses a pair of rails, one on the ceiling and one on the floor, for longitudinal positioning. Rooms with extremely high ceilings may use an overhead rail suspended from a wall.

FIGURE 5-2 A C-arm tube suspension system.

FIGURE 5-3 An upright Bucky unit.

A **floor suspension system** uses a tube-support column mounted on the floor. The system must be carefully counterbalanced to avoid tipping. This is usually accomplished by adding a counterweight to the back of the telescoping tube arm and requires that both tube system and table be installed further from the back wall than other systems.

There are many types of **mobile systems** as well. The tube suspension systems for mobile units vary tremendously but most are based on the floor suspension system.

A **C-arm tube suspension system** utilizes a C-shaped arm to support the tube and image receptor (Figure 5–2). The tube and image receptor are fixed to opposite ends of the C-arm. When the clamp or lock holding the C-arm in position is released, it permits both tube and image receptor to be rotated to a new position. C-arms (or U-arms) are used in head units, mobile fluoroscopy units, and ceiling-suspended angiography and surgical units.

Upright Units

An upright cassette holder or Bucky unit is a common and useful ancillary piece of equipment in any radiographic room (Figure 5-3). Chest radiography should routinely be done in an upright position and there are numerous other procedures that are best done upright (for example, acromioclavicular joints, abdominal obstructive procedures, cervical spine, etc.). Upright cassette holders may or may not include a radiographic grid. Upright Bucky units may include the same equipment as the Bucky tray located in a table (movable radiographic grid, cassette tray and automatic exposure control sensors).

Other Specialized Diagnostic Equipment

Other types of equipment have been developed to meet specialized needs. They include chest units designed to automate chest radiography by combining an upright Bucky unit with an automatic film handling mechanism, **mammography units** for breast studies, **tomography units** with tubes that move in an arc during exposure, **head units** for cranial stud-

FIGURE 5-4   Three-phase, 60 Hz, 240 V incoming-line current.

FIGURE 5-5   Single-phase power: (A) incoming line; (b) full-wave rectified.

ies, **panoramic dental and facial units** for combined tomography of facial structures, **computed tomography units** for computerized sectional images, radiation therapy **simulator units** to verify radiation therapy treatment set-ups prior to actual treatment, **urologic units** to facilitate urological and genital studies, and units custom built to nearly any specifications.

POWER FOR X-RAY GENERATION

A diagnostic x-ray generator is composed of numerous basic electrical devices. An x-ray circuit is established when these devices are connected in a sequence capable of accelerating electrons to the speed necessary to cause the production of x-ray photons within an x-ray tube. The incoming line power may be modified in several ways to establish these conditions.

Incoming Line Current

Electricity is usually supplied to buildings in the United States by 60 Hz alternating current with a nominal rms of 200–240 volts. These are termed nominal because, as users operate various resistances, the voltages constantly fluctuate, as illus-

trated by Ohm's law. This power is called the **incoming-line current** (sometimes called the **mains**) and is supplied in the form of a three-phase power cycle (Figure 5-4). One of the "hot" wires is always half the incoming voltage above-ground potential, while the other is always the same voltage below-ground potential. In the United States each carries 110–120 volts. With 60 Hz alternating current, the two hot wires reverse their polarity 120 times per second. Bringing incoming line current from the neutral (or ground) wire and one of the hot wires produces a potential difference of 110–120 volts. Because the two lines are not in phase with one another, using incoming current from both hot wires produces a potential difference that is less than the sum of the two single phases. The usual result is about 210 volts. Nearly all x-ray equipment operates from an incoming line of 210–220 volts.

Single-Phase Power

Single-phase power permits the potential difference to drop to zero with every change in the direction of current flow (Figure 5-5A) and is represented by the symbol 1ɸ. In a full-wave rectified circuit (direct pulsating current), this means

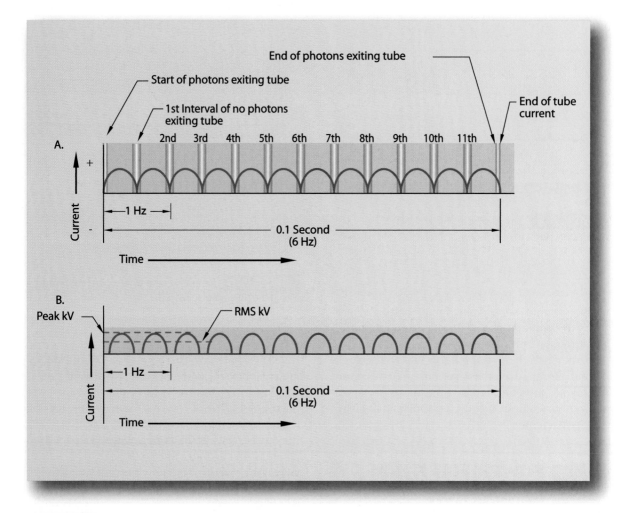

End of photons exiting tube

Start of photons exiting tube

1st Interval of no photons exiting tube

2nd 3rd 4th 5th 6th 7th 8th 9th 10th 11th

End of tube current

A.

Current

+

−

1 Hz

0.1 Second (6 Hz)

Time

B.

Peak kV

RMS kV

Current

1 Hz

0.1 Second (6 Hz)

Time

FIGURE 5-6 The difference between the photons produced inside the x-ray tube during an exposure and the photons emitted from the tube during the same exposure. (A) X-ray production during an exposure of 0.1 second with a 1ɸ full-wave rectified unit. (B) Emission of photons from an x-ray tube during an exposure of 0.1 second with a 1ɸ full-wave rectified circuit.

the x-ray tube is experiencing no potential difference and is producing no x-ray photons 120 times each second on a 60 Hz line (see Figure 5-5B). With the 60 Hz line, an exposure of 0.1 second with a single-phase full-wave rectified unit results in twelve intervals of no photon production (Figure 5-6). In addition, the photons produced during the low-voltage periods are of such low energy that they may not exit the tube, or they do not contribute to the radiographic image because they are absorbed before reaching the image receptor. The

root mean square (rms) voltage of a single-phase sinusoidal wave is usually given as 70.7 percent of the peak voltage.

EXAMPLE: What is the approximate rms voltage of a single-phase sine wave with a peak of 80 kVp?

Answer:

rms voltage = 70.7% peak kVp
rms voltage = 70.7% x 80 kVp
rms voltage = 56.6 kVp

FIGURE 5-7 (A) Three-phase incoming-line current. (B) Full-wave rectified three-phase current.

Obviously this is not as efficient as desired. A solution is to combine several waveforms of current slightly out of step with one another to create **three-phase power.**

Three-Phase Power

Three-phase power is produced by the generator and is the common form in which power is supplied to users by power companies. Three-phase power is generated as is shown in Chapter 4 by Figure 4-16 and is represented by the symbol 3ϕ. As each wave peak begins to drop toward zero, the overall potential difference is boosted back to peak by the next phase wave. The result is that the sum of the phasing never drops to zero (Figure 5-7A). When full-wave rectification is applied, the net voltage produces a **voltage ripple.** Three-phase current produces a voltage ripple of 3 pulses per half cycle,

which is 6 pulses per Hz and 360 pulses per second. (see Figure 5-10.)

Whenever any of the phases is at zero, the other two phases are of equally opposite values so that the sum of the three currents is always zero. This fact is used in connecting the generator windings to combine the current.

 A BASIC X-RAY CIRCUIT

The basic x-ray circuit can be divided into the **main** and **filament circuits. The main circuit supplies the x-ray tube with properly modified power.** Its purpose is to produce x-rays. **The filament circuit supplies the filament of the x-ray tube with properly modified power.** Its purpose is to create the appropriate thermionically emitted electron cloud at the filament. These two circuits are distinct from each other although they are interconnected (Figure 5-8).

The Main X-Ray Circuit

The main x-ray circuit modifies the incoming-line power to produce x-rays by a sequence of devices, as shown in Figure 5-9. The circuit must boost the voltage to the range necessary to produce x-rays and to permit the radiographer to adjust the amperage, voltage, and length of exposure, as well as incorporate appropriate circuitry to increase the efficiency of x-ray production.

The **main switch** and circuit breakers are usually enclosed in an electrical power box. The **exposure switch** is simply a remote control switch that permits current to flow through the circuit. Diagnostic x-ray control exposure switches are designed to begin but not end exposures. The **timer** circuit is intended to end the exposure at an accurately measured, preset time. For this reason, whenever the exposure switch is depressed it must be held until both the audible and visible indicators (usually a buzzer and a light) have ceased. For example, if a radiographer is accustomed to making short exposures of less than 0.5 second, failure to hold the exposure switch for a 2.5-second exposure of a large abdomen would prematurely terminate the exposure.

Incoming line current

Main circuit

Filament circuit

FIGURE 5-8 Main and filament circuits.

The Exposure Switch

The exposure switch can be connected to the switch that activates the rotating anode of the x-ray tube. The anode must be turning at a sufficiently high speed to avoid melting of the target area by the high kilovoltage exposure. To avoid the possibility of error, all x-ray units that utilize rotating anodes have circuitry that prevents an exposure until the anode is turning at the correct speed. It is usually convenient to combine the anode rotor and the exposure switch in a two-step button. Therefore, most exposure switches are depressed halfway to activate the anode rotation and then depressed completely to initiate the x-ray exposure. Tube manufacturers recommend that these buttons be depressed completely in one motion. This helps to extend the life of the x-ray tube.

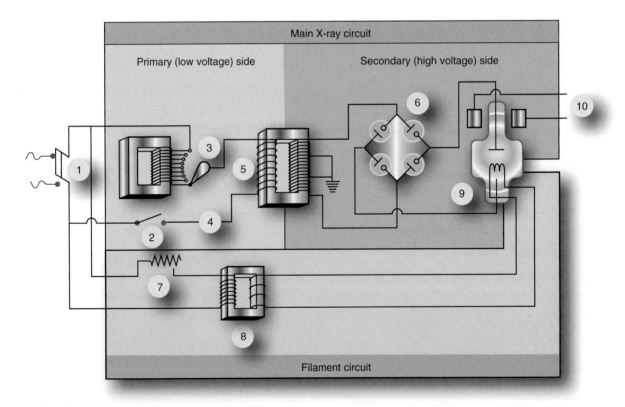

FIGURE 5-9 The complete basic x-ray circuit: (1) main breaker; (2) exposure switch; (3) autotransformer; (4) timer circuit; (5) high-voltage step-up transformer; (6) four-diode rectification circuit; (7) filament circuit variable resistance; (8) filament step-down transformer; (9) x-ray tube; and (10) rotor stator.

The exposure switch must be attached to the control console in such a manner that it is impossible for the operator to be exposed. In addition, the equipment must be designed to prohibit the x-ray tube from being manipulated into a position where it could expose the user. On mobile equipment the switch must be on a cord with a minimum length of 6 feet. This is to permit the radiographer to move as far as possible from the x-ray tube during an exposure. All exposure switches must be of the "dead-man" type, in which x-ray exposure may occur only while the switch is depressed. Release of the switch must terminate the exposure. This prevents the exposure from continuing when the operator enters the radiation area.

The Timer Circuit

Electronic timers are the most common timers in use today. They are capable of accurate exposures as short as 0.001 second with only a 1 msec delay. Most electronic timers operate by charging a silicon-controlled rectifier (SCR), which then triggers the exposure. It is linked with a microprocessor that calculates the length of time the current will need to reach a trigger value. This level is set by the variation of the timer controls on the console unit by the radiographer.

Milliampere-Second Timers. Milliampere-second timers are used in falling load generators as well as some capacitor discharge units. They monitor the product of mA and time on the secondary side of the high-voltage step-up transformer. When the desired mAs level is reached, these timers interrupt the circuit to stop the exposure. Because the high-voltage capacitor, timer, and x-ray tube are operating on the same circuit, mAs value remains constant even when there is a slight fluctuation in the capacitor charging current.

Automatic Exposure Control Timers. Automatic exposure controls or automatic exposure devices are also used, as described later in this chapter. The autotransformer, with its taps controlled by the kVp selectors on the control console, modifies the incoming-line voltage in anticipation of the kilovoltage that will be produced by the step-up transformer. Some units divide the kVp adjustments into major and minor regions. Usually a major adjustment will change in units of 10 kVp, while minor adjustments will change in units of 1 or 2 kVp.

The Filament Circuit

The filament circuit modifies the incoming-line power to produce the thermionic emission from the filament wire of the x-ray tube by a sequence of devices (see Figure 5-9). The incoming line must be modified to about 3–5 amperes and 6–12 volts. The filament circuit's supply is drawn directly from the main circuit's supply. Current control devices regulate the amperage supplied to the filament in the x-ray tube. This control device can be adjusted by the radiographer at the control console. It is not labeled by the actual amperage it controls. Instead it is marked in increments representative of the mA that will be available at the filament when the high-voltage supply is released at exposure. Filament circuits are usually adjustable to the equivalent of mA ratings of 50, 100, 200, 300, 400, 500, 600, 800, 1,000, and 1,200. Not all equipment will have all mA settings and some may have other unusual settings, as discussed in the section on timers. Most 1ϕ units do not go beyond 500 mA. Specialized tomographic equipment generators may also include 10, 15, 20, 25, 30, and 40 mA stations.

Many units include a meter at this point to provide an accurate reading of the amperage delivered. After regulation, the current is then sent to a step-down transformer that modifies it to the appropriate amperage that will reach the filament itself. A very slight shift in the quantity of electrons in the thermionic cloud around the filament can have a dramatic effect on the quantity of x-ray photons produced when the kilovoltage exposure occurs. Therefore, filament circuits also incorporate several types of current stabilization devices, including frequency compensators, voltage stabilizers and space charge compensators.

The main and filament circuits are combined to form the complete basic x-ray circuit (see Figure 5-9). The radiographer adjusts the various factors from a control console, which must be located in a radiation-shielded location outside the radiographic exposure room. **All of the radiographer-operated controls are located on the low-voltage side of the circuit to protect operators from high-voltage shock hazards.** The controls that are likely to be located on this console are included in Table 5-1.

TABLE 5-1. Common Diagnostic X-Ray Console Controls

Control	Factor	Electrical Device and Location in Circuit
kVp selection	kVp level	Autotransformer (between incoming line and exposure switch)
mA selection	Filament current	Variable resistor (in filament circuit between incoming line and step-down transformer)
Time selection	Length of exposure	Timer circuit (between exposure switch and step-up transformer)
Rotor switch	Speed of rotating anode	Stator (separate circuit from stator of anode motor)
Exposure switch	Moment of exposure	Switch (between autotransformer and timer circuit)

GENERATORS

Single-Phase Generators

Single-phase generators with full-wave rectification produce a voltage ripple of 2 pulses per Hertz or 120 pulses per second. This produces two usable pulses per cycle (1φ 2P waveform) with a ripple of 100 percent. This means the voltage in the tube drops to 0 twice per period or cycle. These relationships are shown in Figure 5-10.

Three-Phase Generators

When full-wave rectification is applied to 3φ current, it produces a voltage ripple of 6 pulses per hertz or 360 pulses per second. This produces six usable pulses per cycle, which is known as a **three-phase, six-pulse** (3φ 6P) waveform. Three-phase, six-pulse power produces a ripple of 13–25 percent. This means the voltage in the x-ray tube never falls below 75–87 percent of the peak kilovoltage setting on the console. These relationships are shown in Figure 5-10. **A full-wave rectified, three-phase, six-pulse waveform produces approximately 35 percent more average photon energy than full-wave rectified, single phase.** This will be-

come an important point to remember when setting technical factors.

Equipment is also available with a **three-phase, 12-pulse** waveform. This is accomplished by a complicated combination of 12 diodes. When full-wave rectified, this configuration produces a voltage ripple of 4–10 percent, with tube voltage never dropping below 90–96 percent of the peak kilovoltage setting. These relationships are shown in Figure 5-10. **A full-wave rectified, three-phase, 12-pulse waveform produces approximately 40 percent more average photon energy than full-wave rectified, single-phase.** This is also an important point to remember when setting technical factors. Voltage ripple varies as higher voltage loads are applied; the percentage figures given are approximations under average loads.

Generator power ratings are determined by the greatest load the generator is capable of sending to the x-ray tube. Power is calculated as voltage times amperage. The unit of power is the watt, so V × A = W. This formula applies to a 3φ generator. Because 1φ generators have a lower average photon emission energy, the formula must be corrected by using a constant. For a 1φ generator the power rating formula is V × A × 0.7 = W. Since x-ray generators operate in the kilovoltage and milliamperage range, their power ratings are stated in kilowatts.

FIGURE 5-10   The relationships between (A) relative value radiation output and approximate ripple; (B) tube kVp and approximate ripple; and (C) tube average mA. Each relationship is shown for one cycle of 1ϕ 2P, 3ϕ 6P, 3ϕ 12P, and high-frequency generator configurations.

EXAMPLE: What is the power rating for a 3ϕ generator capable of delivering 150 kVp at 1,000 mA to the tube?

Answer:

$$V \times A = W$$
$$150 \text{ kV} \times 1,000 \text{ mA} = W$$
$$150,000 \text{ V} \times 1.0 \text{ A} = 150,000 \text{ W}$$
$$= 150 \text{ kW}$$

EXAMPLE: What is the power rating for a 1ϕ generator capable of delivering 120 kVp at 300 mA to the tube?

Answer:

$$V \times A \times 0.7 = W$$
$$120 \text{ kV} \times 300 \text{ mA} \times .07 = W$$
$$120,000 \text{ V} \times 0.3 \text{ A} \times 0.7 = 25,200 \text{ W}$$
$$= 25.2 \text{ kW}$$

These ratings serve as a guideline for comparing the capability of various generators. Generator power often varies as kilovoltage changes so a high-power generator at 150 kVp may not be as powerful when the kVp is lowered into the middle diagnostic range.

High Frequency

High-frequency generators use AC and DC power converters to change the incoming-line voltage frequency from 60 Hz to the 6,000 Hz range (Figure 5-11A). When a high-frequency current is supplied with full-wave rectified power, a 12–13 kHz waveform can be produced. An oscillator or invertor unit controls the pulses sent through the circuit, sending them at a much higher frequency (closer together), as shown in Figure 5-11B. When this wave is applied to the x-ray tube, the peak kilovoltage is achieved in about 10 percent of the time necessary for 3ϕ generators and with only 3–4 percent voltage ripple. Figure 5-10 illustrates the complex conversions used in a high-frequency generator to create the various waveforms prior to achieving the final multipulsed radiation beam. Full-wave rectified high-frequency generator ripple ranges from 4–15 percent, depending on the total load, which is comparable to 3ϕ 12P generators. These relationships are shown in Figure 5-10. Because of the higher-frequency current, transformers for these units are significantly smaller.

Capacitor Discharge Mobile Units

It is also possible to operate an x-ray tube with the power generated from the discharge of a high-voltage capacitor. The capacitor operates exactly as explained in Chapter 4 but in the kilovoltage range necessary to produce x-rays. In these units, depression of a charge button causes the rectification circuit to charge a capacitor instead of the x-ray tube. A signal indicates readiness when the capacitor fills to the appropriate level, and depression of the exposure switch triggers a discharge to the x-ray tube.

The disadvantage of a capacitor discharge unit is that the capacitor may continue to discharge after the usable exposure. Figure 5-12A shows the charging curve, the exposure period, and the discharging curve. Exposure begins at the peak voltage and then decreases (see Figure 5-12B). This is sometimes called wavetail cutoff. **Capacitor discharge units provide an rms voltage significantly lower than the peak voltage.** The ending kV is approximately 1 kV per mAs lower than the initial kVp. Therefore, the rms voltage is about 0.5 kV/mAs lower than the initial kVp. Because capacitors discharge more slowly as potential difference decreases, considerable residual kV may exist after the desired exposure time. This can create a leakage of radiation, although several devices help avoid the problem. Grid-biased x-ray tubes can be used to cut the photon emission at a set time by reversing the charge polarity of a wire grid in front of the filament. Additionally, the tube collimator can be designed to automatically close its lead shutters after the desired exposure, thus stopping radiation leakage.

Capacitor discharge units are most commonly used for mobile equipment. The capacitor circuit is supplied from batteries which are charged from line current. This permits the unit to be mobile without having to be plugged into a wall outlet. Instead, the batteries can be recharged periodically when the unit is parked.

FIGURE 5-11 High–frequency waveforms; (A and B) Conversion of 1ϕ 2P to 3ϕ 6P to high frequency; (C and D) comparison of time interval necessary to reach peak kV on 3ϕ 6P and high-frequency generators. *(Courtesy of Siemens Medical Solutions USA, Inc.)*

Battery-Operated Mobile Units

Mobile units are also available that operate on nickel-cadmium (NiCd) battery-supplied AC current. The batteries supply nonpulsating direct current to a rotary converter, which provides current similar to 3ϕ 12P or even greater frequencies. Compared to capacitor discharge machines, these units have the obvious advantage of 3ϕ exposure consistency, higher rms voltage, and no leakage possibility. They also have all the advantages of mobility, with recharging capabilities, and for these reasons they have become extremely popular.

Falling Load Generators

Falling load generators usually are specially designed 3ϕ or high-frequency generators. They take full advantage of the current loading capability of the x-ray tube by beginning the exposure with a high amperage and then allowing it to fall during the exposure. This can be accomplished with a constant potential generator. It requires that both the mA and the kV be regulated independently.

Falling load generators are a solution to this problem as they permit greater use of the acceptable tube limits. They do so without requiring a

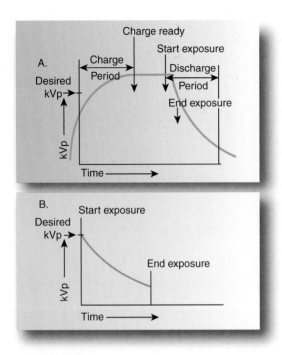

FIGURE 5-12 (A) Capacitor discharge unit waveform; (B) wavetail cutoff.

by comparing the falling load of the 240 mAs example with a constant-potential load for the same mAs. In actual practice a margin of error is allowed for the tube loading. Most falling load generators will step down the mA at 70–80 percent of the tube loading capacity. This feature has a disadvantage in that constant-potential generators may actually make better use of tube loading capacity on very short exposures, where they may use 80–90 percent of the tube loading capacity.

Falling load generators begin exposures at the highest possible mA. This removes control of the mA from the radiographer, and there are instances when this is undesirable. For example, some examinations, such as those for the lateral thoracic vertebra (spine) and sternum, require a "breathing technique" in which low mA and long-time exposures are used to blur superimposing structures from the image. Unless falling load consoles are equipped with special controls (often as tomographic options) to permit starting exposures at low mA, these examinations cannot be performed correctly.

There are several factors that should be understood before using falling load generators. Because they function with an mA that is unknown to the operator, it is impossible for the operator to set the correct time to achieve the desired mAs. Therefore, falling load generators must be used with automatic exposure controls, or rely on an mAs timer, instead of independent mA and time controls. The kVp across the tube varies for a brief moment as the mA is adjusted. This is an Ohm's law effect during the continuous mA reductions and results in a slightly lower average kVp. Falling load generators can shorten x-ray tube life considerably as they use higher mA settings, thus causing the filament to wear out more quickly. The advantages of falling load generators are shorter times in heavy-load situations, and simpler operation.

When comparing the various types of generators it is most important to evaluate the radiation output from the tube as this is the factor that influences both patient exposure and image quality. Figure 5-10 assists in this process by illustrating the various transformations that occur in the x-ray tube milliamperage and kilovoltage as well as the all-important relative value of radiation output.

higher-power (and more expensive) generator that would permit higher mA loading. For example, in Figure 5-13, a constant potential generator exposure of 240 mAs is compared to the same falling load exposure. A falling load generator permits the same tube to achieve 240 mAs in 0.5 second. This is accomplished by beginning the exposure at 600 mA for the first 0.1 second. At this time the 600 mA tube limit is reached and the generator is programmed to automatically reduce the mA to 500 until the tube limit is again reached (0.2 second later, or 0.3 second from exposure start). Once again the generator reduces the mA to 400 until the limit is reached (0.2 second later, or 0.5 second from exposure start). This produces 240 total mAs.

A falling load generator utilizes the tube's loading potential to a much greater extent than the constant-potential generator. This is made evident

FIGURE 5-13   Falling load generator versus constant-potential tube limit curve. In the example shown, the mAs is calculated as follows:

mA	Time in sec	mAs achieved
600	0.1	60
500	0.2	100
400	0.2	80
Total	0.5	240

AUTOMATIC EXPOSURE CONTROLS

All automatic exposure controls do exactly what their name indicates; they are programmed to terminate the radiographic exposure time. It is important to remember that automatic exposure controls do not control any factor except time. Milliampere-seconds and kVp remain under the control of the radiographer in all but falling load generators. Even falling load units leave the kVp under the radiographer's control.

There are two types of automatic exposure controls: **phototimers** and **ionization chamber devices. The term phototimer is often used to refer to all automatic exposure controls.** They are also referred to as automatic exposure devices, and the acronyms AEC and AED occasionally appear in professional literature. Actually, phototimers are seldom utilized in modern radiography. Most of the devices that are called phototimers today consist of ionization chambers.

All automatic exposure controls function by measuring a preset quantity of radiation and breaking the timer circuit when a dose sufficient to produce the desired exposure has been reached.

Phototimers

Old-fashioned phototimer devices used a thyratron to regulate exposure automatically. The x-ray beam would pass through the patient, tabletop, and cassette before it struck a fluorescent screen that had the ability to absorb the x-rays and produce light photons. The light photons were then directed toward a photomultiplier tube. A photomultiplier tube had the ability to produce multiple electrons from each light photon. The electrons then established a charge on the capacitor. When the capacitor reached its preset value, it discharged, triggering a thyratron and opening the relay to terminate the exposure. Phototimers were calibrated by setting the capacitor-discharge point (usually controlled by a set screw in the electronics cabinet) at a level that produced a satisfactory exposure to the image receptor.

This was done by a trial-and-error procedure with a radiographic phantom. Radiographs were exposed at various combinations of kVp, time, and mAs until a satisfactory diagnostic quality image was consistently obtained.

Ionization Chambers

Ionization chamber automatic exposure control is quite different (Figure 5-14). The x-ray beam passes through the patient and tabletop before striking the ionization chamber. Unlike with the old photo-

FIGURE 5-14 Ionization chamber AEC circuit.

timers, the image receptor is positioned under the ion chamber. Until the development of a thin, parallel-plate ionization chamber, it was impossible to locate the chamber in this position because it would cast an objectionable shadow artifact on the film. Because thin, parallel-plate chambers are only about 5 mm in thickness, this is not a problem (Figure 5-15). It is critical that the exact size, shape and position of the ionization chamber be known to the radiographer.

Minimum Reaction Time

All automatic exposure controls have a **minimum reaction (or response) time,** which is determined by the length of time necessary for the AEC to respond to the radiation and for the generator to terminate the exposure. This delay is caused primarily by the turn-off delay in the high-voltage circuits. Old phototimers had a minimum reaction time of 0.05 second or less. Modern ionization chambers with SCRs may have a minimum reaction time of less than 0.001 second. Automatic exposure controls are sometimes incapable of terminating exposures quickly enough, especially with extremely high-speed films and intensifying screens during high kVp chest radiography. In this instance, radiographic technology has outstripped itself and either a manual time or a slower film and screen combination must be used, although some manufacturers use an exposure-monitoring circuit to terminate low dose rate exposures quickly.

FIGURE 5-15 Parallel-plate ionization chamber AEC. *(Courtesy of Siemens Medical Solutions USA)*

Backup Time

Nearly all automatic exposure equipped units permit (and may have electronic interlocks that require) a manual backup time to be set. There are numerous reasons why an automatic exposure control may be improperly set. For example, if one forgets to activate the AEC in a wall unit, this may leave an AEC in a table unit waiting for exposure by a tube that is directed toward the wall (and through a patient). Because the wall AEC is not receiving any radiation dose, the exposure would not cease until the tube overload protector activated. Not only is this an ex-

pensive waste of tube life, but the radiographer error causing excessive radiation dose to the patient is completely unwarranted. The fact that the image would be overexposed, requiring it to be repeated, adding to the patient's dose again, simply makes matters worse. **Backup times cannot exceed the tube limit and should be set at 150 percent of the anticipated manual exposure mAs.** According to U.S. Public Law 90–602, generators must terminate the exposure at 600 mAs for exposures above 50 kVp and 2,000 mAs for exposures below 50 kVp (primarily during mammography).

SUMMARY

Medical x-ray units can be classified as diagnostic or therapeutic. Diagnostic units operate within a range of 10–1,200 milliamperes (mA), 0.001–10 seconds, and at a peak kilovoltage (kVp) of approximately 25–150.

Radiographic equipment includes a wide variety of units with different tube stand configurations, including ceiling suspension, floor-to-ceiling, floor mounted and C-arms. Nearly all x-ray equipment operates from an incoming line of 210–220 volts, which is then used for single-phase or three-phase power.

The basic x-ray circuit can be divided into the main and filament circuits. The main circuit supplies the x-ray tube with properly modified power, while the filament circuit supplies the filament of the x-ray tube with properly modified power. The basic circuit includes the exposure

switch, timer, high-voltage step-up transformer, and rectifier circuit.

Although waveforms differ depending on incoming line and rectification, differences occur in both voltage ripple and the interval between initiation of the exposure and the peak kilovoltage.

Generator power ratings are determined by the greatest load the generator is capable of sending to the x-ray tube. Power is expressed in watts and varies by incoming-line current and rectification. Falling load generators permit more effective use of the tube loading capacity but eliminate mA and time settings from consideration.

Although often called phototimers, automatic exposure controls (AECs) today are almost always ionization chambers. When using an AEC, problems may be avoided by considering the minimum reaction time and the backup time.

REVIEW QUESTIONS

1. Name three types of diagnostic radiographic tube-support systems.
2. What are the two types of incoming-line current?
3. How many pulses are there per Hz for 1φ and 3φ power?
4. What device in the x-ray circuit controls kVp? mA? time? rectification?
5. What is the approximate voltage ripple for 1φ 2P equipment? 3φ 6P? 3φ 12P?
6. What happens to the tube mA during an exposure using a falling load generator?
7. What is the difference between an ionization chamber and a phototimer?
8. What factor determines the minimum reaction time?

REFERENCES AND RECOMMENDED READING

Ball, J., & Price, T. (1989). *Chesneys' radiographic imaging.* Oxford: Blackwell Scientific.

Braun, M. (1976). Considerations on the falling load principle. *Optical Engineering, 15*(4), 338–343.

Curry, T. S., Dowdey, J. E., & Murry, R. C. (1990). *Christensen's introduction to the physics of diagnostic radiology* (4th ed.). Philadelphia: Lea and Febiger.

Evans, S. A., Harris, L., Lawinski, C. P., & Hendra I. R. F. (1985). Mobile x-ray generators: A review. *Radiography, 51*(595), 89.

Gray, J. E., Winkler, N. T., Stears, J., & Frank, E. D. (1983). *Quality control in diagnostic imaging.* Baltimore: University Park Press.

Morgan, J. A. (1968). The development and application of multi-phase x-rays in medical radiography. *Radiologic Technology, 40*(2), 57.

Morgan, R. H. (1943). The automatic control of exposure in photofluorography. *Public Health Reports, 58*(42), 1533–1541.

Nadon, J. M., Gelmine, B. J., & McLaughlin, E. D. (1989). *Industrial electricity* (4th ed.). Clifton Park, NY: Thomson Delmar Learning.

Seeram, E. (1985). *X-Ray imaging equipment.* Springfield, IL: Charles C Thomas.

Selman, J. (2000). The *fundamentals of imaging physics and radiobiology for the radiologic technologist.* (9th ed.). Springfield, IL: Charles C Thomas.

Sobol, W. T. (2002). High frequency x-ray generator basics. *Medical Physics, 29*(2), 132–44.

Stears, J. G., Gray, J. E., Webbles, W. E., & Frank, E. D. (1988). Radiologic exchange (automatic exposure control function). *Radiologic Technology, 59*(6), 521–522.

Sterling, S. (1988). Automatic exposure control: A primer. *Radiologic Technology, 59*(5), 421–427.

Thornburn, D. S. *Physical characteristics of falling load generators.* Shelton, CT: Philips Medical Systems, Inc.

Weigl, W. (1989). A new high-frequency controlled x-ray generator system with multi-pulse wave shape. *Journal for Radiological Engineering, 1*(1), 7–19.

Weigl, W. (1988). *Design of falling load generators.* Unpublished paper presented at American Association of Physicists in Medicine seminar.

Wilks, R. J. (2003). *Principles of radiological physics* (4th ed.). Edinburgh: Churchill Livingstone.

Wolbarst, A. B. (1993). *Physics of radiology.* Norwalk, CT: Appleton & Lange.

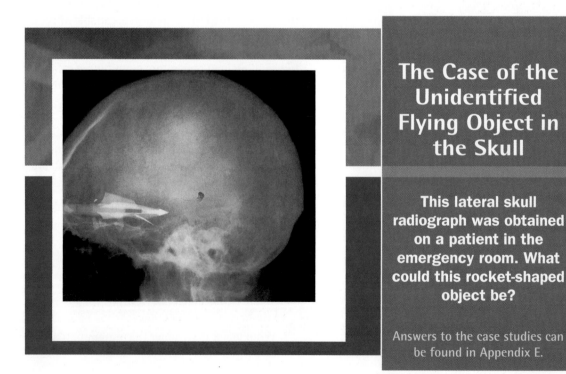

The Case of the Unidentified Flying Object in the Skull

This lateral skull radiograph was obtained on a patient in the emergency room. What could this rocket-shaped object be?

Answers to the case studies can be found in Appendix E.

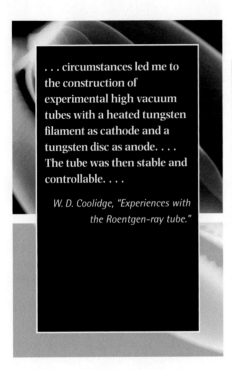

CHAPTER 6

The X-Ray Tube

> . . . circumstances led me to the construction of experimental high vacuum tubes with a heated tungsten filament as cathode and a tungsten disc as anode. . . . The tube was then stable and controllable. . . .
>
> *W. D. Coolidge, "Experiences with the Roentgen-ray tube."*

KEY TERMS

actual focal spot
anode
anode assembly
anode cooling chart
anode heel effect
cathode
cathode assembly
dual focus
effective focal spot
envelope
extrafocal radiation
filament
focal point

focal spot
focal track
focus
focusing cup
fractional focal spot
grid–biased
grid–controlled
grid–pulsed
housing cooling chart
leakage radiation
line-focus principle
off-focus radiation
protective housing

radiographic tube
  rating chart
rotating anode
rotor
saturation current
space charge effect
stationary anode
stator
target
tube rating chart
window
wiring

OBJECTIVES

Upon completion of this chapter, the student should be able to:

- Draw a complete dual-focus cathode assembly.

- Discuss the necessary characteristics of filament metals and construction.

- Describe the control of thermionic emission from the filament.

- Select exposure factors and techniques that will extend tube life.

- Explain the function and design of a grid-biased focusing cup.

- Draw a complete rotating anode assembly.

- Discuss the characteristics of anode targets.

- Explain the line-focus principle and its effect on anode target design.

- Explain the anode heel effect and its effect on primary beam intensity.

- Explain the production of off-focus radiation.

- Describe the function of a rotating anode induction motor, stator, and rotor.

105

- Discuss the construction of the envelope and protective housing.

- Calculate safe exposures when provided with a tube rating chart, anode cooling curve, and housing cooling curve.

The electrical production of x-rays is only possible under very special conditions including a source of electrons, an appropriate target material, a high voltage, and a vacuum. The x-ray tube is the device that permits these conditions to exist, and it is within the tube that x-ray photons come into existence. The tube consists of a **cathode** and an **anode** enclosed within an **envelope** and then encased in a **protective housing** (Figure 6-1). X-ray tubes, whose useful life can be significantly extended by proper care and handling by professional radiographers, can cost over $10,000.

THE CATHODE ASSEMBLY

The cathode is the negative side of the x-ray tube. The function of the cathode is to produce a thermionic cloud, conduct the high voltage to the gap between cathode and anode, and focus the electron stream as it heads for the anode. The cathode is

a complex device and can be referred to as the **cathode assembly**. This assembly consists of the **filament** or filaments, **focusing cup,** and associated **wiring** (Figure 6-2).

The Filament

The filament is a small coil of thin thoriated tungsten wire. The wire is about 0.1–0.2 mm thick and the coil 1–2 mm wide by 7–15 mm long. It is set in the cathode assembly within the focusing cup (Figure 6-3). Tungsten is the material of choice because of its high melting point (3,370° C) and because it is difficult to vaporize (turn into a gas). Rhenium (melting point of 3,170° C) and molybdenum (melting point of 2,620° C) are also desirable materials. The high melting point permits the filament to operate at the high temperatures required of an x-ray tube. In addition, tungsten is not easily vaporized. Vaporization produces particles that deposit on other surfaces and reduce the vacuum within the tube. The length and width of the filament have a great effect on the ability of the particular x-ray tube to image fine details.

FIGURE 6-1 A rotating anode x-ray tube.

FIGURE 6-2   A cathode assembly.

FIGURE 6-3   Dual filaments in a focusing cup.
(Photography courtesy of Dunlee, Division of Philips Medical Systems)

FIGURE 6-4   Dual-filament wiring.

Most diagnostic x-ray tubes have dual filaments called a **dual focus** arrangement (see Figure 6-3). The wiring for dual filaments does not require separate ground conductors. Instead a common ground is used (Figure 6-4).

As we have discussed previously, the function of the filament is to provide sufficient resistance to the flow of electrons so that the heat produced will cause thermionic emission to occur. (A tungsten filament will not exhibit significant thermionic emission below 2,200° C.) This process causes electrons to leave the surface of the filament wire and form a thermionic cloud. When the high voltage is released

at exposure the entire cloud is available to be driven toward the anode target where x-ray photons will be produced. This provides many more times the number of electrons than would be available from a cold cathode.

Not all of the electrons that are thermionically emitted from the filament are driven to the anode or return to the filament. A very small percentage of the electrons are permanently vaporized from the filament and they contribute to reducing the vacuum, thus making the tube gassy. Vaporized tungsten (from both filament and anode) is also gradually deposited on the inner surface of a glass envelope. This deposit causes old tubes to have a mirrored appearance and can eventually cause high-voltage arcing when sufficient current is attracted to a deposit during an exposure. Arcing of this type immediately destroys the tube. Evaporization deposits on the glass envelope also cause increased filtration of the primary beam and this decreases tube efficiency. Tubes with a metal envelope can be grounded to significantly reduce this problem.

Another major cause of tube failure is the breaking of the filament itself. Filaments become increasingly thin as vaporization continues. When about 10 percent of the diameter has vaporized, a filament becomes subject to breaking, exactly the way a light bulb filament will burn out. However, older tubes are much more sensitive to rough handling and a thin filament that is jarred can break prematurely.

When the x-ray machine is first turned on, a mild current is sent to the filament. The filament remains in this preheated mode until immediately prior to an exposure. When the switch labeled "rotor" is activated prior to an exposure, not only does the rotor begin to turn but a higher current is sent to the filament to bring the thermionic cloud to the proper size for the mA selected. This increase in filament heating is what causes most of the vaporization of the filament. An average diagnostic x-ray tube filament life is only about 6–9 hours (10,000–20,000 exposures) at this heating level. One of the primary causes of premature tube failure is the radiographer's habit of holding the rotor switch prior to making exposures. Every second the rotor switch is depressed, life is removed from the filament. Routinely delayed exposures while the filament is enduring maximum current can shorten tube life by 50–60 percent (to 5,000–6,000 exposures).

Most tube manufacturers recommend that two-step exposure switches be **fully depressed in one motion.** All units have electronic interlocks that will not permit the exposure to occur until the rotor has brought the anode up to the proper speed. Holding the rotor switch (and filament heat) can be justified in cases where the patient is unable to cooperate. In these instances (such as with pediatric patients) the rotor and filament must be readied to permit an instant exposure to avoid patient breathing and motion. Single-phase generators are usually capable of initiating exposure within 10 milliseconds (0.01 second), and 3φ and high-frequency generators may be a quick 1 millisecond (0.001 second). Routine clinical examinations seldom need to be timed closer than these limitations.

Historical Notes. In the earliest days of radiography a cold cathode with an unheated filament was used. It was not until the American physicist William D. Coolidge (1873–1975) developed the Coolidge tube for the General Electric Corporation in 1915 that the hot filament became available. Prior to the development of the Coolidge tube, the radiographer kept a selection of tubes of various mA values on a rack, usually in the darkroom (Figure 6-5).

FIGURE 6-5 A selection of cold filament tubes as displayed at the Deutsches Röntgen Museum, Remscheid–Lennep, Germany. *(Photograph courtesy of Philip W. Ballinger)*

When a change of mA was required, the radiographer disconnected the tube and replaced it with a different one from the rack. Coolidge's contributions to radiography included not only the hot filament, but also the focusing cup, the imbedded anode target, and various anode cooling devices (including the unique water-cooled tube).

The Focusing Cup

The focusing cup is a shallow depression in the cathode assembly designed to house the filament (see Figure 6-2). It is made of nickel and its purpose is to narrow the thermionic cloud as it is driven toward the anode. Because electrons all possess negative charges, their tendency is to diverge rather than to travel in straight lines. The focusing cup is provided with a low negative potential, which, because of its geometry, focuses the electrons toward one another in a convergence pattern (Figure 6-6). Most x-ray tubes have the focusing cup at the same potential as the filament. It is possible to decrease the size of the focal spot by using a biased focusing cup. A biased focusing cup maintains the cup at a more negative voltage than the filament. This causes the exiting electron beam to be focused into a narrower stream as it heads toward the anode. In mammographic x-ray tubes focusing cup biasing is used when the small focal spot is selected.

FIGURE 6-6 The geometry of the negative charge on the cathode focusing cup.

FIGURE 6-7 A filament emission chart showing saturation as a function of filament amperage, tube voltage, and tube current. *(Courtesy of Varian EIMAC)*

As more and more electrons build up in the area of the filament, their negative charges begin to oppose the emission of additional electrons. This phenomenon is called the **space charge effect** and it limits x-ray tubes to maximum mA ranges of 1,000–1,200.

Saturation current is another filament phenomenon that affects the efficiency of the x-ray tube. As kVp increases, a greater percentage of the thermionically emitted electrons are driven toward the anode. This relationship is shown by a filament emission chart (Figure 6-7). The filament amperage curve flattens out when the kVp is driving the entire thermionic cloud toward the anode. The filament saturation current has been achieved when there are no further thermionic electrons to be driven toward the anode. At this point an increase in kVp will not increase the tube mA. Further mA increases must be achieved by increasing the filament amperage. Close examination of a filament emission chart demonstrates that something must be done to compensate for the tube mA increase when kVp is changed. For example, an exposure at 100 kVp will produce a significantly greater tube mA than the same exposure at 60 kVp. The filament amperage must be adjusted to compensate for these changes and the x-ray circuitry does this automatically whenever factors are changed by the operator.

Grid-Biased Tubes. In some applications, such as digital angiography or capacitor discharge generators, it is desirable to quickly regulate the flow of electrons producing x-ray photons. The addition of a more negative potential difference (approximately 2,000 volts) at the focusing cup causes the cup to attract the thermionic cloud. This attraction very cleanly removes electrons from use for x-ray production when the focusing cup charge is pulsed from negative to positive in synchrony with another device, it becomes possible to regulate, pulse, and synchronize x-ray production very precisely. These types of tubes are sometimes called **grid-pulsed, grid-biased,** or **grid-controlled.**

THE ANODE ASSEMBLY

The anode is the positive side of the x-ray tube and has three functions: it serves as a target surface for the high-voltage electrons from the filament, thereby

FIGURE 6-8 The anode assembly with anode, target, rotor, bearings, and stator.

becoming the source of the x-ray photons; it conducts the high voltage from the cathode back into the x-ray generator circuitry; and it serves as the primary thermal conductor. The anode target surface is where the high-speed electrons from the filament are suddenly stopped, resulting in the production of x-ray photons. The entire anode is a complex device referred to as the **anode assembly.** This assembly consists of the anode, **stator,** and **rotor** (Figure 6-8) and serves as the path for the high-voltage flow during exposure.

The Anode

Anodes are divided into two types: **stationary** and **rotating** (Figure 6-9). Rotating anodes, developed in 1936, turn during the exposure, thus presenting a much larger target area. Modern rotating anodes permit bombardment of a given area of the target for only 7–50 microseconds. The faster the anode rotates, the better the heat dissipation. The use of stationary anode x-ray tubes has become limited to low-power functions, such as those of dental units. Nearly all units designed for diagnostic radiography utilize rotating anodes because of their greater efficiency.

The anode is composed of several different metals, each designed to contribute the maximum to the overall function of the anode. Stationary anodes are composed of rhenium-alloyed tungsten imbedded in a 45° angled end of a copper rod. Rotating anode disks range from 5–13 cm in diameter and are composed of molybdenum. The anode's function as the source of x-ray photons and as the primary thermal conducting device is enhanced by the use of rhenium-alloyed tungsten as the target focal track material (Figure 6-10). Tungsten is the metal of choice for the source of x-ray photons for three primary reasons:

1. High atomic number
2. High melting point
3. Heat-conducting ability

Tungsten's atomic number (74) enhances the production of diagnostic-range photons. During normal use, the focal track reaches a temperature between 1,000°C and 2,000°C but the temperature can go higher if the tube load increases. Because of tungsten's high melting point, it can withstand nor-

FIGURE 6-9 A stationary and a rotating anode.

Tungsten-rhenium alloy

Graphite

Molybdenum

FIGURE 6-10   Rotating anode construction.

FIGURE 6-11   Pitting of a rotating anode focal track from extended use.

mal operating temperatures. Tungsten also conducts heat very well. The rhenium provides greater elasticity when the focal track expands rapidly due to the intense heat. To assist in the dissipation of heat in heavy load situations, specialized anodes may have the anode disk backed by a thicker layer of molybdenum or graphite. Graphite-backed anodes can double heat-loading capabilities without increasing bearing wear.

Specialized x-ray tubes for mammography utilize molybdenum (atomic number 42) as the primary target material due to its ability to emit a more uniform range of lower energy photons. The lower characteristic energy photons permit a better soft tissue image. Molybdenum also has a high melting point, as discussed above. These tubes also utilize a specialized glass envelope window made of beryllium because the glass used in most x-ray tubes absorbs too much of the low-energy beam.

Normal use of a rotating anode will eventually vaporize sufficient target focal track material to roughen or pit the target area (Figure 6-11). Pitting reduces the efficiency of the tube; the term *pitted*, or *pitting*, is often used to describe an older tube's focal track.

When first activating an x-ray unit, it is important to use an **anode warm-up procedure**. These procedures are specified by the tube manufacturers and are designed to bring the anode heat from room temperature to near the range of operation. The proce-

dure also permits the heat from the hot anode to serve as a "vacuum pump" to maintain a strong vacuum inside the envelope. This is why x-ray tubes should be warmed up regularly, even when the unit is not being used for patients. A normal procedure might require an average kVp and mA station for a 1-second exposure to be followed by two more 2-second exposures. Failure to follow the warm-up procedure can cause the entire anode to crack if the molybdenum absorbs the heat too rapidly and exceeds its expansion capability. Many anodes are stress relieved (Figure 6-12). A stress-relieved anode dissipates heat much more efficiently and does not require an elaborate tube warm-up procedure.

The Target Area.   The portion of the anode where the high-voltage electron steam will impact is called by various names: the **target,** the **focus,** the **focal point,** the **focal spot,** or the **focal track** (although this last term has a more specific definition, it is the target area). This is the precise point at which the

FIGURE 6-12 The back of a stress-relieved anode.

x-ray photons are created. The target is considered to be a point source of x-ray photons and it is from this point that all tube-to-object and image-receptor distances are measured. Some x-ray tube housings have a line drawn on them to indicate the exact level of the target within. All measuring devices have their zero point at this level. This is why a tape measure attached to the side or bottom of a tube collimator may begin at 12 cm. It is attached 12 cm from the target but is calculated to measure target-to-image-receptor distances.

Stationary anodes have a static target area. Rotating anodes have a dynamic target area and are designed to greatly increase the target area (see Figure 6-9). A rotating anode can increase the target area up to 300 times, depending on the diameter of the anode disk. Rotating anodes have much greater heat loading capacities than stationary anodes. High-speed anodes have higher heating capacities than regular-speed anodes (often 50 percent greater).

When discussing a rotating anode target area, the term **focal track** is used to represent the circular path that will be impacted by the electron beam. The terms **target, focus, focal point,** and **focal spot** refer to the area of the focal track that is impacted by the electron beam at one time. In addition, the term **actual focal spot** is used to describe the physical area of the focal track that is impacted. The term **effective focal spot** is used to describe the area of the focal spot that is projected out of the tube toward the object being radiographed (Figure 6-13).

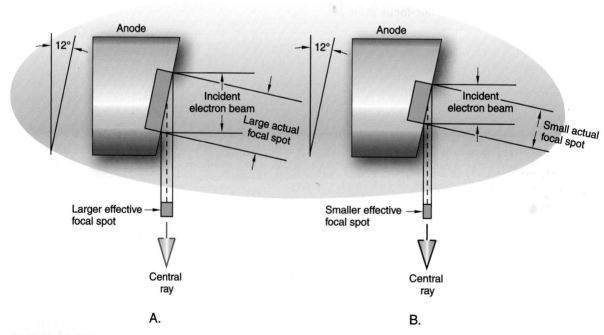

FIGURE 6-13 Effect of actual focal-spot size on effective focal-spot size.

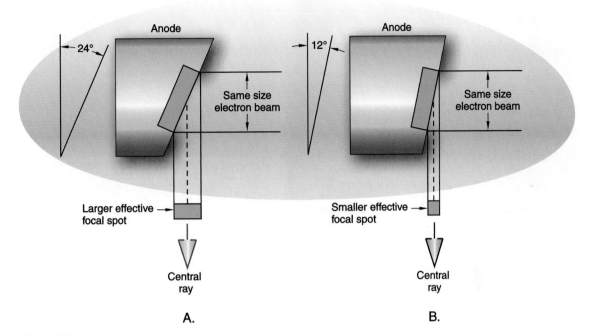

Anode

24°

Same size
electron beam

Larger effective
focal spot

Central
ray

A.

Anode

12°

Same size
electron beam

Smaller effective
focal spot

Central
ray

B.

FIGURE 6-14   Use of the line-focus principle to obtain an effective focal spot smaller than the actual focal spot.

Line-Focus Principle. The **line-focus principle** is used to reduce the effective area of the focal spot. This permits the best resolution of detail while permitting as large an actual area as possible (to increase thermal conductivity). **The effective focal-spot size is controlled by the size of the actual focal spot (which is controlled by the length of the filament) and the anode target angle.** As the actual focal-spot size increases, the effective focal-spot size also increases (see Figure 6-13).

When the target angle is less than 45°, the effective focal spot is smaller than the actual focal spot (Figure 6-14). This is accomplished by the line-focus principle. This principle can best be understood by holding a pencil straight up and then sloping it towards oneself so that the pencil is seen end on. The perceived dimensions of the pencil change as the angle changes. In the x-ray tube, changing the angle of the target changes the effective focal spot.

The most common diagnostic radiography target angle is 12°. However, tubes are available with an-gles ranging from 7° to 17°. When the angle is decreased, smaller focal spots can be achieved. A disadvantage of extremely small target angles is that the geometry of the angle can limit the size of the primary beam field at short source-to-image receptor distances (Figure 6-15). To cover a 14″ × 17″ field at 40″, a minimum of a 12° target angle is required. It has been shown that at large heat loads, target angles can decrease due to "warping" of the anode. In these instances, the anode end of the primary beam field can be reduced enough to cut off structures near the collimated edge. A slight angle of the tube will compensate for this effect. Target angles of less than 14° have been shown to produce some degree of cut-off as they age. Some tubes have offset filaments with two different focal tracks, which can be set at different target angles.

X-ray tube focal spots are rectangular because the line-focus principle applies only in the direction of the angle. It does not apply horizontally across the anode focal track because there is no angle in this direction. X-ray tube targets must be narrow to

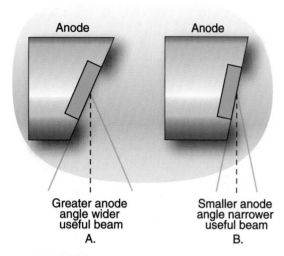

A. Greater anode angle wider useful beam

B. Smaller anode angle narrower useful beam

FIGURE 6-15 Anode target angle as a function of maximum primary beam field size.

75 80 90 100 105 110 120
% of central ray intensity

FIGURE 6-16 The anode heel effect.

maintain the small effective focal-spot size in the horizontal direction, usually not over 2 mm. The line-focus principle permits the actual focal spot's vertical dimension to be as much as 6 mm to gain the maximum thermal conductivity. **The effective focal spot's vertical dimension is the one that is stated as the focal-spot size.**

The National Electrical Manufacturers Association (NEMA) establishes standards for focal-spot size. These standards provide tolerance ranges for 23 focal-spot sizes. For example, a 1.0 mm focal spot is within tolerance if it measures up to 1.4 mm in width and 2.0 mm in length. It is important to remember that, in some instances, focal spots may be considerably larger than their stated size. Diagnostic tubes are available with focal spots of 0.1 mm to 3.0 mm. Occasionally, the term **fractional focal spot** is used to refer to a very small focal spot, one that is a fraction of a millimeter in size.

In normal usage, the term *focal-spot size* refers to the effective focal-spot size. Most diagnostic x-ray tubes have dual focal spots to include one for fine detail studies and the other for heavy tube loads. The small focal spot will not permit the use of higher mA stations. If the x-ray unit allows the radiographer to choose the focal-spot size, an exposure cannot be

made with a high mA station and the small focal spot. Automatic systems link the focal-spot size selection with the appropriate mA station. Therefore, the radiographer should realize that the focal-spot size may be mandated by the mA station. When a small focal spot is desired, it is important to use only low mA stations, even though this may require a longer exposure time.

Focal-spot size increases, or blooms, as milliamperage is increased. For example, the focal spot is slightly larger during an exposure of 80 kVp, 800 mA, and 0.1 second than it is during an exposure of 80 kVp, 100 mA, and 0.8 second. Although originally considered to be a significant factor, recent research has indicated that focal-spot blooming does not have a resounding effect on recorded detail.

Anode Heel Effect. The use of the line-focus principle causes a problem that is known as the **anode heel effect** (Figure 6-16). Because of the geometry of an angled anode target, the **radiation intensity is greater on the cathode side.** As electrons bombard the target, x-rays are produced and most are emitted at angles between 45° and 90° in the direction of the electron travel. These are absorbed by the anode itself or by the tube housing. Those photons

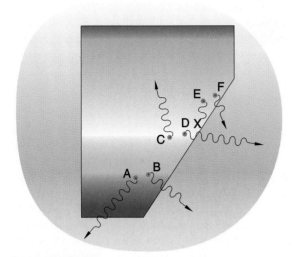

FIGURE 6-17 A–F represent photons created in the target. A exits at anode end of the tube, while B exits at cathode end of the tube. Notice the greater distance that photon A must travel through the target material itself as compared to photon B. Most photons are absorbed as in C. C is absorbed in the anode D, which exits the anode but is absorbed in the housing, and E, which is heading toward the anode end but does not exit the anode. F exits at the cathode end because it has a shorter distance to travel through the anode.

FIGURE 6-18 Variation in intensity of x-ray emissions parallel and perpendicular to anode–cathode axis. *(Note. From Quality Control in Diagnostic Imaging, by the Mayo Foundation, 1983, Rockville, MD: Aspen. Reprinted by permission of the Mayo Foundation for Medical Education and Research. All rights reserved.)*

that are emitted from the surface of the target are emitted in all directions. The intensity of the radiation which is emitted will vary between the cathode end of the tube and the anode end of the tube. This is because photons that are emitted toward the anode end are more likely to be absorbed by the target material itself than those that are emitted toward the cathode end (Figure 6-17). This can cause as many as 20 percent more photons at the cathode end of the tube and 25 percent fewer photons at the anode end (Figure 6-18). A total variation of approximately 45 percent exists parallel to the anode-cathode axis. No significant variation occurs perpendicular to the anode-cathode axis.

The 45 percent variation is significant enough to cause a visible difference in exoposure during radiographic examinations **when large film sizes are used at short distances.** The anode heel effect is

the reason why each radiographic table has a standard or natural "head" end. The tube anode is established at the head of the table to utilize the anode heel effect to best advantage. No significant variations will be seen in exposure from side to side.

Because the cathode end of the x-ray tube has a more intense beam, it should be positioned toward the denser (thicker) part of the body.

EXAMPLE: In which direction should the cathode be placed for an anteroposterior examination of the thoracic vertebral column?

Answer: Because the inferior thoracic region is more dense, the cathode's more intense beam should be positioned inferiorly to help increase the exposure in that region.

The Stator

The induction-motor electromagnets comprise the stator that turns the anode. The stator is the only part of cathode or anode assemblies that is located *outside* the vacuum of the envelope (see Figure 6-8). The electromagnetic effect that causes the rotor to turn can function through the envelope, permitting electrical isolation of the stator coils from the high voltage of the exposure. The kilovoltage range of the exposure would destroy the stator's electromagnets. The switch labeled "rotor" that must be activated prior to an exposure actually sends current to the

FIGURE 6-19 Anode melt due to rotor-bearing failure.

stator, which then causes the rotor to turn the anode. If the stator fails, the rotor will cease to turn the anode, resulting in the immediate melting of a spot on the target because rotating anode targets are not designed to absorb the heat of a high-voltage exposure while stationary (Figure 6-19).

The Rotor

The rotor is located inside the stator and inside the envelope. It is composed of a hollow copper cylinder or cuff that is attached to the anode disk by a molybdenum shaft. The cuff is the true rotor that is affected by the electromagnetic field of the stator, causing it to turn. Common rotating anodes revolve at 3,200–3,600 revolutions per minute (rpm). High-speed rotating anodes that operate at 10,000–12,000 rpm are also available to assist in dissipating heat.

The inside of the rotor contains silver-plated steel ball bearings around a shaft that is anchored to the envelope (see Figure 6-8). The ball bearings use silver plating as a high-temperature lubricant between the cuff and the anode shaft. Liquids tend to produce gas at high temperatures and this would reduce the vacuum in the tube. When the rotor switch is depressed prior to an exposure, the sound that is heard from the tube is actually the sound of the ball bearings turning at high speed. A new tube rotor with fresh bearings should coast for about 60 seconds after a 3,000 rpm exposure before stopping. When the coasting time slows to less than 20 seconds, the bearings are usually near binding.

High-speed anodes have a particular problem that is caused by the tone produced by their rotating. At between 5,000 and 7,000 rpm, the harmonics produced by the rotating cuff are at a frequency capable of shattering the glass envelope. Consequently, at the end of an exposure, direct current is run through the stator to quickly slow the rotor safely through the dangerous harmonic range. Another problem associated with high-speed anodes is the gyroscopic effect produced by the centrifugal force of the rotation. This force is great enough that if a high-speed anode tube housing is quickly rotated from one position to another (for example, from horizontal to perpendicular), the gyroscopic effect can cause trauma to the anode disk and bearing, causing the destruction of the tube. Usually the reversal of the stator prevents this problem but constant rough handling of this sort can cause undue wear on the rotor bearings. Any rough or extremely fast movement of the housing is not healthy for an x-ray tube and should be avoided.

A common cause of tube failure is bad bearings caused by long use at high temperatures. Although the molybdenum shaft that attaches the anode disk is designed to conduct a minimal amount of heat, the ball bearings eventually become imperfectly round. This leads to a grinding noise and wobbling of the rotor. Rotor wobble throws the focal track off center and tube efficiency drops dramatically.

Another effect of stator or rotor failure is that the electron stream overheats the target area of the anode focal track. When the temperature exceeds the melting point of tungsten, melting will occur. Superheated melted tungsten that drips onto the envelope will destroy the tube.

Any tube is dangerous to use when these events occur. A wobbling or melting anode disk can crack from the heat of exposure. A cracked anode can divert the electron and/or photon stream toward the envelope. Either instance will crack the envelope, permitting implosion of the vacuum, which can suck the insulating oil into contact with the superheated anode assembly. This can cause vaporization of the oil in a violent explosion that can blow out the rubber expansion seals of the housing, permitting hot oil to drop from the tube housing. Superheated oil is a severe hazard to the patient and the normal response should be emergency removal of the patient from under the tube. In nearly all instances, it is quicker to pull the patient from under the tube than to release the locks necessary to manipulate the tube away from the patient. In an angiographic laboratory or surgical situation, the breaking of sterile aseptic technique would be justified. A blown tube is a rare event and should never occur if proper tube loading, quality control and maintenance procedures are followed.

THE ENVELOPE

The entire cathode assembly and all of the anode assembly except the stator are enclosed within a glass or metal envelope commonly called the tube

FIGURE 6-20 A complete diagnostic x-ray tube with envelope, cathode assembly, anode disk, and rotor. A. Glass envelope B. Metal envelope *(Photo courtesy of Dunlee, Division of Philips Medical Systems)*

(Figure 6-20). A common glass envelope is made by sculpting several different types of heat-resistant Pyrex glass together to form a tube about 10″ long, 6″ in diameter at the center and 2″ in diameter at the ends. The glass is joined to the metal of the cathode assembly at one end and the anode assembly at the other.

The Envelope

Metal envelopes are increasingly becoming more common. They prolong tube life because they eliminate the problem of tungsten vaporization, as discussed earlier. The vast majority of high-output x-ray tubes are now made with metal envelopes.

The envelope is constructed around both the cathode and anode assemblies and must be sealed tight to maintain a high vacuum. At the point where the primary x-ray beam exits the envelope, a **window** segment is constructed. In some tubes this is simply a thinner section of the envelope to allow less absorption or scatter of the photons. Some special application tubes have other types of windows. For example, a molybdenum target tube for mammography uses a special metallic beryllium window to avoid attenuating the lower-energy photons, as discussed earlier.

The Vacuum

The primary function of the envelope is to maintain the vacuum between the cathode and anode. After construction, the air is removed from the tube until a pressure of less than 10^{-5} mm mercury (Hg) is achieved. This is done by use of a vacuum pump through a special vent, which is then permanently sealed. **The removal of the air permits electrons to flow from cathode to anode without encountering the gas atoms of air** and greatly increases the efficiency of the tube's operation.

Historical Notes. Röntgen discovered x-rays with a Crookes or Hittorf tube, which did not enclose a vacuum but instead contained known volumes of various gasses. Specialized tubes were quickly developed to meet the increasing need for x-ray production, and the vacuum tube was an early improvement. The x-ray pioneers simply placed the glass envelope within a leaded glass bowl. This was convenient when tubes had to be changed manually during the era of cold cathodes. Rapidly increasing awareness of the biological effects of ionizing radiation led to the development of metallic housings for x-ray tubes.

PROTECTIVE HOUSING

Modern x-ray tubes must be mounted inside a protective housing (Figure 6-21). **The housing controls leakage and scatter radiation, isolates the high voltages, and provides a means to cool the tube.**

Control of Leakage Radiation and Scatter Radiation

When x-ray photons are produced at the anode, they are emitted isotropically (in all directions). The primary beam consists of photons emitted through the window. The remaining photons are unwanted and the tube housing is designed to absorb them. The protective housing is composed of cast steel and is capable of absorbing most of the unwanted photons. The housing is usually lined with lead for additional absorption only at the cathode end because of the direction of the photons being emitted from the anode. The housing is equipped with a window to permit unrestricted exit for the useful photons from the envelope window. Any photons that escape from the housing except at the port are **leakage radiation. Leakage radiation must not exceed 100 mR/hr at 1 meter.** The housing also serves to cushion the x-ray tube from rough handling by operators.

High-Voltage Isolation and Tube Cooling

A special dielectric oil is used to fill the space between the envelope and the tube housing. The dielectric property of the oil insulates the high-voltage components from the tube housing, which is handled by the radiographer. In addition, the oil absorbs much of the heat that is produced by x-ray production. One end of the tube housing is sealed with an expandable gasket to permit the oil to expand as it is heated (see Figure 6-21). This gasket can be blown out by an imploded tube that has vaporized some of the insulating oil, thereby presenting a hazard to the patient. Many tube housings include a small air fan to remove heat from the

FIGURE 6-21   A diagnostic x-ray tube housing.

housing itself. In tubes that are subjected to extremely high loads, such as computed tomography tubes, the oil may be routed through a recirculation system (heat exchanger) to further cool it. Under no circumstances should anyone be in contact with a tube housing during an exposure.

OFF-FOCUS RADIATION

An often overlooked factor that can cause serious degradation of radiographic image quality is **off-focus,** or **extrafocal radiation. Off-focus radiation is composed of photons that were not produced at the focal spot.** It occurs when the high-voltage electrons striking the focal spot produce scattered electrons or photons. In some cases these scattered electrons or photons have sufficient energy remaining that when they strike another object in the tube (the cathode assembly, vaporized metal on a glass envelope, off-target sites on the anode, etc.) they produce photons. These photons are produced away from the focal spot and are therefore considered off-focus. The tube housing will absorb the majority of off-focus radiation but enough will be produced at a proper angle that they will exit through the tube window, housing port, and colli-

mator (Figure 6-22). These photons can cause "ghosting" of structures adjacent to the edge of the primary beam (Figure 6-23). This is not the result of scatter from the patient. Patient scatter is not capable of creating a diagnostic image of anatomical structures. Off-focus radiation may contribute as much as 25–30 percent of the total primary beam. However, all off-focus radiation is of significantly lower energy than the primary beam itself. X-ray tubes are available with a grounded metal and ceramic envelope to absorb off-focus radiation. These tubes may also use two sets of bearings to increase the heat-loading capacity. They have received limited acceptance because of their cost and the fact that they will not fit most existing tube housings. However, they can increase the total tube life by up to three times.

RATING CHARTS AND COOLING CURVES

Three types of rating charts are available to help radiographers avoid thermal damage to x-ray tubes: **radiographic tube rating charts, anode cooling charts,** and **housing cooling charts.** Radiographic

FIGURE 6-22 The production of off-focus radiation.

FIGURE 6-23 Off-focus radiation producing an image of the nose on a collimated sinus radiograph.

rating charts, sometimes called **tube rating charts,** are the most valuable because they provide a guide regarding the maximum technical factor combinations that can be used without overloading the tube. All radiographic tube rating charts plot milliamperage, kilovoltage, and time (the three most important factors set by the radiographer). Various manufacturers plot these factors in different ways (Figure 6-24). In most instances, any combination of factors at or under the curve is safe. However, the radiographer should verify this fact by establishing that lower technical combinations lie under the curve. (If both the x and the y axes have lower values at the lower left corner of the chart, safe factors are under the curves.) **Each filament of each tube has a unique radiographic tube rating chart.** The radiographer must ascertain that the correct chart for the **tube and filament** is being used.

FIGURE 6-24 Example tube rating chart for 1φ full-wave rectification. *(Courtesy of Varian EIMAC)*

> **EXAMPLE:** Is an exposure of 80 kVp, 0.1 second, and 200 mA within the limits of the 1φ, 0.6 mm focal-spot tube rating chart shown in Figure 6-24?

> **Answer:** When the intersection of the 80 kVp and 0.1-second lines is located on the tube rating chart, it is below the 200 mA line. Since the lower technical combinations lie below the mA lines, this is within limits.

60 Hertz stator operation

FIGURE 6-25 Example tube rating chart for 3φ full-wave rectification. *(Courtesy of Varian EIMAC)*

FIGURE 6-26 Example anode cooling chart.

EXAMPLE: Is an exposure of 90 kVp, 0.08 second, and 600 mA within the limits of the 3φ, 1.2 mm focal-spot tube rating chart shown in Figure 6-25?

Answer: When the intersection of the 90 kVp and 0.08-second lines is located on the tube rating chart, it is above the 600 mA line. Since the higher technical combinations lie above the mA line, it is not within limits.

Anode cooling charts permit the calculation of the time necessary for the anode to cool enough for additional exposures to be made (Figure 6-26). All cooling charts are calculated in terms of radiographic heat units. **A heat unit is calculated as kVp × mA × time × rectification constant.** The heat unit (HU) constants are given in Table 6-1. (Radiographic heat units are based on 1 kVp × 1 mA = 1 watt × 1 sec = 1 watt/sec × 0.71 rms voltage = 1 heat unit. Technically, 1 radiographic heat unit = 0.78 joule.)

TABLE 6-1. Heat Unit Rectification Constants

Rectification	Constant
1φ	1.00
3φ	1.35
High frequency	1.40

EXAMPLE: How many heat units are generated by an exposure of 80 kVp, 200 mA, and 0.2 second on a 1φ rectified unit?

Answer:
80 kVp × 200 mA × 0.2 sec
   × 1.00 = 3,200 hu

EXAMPLE: How many heat units are generated by an exposure of 70 kVp, 300 mA, and 0.15 second on a 3φ rectified unit?

Answer:
70 kVp × 300 mA × 0.15 sec
   × 1.35 = 4,253 HU

EXAMPLE: How many heat units are generated by two exposures of 65 kVp, 400 mA, and 0.05 second on a high-frequency unit?

Answer:
65 kVp × 400 mA × 0.05 sec
　　× 1.40 × 2 exposures
　　= 3,640 HU

To use the chart, the exposure factors must first be calculated in heat units. The length of time for the anode to cool can then be calculated by the following steps:

1. Find the total heat units applied on the vertical scale.

2. Read from the heat units over to the cooling curve and then down to read the corresponding time.

3. Calculate the time necessary for the anode to cool to any desired level and subtract the corresponding time of the initial exposure. (Or make the corresponding time of the initial exposure zero and calculate the time necessary for the anode to cool to any desired level from this point.)

For example, with the anode cooling chart in Figure 6-26, if a series of exposures produces 200,000 HU, the corresponding time is 2 minutes. The anode will cool to 150,000 HU in 2.5 minutes, so it will take 0.5 minute for the anode to cool from 200,000 HU to 150,000 HU. Similarly, the anode will cool to 100,000 HU in 1.5 minutes, to 50,000 HU in 4 minutes, and to room temperature (0) in 13 minutes.

EXAMPLE: Use the anode cooling curve in Figure 6-26 to calculate the length of time necessary for the anode to cool to 50,000 HU after five exposures of 80 kVp, 500 mA, and 0.5 second on a 1ϕ unit.

Answer:
　　80 kVp × 500 mA × 0.5 sec × 1.00
　　　　× 5 = 100,000 HU
　50,000 HU = 6 minutes on cooling curve
100,000 HU = 3.5 minutes on cooling curve,
　　　　so 6 min − 3.5 min = 2.5 min to
　　　　cool from 100,000 to 50,000 HU

A more practical application of an anode cooling curve is to solve a problem regarding whether a desired exposure will overload the anode. For example, again using Figure 6-26, how long would it be after a load of 250,000 HU before a series of exposures equal to 150,000 HU could be made? Since the total HU capacity of the anode is 350,000 HU, it must cool to 200,000 HU in order to take the additional 150,000 HU. The question becomes "How long will it take the anode to cool from 250,000 to 200,000 HU?" It will take 0.75 minute (2–1.25 min), or 45 seconds, before the new series of exposures can be made because 250,000 HU corresponds to 1.25 minutes and 200,000 HU corresponds to 2 minutes.

EXAMPLE: Use the anode cooling curve in Figure 6-26 to calculate the length of time necessary for the anode to cool sufficiently from 350,000 HU to accept a series of exposures totaling 150,000 HU on a 1ϕ unit.

Answer:
350,000 HU − 150,000 HU = 200,000 HU as level to which anode must cool
350,000 HU = 0 minute
200,000 HU = 2 minutes
It will be 2 minutes (2 − 0 min) before the series of exposures can be made.

After working through several of these problems for most tube anodes, it becomes apparent that modern x-ray tubes are designed to withstand most exposures within the diagnostic range for average patients. It is when a series of exposures must be made (as occurs routinely in angiographic procedures) that most radiographic tube rating and anode cooling charts must be consulted.

Housing cooling charts permit the calculation of the time necessary for the housing to cool enough for additional exposures to be made (Figure 6-27). As with anode cooling charts, they are calculated in terms of radiographic heat units. They are used in exactly the same manner as an anode cooling chart. In actual practice the anode will usually reach its limits long before the housing. However, there are instances, as when the forced-air fan for the housing is not functioning, when these charts can be useful.

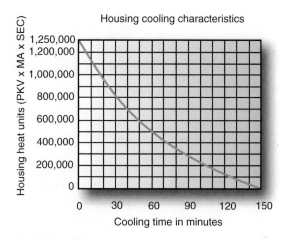

Housing cooling characteristics

FIGURE 6-27   Example housing cooling chart.
(Courtesy of Varian EIMAC)

TABLE 6-2.	Recommendations for Extending Tube Life

1. Warm up the anode following manufacturer's recommendations.

2. Do not hold the rotor switch unnecessarily. Double-press switches should be completely depressed in one motion. Dual switches should have exposure switch depressed first, followed by rotor switch.

3. Use lower mA stations when possible.

4. Use lower-speed rotor when possible.

5. Do not make repeated exposures near tube loading limits.

6. Do not rotate the tube housing rapidly from one position to another.

7. Do not use a tube when you can hear loud rotor bearings (unless it has been checked by a qualified service person).

RECOMMENDATIONS FOR EXTENDING TUBE LIFE

There are many things that the professional radiographer can do to extend the life of an x-ray tube. Warming up the anode according to the manufacturer's recommendations prevents thermal shock (cracking of a cold anode). Cracking can occur when a nonstress-relieved anode is unable to expand rapidly enough to absorb a room temperature-to-operating heat level exposure. Holding the rotor switch unnecessarily should be avoided. The rotor switch increases the filament's thermionic emission to exposure levels. Thermionic emission removes the electrons from the filament, deposits vaporized electrons on tube surfaces and decreases the tube vacuum, all of which can cause tube failure. In addition, the rotor switch causes stress to the rotor bearings, which can also decrease tube life. To avoid these problems, double-press switches should be completely depressed in one motion and dual switches should have the exposure switch depressed first, followed by the rotor switch. Lower mA stations should be used when possible because high mA increases filament thermionic emission. The lower-speed rotor should be used when possible because the high-speed rotor increases rotor bearing wear. Repeated exposures near tube loading limits should not be made as total heat units may approach anode or housing loading limits. Rotating the tube housing rapidly from one position to another should be avoided because the gyroscopic effect may crack or otherwise damage the rotor. A tube should not be used when loud rotor bearings can be heard (unless it has been checked by a qualified service person) because a wobbling anode disk can cause tube failure. These recommendations are summarized in Table 6-2.

SUMMARY

X-ray production requires a source of electrons, an appropriate target material, a high voltage, and a vacuum. The x-ray tube is the device that permits these conditions to exist. It consists of a cathode and an anode enclosed within an envelope and then encased in a protective housing.

The cathode is the negative side of the x-ray tube. The function of the cathode is to produce a thermionic cloud, conduct the high voltage to the gap between cathode and anode, and focus the electron stream as it heads for the anode. The cathode assembly consists of the filament or filaments, focusing cup, and associated wiring. The filament is a small coil of thin, thoriated tungsten wire. The focusing cup serves to narrow the thermionic cloud as it is driven to the anode.

The anode is the positive side of the x-ray tube. Anodes are divided into two types: stationary and rotating. Anodes are made using tungsten because of its high atomic number, high melting point, and good heat-conducting ability. The anode assembly consists of the anode, the stator, and the rotor. The portion of the anode where the high-voltage electron stream impacts is called the target, focus, focal point, focal spot, or focal track. The term actual focal spot is used to describe the physical area of the focal track that is impacted. The term effective focal spot is used to describe the area of the focal spot that is projected out of the tube toward the object being radiographed.

The line-focus principle is used to reduce the effective area of the focal spot. This permits the best resolution of detail in as large an actual area as possible. The effective focal-spot size is controlled by the filament size and the anode target angle. When the target angle is less than 45°, the effective focal spot is smaller than the actual focal spot.

The anode heel effect states that radiation intensity is greater on the cathode side than on the anode side.

An often overlooked factor that can cause serious degradation of radiographic image quality is off-focus or extrafocal radiation. Off-focus radiation is composed of photons that were not produced at the focal spot.

Three types of heating charts are available to help radiographers avoid thermal damage to x-ray tubes: radiographic tube rating charts, anode cooling charts, and housing cooling charts. Radiographic rating charts, sometimes called tube rating charts, are the most valuable because they provide a guide regarding the maximum technical factor combinations that can be used without overloading the tube. There are many things a radiographer can do to extend the life of an x-ray tube.

REVIEW QUESTIONS

1. What conditions must exist for x-rays to be produced?

2. What are the basic parts of a cathode assembly?

3. What is the purpose of the focusing cup?

4. Explain the space charge effect.

5. Why is tungsten the best metal for the x-ray source?

6. Explain the line-focus principle.

7. How does the anode heel effect affect radiation intensity?

8. What is the advantage of a high-speed rotor?

9. Why is it necessary for a vacuum to exist within the envelope?

10. Define leakage radiation.

11. How is off-focus radiation produced?

12. What is the function of rating charts and cooling curves?

13. Define a heat unit.

14. Name five things a radiographer can do to extend the life of an x-ray tube.

REFERENCES AND RECOMMENDED READING

Bushberg, J. T., Seibert, J. A., Leidholdt, E. M., & Boone, J. M. (2003). *The essential physics of medical imaging* (2nd ed.). Philadelphia: Lippincott Williams & Wilkins.

Coolidge, W. D. (1913). A powerful Röntgen ray tube with a pure electron discharge. *The Physical Review, 2*(6).

Coolidge, W. D. (1945). Experiences with the Röentgen-ray tube. *American Journal of Roentgenology, 54,* 583–589.

Curry, T. S., Dowdey, J. E., & Murry, R. C. (1990). *Christensen's introduction to the physics of diagnostic radiology* (4th ed.). Philadelphia: Lea and Febiger.

Dendy, P. P. & Heaton, B. (1999). *Physics for diagnostic radiology* (2nd ed.). Institute of Physics. Bristol, England.

Eisenberg, R. L. (1992). *Radiology: An illustrated history.* St. Louis, MO: Elsevier/C. V. Mosby.

Engel, T. L. (1979). Effect of kilovoltage and milliamperage on focal spot size. *Radiologic Technology, 50*(5), 559–561.

Everson, J. D., & Gray, J. E. (1987). Focal-spot measurement: Comparison of slit, pinhole, and star resolution pattern techniques. *Radiology, 165*(1), 261–264.

Fairbanks, R., & Doust, C. (1979). Methods for studying the focal spot size and resolution of diagnostic x-ray tubes. *Radiography, 45*(533), 89.

Fuchs, A. W. (1947). The anode 'heel' effect in radiography. *The X-Ray Technician, 18,* 158–163.

Glasser, O. (1936). What kind of tube did Röntgen use when he discovered x-ray? *Radiology, 27,* 138–140.

Glasser, O. (1958). *Dr. W. C. Röentgen* (2nd ed.). Springfield, IL: Charles C Thomas.

Grigg, E. R. N. (1965). *The trail of the invisible light: From x-Strahlen to radio(bio)logy.* Springfield, IL: Charles C. Thomas.

National Electrical Manufacturers Association. (1985). *Measurements of dimensions and properties of focal spots of diagnostic x-ray tubes* (NEMA Standards Publication No. XR-5-1984). Rosslyn, VA: Author.

Selman, J. (2000). *The fundamentals of imaging physics and radiobiology: For the radiologic technologist.* (9th ed.). Springfield, IL: Charles C Thomas.

Stears, J. G., Gray, J. E., & Frank, E. D. (1986). Half-value layer increase owing to tungsten buildup in the x-ray tube: Fact or fiction? *Radiology, 837.*

Stears, J. G., Gray, J. E., Webbles, W. E., & Frank, E. D. (1988). Radiologic exchange (tube warm-up and leaving x-ray units on). *Radiologic Technology, 59*(4), 325–326.

Stears, J. G., Gray, J. E., Webbles, W. E., & Frank, E. D. (1989). Radiologic exchange (resolution according to focal spot size). *Radiologic Technology, 60*(5), 429–430.

Thompson, T. T. (1985). *A practical approach to modern imaging equipment* (2nd ed.). Boston: Little, Brown, & Co.

Trigg, C. N. (1979). X-ray tube failures and prevention: A preliminary report. *Radiologic Technology, 50*(4), 430.

Wilks, R. J. (2003). *Principles of radiological physics.* (4th ed.) Edinburgh: Churchill Livingstone.

Wolbarst, A. B. (1993). *Physics of radiology.* Norwalk, CT: Appleton & Lange.

CHAPTER 7 X-Ray Production

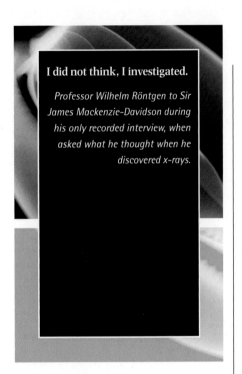

I did not think, I investigated.

Professor Wilhelm Röntgen to Sir James Mackenzie-Davidson during his only recorded interview, when asked what he thought when he discovered x-rays.

KEY TERMS

bremsstrahlung interaction
characteristic cascade

characteristic interaction
characteristic peak

incident electron
target interaction

OBJECTIVES

Upon completion of this chapter, the student should be able to:

- State the percentage of electron energy that is converted to x-ray photon energy in the x-ray tube.

- Describe a bremsstrahlung target interaction.

- Describe a characteristic target interaction.

- Identify factors affecting characteristic K-shell photon production.

- Explain the shape of the x-ray photon emission spectrum curve.

CONDITIONS

X-ray photons are produced when the high-speed electrons from the cathode strike an anode target. The fact that they are man-made is the only difference between x-rays and gamma rays (which are products of nuclear radioactive decay). An understanding of how x-ray photons are created from the atoms of the target material permits the radiographer to assert full control over the production of the primary beam.

The electrons that form the thermionic cloud around the filament arrive at the anode target (2 cm distant) traveling at nearly half the speed of light. A true understanding of the force contained in a kilovoltage-level exposure can be obtained by realizing that these electrons were accelerated from zero to half the speed of light in about 2 cm. These incoming electrons are called **incident electrons** and are represented in drawings by a solid arrow. In contrast, photons are represented by a wave arrow.

When incident electrons strike the target, they convert their tremendous kinetic energy to the atoms of the target material, and this interaction produces x-ray photons. The greater the mass or speed of the incident electrons, the greater the quality (energy) and quantity (number) of photons produced. This process occurs through two very different **target interactions.** All target interactions occur within 0.25 to 0.5 mm of the surface of the target. After giving up their energy to the target atoms, the electrons slow down enough to be conducted through the anode and the remainder of the high-voltage circuit. However, the incident electrons often experience 1,000 or more interactions before reaching this state.

TARGET INTERACTIONS

Heat Production

The target interactions that produce the x-ray photons consist of **less than 1 percent** of the total kinetic energy of the incident electrons. **Over 99 percent** of the kinetic energy of the incident electrons is converted to heat. This is the reason why so much technical research has gone into the development of the thermal aspects of x-ray tubes. In spite of the cost and performance capabilities of modern x-ray tubes, they are tremendously inefficient because they waste over 99 percent of the energy they use. This is true only in the range of diagnostic x-rays. As the kinetic energy of the incident electrons increases, so does the efficiency of photon production. By the time the therapeutic MeV range is reached, the majority of the energy is producing photons instead of heat.

Because they have such high kinetic energy, incident electrons seldom transfer enough energy to the outer shells of target atoms to cause ionization. Instead, they transfer enough energy to excite the outer-shell electrons to the point where they will emit infrared radiation as heat. These electrons then return to their normal state—where they will be re-excited again and again, each time emitting infrared radiation as heat.

There are two types of target interactions that can produce diagnostic-range x-ray photons: **bremsstrahlung interactions** and **characteristic interactions.** The interaction which will occur depends on the **electron kinetic energy** and the **binding energy of the electron shells** of the atom. Tungsten and rhenium are used as target materials in an effort to provide appropriate atomic number atoms and a maximum number of similar electron shell binding energies.

Bremsstrahlung Interactions

Bremsstrahlung interactions are named by the German word for braking or slowing. The abbreviation "brems" is also used. **Brems interactions may occur only when the incident electron interacts with the force field of the nucleus.** The incident electron must have enough energy to pass through the orbital shells and approach the nucleus of the atom. Because atomic nuclei have a positive charge and the incident electron has a negative charge, there is a mutual attraction between them. When the incident electron gets close to the nucleus, the powerful nuclear force field is much too great for the electron to penetrate. Instead, the force field causes the incident electron to slow down (or brake) and

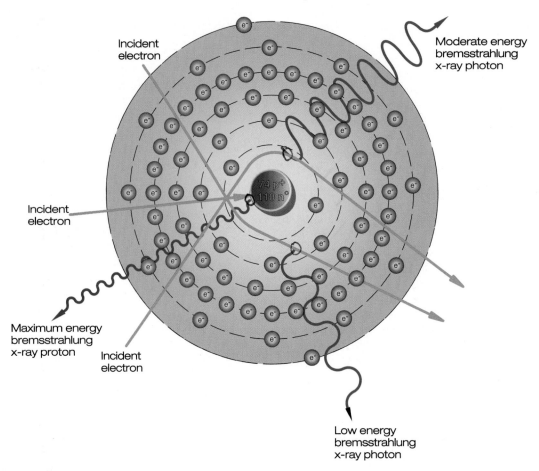

FIGURE 7-1 The bremsstrahlung interaction in a tungsten atom.

then it diverts the electron's course. As a result, the electron loses energy and changes direction. The energy that is lost during the braking (or bremsstrahlung) is emitted as an x-ray photon. **These emissions are called bremsstrahlung photons and their energy is exactly the difference between the entering and exiting kinetic energy of the electron** (Figure 7-1). The amount of kinetic energy lost by the incident electron in a brems interaction is determined by the distance the electron is from the nucleus. At larger distances very little kinetic energy is lost, resulting in low-energy brems radiation. At closer distances more energy is lost, resulting in higher-energy brems radiation. The incident electron can also have a direct impact with the nucleus, resulting in the loss of all

of the electron's kinetic energy. Because of the relatively small size of the nucleus, the chance of a direct impact is very low.

These energies are individually unpredictable and can range from the total value of the incident electron (which could be as high as the peak kilovoltage) to such a minimal amount of energy that it is immeasurable. Statistically, it is possible to predict their energies quite accurately by a study of the x-ray emission spectrum, as will be discussed later in this chapter. Only when the incident electron loses all of its excess kinetic energy would the electron drift away to join the current flow. A single incident electron can cause numerous brems interactions in many different atoms before losing enough energy to become included in the current flow.

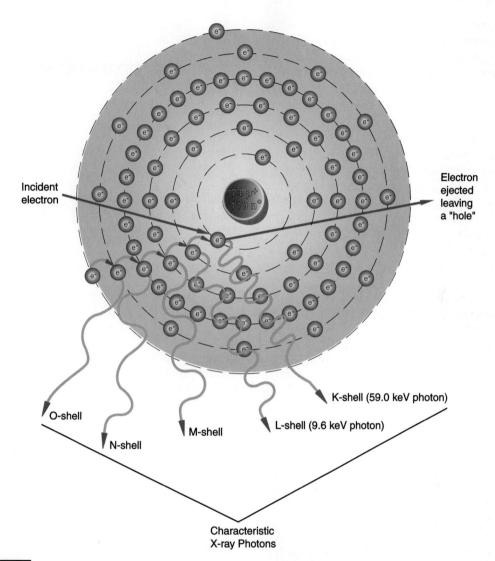

Incident electron

Electron ejected leaving a "hole"

K-shell (59.0 keV photon)

L-shell (9.6 keV photon)

M-shell

N-shell

O-shell

Characteristic X-ray Photons

FIGURE 7-2 The characteristic interaction in a tungsten atom. Only the K–shell characteristic photon has sufficient energy to be a part of the useful beam.

Characteristic Interactions

Characteristic interactions may occur only when the incident electron interacts with an inner-shell electron (Figure 7-2). The incident electron must have enough energy to knock an inner-shell electron from orbit, thereby ionizing the atom. The incident electron will usually continue but in a slightly different direction. More important is the fact that the electron "hole" that has been cre-

ated in the inner shell makes the atom unstable. An electron from another shell will immediately drop into the "hole." This dropping of an electron from an outer, higher-energy state into an inner, lower-energy state results in the energy difference between the two shells being emitted as an x-ray photon. **These emissions are called characteristic photons because their energy is exactly the difference between the binding energy of the outer and inner shells between which the**

electron dropped. After an outer shell electron has dropped to fill the "hole," another electron will drop to fill the "hole" it left and so on until only the outermost shell is missing an electron. This process is called a **characteristic cascade** and it can produce numerous x-ray photons for each electron that leaves the atom.

The first electron that was knocked from position in an inner orbital shell often has sufficient energy that it, too, may cause further interactions before it loses enough energy to become part of the current flow. Of course, this will also contribute to the total number of photons created.

Unlike brems photons, characteristic photon energies are so predictable that the science of x-ray spectroscopy uses measurements of these photon energies to determine what types of atoms make up the sun, stars, and other celestial bodies.

A tungsten atom, with its high atomic number of 74, has sufficient electron shells to produce relatively high-energy characteristic photons. Tungsten has a total of 74 electrons, with 2 electrons in the K-shell, 8 in L, 18 in M, 32 in N, 12 in O, and 2 in the P-shell (see Figure 2-5). The binding energies of the electrons in these shells are 69.5 keV for the K-shell electrons, 12.1 keV for L-shell electrons, 2.8 keV for M, 0.6 keV for N, and 0.08 keV for the O-shell electrons. The electron that drops into the "hole" may be from any shell further away from the nucleus. Of course, the further out the dropping electron's original position, the greater the energy imparted to the characteristic photon.

Characteristic photons can be created from incident electron ionization of any shell and "hole" filling from any shell. For example, K-shell ionizations can result in characteristic photons from electron drops between shells L and K, M and K, N and K, etc. Characteristic photons can also result from L-shell ionizations with electron drops between shells M and L, N and L, and so on. A wide variety of characteristic photon energy levels are thus produced (Table 7-1). The filling of a "hole" from an adjacent shell results in a lesser energy photon than nonadjacent shell transitions. For example, a K-shell vacancy filled by an L-shell electron will result in a weaker characteristic photon than the same vacancy filled by an M-shell electron. That is the result of the lower binding energy for the M-shell elec-

TABLE 7-1.	Characteristic Photon Emissions from X-Ray Target Materials		
Tungsten			
K–Shell Characteristics Photons		L–Shell Characteristics Photons	
L to K	59.0 keV		
M to K	67.2 keV	M to L	9.6 keV
N to K	69.1 keV	N to L	11.0 keV
Effective energy	69.5 keV	Effective energy	12.1 keV
Molybdenum			
K–Shell Characteristics Photons			
L to K	17 keV		
M to K	20 keV		
Effective energy	18 keV		

trons. In addition, within each shell there are discrete energy states for individual electrons. As a result, slightly different energies can result from an L to K transition depending on the specific energy state of the electron involved in the transition. Note that only electron drops into the K-shell will produce characteristic photons within the diagnostic x-ray range. Characteristic photons from the other shells (L, M, N, etc.) have energies that are too low to be significant in diagnostic radiology.

A single incident electron can cause a variety of interactions in many different atoms before losing enough energy to become included in the current flow (Figure 7-3). Remember, most of these interactions will result in the production of heat.

 EMISSION SPECTRUM

Within the diagnostic x-ray range most photons are produced by bremsstrahlung target interactions. Characteristic photons will not comprise any of the useful beam until the kVp is above 70 because removal of a K-shell electron from tungsten requires 69.5 keV. Between 80 and 100 kVp, about 80–90 percent of the primary beam is produced by brems interactions and 10–20 percent by characteristic interactions.

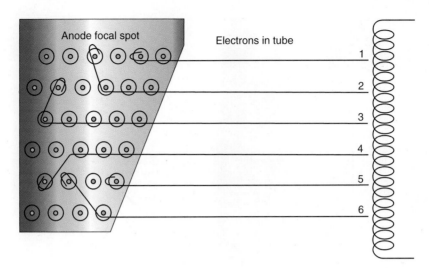

FIGURE 7-3 Sample paths of interactions for incident electrons striking the tube target.

As mentioned previously, the K-shell emissions are the only ones within the diagnostic x-ray range, although the L-shell emissions form a similar group and the M- to P-shell emissions form a third group. Both brems and characteristic emissions combine to form the complete primary beam spectrum (Figure 7-4). The L-shell characteristic emissions are included within the total spectrum, but when filtration is added to the tube these photons do not have sufficient energy and are absorbed by the filter. The K-shell emissions form a **characteristic peak** at their effective energy range of 69 keV. This characteristic peak is worthy of special note as it can cause strange results for the radiographer who is operating the x-ray tube slightly above the K-shell peak and needs a slight decrease in radiation output. A slight decrease that sets the tube potential directly on the 69 keV K-shell peak would greatly increase the tube output instead of decrease it, as anticipated. Modern x-ray equipment is capable of somewhat overcoming these fluctuations by programmed switching and the use of tungsten alloys (such as molybdenum) in the target to smooth out characteristic peaking. However, characteristic peaks are a point of consideration, not only in the target material but in the construction of x-ray tabletops, grids, cassettes, intensifying screens, and any other object through which the primary beam must pass.

The kilovoltage peak of the exposure is the maximum possible energy for any photon that exits the x-ray tube.

EXAMPLE: At what kVp was the exposure made that produced the graph in Figure 7-4?

Answer: As the maximum brems photons were at 80 keV, the kVp was set at that level.

What is interesting about Figure 7-4 is that it clearly demonstrates an often overlooked fact about radiographic exposures. **The average primary beam photon has a keV energy of only about 30–40 percent of the kVp.**

The emission spectrum for a mammographic molybdenum target is quite different from that of a tungsten target. The K-shell characteristic peak is about 18 keV and the average photon energy range is between 20 and 40 keV, which is perfect for soft-tissue visualization.

It is very useful to examine the effect on the primary beam emission spectrum of various factors under the control of the radiographer. When **mA time,** or **mAs** is changed, all of which control the quantity (number) of electrons striking the target, the result is a change in the **amplitude** of the emission graph (Figure 7-5). Note that each point on the higher curve represents exactly twice the number of photons on the lower curve. When **kVp,** which controls

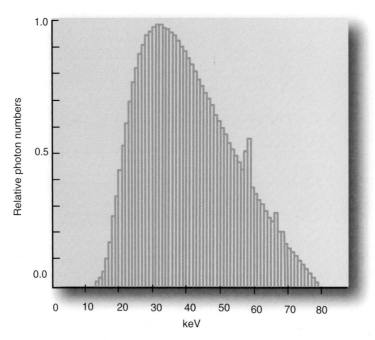

FIGURE 7-4 The x-ray emission spectrum with a tungsten target. This graph is the result of an exposure made with 2.8 mm Al/Eq filtration at constant potential, producing 17.8 mR/mAs at 30 in. (75 cm). The effective photon energy was 31 keV. *(Courtesy of Raymond P. Rossi, University of Colorado Health Science Center)*

FIGURE 7-5 The effect of mA changes on the x-ray emission spectrum.

FIGURE 7-6 The effect of kVp on the x-ray emission spectrum.

the quality (energy) of electrons striking the target, is changed, the result is a change in the **number of higher-energy photons as well as in the amplitude** of the emission graph (Figure 7-6). Note that there are more higher-energy photons on the higher curve, as well as an increase in the number of photons (seen in the increased amplitude). There was no increase in the total number of electrons striking the

target. The increase in amplitude represents more emitted photons due to the higher energy of each incident electron striking the target.

The x-ray emission spectrum is affected by the quantity and composition of the materials through which it must pass to exit the x-ray tube and housing. This is the filtration, which is the subject of Chapter 10. As the x-ray beam passes through the

x-ray photon energy (keV)

FIGURE 7-7 The effect of generator phase on the x-ray emission spectrum.

filtering materials, some of the lower-energy photons are absorbed. This **decreases** the intensity of the beam but at the same time **increases** the average photon energy. Increased filtration decreases image receptor exposure, and vice versa.

The generator phasing also has an effect on the emission spectrum. As the efficiency of x-ray production increases—from 1φ to 3φ to constant potential—the emission spectrum changes (Figure 7-7). As generator phasing efficiency increases, the x-ray beam increases in intensity, and there is also an increase in the average photon energy. Decreased phasing efficiency decreases both intensity and average photon energy.

SUMMARY

X-ray photons are produced when the high-speed electrons from the cathode strike an anode target. When incident electrons strike the target, they convert their tremendous kinetic energy to the atoms of the target material and this interaction produces x-ray photons. The greater the mass or speed of the incident electrons, the greater the quality (energy) and quantity (number) of photons produced.

The two target interactions that produce x-ray photons are bremsstrahlung (brems) and characteristic interactions. Less than 1 percent of the total kinetic energy of the incident electrons produces these interactions. Over 99 percent of the kinetic energy of the incident electrons is converted to heat.

Brems interactions occur when the incident electron interacts with the force field of the nucleus. This force field causes the incident electron to slow down (or brake), and then it diverts the electron's course. As a result, the electron loses energy and changes direction. The energy that is lost during the braking is emitted as a bremsstrahlung photon, and the photon energy is exactly the difference between the entering and exiting kinetic energy of the electron.

Characteristic interactions occur when the incident electron interacts with an inner shell electron. The incident electron knocks out an inner shell electron and continues in a slightly different direction. An electron "hole" is created in the inner shell, making the atom unstable. An electron from another shell will immediately drop into the "hole," which results in the emission of an x-ray photon. This emission is called a characteristic photon because the energy is exactly the difference between the binding energy of the outer and inner shells between which the electron dropped.

Within the diagnostic x-ray range most photons are produced by bremsstrahlung target interactions. An x-ray emission spectrum graph illustrates the relationship between the two target interactions within the primary beam. The average primary beam photon has a keV energy of only about 30–40 percent of the kVp.

When mA, time, or mAs is changed, all of which control the quantity (number) of electrons striking the target, the result is a change in the amplitude of the emission spectrum graph. When kVp is changed, which controls the quality (energy) of electrons striking the target, the result is a change in the number of higher-energy photons, as well as in the amplitude of the emission spectrum graph.

REVIEW QUESTIONS

1. What is the approximate percentage of electron energy that is converted to x-ray photon energy in the x-ray tube?
2. The majority of the electron energy in the x-ray tube is converted to what form of energy?
3. Describe a bremsstrahlung target interaction.
4. Describe a characteristic target interaction.
5. What is a characteristic cascade?
6. What is the average keV of the primary beam as compared to the kilovoltage peak?
7. What effect does increasing mAs and kVp have on the total x-ray emission spectrum?

REFERENCES AND RECOMMENDED READING

Bushberg, J. T., Seibert, J. A., Leidholdt, E. M., & Boone, J. M. (2002). *The essential physics of medical imaging* (2nd ed.). Philadelphia: Lippincott Williams & Wilkins.

Bushong, S. C. (2004). *Radiologic science for technologists: Physics, biology, and protection* (8th ed.). St. Louis, MO: Elsevier/C. V. Mosby.

Coolidge, W. (1945). Experiences with the Roentgen ray tube. American Journal of Roentgenology, 54, 583–589.

Dendy, P. P., & Heaton, B. (1999). *Physics for diagnostic radiology* (2nd ed.). Institute of Physics. Bristol, England.

Irfan, A. Y., Pugh, V. I., & Jeffery, C. D. (1985). Some practical aspects of peak kilovoltage measurements. *Radiography, 51*(599), 251–254.

Johns, H. E., & Cunningham, J. R. (1983). *The physics of radiology* (4th ed.). Springfield, IL: Charles C. Thomas.

Stears, J. G., Gray, J. E., Webbles, W. E., & Frank, E. D. (1989). Radiologic exchange (kVp measurements). *Radiologic Technology, 60*(3), 233–236.

Storm, E., & Israel, H. I. (1970). *Photon cross sections from 1 keV to 100 MeV. Nuclear Data Tables.* Boca Raton, FL: CRC Press.

Wolbarst, A. B. (1993). *Physics of radiology.* Norwalk, CT: Appleton & Lange.

UNIT II Protecting Patients and Personnel

A critical skill of the radiographer is the ability to protect both patients and other personnel from excessive exposure to ionizing radiation. This includes the radiographer as well. A thorough knowledge of basic radiation physics, personnel monitoring procedures, and advanced procedures for reducing exposure are expected of all radiographers.

Prior to beginning to function in a clinical setting, the radiographer must learn the **basics of radiation protection concepts and equipment.** The critical skill is the ability to apply this information to the **radiation protection procedures for patients and personnel.**

The chapters on **filtration** and the **prime factors** explain how to shape and mold the beam to minimize radiation exposure while obtaining maximum diagnostic information. **X-ray interactions** open the door to exactly what occurs to the biological systems that are being imaged as well as laying groundwork for future understanding of problems in image production.

Finally, advanced procedures for **minimizing patient dose** are covered to provide the practicing radiographer with real clinical skills that will achieve the theory presented in this unit.

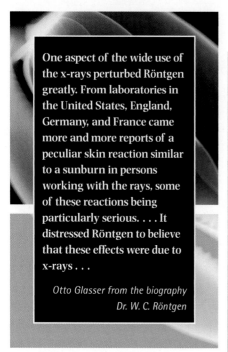

CHAPTER 8

Radiation Protection Concepts and Equipment

One aspect of the wide use of the x-rays perturbed Röntgen greatly. From laboratories in the United States, England, Germany, and France came more and more reports of a peculiar skin reaction similar to a sunburn in persons working with the rays, some of these reactions being particularly serious. . . . It distressed Röntgen to believe that these effects were due to x-rays . . .

Otto Glasser from the biography
Dr. W. C. Röntgen

KEY TERMS

activity
air kerma
alpha particle
becquerel
beta particle
Compton scattering
Curie (ci)
dosimeter
effective dose
electromagnetic
   radiation
field survey
   instrument

film badge dosimeter
genetic
gray (Gy)
integral dose
kerma
optically stimulated
   luminescence
   (OSL) dosimeter
particulate radiation
personnel monitoring
   device
photoelectric
   absorption

pocket dosimeter
quality factor
rad
rem
roentgen (R)
sievert (Sv)
somatic
Système
   Internationale
   d'Unites (SI units)
thermoluminescent
   dosimeter (TLD)

OBJECTIVES

Upon completion of this chapter, the student should be able to:

- Describe the nature of ionizing radiation.
- Identify the types of biological effects of ionizing radiation.
- Identify the principle sources of ionizing radiation.
- Define the quantities and units used for measurement of radiation.
- Describe devices used to detect and measure radiation, including field survey instruments and personnel monitoring devices.

CHAPTER 8

Radiation Protection Concepts and Equipment

One aspect of the wide use of the x-rays perturbed Röntgen greatly. From laboratories in the United States, England, Germany, and France came more and more reports of a peculiar skin reaction similar to a sunburn in persons working with the rays, some of these reactions being particularly serious. . . . It distressed Röntgen to believe that these effects were due to x-rays . . .

Otto Glasser from the biography
Dr. W. C. Röntgen

KEY TERMS

activity
air kerma
alpha particle
becquerel
beta particle
Compton scattering
Curie (ci)
dosimeter
effective dose
electromagnetic radiation
field survey instrument
film badge dosimeter
genetic
gray (Gy)
integral dose
kerma
optically stimulated luminescence (OSL) dosimeter
particulate radiation
personnel monitoring device
photoelectric absorption
pocket dosimeter
quality factor
rad
rem
roentgen (R)
sievert (Sv)
somatic
Système Internationale d'Unites (SI units)
thermoluminescent dosimeter (TLD)

OBJECTIVES

Upon completion of this chapter, the student should be able to:

- Describe the nature of ionizing radiation.
- Identify the types of biological effects of ionizing radiation.
- Identify the principle sources of ionizing radiation.
- Define the quantities and units used for measurement of radiation.
- Describe devices used to detect and measure radiation, including field survey instruments and personnel monitoring devices.

136

THE BASICS OF RADIATION PROTECTION PRINCIPLES AND PRACTICE

In medical applications exposure to ionizing radiation carries with it both a benefit and a risk. The benefit of information from an x-ray examination regarding the clinical management of the patient examination is weighed against the small, but nonetheless finite, risk when a physician requests the examination. The diagnostic benefit of a radiologic procedure far outweighs the risk resulting from the associated x-ray exposure. The information about the clinical condition of a patient received by the physician from a radiologic examination is an essential part of the practice of modern medicine.

It is the responsibility of the radiographer to ensure that each patient receives the minimal dose of radiation that will produce a diagnostic image consistent with the requirements of the examination. Radiographers must also ensure that all individuals are properly protected from unnecessary radiation exposure.

The Nature of Ionizing Radiation

Ionizing radiation is capable of creating positively and negatively charged particles when it interacts with matter. It arises from both natural and man-made sources and has the ability, as a consequence of its interactions with matter, to affect the various organs and tissues within the body. The energy possessed by ionizing radiation is capable of displacing atomic electron bonds and breaking the electron bonds that hold the molecules of matter together resulting in chemical changes, which can lead to harmful effects.

Ionizing radiations are grouped as either **particulate** or **electromagnetic radiations.** Particulate radiations include high energy electrons, neutrons, and protons that produce ionization in matter by direct atomic collisions. There are two principal types of particulate radiation that are associated with radioactive decay, **alpha particles** and **beta particles.** An alpha particle contains two protons and two neutrons and, as a result, is equivalent to a helium nucleus. Alpha particles are emitted from the nuclei of very heavy elements as they undergo radioactive decay. Compared to other types of particulate radiation, alpha particles have great mass and a positive charge. The energy of an alpha particle is transferred over a very short range in matter. In air, alpha particles can travel about 5 cm. As a result, alpha particles from external sources are essentially harmless. Beta particles are identical to electrons with the exception of their origin. Beta particles are emitted from the nuclei of radioactive material, while electrons exist in shells around the nucleus. Beta particles are negatively charged and very light. As a result, they travel farther in matter than alpha particles. Beta particles are capable of traveling approximately 10–100 cm in air.

Electromagnetic radiations include x-rays and gamma rays, which produce ionization in matter by other types of interactions. X-ray and gamma rays are essentially the same with the exception of their origin. Gamma rays are emitted by the nuclei of radioactive materials, while x-rays are man-made in an x-ray tube. For electromagnetic radiation in the medically useful x-ray energy range (<200 keV) the transfer of energy from the photon to matter, resulting in ionization, occurs by processes known as **photoelectric absorption** and **Compton scattering.**

During such interactions with matter, photon energy is transferred by a two-step process. First, the incident photon interacts with an atom causing an electron to be set in motion, which results in kinetic energy being released in the material. Second, the absorption of the released kinetic energy from the electron occurs via excitation and ionization. The excitations and ionizations that occur along the tracks of the charged particles set in motion give rise to biological damage in tissue. The biological damage may be a result of a direct interaction between the charged particle set in motion by the photons, in which cellular macromolecules are directly excited or ionized, or may be a result of an indirect interaction in which the absorption of radiation occurs in a water molecule, producing highly reactive species such as free radicals, which diffuse from the site of origin and subsequently cause biological damage. For x-rays and gamma rays approximately two-thirds of the biological effects on tissue are the result of indirect actions.

Biological Effects of Ionizing Radiation

Exposure to ionizing radiation affects various organs and tissues in the body and may result in a finite probability for radiation-induced disease in persons exposed to the radiation, and in their descendants. Health effects are known to be influenced by radiation characteristics and biological factors and include cancer induction, genetically determined ill health, nonspecific life shortening, developmental abnormalities, and degenerative diseases. The effects from the exposure to ionizing radiation may be classified as either **somatic** or **genetic.**

Somatic effects may become evident in the irradiated individual. Such effects are not usually to be expected in individuals exposed in the course of their work in the medical environment. To demonstrate a radiation response in humans within a few days to weeks, the dose must be quite high. Among the somatic effects of radiation are skin erythema, cataracts, and radiation-induced malignancies.

Genetic effects do not produce any significantly observable effect in the exposed individual but may appear in descendants of the exposed individual. They may not be manifest in the children of the exposed individual but may lie dormant for several generations and, eventually, may be eliminated completely from the genetic pool. Such effects result from alterations in the reproductive cells that can lead to defects in the offspring. Detectable radiation-induced mutations can result if the individual's reproductive cells have been exposed to an appreciable amount of radiation. It is unlikely that any worker in the medical environment would be exposed to ionizing radiation at a level high enough to cause the transmission of appreciable genetic effects.

Among the many factors that will influence the effect of exposure to ionizing radiation are the total dose received, the rate at which the dose was received, the age at exposure, the type of radiation, the sensitivity of the irradiated cells, and the portion of the body that was irradiated.

When x-rays were initially investigated, scientists were unaware of any harmful effects of their use and a number of the early radiation workers suffered injuries that are easily prevented today. Injuries from exposure were reported in Europe within the first year of investigation of x-radiation. In 1904 the first radiation fatality, a radiation-induced cancer, was reported in the United States. Over the next decade blood disorders such as leukemia and anemia, cancerous skin lesions, and cancer deaths were reported among radiation workers and linked to x-ray exposure. As a result of the high rate of documented radiation-related injuries, the British X-Ray and Radium Protection Committee was formed in 1921 to study ways to reduce radiation exposure to patients and medical personnel.

The goal of radiation protection is to limit human exposure to ionizing radiation to a degree that is reasonable and acceptable in relation to the benefit gained from the activities that involve the exposure, thereby reducing the likelihood of occurrence of somatic and genetic effects.

Sources and Magnitude of Ionizing Radiation Exposure

Everyone is exposed to sources of ionizing radiation. Some individuals will be exposed to a wide variety of such sources, while others will be exposed to only a few. The sources include those of **natural origin** either undisturbed by human activities or that have somehow been affected by human activities and **man-made** sources.

Natural sources include cosmic radiation, terrestrial radiation from naturally occurring radioactive sources in the ground, radionuclides naturally present in the body, and inhaled and ingested radionuclides of natural origin, such as radon. Human exposure to these natural sources varies depending on locality and other circumstances. When human exposure to natural sources increases as a result of human's actions, deliberate or otherwise, the natural sources are enhanced.

Man-made sources of radiation result from various man-made materials and devices and include such sources as x-rays and radiopharmaceuticals in medicine; consumer products containing radioactive materials, such as some smoke detectors and static eliminators; nuclear fuel production for power, air travel; and such catastrophic events as atmospheric fallout from nuclear weapons testing and accidents in nuclear power plants.

TABLE 8-1.	Annual Effective Dose Equivalent and Genetically Significant Dose in the U.S. Population			
Source	**Average Annual Effective Dose Equivalent**		**Average Annual Contribution to the GSD**	
	mSv	mrem	mSv	mrem
Natural sources				
Radon	2.0	200	0.1	10
Other	1.0	100	0.9	90
Occupational	0.009	0.9	≈0.006	≈0.6
Nuclear fuel cycle	0.0005	0.05	<0.005	<0.5
Consumer products				
Tobacco	—		—	
Other	0.05–0.13	5–13	≈0.05	<5
Miscellaneous				
Environmental sources	0.0006	0.06	<0.001	<0.1
Medical				
Diagnostic x–ray	0.39	39	0.2–0.3	20–30
Nuclear medicine	0.14	14	0.02	2
Rounded Total	3.6	360	1.3	130

Adapted with permission of the National Council on Radiation Protection and Measurements, NCRP Report No. 93.

The magnitude of exposure from these sources for the average member of the United States population has been studied and the results are summarized in Table 8-1 as the average annual effective dose equivalent. Also listed in Table 8-1 is the average annual contribution to the genetically significant dose (GSD). The genetically significant dose to a population is a measure of the average annual gonadal dose to members of the population, adjusted for the expected number of children conceived by each individual after exposure to radiation.

QUANTITIES AND UNITS RELEVANT TO RADIATION PROTECTION

Various quantities, units, and radiation dosimetry concepts have been developed and defined to quantify the amount of radiation received by individuals. Historically the quantities and units associated with radiation dosimetry have included the **roentgen (R),** used for specifying exposure; the **rad** (radiation absorbed dose), used for specifying energy absorbed; and the **rem** (radiation equivalent in man), used for specifying biologically equivalent dose.

Other radiation quantities of importance are the **kerma,** used to describe the kinetic energy released per unit mass; the **air kerma,** used to describe the kinetic energy released per unit mass of air; **integral dose,** used to describe the total radiation energy imparted to matter; **effective dose** used to measure the radiation and organ system specific damage in man; and **activity** used to measure the amount of a radioactive material as it undergoes decay.

In 1948, the International Committee for Weights and Measures was charged with developing an international system of units based on the metric system. The committee developed the **Système Internationale d'Unites,** or **SI,** units. In recent years the international system of units has been adopted for radiation protection, and within this system of units the older units are no longer applicable. Although the National Council on Radiation Protection and Measurement (NCRP) adopted the SI units for use with ionizing radiation in 1985, traditional units are still very much in use. The following discussion will serve to review

TABLE 8-2.	Conversions between Conventional and SI Units	
Conventional Unit (Column A)	Conversion Factor (Column B)	SI Unit (Column C)
roentgen	2.58×10^{-4}	coulomb/kilogram
rad	0.01	gray
rem	0.01	sievert
curie	3.7×10^{10}	becquerel

Column A amount multiplied by Column B equals Column C amount.

Column C amount divided by Column B equals Column A amount.

Adapted with permission of the National Council on Radiation Protection and Measurements, NCRP Report No. 93.

the conventional and more familiar units and SI units. Table 8-2 provides conversion between conventional units and SI units.

Exposure

The roentgen (R) represents a unit of exposure in air and was defined as that quantity of x-rays or gamma rays required to produce a given amount of ionization (charge) in a unit mass of air. One roentgen creates 2.08×10^9 ion pairs per cubic centimeter of air to produce a total ion charge of 2.58×10^{-4} coulomb (C) per kilogram (kg). The roentgen is limited to the measurement of exposure in air only and is not applicable to photons of energy above 3 Mev or to particulate radiations. The roentgen has no direct equivalent or special unit in the SI system of units and is no longer used. Exposure may be expressed directly in C/kg.

Absorbed Dose

The rad was developed as a unit of absorbed energy or dose and is applicable to any material. The rad was defined as 100 ergs of energy absorbed in one gram of absorbing material. In the SI system of units the rad has been replaced by the **gray (Gy)**, which is defined as 1 joule (J) of energy absorbed in each kilogram (kg) of absorbing material. One gray is equivalent to 100 rads; therefore, 1 rad equals 10 mGy. This unit is not restricted to air and can be measured in other absorbing materials.

Kerma/Air Kerma

The rad is also a unit of kerma, an acronym for *kinetic energy released in matter*. As radiation passes through matter it interacts and the energy carried by the photons is transformed to kinetic energy of charged particles such as the electrons in the photoelectric and Compton interactions. The energy imparted directly to the electrons, per unit mass, is the kerma. Some of the kerma may be radiated away as bremsstrahlung if any of these electrons interact with the nuclei of the atoms in the matter. In these instances, kerma and absorbed dose would not be identical. At diagnostic energies, however, practically no brems is produced in the tissues and, as a result, kerma will equal dose. The SI unit for the kerma is the gray.

Air kerma is the kinetic energy released per unit mass of air. X-ray tube outputs and inputs to image receptors are sometimes described in air kerma. An air kerma of 1 cGy (1 rad) corresponds to an exposure of about 1 R.

Integral Dose

The integral dose describes the total amount of energy imparted to matter. It is a product of the dose and the mass over which the energy is imparted. For example, when a patient has a CT scan of the abdomen, the dose per section (irradiated volume) might be 1 rad (10 mGy). Regardless of the number of scan sections, the dose to the irradiated volume would be defined as 1 rad (10 mGy). If the patient has 20 scan sections, the integral dose would be approximately 20 rad (200 mGy).

Equivalent Dose

Different types of radiation, such as alpha and beta particles and neutrons, produce different degrees of biological damage as compared to gamma or x-radiation. To account for the fact that the same absorbed dose of radiation may result in different biological responses for different types of radiation, a unit known as the rem (radiation equivalent man) was developed. The rem is the conventional unit for equivalent dose (H_T). **In NCRP Report No. 116, Limitations of Exposure to Ionizing Radiation (which replaces NCRP Report No. 91), the term equivalent dose replaces the previously**

TABLE 8-3.	Comparison between SI and Conventional Units							
Quantity	Symbol for Quantity	Expression in SI Units	Expression in Symbols for SI Units	Special Name for SI Units	Symbol Using Special Name	Conventional Unit	Symbol for Conventional Unit	Value of Conventional Unit in SI Units
Activity	A	1 per second	s^{-1}	becquerel	Bq	curie	Ci	3.7×10^{10} Bq
Absorbed Dose	D	joule per kilogram	J/kg	gray	Gy	rad	rad	0.01 Gy
Dose Equivalent	H	joule per kilogram	J/kg	sievert	Sv	rem	rem	0.01 Sv
Exposure	X	coulomb per kilogram	C/kg			roentgen	R	2.58×10^{-4} C/kg

used term, **dose equivalent (H), in defining dose limits.** These two terms are conceptually different. Dose equivalent (H) is based on the absorbed dose at a "point" in tissue and equivalent dose (H_T) is based on the average absorbed dose in the tissue or organ.

Equivalent dose (H_T,R) is the product of the average-absorbed dose (D_T,R), in a tissue (T) due to radiation (R) and a radiation weighting factor (W_R), previously known as the **quality factor** (Q), which is specific to specific types of radiation and accounts for the biological effectiveness of the specific radiation. The radiation weighting factor for gamma or x-radiation equals 1. This means that 1 rad equals 1 rem for gamma or x-radiation. For alpha particles, however, the radiation weighting factor is 20. This means that 1 rad equals 20 rem for alpha particle absorption. In the SI system of units the rem has been replaced by the **sievert (Sv),** which is defined as the product of the absorbed dose in gray and the radiation weighting factor. One sievert is equal to 100 rem, and 1 rem is equal to 10 mSv.

Effective Dose

Effective dose (E) is the sum of the weighted equivalent doses for all irradiated tissues and organs. It takes into account the fact that not all tissues are equally sensitive to the effects of ionizing radiation. As was seen with equivalent dose and dose equivalent, in NCRP Report No. 116, Limitations of Exposure to Ionizing Radiation, the term *effective dose* (E)

replaces the previously used term, *effective dose equivalent* (H_E), in defining dose limits.

Since exposure received from ionizing radiation is rarely uniform over the whole body, the concept of effective dose is used to compare the detriment from irradiation of a limited portion of the body with the detriment from irradiation of the entire body and employs weighting factors for the relative risks associated with irradiation of various body tissues. The effective dose is defined as the sum over specified tissues of the products of the equivalent dose in a tissue (T) and the weighting factor for that tissue.

Activity

Activity (A) describes the quantity of radioactive material. It is expressed as the number of radioactive atoms that undergo decay per unit time. The unit of activity has traditionally been the **curie (Ci).** The curie is defined as 3.7×10^{10} disintegrations per second (dps). One curie is a very large amount of radioactive material. In a typical nuclear medicine procedure, activities from 0.1–30 millicuries (mCi) are used. The SI unit for activity is the **becquerel.** The becquerel is defined as 1 dps.

Further information regarding international system of units and its application in radiation protection and measurements may be found in **NCRP Report No. 82, SI Units in Radiation Protection and Measurements.** A comparison between SI units and conventional ones is displayed in Table 8-3.

DETECTION AND MEASUREMENT OF IONIZING RADIATION

A number of different dose-measuring devices, known as dosimeters, are employed for detection and measurement of radiation exposure from x-rays. These **dosimeters** may be classified as either **field survey instruments** or **personnel monitoring devices**.

Field Survey Instruments

A number of portable field survey instruments are available for use in radiation detection and measurement. They include the Geiger-Mueller (GM) survey instruments, scintillation detection devices, and ionization chamber instruments. Regardless of the type, field survey instruments should be calibrated at least annually.

Geiger-Mueller Survey Instruments. Geiger-Mueller survey instruments or counters are primarily used to detect the presence of radiation rather than provide exact measurements. A GM counter is a gas-filled detector. It consists of a volume of gas between two electrodes. Ionizing radiation produces ion pairs in the gas that can be collected and measured. GM counters are very efficient at detecting charged particles, such as beta particles, but are relatively inefficient at detecting x- and gamma radiation. GM counters are most commonly used in nuclear medicine as radioactive contamination survey instruments.

Scintillation Detection Devices. Scintillation detectors combine the use of a scintillator with a device that can convert light to an electric signal. Scintillators are materials that emit visible or ultraviolet light when exposed to ionizing radiation. In a scintillation detector, this light is converted to an electric signal and is measured. The most common applications for scintillation detectors are in gamma cameras in nuclear medicine and in some CT scanner detectors.

Ionization Chamber Instruments. Ionization chamber instruments are commonly employed for the measurement of the primary and secondary radi-

FIGURE 8-1 An ionization chamber dosimeter. The chamber encloses a known volume of air, inside of which a chargeable electrode is positioned to attract electrons freed by the ionization of the gas by the radiation. The difference in the electrode's charge before and after exposure is measured by an electrometer and displayed in radiation units.

ation beam for purposes of evaluation of equipment performance, environmental exposure assessment of scatter and leakage radiation, and for measurement of patient exposure. An ionization chamber works on the principle that when radiation interacts with air electrons, positive ions are produced giving rise to an electrical charge that can be measured.

A typical ionization chamber dosimeter consists of a chamber with a known volume of air and an electrode (Figure 8-1). A small voltage is applied between the electrode and the wall of the chamber, so the electrode is positive and the chamber wall is negative. As x-ray photons pass through the chamber they ionize the air. The free electrons from these ionizations are attracted to the positive electrode, where they can be measured with an electrometer. The intensity of the signal that is produced on the electrode is proportional to the radiation exposure that occurred in the air volume of the chamber. This relationship can be displayed on a digital readout in R or C/Kg units. Ionization dosimeters can be designed to measure specific ranges of radiation intensity.

Personnel Monitoring Devices

Individuals who are regularly exposed to ionizing radiation should be supplied with personnel monitoring devices that will provide an estimate of the exposure they received. Personnel monitoring is recommended whenever a possibility exists that an individual will receive more than 1/10 of the recommended dose limit as a result of his or her occupational activities. A personnel monitoring device measures the quantity of exposure it has received. It is not a radiation protection device.

When only one personnel monitoring device is issued, it should be worn on the anterior surface of the body between the chest and waist level. When a lead apron is worn and only one personnel monitoring device is issued, it is recommended that it be worn outside the apron at the collar level. Because of the considerable controversy regarding the proper location of the dosimeter when a lead apron is worn, the local radiation safety officer should be contacted for specific guidance. It is important that all persons wear their dosimeters at the same locations.

An additional dosimeter, usually designated as a whole body dosimeter, may be worn in addition to the collar dosimeter when the potential for significant exposure to the thyroid or eyes exists. This dosimeter is usually positioned near the waist under the lead apron and may be used in conjunction with the collar dosimeter to determine the effective dose. The whole-body dosimeter and collar dosimeter must never be interchanged.

The most common types of personnel monitoring devices are the **optically stimulated luminescence (OSL) dosimeter, film badge dosimeter, thermoluminescent dosimeter (TLD),** and **pocket dosimeter.**

Optically Stimulated Luminescence (OSL) Dosimeter.

The most common type of radiation monitoring device is the optically stimulated luminescence (OSL) dosimeter. The OSL dosimeter measures radiation that passes through a thin strip of aluminum oxide (Al_2O_3). A laser light is used to stimulate the aluminum oxide, which becomes luminescent in proportion to the amount of radiation exposure it has received.

The OSL dosimeter has distinct advantages over both the film badge or the TLD. It can report doses along a wide range from as low as 1 mrem with a precision of $\pm$ 1 mrem. In addition, it can undergo complete reanalysis to confirm the radiation exposure received with no loss of information. It also has excellent

FIGURE 8-2A   The Luxel Dosimeter. *(Courtesy of Landover, Inc.)*

FIGURE 8-2B   The Luxel Filter Pack. *(Courtesy of Landover, Inc.)*

long-term and environmental (temperature and humidity) stability.

Laudauer, Inc. offers the Luxel® OSL Dosimeter with a variety of color coding options for both department/series and exchange frequencies. The Luxel® dosimeter is a self-contained packet that contains an aluminum oxide strip located between three filters and an open window (Figure 8-2). The open window and the copper and tin filters are used to determine the energy levels of the exposure to the dosimeter. The imaging filter is used to determine whether the exposure was a static or dynamic exposure. A static image indicates that the dosimeter was not moving at the time of exposure. This may imply that the dosimeter was not worn during the time of exposure and an accidental exposure may have occurred. A dynamic exposure image will have a blurred appearance and indicates that the dosimeter was being worn during the time of exposure and the dose is valid.

Film Badge Dosimeter.
Film badge dosimeters are usually issued on a monthly basis and consist of two pieces of film having different sensitivities to x-rays and contained within a light, tight envelope. This film packet is placed within a holder, which contains a number of different filter elements held in a fixed position with respect to the film. Printed on the front of the film packet is the name of the individual, the beginning date for which the film badge is issued, and other coded information.

When the badge is exposed to ionizing radiation, the film emulsion darkens in proportion to the degree of radiation exposure received. The resultant optical density can be measured with a densitometer and calibrated to the degree of radiation exposure received.

The filters in the film badge holder provide a means of determining the energy of the incident radiation. Because the absorption of radiation by a specific thickness of given material will depend on the energy of the radiation, the measurement of the relative film densities under the different filters provides a means of estimating the energy of the exposing x-ray beam. Typically copper, cadmium, and aluminum are used as filtering metals.

Film badges are capable of measuring exposures over the range of approximately 10 mrem (0.1 mSv) to 2,000 rem (20 Sv) and are most commonly used to measure the total body exposure of the individual. Readings of less than 10 mrem (0.1 mSv) are generally not detectable and may be reported as minimal (M).

Thermoluminescent Dosimeter (TLD).
Personnel monitoring devices using thermoluminescent dosimeters contain small chips of a thermoluminescent material, usually lithium fluoride (LiF). When exposed to radiation, a portion of the absorbed energy is stored in the crystal structure of the LiF chips in metastable states. This absorbed energy will remain in these states for long periods of time. If the LiF chips are heated, the absorbed energy is released as visible light. The heating and measurement of the LiF chips are carried out in a device called a reader, and the amount of measured light is proportional to the absorbed radiation dose. TLDs provide approximately

FIGURE 8-3   A pocket ionization chamber.
(Courtesy of Fluke Biomedial RMS)

the same measurement range as film badges and can be used as whole-body badges or collar badges. Because of their small size, TLDs are commonly used for monitoring exposure to the extremities in the form of ring badges.

Pocket Dosimeter.
A special type of ionization chamber used for personnel dosimetry is known as a pocket dosimeter (Figure 8-3). When irradiated, the radiation ionizes the air in the chamber, which partially neutralizes a previously positively charged electrode (quartz fiber on a wire frame), causing the hairline fiber to move on an exposure scale (Figure 8-4). The amount of ionization and movement of the fiber is proportional to the radiation exposure to the chamber. Such devices are usually charged and read out on a special charger-reader device. Pocket dosimeters are occasionally used for personnel monitoring in situations in which the convenience of an immediate readout is desired (for example, after each procedure in a cardiac catheterization laboratory). However, they provide no permanent record of personnel exposure and are not routinely used.

Care of Personnel Monitoring Devices.
The proper care and handling of personnel monitoring devices is essential to obtaining accurate results. The personnel monitoring device must be worn only by the individual to whom it is assigned, must be worn in the proper location for the prescribed time period, and must be turned in for processing when due.

The OSL dosimeter has distinct advantages because it can report a wide range of doses from as low as 1 mrem with precision, and it has excellent long-term environmental stability.

Both film badge dosimeters and TLD dosimeters may be adversely affected by heat, humidity, mechanical pressure, inadvertent exposure to light, and prolonged delay between exposure and process-

FIGURE 8-4   **Cross section of a pocket ion chamber (dosimeter).** *(Courtesy of Bushberg, J. T., Seibert, J. A., Leidholdt, E. M., & Boone, J. M. [1994]. The essential physics of medical imaging. Baltimore: Lippincott Williams & Wilkins.)*

ing. Exposure from the rear or from oblique angles may also result in inaccurate results.

Generally, groups of personnel dosimeters are provided with a control that must be stored in an unexposed area at the facility and returned with the group for processing. This control provides an unexposed level against which the personnel dosimeters are evaluated.

Personnel monitoring devices should not be worn during medical or dental exams and should never be intentionally exposed to the primary radiation beam. Individuals should be aware of the exposure they receive by reviewing their exposure readings on the reports posted in the facility on a routine basis. Should any aspect of the reported exposure be unclear or cause concern, the individual

should seek the counsel of the facility radiation safety officer.

Dosimetry Reporting

After each wear date period, the dosimeters are returned to the company's laboratory for analysis. Wear date periods can range from weekly to biweekly to monthly to bimonthly to quarterly. A report is generated for the facility and includes a wide variety of information (Figure 8-5). For the Luxel® OSL dosimeters, Landauer, Inc. provides participant identification information, the type of dosimeter used, the radiation quality that exposed the dosimeter (e.g., x or gamma photons, beta, neutrons), and the radiation exposures that were received. The radiation exposure is expressed as the dose equivalent in millirem for the wear period, a quarterly accumulated dose equivalent, a year-to-date dose equivalent, and a lifetime dose equivalent for each participant. In addition, for each column, exposures are provided for deep dose, lens of the eye dose, and shallow dose equivalents. The deep dose equivalent applies to the external whole body exposure at a tissue depth of 1 cm, the eye dose equivalent applies to the external lens of the eye at a tissue depth of 0.3 cm, and the shallow dose equivalent applies to the external exposure of the skin at a tissue depth of 0.007 cm. Participants should check their dosimetry report for each wear period.

SUMMARY

Exposure to ionizing radiation carries with it both a benefit and a risk. With few exceptions, the diagnostic benefit of a radiologic procedure far outweighs the minimal risk resulting from the x-ray exposure. The information received by the physician from a radiologic examination about the clinical condition of the patient is an essential part of the practice of modern medicine.

Ionizing radiation is any form of radiation that possesses energy capable of displacing atomic electron bonds and breaking the electron bonds that hold the molecules of matter together. The potential biological damage from the ionization process is the reason for the need to understand proper radiation protection practices. Ionizing radiation comes from two major sources: natural background radiation and man-made radiation.

The biological effects of radiation exposure are either somatic, occurring in the individual exposed, or genetic, occurring in the descendants of the individual exposed. It is the responsibility of the radiographer to ensure each patient receives the minimal dose of radiation necessary to produce a diagnostic image. Radiographers must also be properly shielded from unnecessary radiation exposure.

Radiation quantities and units that are important in radiation protection are exposure, absorbed dose, and equivalent dose. The SI units that correspond to these quantities are the coulomb per kilogram (C/kg), the gray (Gy), and the sievert (Sv). The corresponding traditional units are the roentgen (R), the rad, and the rem. Other radiation quantities of importance are the kerma, the air kerma, integral dose, effective dose, and activity.

Various devices are available to detect and measure exposure to ionizing radiation. Portable field survey instruments include the Geiger-Mueller (GM) survey instruments, scintillation detection devices, and ionization chamber instruments. Personnel monitoring devices include the optically stimulated luminescence dosimeter, film badge dosimeter, thermoluminescent dosimeter, and pocket dosimeters.

REVIEW QUESTIONS

1. Explain the differences between alpha and beta particles.
2. Differentiate between somatic and genetic effects.
3. What are the primary sources of ionizing radiation? Give examples of each.
4. What are the three basic quantities of radiation measurement and their associated conventional and SI units?
5. What is the kerma?
6. Describe the function of a GM survey instrument.
7. List the four types of personnel-monitoring devices.
8. Explain the function of the filters in a dosimeter.

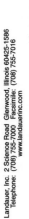

FIGURE 8–5 A sample Radiation Dosimetry Report. *(Courtesy of Landover, Inc.)*

REFERENCES AND RECOMMENDED READING

Bednorck, D. R., Rozenfeld, M., Lanzl, L. H., & Sabau, M. (1981). A protocol for exposure limitations in radiography. *Radiologic Technology, 53*(3) 229.

Bushberg, J. T., Seibert, J. A., Leidholdt, E. M., & Boone, J. M. (2002). *The essential physics of medical imaging* (2nd ed.). Baltimore: Lippincott Williams & Wilkins.

Bushong, S. C. (2004). *Radiologic science for technologists: Physics, biology, and protection* (8th ed.). St. Louis: Elsevier/C. V. Mosby.

Curry, T. S., Dowdey, J. E., & Murry, R. C. (1990). *Christensen's introduction to the physics of diagnostic radiology* (4th ed.). Philadelphia: Lea and Febiger.

Dowd, S. B. (1994). *Practical radiation protection and applied radiobiology.* Philadelphia: W. B. Saunders.

Elsberry, J. S. (1979). A technique for scatter dose calculations. *Radiologic Technology, 51*(1), 51.

Hall, E. J. (2000). *Radiobiology for the radiologist* (5th ed.). Philadelphia: J. B. Lippincott.

Hendee, W. R. (Ed.) (1984). *Health effects of low-level radiation.* Norwalk, CT: Appleton-Century-Crofts.

International Commission on Radiation Protection. (1970). *Protection of the patient in x-ray diagnosis publication number 16.* Oxford: Pergamon Press.

Mettler, F. A., & Moseley, R. D. (1985). *Medical effects of ionizing radiation.* Orlando, FL: Grune & Stratton.

Morgan, K. Z. (1973). The need for radiation protection. *Radiologic Technology, 44*(6), 385.

National Council on Radiation Protection and Measurements (NCRP). (1976). *Structural shielding design and evaluation for medical use of x-rays and gamma rays of energies up to 10 mev* (NCRP Report No. 49). Bethesda, MD: Author.

National Council on Radiation Protection and Measurements (NCRP). (1977). *Medical exposure of pregnant and potentially pregnant women* (NCRP Report No. 54). Bethesda, MD: Author.

National Council on Radiation Protection and Measurements (NCRP). (1985). *SI units in radiation protection and measurements* (NCRP Report No. 82). Bethesda, MD: Author.

National Council on Radiation Protection and Measurements (NCRP). (1987). *Ionizing radiation exposure of the population of the United States* (NCRP Report No. 93). Bethesda, MD: Author.

National Council on Radiation Protection and Measurements (NCRP). (1989). *Medical x-ray, electron beam and gamma-ray protection for energies up to 50 mev (equipment design, performance and use)* (NCRP Report No. 102). Bethesda, MD: Author.

National Council on Radiation Protection and Measurements (NCRP). (1989). *Radiation protection for medical and allied health personnel* (NCRP Report No. 105). Bethesda, MD: Author.

National Council on Radiation Protection and Measurements (NCRP). (1990). *Implementation of the principle of ALARA for medical and dental personnel* (NCRP Report No. 107). Bethesda, MD: Author.

National Council on Radiation Protection and Measurements (NCRP). (1993). *Limitations of exposure to ionizing radiation* (NCRP Report No. 116). Bethesda, MD: Author.

National Council on Radiation Protection and Measurements (NCRP). (2000). *Radiation protection for procedures performed outside the radiology department* (NCRP Report No. 133). Bethesda, MD: Author.

National Council on Radiation Protection and Measurements (NCRP). (2001). *Evaluation of the linear-nonthreshold dose-response model for ionizing radiation* (NCRP Report No. 136). Bethesda, MD: Author.

Noz, M. E., & Maguire, G. Q. (1985). *Radiation protection in the radiologic and health sciences* (2nd ed.). Philadelphia: Lea & Febiger.

Seeram, E., & Travis, E. L. (1997). *Radiation protection.* Baltimore: Lippincott Williams & Wilkins.

Statement from the 1985 Paris meeting of the International Commission on Radiological Protection. (1985, September). *Radiology.*

Upton, A. C. (1982). The biological effects of low-level ionizing radiation. *Scientific America, 246*(2).

Watkins, G. L. (1988). Public health risks from low dose medical radiation. *Radiologic Technology, 59*(2), 160.

CHAPTER 9

Radiation Protection Procedures for Patients and Personnel

Röntgen almost from the beginning had conducted all his experiments in his big zinc box. . . . Then he had added a lead plate to the zinc between the tube and himself, and in doing so he had unknowingly protected himself completely. With an accurate appreciation of the import of these unexplained effects, Röntgen foresaw the suffering consequent to the careless handling of the rays.

Otto Glasser from the biography
Dr. W.C. Röntgen

KEY TERMS

10-day rule
ALARA
deterministic effect
dose limit
occasionally exposed
 worker

occupationally
 exposed worker
primary barrier
protective device
radiation worker
secondary barrier

stochastic effect
structural protective
 barrier

OBJECTIVES

Upon completion of this chapter, the student should be able to:

- Differentiate between the various advisory groups and regulatory agencies involved in developing radiation protection standards.

- Explain the concept of dose limits related to the use of radiation.

- Describe the ALARA concept.

- Explain the basic principles of reducing exposure to radiation.

- Describe techniques used to minimize radiation exposure to patients and personnel.

- Discuss the precautions that should be taken to minimize potential fetal exposures.

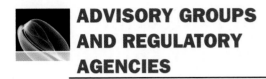

ADVISORY GROUPS AND REGULATORY AGENCIES

A number of different organizations and agencies are involved in the development of standards for radiation protection and the establishment of regulations for the protection against the hazards that can result from the use of ionizing radiation.

The advisory groups that have shared in the establishment of radiation protection standards include: the **International Commission on Radiological Protection (ICRP)**; the **National Council on Radiation Protection and Measurements (NCRP)**; the **National Academy of Sciences Advisory Committee on the Biological Effects of Ionizing Radiation (NAS-BEIR)**; and the **United Nations Scientific Committee on the Effects of Atomic Radiation (UNSCEAR).**

The ICRP was formed in 1928 and has an international membership. It provides a variety of perspectives on radiologic health issues. In 1929 the ICRP established the National Committee on Radiation Protection and Measurements, which was later chartered by Congress in 1964 as the National Council on Radiation Protection and Measurements (NCRP). The NCRP is a nonprofit organization that is charged with collecting, analyzing, developing, and disseminating in the public interest, information, and recommendations about radiation protection, radiation measurements, quantities, and units. It works cooperatively with the ICRP and other agencies to accomplish its mission.

The NAS-BEIR and UNSCEAR are two additional advisory groups that study and report on the risks from exposure to ionizing radiation.

In addition to the advisory groups, there are a number of regulatory agencies responsible for protecting the public and occupationally exposed individuals from the effects of ionizing radiation. Regulatory agencies carry the force of law and can inspect facilities, issue fines, and revoke radiation use authorizations. Two such agencies are the **U.S. Nuclear Regulatory Commission (NRC)** and the **U.S. Food and Drug Administration (FDA).** The NRC has been given the regulatory authority for special nuclear materials and by-products. In a number of instances, the NRC has entered into agreements with the states to oversee and enforce the regulations. In these "agreement states," it becomes the state's responsibility to enforce NRC regulations. The FDA regulates radiopharmaceuticals as well as the performance and radiation safety requirements of commercial x-ray equipment.

The two primary sources of radiation protection standards in the United States are the NRC, which is a U.S. federal agency charged with licensing facilities and controlling the use of radioactive materials, and the NCRP, an advisory group that makes recommendations for radiation protection. Both sources are used when setting radiation protection policies and procedures. The NRC regulations are available on the Internet at *www.nrc.gov*, and the NCRP reports are available at *www.ncrp.com*.

LIMITING EXPOSURE TO IONIZING RADIATION

It is important to set limits for the protection of the radiation worker and the general public because of the known biological effects of exposure to ionizing radiation. The primary purposes for establishing dose limits are to limit the risks of **stochastic effects** and to prevent **deterministic effects** (also known as nonstochastic effects). Stochastic effects are those for which no threshold dose of radiation exists, such as cancer and genetic effects. They are random in nature. Regardless of dose, some will experience an effect. As dose goes up, the chance of experiencing an effect also goes up. Deterministic effects such as cataracts, skin erythema, and sterility, are those for which a threshold dose is assumed. As dose increases, the severity of the effect increases. Although the dose has to be high to demonstrate the effect, once that dose is reached, the probability of demonstrating the effect is very high.

For radiation protection purposes, individuals may be divided into two groups. First are those classified as **radiation workers,** who incur, as an occupational risk, a certain likelihood of exposure to ionizing radiation in the course of their normal duties. The second group includes members of the general public.

Radiation workers may be further classified as **occupationally exposed workers** and **occasionally exposed workers.** Occupationally exposed workers are individuals who have a significant potential for exposure to radiation in the course of their employment. Occasionally exposed workers are individuals whose duties may occasionally bring them into areas where radiation exposure may occur. Both occupationally exposed workers and occasionally exposed workers should receive instruction and training regarding hazards of radiation exposure and radiation protection practices.

Dose Limits

Radiation exposure limits pertinent to the protection of radiation workers are known as **dose limits** and are specified for both **whole body** exposure and for exposure to **certain tissues and organs.** Several terms have been used to describe dose limits, including maximum permissible dose, dose equivalent limits, and equivalent dose limits. Prior to 1987, the term *maximum permissible dose* (MPD) was used to describe dose limits; this is no longer acceptable terminology because no dose is considered permissible.

Dose equivalent limits and *cumulative effective dose equivalent* replaced MPD, and this philosophy was described in NCRP Report No. 91: Recommendations on Limits for Exposure to Ionizing Radiation. In 1993, **NCRP Report No. 116, Limitation of Exposure to Ionizing Radiation** replaced NCRP Report No. 91. This new report follows the same basic framework to dose limits as the previous report but incorporated some changes as provided in ICRP Publication 60. Of particular note is the change in terminology, from effective dose equivalent limits (Report No. 91) to effective dose limits (Report No. 116) and dose equivalent limits for tissues and organs (Report No. 91) to equivalent dose limits for tissues and organs (Report No. 116). Equivalent dose (H_T) replaces the previously used term, *dose equivalent* (H), in defining dose limits. These two terms are conceptually different. Dose equivalent (H) is based on the absorbed dose at a "point" in tissue and

TABLE 9-1.	Effective Dose Limit Recommendations	
Occupational Exposures		
Effective dose limits		
Annual	50 mSv	(5 rem)
Cumulative	10 mSv × age	(1 rem × age)
Dose equivalent annual limits for tissues and organs		
Lens of eye	150 mSv	(15 rem)
Skin, hands, and feet	500 mSv	(50 rem)
Public Exposures (Annual)		
Effective dose limit		
continuous or frequent exposure	1 mSv	(0.1 rem)
infrequent exposure	5 mSv	(0.5 rem)
Equivalent dose limits for tissues and organs		
lens of eye	15 mSv	(1.5 rem)
skin, hands, and feet	50 mSv	(5 rem)
Embryo–Fetus Exposures (Monthly)		
Equivalent dose limit	0.5 mSv	(0.05 rem)
Education and Training Exposures (Annual)		
Effective dose limit	1 mSv	(0.1 rem)
Dose equivalent limit for tissues and organs		
Lens of eye	15 mSv	(1.5 rem)
Skin, hands, and feet	50 mSv	(5 rem)

Adapted from NCRP Report No. 116:*Limitations of Exposure to Ionizing Radiation,* Table 19.1

equivalent dose (H_T) is based on the average absorbed dose in the tissue or organ.

Currently recommended values for occupational and public dose limits are given in Table 9-1 and reflect the recommendations of the NCRP as put forth in Report No. 116. The effective dose limit for whole body exposure of a radiation worker is 5 rem (50 mSv) per year.

The cumulative effective dose (E) limit is age in rem, which is determined in SI units by the formula:

where   E = 10 mSv × N
      E = effective dose limit
      N = age in years

EXAMPLE: What is the dose limit for a 19-year-old radiation worker?

Answer:

E = 10 mSv × N
E = 10 mSv × 19
E = 190 mSv (19 rem)

EXAMPLE: What is the dose limit for a 35-year-old radiation worker?

Answer:

E = 10 mSv × N
E = 10 mSv × 35
E = 350 mSv (35 rem)

Irradiation at the upper level of the dose limits is not to be considered as desirable, and in every case efforts to reduce exposures to the lowest possible level should be taken.

Individuals not classified as radiation workers are considered members of the **general public.** For purposes of protection of these individuals, the level of recommended dose limits, exclusive of any exposure received as the result of a medical procedure, has been established as one-tenth of the effective dose limit for radiation workers. That is, 0.5 rem (5 mSv) per year for infrequent exposure and one-fiftieth of the effective dose limit for radiation workers, which is 0.1 rem (1 mSv) per year for continuous exposure. Individuals in education and training have the same effective dose limit (for continuous or frequent exposure) as the general public, that is 0.1 rem (1 mSv).

Nuclear Regulatory Commission (NRC)

The Nuclear Regulatory Commission regulations for radiation protection are known by their Code of Federal Regulations (CFR) No. 10CFR20. Unlike the NCRP, which is an advisory body, the NRC is a U.S. federal government agency and its regulations are law in the United States. NRC licensees are required to implement these standards. The standards for occupational dose limits for adults are shown in Table 9-2.

The most critical of the NRC regulations is the whole body exposure regulation that limits exposure to 500 mSv (50 rem)/year to any organ or 50 mSv (5 rem)/year whole body. Also worthy of note are the regulations for exposure to the extremities, lens of the eye, and pregnancy (which is discussed in detail later in this chapter).

Maintaining Exposure as Low as Reasonably Achievable (ALARA)

A basic philosophical principle of radiation protection concerning the use of ionizing radiation emphasizes the need to maintain exposure to ionizing radiation at a level **A**s **L**ow **A**s **R**easonably **A**chievable **(ALARA),** with economic and societal factors being taken into consideration. This premise has been accepted by advisory and regulatory agencies and requires that radiologic personnel take on the responsibility of minimizing the exposure to their patients and any other individuals involved in a ra-

TABLE 9-2.	Occupational Dose Limits for Adults–NRC Regulation IOCFR20
Whole body definition	Head, trunk, gonads, arms above elbow, legs above knee
Extremities definition	Arms elbows and below, legs knees and below
Whole body exposure limits	Most limiting of: 500 mSv (50 rem)/yr to any organ **or** 50 mSv (5 rem)/yr whole body
Lens of the eye	150 mSv (15 rem)/yr
Skin of the whole body	500mSv (50 rem)/yr
Extremities	500 mSv (50 rem)/yr applied to each extremity
Embryo/fetus/pregnancy	5 mSv/term (0.5 rem or 500 mrem)

diologic procedure. Implementation of the ALARA principle is achieved by application of the basic principles of radiation protection and a thoughtful approach to all work involving exposure to ionizing radiation.

PROTECTION OF PERSONNEL

When radiological procedures are performed, there is a possibility that individuals other than the patient will receive some radiation exposure. While the patient should be the only person exposed to the primary beam, others involved in the procedure may be exposed to radiation scattered from the primary beam or to leakage radiation from the x-ray tube. This occurs particularly during fluoroscopy, mobile examinations, interventional special procedures, and cardiac catheterization. For most radiographic exposures, personnel should be behind protective barriers. Radiologic personnel should not be involved in holding patients who are unable to cooperate during an x-ray exposure. Immobilization devices should be used or, if absolutely necessary, assistance should be requested from the patient's family or friends.

Figure 9-1A and B represent diagrams of two iso-exposure curves that illustrate the percentage of scattered radiation that personnel are exposed to during a single exposure of 20 mAs to a chest phantom. The curves represent the percentage of the exposure to the skin at various distances from the patient using two different kilovoltages (60 kVp and 80 kVp) and two different field sizes (20 × 20 cm and 28 × 32 cm). The effect of kVp is illustrated in Figure 9–1A for the transverse plane. The effect of beam restriction (collimation) is shown in Figure 9–1B for the coronal plane. In both instances, an obvious reduction in exposure to scattered radiation occurs as the distance away from a patient increases. In addition, the amount of scatter around a patient is affected to a greater extent by changes in collimation rather than changes in kVp.

Principles of Personnel Exposure Reduction

Reduction of an individual's exposure to ionizing radiation may be accomplished by application of three basic principles: (1) reduce the amount of **time** spent in the vicinity of the radiation source while it is operating; (2) increase the **distance** between the radiation source and the individual to be protected; and (3) interpose a **shielding** material, which will attenuate the radiation from the source. These three basic principles are sometimes referred to as the three cardinal rules of radiation protection.

Time. X-ray imaging equipment produces radiation only during the actual exposure used to form the image during a procedure. The time of exposure on a per-image basis is very short (typically much less than 1 second) during radiographic procedures. During fluoroscopic procedures, which are used when dynamic information is required, the x-ray source may be on (usually intermittently) for several minutes to as long as an hour or more. To minimize exposure to radiation, individuals should reduce the amount of time they spend in the vicinity of an operable radiation source. The simplest way to do this is to ascertain whether their presence is needed during the procedure. Whenever possible, individuals should remain behind protective barriers.

Distance. Increasing the distance between the individual and the source of radiation is an effective method to reduce exposure to radiation. As distance from the source of radiation is increased, the radiation level will decrease significantly. Maximizing the distance from an operable source of radiation is a particularly effective method of exposure reduction during mobile radiographic and fluoroscopic procedures.

The amount of exposure reduction can be calculated using the inverse square law, which describes the relationship between distance and radiation intensity. The inverse square law states that the intensity of radiation at a given distance from a point source is inversely proportional to the square of the

Transverse plane

100 cms FSD

200 mA

0.1 sec

2.5 mm A1

60 kVp

80 kVp

0   0.5   1.0

Meters

100%   0.5   0.3   0.1

A.

Coronal plane

100 cms FSD

60 kVp

200 mA

0.1 sec

2.5 mm A1

20 X 20 cms

28 X 32 cms

0   0.5   1.0

Meters

100%

0.5

0.5

0.1

0.05

0.1

B.

FIGURE 9-1 The iso-exposure curves represent the percentage of the exposure to the skin at various distances from the patient using two different kilovoltages (60 kVp and 80 kVp) and two different field sizes (20 × 20 cm and 28 × 32 cm). The effect of kVp is illustrated in (A) for the transverse plane. The effect of beam restriction (collimation) is shown in (B) for the coronal plane. *(Reprinted with permission from Cartwright, P. [1992]. Distribution and relative intensity of scattered radiation. Radiography Today. 58[664], 12–13.)*

distance. For example, if the distance between the individual and the source of radiation is doubled, the exposure to the individual will be reduced by a factor of 4 (2^2); if the distance between the individual and the source of radiation is tripled, the exposure to the individual will be reduced by a factor of 9 (3^2). The relationship between distance and radiation exposure is explained in further detail in Chapter 11.

Shielding. Shielding is used when neither time nor distance is effective in achieving the desired degree of reduction in exposure. By interposing any material between the source of radiation and the point at which it is desired to reduce the exposure, a certain reduction in exposure will be achieved. The degree of exposure reduction will depend on the physical characteristics of the material (atomic number, density, and thickness). For fixed x-ray imaging facilities, the most common materials are lead and concrete. Such facilities are designed in accordance with specific recommendations (NCRP Report No. 49) depending on the configuration of the equipment, its intended use, and the surrounding area. Additional devices, such as mobile shields, lead-equivalent aprons, and lead-equivalent gloves should be used when it is not possible to take advantage of fixed structural barriers.

Protective Barriers

During the design of fixed x-ray imaging facilities it is necessary to ensure that the layout of the equipment and shielding of the room are such that the exposure to personnel and members of the public within adjacent areas is within the recommended equivalent dose limits. This is accomplished through the use of **structural protective barriers** made of materials having effective x-ray attenuating properties and of thicknesses sufficient to reduce exposures to the desired levels. Commonly used materials include lead sheet, concrete, lead glass, steel, and leaded acrylic.

Protective barriers are classified as either **primary barriers** or **secondary barriers.** Primary barriers can be struck by the primary or useful beam exiting the x-ray tube. Secondary barriers can only be struck by scattered and leakage radiation. The primary beam cannot be directed at secondary barriers. Secondary barriers are always thinner than primary barriers.

The design of structural shielding for x-ray imaging facilities is treated in detail in **NCRP Report No. 49, Structural Shielding Design and Evaluation for Medical Use of X Rays and Gamma Rays of Energies Up to 10 MeV.** Barrier requirements are dependent on the type of equipment, its layout within the room, the occupancy of adjacent areas, and other factors. Such shielding should always be designed by a qualified diagnostic radiological physicist.

Protective Devices

When it is not possible for personnel to remain behind a protective barrier, it is the radiographer's responsibility to ensure that **protective devices** are worn by all personnel, including physicians, nurses, aides, etc. These situations arise frequently during fluoroscopy and some mobile procedures. The most common protective devices are lead aprons and lead gloves. Special devices include leaded glasses and thyroid shields.

During fluoroscopy and mobile radiography, personnel should always wear a protective apron. Lead gloves should also be worn if the hands will be in close proximity to the primary beam. Protective aprons and gloves are usually made of lead-impregnated vinyl within the range of 0.25–1.0 mm of lead equivalency. The greater the lead equivalence, the greater the protective ability and the weight of the item. Aprons vary in weight from a few pounds to over 20 pounds depending on design and lead content. For example, a lead apron that wraps completely around the body, extending from shoulders to knees with a 1 mm lead equivalent, will possess a significant weight. This weight can be a serious consideration if personnel are expected to wear the apron for long periods of time. The protective aprons must possess a minimum of 0.5 mm lead equivalent if the peak energy of the x-ray beam is 100 kVp. Most departments use aprons with 0.5 mm lead equivalent to provide personnel with a balance between protection and weight. Lead gloves usually possess 0.25 mm of lead equivalency.

PROTECTION OF THE PATIENT

Proper radiation protection of the patient is achieved through both medical and technical decisions. Medical decisions lie with the patient and are based on the professional judgment of physicians and other practitioners of the healing arts in consultation with the patient.

Technical decisions include a number of factors that affect the amount of radiation a patient receives during a diagnostic x-ray examination. Many of these factors are under the direct control of the radiographer. It is a radiographer's responsibility to understand these factors and to minimize patient exposure while producing a satisfactory diagnostic image.

While it is desirable to minimize the exposure to a patient undergoing a radiologic procedure, it must be kept in mind that the goal of any radiologic imaging procedure is to provide information about the medical condition of the patient to aid in clinical management. Overzealous attempts to reduce patient exposure may significantly compromise the information to be obtained from the examination. Keeping these concepts in mind, the following principles should be applied to minimize exposure to the patient.

Beam Limitation

The size of the x-ray beam should always be restricted to the area of clinical interest and should never exceed the size of the image receptor. Proper collimation not only reduces patient dose but also improves the overall quality of the radiographic image because less scatter radiation is created with smaller field sizes. Ideally, evidence of proper collimation, as demonstrated by an unexposed border on all sides of the radiographic image, should be present.

Technique Selection

Technique factors for a given examination should be selected to minimize dose to the patient. High kVp/low mAs techniques are preferred to decrease patient dose. However, the selected kVp should be chosen so the required contrast in the radiographic image is not compromised as a result of a more penetrating x-ray beam or because of an increase in the amount of scatter radiation reaching the image receptor, which can impair image quality. Tube current and exposure time should be chosen to minimize the degrading effects of anatomical motion. Proper technical factor selection is the responsibility of the radiographer. This decision must take into account the information needed to make a proper diagnosis. It is important to remember that increasing kVp alone does not decrease patient dose but instead will increase patient dose. To reduce patient dose, the increase in kVp must be accompanied by a reduction in mAs to maintain an acceptable exposure.

Filtration

Filters are placed at the x-ray port to selectively absorb low-energy photons that would be absorbed by the patient and not contribute to the image. These low-energy photons would be absorbed by the patient, resulting in an increase in the patient dose. Specialized filtration is also available. It allows for additional exposure reduction by the selective removal of photons from the beam.

Aluminum is the most common filtering material used and filtration is expressed in terms of the thickness of aluminum equivalency (Al/Eq). The NCRP recommends a minimum total filtration of 2.5 mm Al/Eq for x-ray equipment operating above 70 kVp. When filtration is increased, technical factors do need to be increased to compensate for the reduction in exposure associated with the filtration. Despite the need to increase exposure to maintain exposure, the overall dose to the patient decreases with the use of filtration.

Grids

Radiographic grids are placed between the patient and the image receptor to preferentially absorb scatter radiation. Because grids absorb primary as well as scatter radiation, technical factors must be increased to produce an image of acceptable exposure. This increase in technical factors results in an increase in patient dose but image quality is significantly improved. The lowest possible grid ratio consistent with effective scatter removal should be utilized to keep patient dose as low as reasonably achievable.

A

B

FIGURE 9-2   Gonadal shields: A. flat shield, B. shadow shield.

Gonadal Shielding

Shielding the gonads (ovaries or testes) is especially important to minimize the possibility of any genetic effect on the future children of an exposed individual. Special attention should be paid to shielding the gonads of children and adults of childbearing age.

Proper collimation is important when decreasing gonadal dose, but special gonadal shields should be used any time the gonads are within 4 to 5 cm of the primary beam. The three basic types of gonadal shields are **flat contact shields, shaped contact shields,** and **shadow shields** (Figure 9-2).

Flat contact shields are usually made of various sizes of lead-impregnated vinyl and are placed between the patient's gonads and the source of radiation. During fluoroscopy, the shield usually needs to be placed underneath the patient because that is where the source of radiation is most often located. Flat contact shields may need to be secured in place to ensure correct placement for a variety of patient positions.

Shaped contact shields are cup-shaped and designed to enclose the male gonads. These shields provide maximum protection in a number of patient positions.

Shadow shields are mounted to the tube and are placed in the x-ray beam near the collimator. The collimator's light field must be precise for accurate shield placement. The device is adjusted to cast a shadow over the patient's gonads.

Image Receptors

The speed of the image receptor should be chosen to be as high as possible, consistent with the required information of the radiologic procedure. The use of film/screen image receptor systems greatly reduces patient dose by reducing the quantity of x-ray photons needed to create an image. Intensifying screens convert x-ray photons to light photons, which expose the film within the cassette. The speed of the image receptor is influenced by the type of intensifying screen and film. Intensifying screens, which provide efficient absorption of the incident radiation, allow the production of a satisfactory image with less dose to the patient. As the speed of the film/screen system is increased, patient dose is reduced; however, image sharpness is decreased as a result.

With digital image receptor systems, the speed of the system is selected based on the specific exam being performed and is not as closely linked to patient dose as film/screen image receptor systems are. With digital systems, it becomes the responsibility of the department to establish exposure ranges based on the image quality desired for a particular examination. A wide range of patient exposures can produce acceptable images, and it is the technologist's responsibility to keep the patient dose for a given exam as low as possible without compromising image quality. Gross over- or underexposure errors are not as obvious to the eye but do significantly affect image quality and require repeating the procedure.

All digital radiography systems have a method for evaluating the image receptor exposure although this varies from company to company.

Projection

The projection used for a particular exam will have an impact on patient dose to specific body tissues. For example, the lens of the eye receives a greater dose during anteroposterior (AP) projections of the cranium than it does if the posteroanterior (PA) projection is used. Or, a contrast-filled bladder will serve as a gonadal shield for females if the exposure is made with the patient in the AP projection but will not shield the ovaries in the PA projection.

Repeat Radiographs

Any time a radiograph must be repeated, patient dose increases as a direct result of the exposure from the poor radiograph. Radiographers must possess a complete understanding of the entire radiographic process to minimize repeat exposures. Radiographs generally need to be repeated for such reasons as improper exposure factor selection, poor positioning (tube/part/film alignment), poor patient instruction, or improper film processing. Radiographs should only be repeated when the quality of the radiograph compromises the diagnostic information of the procedure. It is important for the radiographer to communicate effectively with the patient and provide the patient with clear instructions during the procedure to minimize the possibility of needing to repeat the exposure.

Patient Exposure Estimates

Estimates of the exposure received by patients undergoing radiographic procedures should be available. These estimates should be developed for the average patient based on standard technique charts and measured exposure characteristics of the radiological imaging equipment. Chapter 13 provides information on calculating the patient exposure for a given procedure and describes ways in which the radiographer can minimize the exposure to the patient.

Equipment

All radiologic imaging equipment should be surveyed periodically by a diagnostic radiological physicist to assess its radiation safety characteristics. Such surveys should normally be conducted in conjunction with scheduled preventive maintenance and performance surveys and should be performed at least annually. The results of such surveys should be documented. Any deficiencies should be corrected prior to returning the equipment to clinical service.

RADIATION EXPOSURE AND PREGNANCY

A situation deserving special consideration is the possibility of radiation exposure during the early weeks of pregnancy, generally before the woman is aware of her condition. The dose to the fetus is of concern, particularly in the early stages of development when certain tissues and organs are especially sensitive to radiation. Recent studies, as summarized in the report, BEIR V, suggest the fetus may be particularly radiosensitive during the period of 8 to 15 weeks postconception. As a result, care must be taken to reduce radiation exposure to any pregnant individual, including pregnant (or potentially pregnant) patients and pregnant personnel. It is currently recommended by the NCRP that the monthly equivalent dose limit (excluding medical exposure) for the embryo not exceed 0.05 rem (50 mrem, 0.5 mSv) once the pregnancy becomes known.

NCRP Report No. 54, Medical Exposure of Pregnant and Potentially Pregnant Women, discusses the risks associated with fetal exposure: This risk is considered to be negligible at 5 rad or less when compared to other risks of pregnancy, and the risk of malformations is significantly increased above control levels only at doses above 15 rad. Therefore, the exposure of the fetus to radiation arising from diagnostic procedures would very rarely be cause, by itself, for terminating a pregnancy. If there are reasons, other than the possible radiation effects, to consider a therapeutic abortion, such reasons should be discussed with the patient by the attending physician, so that it is clear that the radiation exposure is not being used as an excuse for terminating the pregnancy (NCRP, 1977).

Pregnant Radiation Worker Exposure Standards

There are two sets of standards that are applied to pregnant radiation workers. These standards include students under the definition of those who are "occupationally" exposed to ionizing radiation because students in radiologic sciences programs are classified as students by occupation, and the exposure occurs during duties in their occupation.

The two standards complement one another. The NRC is a U.S. federal agency charged with licensing facilities and controlling the use of radioactive materials. The NCRP is an advisory group that makes recommendations for radiation protection.

NRC regulations state that the dose equivalent to the embryo/fetus during the entire pregnancy, due to the occupational exposure of a declared pregnant woman, cannot exceed 5 mSv (0.5 rem or 500 mrem). The NCRP recommends that fetal exposure be restricted to an equivalent dose limit of 0.5 mSv (0.05 rem or 50 mrem) per month. These two limits are complementary as a normal human gestation spans a 10-month period. Therefore, 0.5 mSv (0.05 rem) for 10 months equals 5 mSv (0.5 rem) for the entire gestational period. The specific citations (which are often referred to in pregnancy policies and state regulations) are NRC regulation 10CFR20.1208 and NCRP Reports No. 54, No. 116, and No. 128 with the primary recommendation issued in Report No. 116.

Declaring Pregnancy. Pregnant radiation workers are referred to in U.S. federal regulations as "declared pregnant" because a woman has the right to choose whether or not to declare her pregnancy (this was established in a U.S. Supreme Court decision in the case of United Auto Workers vs Johnson Controls). The government currently interprets this as including the right to revoke her declaration at any time. In addition, a female worker can legally declare pregnancy without documented medical proof and there is no limit on how frequently or how long a duration a person can declare she is pregnant.

Although the idea of declaring and undeclaring a pregnancy may sound bizarre, it is legitimate in the light of recent legal decisions that give women the right to choose for their embryo/fetus. This concept requires women to make a decision as to what radiation regulations will be applied to a pregnancy. Therefore, the NRC requires a voluntary declaration of pregnancy to be in writing, dated, and include the estimated month of conception. In addition, **NRC regulation 10CFR19.12 requires that instructions to women assigned to radiation exposure areas must include explanation of the right to declare or not declare pregnancy status as well as requiring that all information in NRC Regulatory Guide 8.13 be discussed.** This mandatory guide has details about the risk of radiation exposure in order to permit women to make an informed decision about declaring a pregnancy. The guide is downloadable at *www.nrc.gov.*

ALARA and Pregnancies

It has become common practice to assign declared pregnant women to areas where exposure is likely to be lower. This approach is now being discouraged in compliance with ALARA concepts of keeping all occupational exposure as low as reasonably achievable. The rationale is that any displacement of normal duties places additional radiation exposure burden on fellow workers, both male and female, which they may find unacceptable. Therefore, reassigning declared pregnant women to lower exposure areas causes increased risk to others.

In addition, because most women are not aware of pregnancy until after the most sensitive first trimester has passed, it is very possible that another as-yet-undeclared pregnant woman could be assigned additional time in a high-exposure area, thus increasing risk to her embryo/fetus at the worst possible time.

Some authors are recommending that if institutions choose to reassign declared pregnant women in opposition to recommended ALARA guidelines, all workers (or students) must clearly understand the ramifications of such a policy. To avoid legal complications, it is recommended that all occupationally exposed persons in the institution agree to the policy in writing and that this documentation include specific statements indicating agreement to be placed in higher exposure areas from time to time as necessary to accommodate those women who have declared pregnancy.

The authors of this book recognize the controversial nature of the above recommendations and acknowledge that administrative ethical beliefs about abortion are often linked to pregnancy policies in institutions. However, we believe that radiologic sciences professionals should have a part in the determination of these policies as it is their bodies and future children that are at risk. Informed decisions cannot be made without the information we have supplied above.

The Pregnant Patient

To minimize the possible exposure to an embryo in the earliest days of a pregnancy, a guideline known as the **10-day rule** was recommended by a number of advisory agencies. This guideline stated that elective abdominal x-ray examinations of fertile women should be postponed until the 10-day period following the onset of menstruation as it would be improbable that a woman would be pregnant during these 10 days. Based on the current understanding of radiobiology, this rule is now considered obsolete, primarily because the egg for the next cycle reaches maximum sensitivity during the 10-day period. The application of this guideline within the radiology department has always proven difficult.

It is now the general belief that postponement of abdominal x-ray examinations is not necessary when the physician requesting the examination has considered the entire clinical state of the patient, including the possibility of pregnancy. The potential pregnancy status of all female patients of childbearing age should always be determined; in the event of known pregnancy, steps should be taken to minimize exposure to the fetus. One way to ensure against irradiating a woman in the early stages of pregnancy is to institute elective scheduling for nonemergency procedures. In many departments, female patients of childbearing ages are asked to provide the date of their last menstrual period (LMP). If there is a concern about a possible pregnancy, the patient's exam may be rescheduled. If a radiologic exam on a pregnant patient is deemed necessary, a diagnostic radiological physicist should perform calculations to estimate the actual fetal dose.

SUMMARY

It is important to set limits for the protection of the radiation worker and the general public because of the known biological effects of exposure to ionizing radiation. Occupational radiation exposure limits pertinent to the protection of radiation workers are known as dose equivalent limits and are specified for both total body exposure and for exposure to certain tissues and organs.

To minimize dose to personnel the basic principles of time, distance, and shielding should be applied. There are two types of fixed x-ray installation protective barriers. Primary protective barriers are designed to protect against the direct exposure of the primary x-ray beam. Secondary protective barriers are designed to protect against exposure from scatter and leakage radiation. When it is not possible for personnel to remain behind a protective barrier, protective devices, such as lead aprons and lead gloves, should be worn.

To minimize patient dose while creating a diagnostic image, the radiographer must understand the factors that have a significant relationship to patient dose, such as beam limitation, technique selection, filtration, grids, gonadal shielding, image receptors, and repeat radiographs.

Care must be taken to reduce radiation exposure to any pregnant individual, including pregnant (or potentially pregnant) patients and pregnant personnel. It is currently recommended by the NCRP that the equivalent dose limit (excluding medical exposure) for the embryo-fetus not exceed 0.05 rem (0.5 mSv) in any month once the pregnancy becomes known.

REVIEW QUESTIONS

1. What is the annual effective dose limit for whole-body exposure of a radiation worker?

2. What is the cumulative effective dose limit for a 28-year-old radiation worker (in rem and mSv)?

3. Explain the ALARA concept.

4. What are the three basic principles used for minimizing an individual's exposure to ionizing radiation?

5. What is the difference between a primary and secondary protective barrier?

6. How can a radiographer minimize radiation exposure to the patient?

7. What is the equivalent dose limit for the embryo-fetus per month?

8. According to NRC regulations, how does a woman declare herself pregnant?

REFERENCES AND RECOMMENDED READING

Barrett, J. (1993). An investigation of radiation dose levels to patients during lumbar spine examinations. *Radiography Today, 59*(675), 19–22.

BEIR V health effects of exposure to low levels of ionizing radiation. (1990). Washington, DC: National Academy Press.

Boice, J. D., Mandel, J. S., & Doody, M. M. (1992). A health study of radiologic technologists. *Cancer, 69,* 586–597.

Boone, J. M., & Levin, D. C. (1991). Radiation exposure to angiographers under different fluoroscopic imaging conditions. *Radiology, 180,* 861–865.

Bushong, S. C. (2004). *Radiologic science for technologists: Physics, biology, and protection* (8th ed.). St. Louis: Elsevier/C. V. Mosby.

Butler, P., Thomas, A. W., Thompson, W. E., Wollerton, M. A., & Rachlin, J. A. (1986). Simple methods to reduce patient exposure during scoliosis radiography. *Radiologic Technology, 57*(5), 411.

Butler, P. F. (1985). Chest radiography: A survey of techniques and exposure levels currently used. *Radiology, 533.*

Caprio, M. L. (1980). The pregnant x-ray tech—providing adequate radiation safety for the fetus. *Radiologic Technology, 52*(2), 161.

Curry, T. S., Dowdey, J. E., & Murry, R. C. (1990). *Christensen's introduction to the physics of diagnostic radiology* (4th ed.). Philadelphia: Lea and Febiger.

Detain, J. (1984). Is it time to question the 10-day rule? *Radiography, 50*(592), 149–150.

Dowd, S. B. (1994). Practical radiation protection and applied radiobiology. Philadelphia: W. B. Saunders.

Dowd, S. B., & Archer, J. (1994). Radiation safety regulations: The evolution and development of standards. *Radiology Management, 16*(1), 39–45.

Floyd, C., Baker, A., Lo, J., & Ravin, C. (1992). Measurement of scatter fractions in clinical bedside radiography. *Radiology, 183*(3), 857–861.

Frank, E., Stears, J., Gray, J., Winkler, N. T., & Hoffman, A. D. (1984). Use of the P. A. projection: A method of reducing x-ray exposure to specific radiosensitive organs. *The Canadian Journal of Medical Radiation Technology, 15*(2), 63.

Fung, K. (1994). Lowering patient dose on single-phase x-ray units. *Radiologic Technology, 66*(3), 159–164.

Glaze, S., LeBlanc, A. D., & Bushong, S. C. (1984). Defects in new protective aprons. *Radiology, 217.*

Gray, J. E., Stears, J. G., & Frank, E. D. (1983). Shaped, lead-loaded acrylic filters for patient exposure reduction and image-quality improvement. *Radiology, 825.*

Gur, D., & Wald, N. (1986). Probability of causation tables and their possible implications for the practice of diagnostic radiology. *Radiology, 158,* 853–854.

Hall, E. J. (2000). *Radiobiology for the radiologist* (5th ed.). Philadelphia: J. B. Lippincott.

Hendee, W. R. (Ed.). (1984). *Health effects of low-level radiation.* Norwalk, CT: Appleton-Century-Crofts.

Hendee, W. R. (1992). Estimation of radiation risks: BEIR V and its significance for medicine. *Journal of the American Medical Association, 268,* 620–624.

Heriard, J. B., Terry, J. A., & Arnold, A. L. (1993). Achieving dose education in lumbar spine radiography. *Radiologic Technology, 65*(2), 97–103.

Hilger, M. T. J. (1983). Radiation exposure to nursing personnel from portable radiographic procedures. *Radiology Management, 6*(2), 16.

Huda, W., & Gordon, K. (1986). Radiation risks to medical radiation technologists during pregnancy. *The Canadian Journal of Medical Radiation Technology, 17*(3), 121.

International Commission on Radiation Protection. (1970). *Protection of the patient in x-ray diagnosis publication number 16.* Oxford: Pergamon Press.

Jankowski, C. B. (1984). Radiation exposure of nurses in a coronary care unit. *The Journal of Critical Care, 13*(1), 55–58.

Jeans, S. P., Faulkner, K., Love, H. G., & Bardsley, R. A. (1985). An investigation of the radiation dose to staff during cardiac radiological studies. *British Journal of Radiology, 58,* 419–428.

Mole, R. H. (1979). Radiation effects on pre-natal development and their radiological significance. *The British Journal of Radiology, 52*(614), 89–101.

Mole, R. H. (1982). Consequences of pre-natal radiation exposure for post-natal development: A review. *International Journal of Radiation Biology, 42*(1), 1–12.

Mole, R. H. (1984). The 10-day rule: A misnomer. *Radiography, 50*(593), 229–230.

National Council on Radiation Protection and Measurements (NCRP). (1976). *Structural shielding design and evaluation for medical use of x rays and gamma rays of energies up to 10 mev* (NCRP Report No. 49). Bethesda, MD: Author.

National Council on Radiation Protection and Measurements (NCRP). (1977). *Medical exposure of pregnant and potentially pregnant women* (NCRP Report No. 54). Bethesda, MD: Author.

National Council on Radiation Protection and Measurements (NCRP). (1985). *SI units in radiation protection and measurements* (NCRP Report No. 82). Bethesda, MD: Author.

National Council on Radiation Protection and Measurements (NCRP). (1987). *Ionizing radiation exposure of the population of the United States* (NCRP Report No. 93). Bethesda, MD: Author.

National Council on Radiation Protection and Measurements (NCRP). (1989). *Medical x-ray, electron beam and gamma-ray protection for energies up to 50 mev (Equipment design, performance and use)* (NCRP Report No. 102). Bethesda, MD: Author.

National Council on Radiation Protection and Measurements (NCRP). (1989). *Radiation protection for medical and allied health personnel* (NCRP Report No. 105). Bethesda, MD: Author.

National Council on Radiation Protection and Measurements (NCRP). (1990). *Implementation of the principle of ALARA for medical and dental personnel* (NCRP Report No. 107). Bethesda, MD: Author.

National Council on Radiation Protection and Measurements (NCRP). (1993). *Limitation of exposure to ionizing radiation* (NCRP Report No. 116). Bethesda, MD: Author.

National Council on Radiation Protection and Measurements (NCRP). (1994). *Considerations regarding the unintended radiation exposure of the embryo, fetus or nursing child* (NCRP Commentary No. 9). Bethesda, MD: Author.

National Council on Radiation Protection and Measurements (NCRP). (1998). *Radionuclide exposure of the embryo/fetus* (NCRP Report No. 128). Bethesda, MD: Author.

National Council on Radiation Protection and Measurements (NCRP). (2000). *Radiation protection for procedures performed outside the radiology department* (NCRP Report No. 133). Bethesda, MD: Author.

National Council on Radiation Protection and Measurements (NCRP). (2001). *Evaluation of the linear-nonthreshold dose-response model for ionizing radiation* (NCRP Report No. 136). Bethesda, MD: Author.

Noz, M. E., & Maguire, G. Q. (1985). *Radiation protection in the radiologic and health sciences* (2nd ed.). Philadelphia: Lea & Febiger.

Osborn, S. B. (1955). Radiation doses received by diagnostic x-ray workers. *British Journal of Radiology, 28,* 650–654.

Parkinson, L. (1991). Assessment of dose in computerised tomography. *Radiography Today, 57*(650), 23–28.

Ragozzino, M. W. (1986). Average fetal depth in utero: Data for estimation of fetal absorbed radiation dose. *Radiology, 158*(28), 513–515.

Rossi, R. P., Harnisch, B., & Hendee, W. R. (1982). Reduction of radiation exposure in radiography of the chest. *Radiology, 144,* 909–914.

Rueter, F. G., Conway, B. J., McCrohan, J. L., & Suleiman, O. H. (1990). Average radiation exposure values for three diagnostic radiographic examinations. *Radiology, 177*(2), 341–345.

Seeram, E., & Travis, E. L. (1997). *Radiation protection.* Baltimore: Lippincott Williams & Wilkins.

Shrimpton, P. (1994). Patient dose in CT and recommendations for reduction. *Radiography Today, 60*(683), 9–11.

Shrimpton, P. C. (1989). Monitoring the dose to patients undergoing common x-ray examinations. *Radiography Today, 54*(619), 38.

Statement from the 1985 Paris meeting of the International Commission on Radiological Protection. (1985, September). *Radiology.*

Stewart, A., & Kneale, G. W. (1970). Radiation dose effects in relation to obstetric x-rays and childhood leukemias. *Lancet, 1,* 1185–1188.

Upton, A. C. (1982). The biological effects of low-level ionizing radiation. *Scientific American, 246*(2).

Wade, P. (1994). Science and practicalities of patient dose measurement procedures. *Radiography Today, 60*(681), 13–16.

Waldron, L., & Wade, J. (1992). Skin dose reduction as part of a regional x-ray dose assessment programme. *Radiography Today, 58*(659), 9–10.

Warner, R. (1993). Using technique factors to predict patient ESE. *Radiologic Technology, 65*(1), 21–26.

Wesenberg, R. L., Blumhagen, J. D., Rossi, R. P., Hilton, S. W., Gilbert, J. M., & Nedeau, D. J. (1980). Low-dose radiography of children. *Radiologic Technology, 51*(5), 641.

Young, A. T. (1986). Surface shield: Device to reduce personnel radiation exposure. *Radiology,* 801.

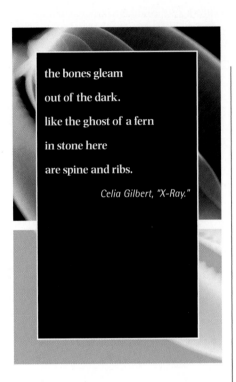

CHAPTER 10

Filtration

the bones gleam

out of the dark.

like the ghost of a fern

in stone here

are spine and ribs.

Celia Gilbert, "X-Ray."

KEY TERMS

added filtration

compensating filter

compound filter

filter

half-value layer (HVL)

inherent filtration

K-edge filter

Thoreaus filter

total filtration

trough filter

wedge filter

OBJECTIVES

Upon completion of this chapter, the student should be able to:

- Define filtration, inherent filtration, added filtration, compound filtration, compensating filtration, and total filtration.

- Explain the concept of half-value layer equivalency measurements of filtration.

- Appraise various types of filters for specific clinical situations.

- Describe the effect of filtration on the entire x-ray beam.

Filtration is the process of eliminating undesirable low-energy x-ray photons by the insertion of absorbing materials into the primary beam. When inserted properly, filtration permits the radiographer to shape the photon emission spectrum into a more useful beam. Filtration is sometimes called **hardening the beam** because it removes the low-energy (soft) photons (Figure 10-1). The primary reason for filtration is the elimination of photons that would cause increased radiation dose to the patient but would not enhance the radiographic image.

At 20 keV, about 45 percent of the incident photons will penetrate 1 cm of soft tissue but only about 0.0006 percent will penetrate 15 cm. At 50 keV, 3.5 percent of the incident photons (a significant percentage) will penetrate 15 cm. Significant soft-tissue penetration occurs between 30 and 40 keV. Although they contribute to the patient dose, low-energy photons have insufficient energy to exit the patient and make any contribution to the image. Therefore, their elimination is desirable.

 ## MEASUREMENT

Any material designed to selectively absorb photons from the x-ray beam is called a **filter.** In diagnostic radiology, filtration is typically added between the source and the patient. Aluminum is the most com-

mon filter material used, although other materials, such as glass, oil, copper, and tin are used or become filters in various instances. **Aluminum is considered the standard filtering material and all filtration can be expressed in terms of the thickness of aluminum equivalency (Al/Eq).** For example, the attachments, mirror and plastic of a collimator might be the equivalent of 0.5 mm of aluminum (Figure 10-2). This would be expressed as 0.5 mm Al/Eq.

Filtration is also expressed in terms of half-value layer. **The half-value layer (HVL) is that amount of absorbing material that will reduce the intensity of the primary beam to one-half its original value.** It is an indirect measure of the total filtration in the path of the x-ray beam. Half-value layers are usually expressed in terms of aluminum filtration equivalency; for example, HVL = 2.0 mm Al/Eq. The federal government specifies the minimum HVLs for all diagnostic x-ray tubes. Table 10-1 outlines this requirement as specified in Title 21 of the Code of Federal Regulation 21 CFR 1020.30. If

FIGURE 10-1   Effect of filtration on the x-ray beam.

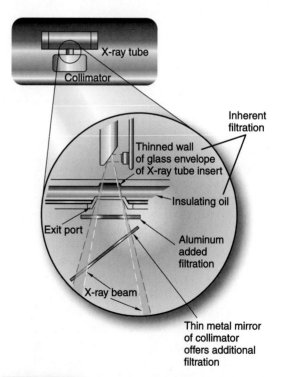

FIGURE 10-2   Total filtration of the x-ray beam.

TABLE 10-1.	Minimum Half-Value Layer (HVL) Requirements for X-Ray Systems in United States (Title 41 of 21 CFR 1020.30)

X-Ray Tube Voltage (Kilovolt Peak)		
Designed operating range	Measured operating potential	Minimum HVL (mm of aluminum)
Below 51	30	0.3
	40	0.4
	50	0.5
51 to 70	51	1.2
	60	1.3
	70	1.5
Above 70	71	2.1
	80	2.3
	90	2.5
	100	2.7
	110	3.0
	120	3.2
	130	3.5
	140	3.8
	150	4.1

the HVL is at the appropriate level, the total filtration in the x-ray tube is adequate to protect the patient from unnecessary radiation.

TYPES OF FILTRATION

Filtration occurs at various points between the x-ray tube and the image receptor. It is either *inherent* in the design of the tube or *added* between the tube and the image receptor.

Inherent Filtration

Filtration that is a result of the composition of the **tube and housing** is often called **inherent filtration** because it is a part of these structures. The thickness of the glass envelope of the tube, the dielectric oil that surrounds the tube, and the glass window of the housing all contribute to the inherent filtration. A

typical x-ray tube might have a total inherent filtration of 0.5–1.0 mm Al/Eq. Most of the inherent filtration comes from the window of the glass envelope.

Because of this, mammographic tubes with special molybdenum targets that are designed to produce lower energy photons for soft-tissue imaging often have special beryllium (atomic number 4) windows in the glass envelope to eliminate the majority of the inherent filtration. Beryllium windows can reduce the inherent filtration to 0.1 mm Al/Eq (see Chapter 42).

As tubes age they become gassy, the anode begins to pit and the glass envelope may gain a mild coating of vaporized metal. All these factors will cause an increase in the inherent filtration, thus reducing the tube efficiency. This is the reason why HVL testing of tubes is a recommended quality control procedure for evaluation of tube efficiency and age.

Added Filtration

Any filtration that occurs outside the tube and housing and before the image receptor is considered **added filtration.** Filtration materials are selected to absorb as many low-energy photons as possible while transmitting a maximum number of high-energy photons. Aluminum, with an atomic number of 13, functions very well as a low-energy absorber.

The collimator device also adds filtration to the beam and is considered to be added filtration. Collimators average 1.0 mm Al/Eq, most of which comes from the silver on the mirror situated in the beam. The mirror is designed to reflect the collimator light to simulate the primary beam field size for positioning purposes. This addition to the inherent filtration is why mammographic units often do not use collimators. The filtering effect would cause absorption of the low-energy photons that are desirable for soft-tissue imaging.

Compound Filtration

A **compound filter** uses two or more materials that complement one another in their absorbing abilities. Most compound filters are constructed so that each layer absorbs the characteristic photons created by the previous layer. For this reason, compound filters are also referred to as **K-edge filters.** Compound filters place the highest atomic number material closest to the tube and the lowest atomic number material closest to the patient. The final layer is usually aluminum, which has an atomic number of 13.

Although aluminum is the most common filtering material, copper, with an atomic number of 29, functions well for slightly higher energies. When a copper filter is used, it must be backed by an aluminum filter to absorb the 8 keV K-shell characteristic radiation produced by the copper. Copper filters should be at least 0.25 mm thick and backed with a minimum of 1 mm of aluminum.

A good example of a compound filter is the **Thoreaus filter** used in radiation therapy. This filter combines tin, copper, and aluminum, in that order. Tin has the highest atomic number (50) and is placed first in the beam. Next, a copper filter is added to absorb the 29.3 keV characteristic photons created by the tin. Finally, aluminum is added to the copper to absorb copper's characteristic photons, which would only contribute to increasing patient dose. The 1.5 keV K-shell characteristic radiation produced by the aluminum filter is absorbed in the air between the filter and the patient.

Compensation Filtration

A **compensating filter** is usually designed to solve a problem involving unequal subject densities. The goal is to add an absorber to compensate for unequal absorption within the subject, thus making the overall absorption of the primary beam more equal. This helps in producing a more uniform image receptor exposure. Compensating filters can be made of aluminum, leaded plastic trademarked under the name ClearPb™ or plastic. Even an ordinary saline solution bag can be a useful compensating filter.

The two most popular compensating filters are the **wedge filter** and the **trough filter** (sometimes called a double wedge). The thicker portions of the filter are matched to the less dense patient body parts (Figure 10-3). A wedge filter can be useful for procedures on the thoracic spine, the feet (Figure 10-4), and the lower extremities, particularly during venography and femoral angiography. A trough filter is useful to even the density differences between the mediastinum and the lungs on a chest radiograph.

Wedge filter   Trough filter

FIGURE 10-3   Compensating filters.

60 kVp	5 mAs	40" SID
No grid	400 RS	

60 kVp	5 mAs	40" SID
No grid	400 RS	

A   B

FIGURE 10-4 (A) Normal AP foot. (B) The use of a compensating wedge filter for an AP foot.

It is also possible to custom design filters by several methods. Aluminum, ClearPb,™ or plastic pieces may be attached by magnets or rods underneath the collimator to permit movement into or out of the primary beam. The advantage of the ClearPb™ is its ability to use the collimator light to project the filter position onto the patient's body. Some plastic filters, such as the boomerang filter, are designed to be placed under the patient. Radiologists may object to the use of compensating filters on the justifiable grounds that they cast artifacts onto the radiographic image.

Explorations have been made into the use of various heavy elements, including some of the rare earths, to utilize K-shell characteristic production to enhance energy ranges that are especially useful. For example, studies have been done using rare earths to increase photon emissions at the energies needed by iodine contrast agents. Difficulties in making these filtration techniques practical have kept them from becoming popular. However, very good results have been obtained for mammography by using a 0.05 mm molybdenum filter and operating the tube at a constant 35 kVp.

| TABLE 10-2. | Percent Attenuation of Monochromatic Radiation by Various Thicknesses of Aluminum Filtration |

Photon Energy (keV)	Photons Attentuated (%)			
	1 mm	2 mm	3 mm	10 mm
10	100	100	100	100
20	58	82	92	100
30	24	42	56	93
40	12	23	32	73
50	8	16	22	57
60	6	12	18	48
80	5	10	14	39
100	4	8	12	35

Reproduced with permission from T. Curry, J. Dowdey, and R. Murry. *Christensen's Physics of Diagnostic Radiology,* 4th ed. Philadelphia: Lea and Febiger, 1990.

Total Filtration

Total filtration is equal to the sum of inherent and added filtration and does not include any compound or compensating filters that may be added later. The thickness of the added filtration varies depending on the anticipated uses of the equipment. The percentage of photons attenuated decreases as photon energy increases, even when filtration is increased (Table 10-2). Note that aluminum filters of 1–3 mm absorb significant percentages of photons below the diagnostic range while permitting the vast majority to pass. The National Council on Radiation Protection and Measurements (NCRP) recommends minimum total filtration levels for diagnostic radiography, as shown in Table 10-3. These filtration levels are commonly used in the United States and correspond to International Council on Radiation Protection (ICRP) recommendations. The importance of the reduction in patient dose, as shown in Table 10-4, must not be overlooked.

EFFECT ON OUTPUT

Not only does filtration reduce the patient exposure dose by eliminating low-energy photons from the primary x-ray beam, it also removes a portion of the

| TABLE 10-3. | Recommended Minimum Total Filtration Levels |

Operating kVp	Total Filtration
Below 50 kVp	0.5 mm aluminum
50 to 70 kVp	1.5 mm aluminum
Above 70 kVp	2.5 mm aluminum

Adapted by permission from Table 3–1, National Council on Radiation Protection and Measurement. *NCRP Report No. 102, Medical X-Ray, Electron Beam and Gamma-Ray Protection for Energies Up to 50 MeV (Equipment Design, Performance and Use).* Bethesda, MD: NCRP, 1989.

| TABLE 10-4. | Comparison of Patient Exposure with Filtration |

Aluminum Filtration in mm	Entrance Skin Exposure in mR	Decrease in Exposure Dose	Increase in Exposure Required to Maintain Same Exposure
60 KVP, 18 CM PELVIS			
none	2,380		
0.5	1,850	22%	14%
1.0	1,270	47%	17%
3.0	465	80%	52%
85 KVP, 18 CM PELVIS			
none	1,225		
0.5	860	30%	0%
1.0	684	44%	12%
3.0	287	77%	34%

From E. Dale Trout, J. P. Kelley, and G. A. Cathey. The Use of Filters to Control Radiation Exposure to the Patient in Diagnostic Roentgenology. *American Journal of Roentgenology 67,* 942, 1952.

useful beam. This has a visible effect on radiographic film density. To compensate for the loss of exposure **when filtration is increased, technical factors must be increased to maintain the same image receptor exposure.**

Note that in Table 10-4 the decrease in patient dose compares very favorably with the increase necessary to maintain image receptor exposure. In other words, although the exposure needs to be increased to maintain exposure, there is a greater decrease in overall exposure to the patient.

Beyond 3.0 mm/Al filtration a point of diminishing returns is reached. The reduction in entrance skin exposure (ESE) does not warrant the tube loading increase.

SUMMARY

Filtration is the process of eliminating undesirable x-ray photons by the insertion of absorbing materials into the primary beam. Any material designed to selectively absorb photons from the x-ray beam is called a filter. Aluminum is the most common filter material used. It is considered the standard filter material and all filtering in diagnostic radiography can be expressed in terms of the thickness of aluminum equivalency (Al/Eq). The half-value layer (HVL) is that amount of absorbing material that will reduce the intensity of the primary beam to one-half its original value.

Filtration occurs at various points between the x-ray tube and the image receptor. It is either inherent in the design of the x-ray tube or added between the tube and the image receptor. Filtration that is the result of the composition of the tube and housing is often called inherent filtration because it is a part of these structures. Any filtration that occurs outside the tube and housing and before the image receptor is considered added. The collimator device adds approximately 1.0 Al/Eq to the beam.

The compound filter uses two or more materials that complement one another in their absorbing ability. A compensating filter is usually designed to solve a problem involving unequal subject density. Two common compensating filters are the wedge and the trough. Total filtration is equal to the sum of inherent and added filtration.

Not only does filtration reduce the patient exposure by eliminating low-energy photons, it also removes a portion of the useful beam and can therefore affect image receptor exposure.

REVIEW QUESTIONS

1. What is filtration?

2. What is the standard filter material used in diagnostic radiography?

3. Define half-value layer.

4. What is inherent filtration?

5. When more than one filtering material is used, as in a compound filter, how are the materials arranged in relationship to the x-ray source?

6. What are the two most common compensating filters?

7. What is total filtration?

8. How does filtration affect patient dose and beam intensity?

REFERENCES AND RECOMMENDED READING

Burns, C. B., & Renner, J. B. (1994). Molybdenum/aluminum filters perform effectively. *Radiologic Technology, 64*(4), 216–219.

Bushberg, J. T., Seibert, J. A., Leidholdt, E. M., & Boone, J. M. (2002). *The essential physics of medical imaging* (2nd ed.). Baltimore: Lippincott Williams & Wilkins.

Curry, T. S., Dowdey, J. E., & Murry, R. C. (1990). *Christensen's introduction to the physics of diagnostic radiology* (4th ed.). Philadelphia: Lea and Febiger.

Dendy, P. P., & Heaton, B. (1999). *Physics for diagnostic radiology* (2nd ed.). Bristol, England: Institute of Physics.

Dilella, D., & Albert, H. (1964). Variable thickness filters for use with 14 × 36 inch film. *Radiologic Technology, 36*(1), 1.

Ekstrand, K. E. (1979). The inverse compensating filter. *Radiology,* 201.

Feczko, P. J. (1983, December). Compensation filtration for decubitus radiography during double-contrast barium enema examination. *Radiology,* 848.

Geissberger, H. (1966). Wedge-shaped filters for improved radiography of the thoracic vertebrae and the foot. *Medical Radiography and Photography, 42*(1), 6.

Gray, J. E., Stears, J. G., & Frank, E. D. (1983). Shaped, lead-loaded acrylic filters for patient exposure reduction and image-quality improvement. *Radiology. 146,* 825–828.

Hart, J. D., Drake, P. A., & Schmugge, M. L. (1986). Plexiglas filtration in cervicocerebrae. *Applied Radiology, 15*(6), 148.

Irvin, R. (1962). Selective filtration: Effect on patient dose and radiographic quality. *Radiologic Technology, 34*(2), 51.

Jacobi, C. A. (1968). Radiation safety: More than filtration. *Radiologic Technology, 40*(2), 97.

James, N. (1983). High kilovoltage radiography using the Cincinnati filter. *Radiography, 49*(585), 210.

Jones, R., & McKenna, A. (1989). The use of saline as a compensating filter. *Radiologic Technology, 62*(2), 134–138.

Kassebaum, M. K. (1949). The use of compensating filters. *Radiologic Technology, 20*(4), 209.

Kelsey, C. A. (1986). Chest radiographs obtained with shaped filters: Evaluation by observer performance test. *Radiology,* 653.

Kohn, M. L., Gooch, A. W., & Keller, W. S. (1988). Filters for radiation reduction: A comparison. *Radiology,* 255.

McEnerney, P. (1951). The value of compensating filters in roentgenography including the double filter technique. *Radiologic Technology, 23*(1), 29.

National Council on Radiation Protection and Measurements (NCRP). (1989). *NCRP Report No. 102: Medical X-ray, electron beam and gamma-ray protection for energies up to 50 MeV (equipment design, performance and use).* Bethesda, MD: Author.

Stears, J. G., Gray, J. E., Webbles, W. E., & Frank, E. D. (1986). The variable filter dial. *Radiologic Technology, 57*(6), 542.

Trout, E. D., Kelley, J. P., & Cathey, G. A. (1952). The use of filters to control radiation exposure to the patient in diagnostic roentgenology. *American Journal of Roentgenology, 67,* 946–963.

Wolbarst, A. B. (1993). *Physics of radiology.* Norwalk, CT: Appleton & Lange.

CHAPTER 11

The Prime Factors

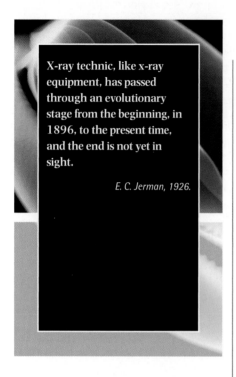

X-ray technic, like x-ray equipment, has passed through an evolutionary stage from the beginning, in 1896, to the present time, and the end is not yet in sight.

E. C. Jerman, 1926.

KEY TERMS

15 percent rule
direct square law
milliamperage (mA)
milliamperage-
     second (mAs)
penetrability
prime factor
reciprocity law
x-ray quality
x-ray quantity

OBJECTIVES

Upon completion of this chapter, the student should be able to:

- Explain the relationships between milliamperage (mA), exposure time, mAs, and x-ray emission.

- State the reciprocity law.

- Calculate mAs when given mA and exposure time, mA when given mAs and exposure time, and exposure time when given mAs and mA.

- Explain the relationship between kVp and x-ray emission.

- State the 15 percent rule.

- Calculate the new kVp value needed to maintain receptor exposure and radiographic film density when changes are made in mAs, using the 15 percent rule.

- Explain the relationship between distance and x-ray emission.

- State the inverse square law.
- Calculate x-ray emission (mR) when distance is changed.

- Calculate the mAs needed to maintain receptor exposure and radiographic film density when changes are made in distance, using the exposure (density) maintenance formula.

THE PRIME FACTORS

The emission of x-ray photons from an x-ray tube is controlled by a number of factors. Those factors related to tube design and construction have been covered in previous chapters and include tube housing, target material, filtration, and voltage waveform. Three factors that affect x-ray emission are under the direct control of the radiographer. These are called the **prime factors.** They are milliamperage-second (mAs), kilovoltage (kVp), and distance (d).

The x-ray beam can be described in terms of both its quantity and its quality. **X-ray quantity** is a measure of the number of x-ray photons in the useful beam. It is also called x-ray output, intensity, or exposure. Recall that the unit of measurement of x-ray quantity is the *roentgen (R)*. The factors that directly affect x-ray quantity are milliamperage-second (mAs), kilovoltage (kVp), distance (d), and filtration. **X-ray quality** is a measurement of the penetrating ability of the x-ray beam. Penetrability describes the distance an x-ray beam travels in matter. High-energy x-ray photons travel farther in matter than low-energy photons and are therefore more penetrating. Highly penetrating x-rays are termed hard x-rays and low penetrating x-rays are called soft x-rays. X-ray quality is numerically represented by the **half-value layer (HVL).** The half-value layer of an x-ray beam is that thickness of absorbing material needed to reduce the x-ray intensity (quantity) to half its original value. The factors that directly affect x-ray quality are kilovoltage and filtration.

The factors that control the quantity and/or quality of x-ray emission are the prime factors and filtration (Table 11-1). Filtration is not something the radiographer controls from exposure to exposure.

TABLE 11-1.	Factors Affecting X-Ray Emission	
Quantitative Factors	**Qualitative Factors**
Milliamperage–second	Kilovoltage
Kilovoltage	Filtration
Distance	
Filtration	

MILLIAMPERAGE-SECOND (MAS)

Milliamperage (mA) is a measurement of x-ray tube current—the number of electrons crossing the tube from cathode to anode per second. Recall that an ampere is equal to an electric charge of 1 coulomb flowing through a conductor per second. The coulomb is equal to 6.3×10^{18} electron charges. Therefore, an ampere equals a flow of 6.3×10^{18} electrons per second and a milliampere would equal 6.3×10^{15} electrons per second. As mA increases, so does the number of electrons which are able to cross the tube to reach the x-ray target. **Milliamperage is directly proportional to tube current.** As the mA doubles, so does the number of electrons able to cross the tube. The number of electrons reaching the target is also controlled by the length of time the tube is energized. Remember that mA is the number of electrons **per second.** This means that changes in the length of time of exposure will affect the total number of electrons flowing from cathode to anode. X-ray exposure time is measured in *seconds.* Like mA, **exposure time is directly proportional to the number of electrons crossing the tube and is therefore directly proportional to the number of x-rays created.** This is the x-ray quantity.

The number of x-rays that will be created at the target is a product of the number of electrons crossing the tube (tube current) and how long the electrons are allowed to cross (exposure time). **Milliamperage-second (mAs)** is the unit used to describe the product of tube current and exposure time. This simple relationship is described by the equation mA $\times$ s = mAs. Milliamperage-second (mAs) is the primary controller of x-ray quantity. X-ray quantity is directly proportional to mAs. This means that as mAs doubles, x-ray exposure (measured in roentgens) doubles; as mAs triples, x-ray exposure triples and so forth.

If an x-ray control panel is set at 100 mA and 0.05 (1/20) second, the mAs would be 100 $\times$ 0.05 or 5 mAs. If either the mA or the exposure time is doubled, the mAs will double, that is, 200 mA at 0.05 second equals 10 mAs, as does 100 mA at 0.1 (1/10) second. This means that a number of possible settings on the x-ray control can all yield the same x-ray exposure. For example, 10 mAs can be set using any of the following technical factors:

$$50 \text{ mA} \times 0.2 \text{ (1/5) second} = 10 \text{ mAs}$$
$$100 \text{ mA} \times 0.1 \text{ (1/10) second} = 10 \text{ mAs}$$
$$200 \text{ mA} \times 0.05 \text{ (1/20) second} = 10 \text{ mAs}$$

Obviously, a number of other possibilities exist as well. This relationship can be described in the equation $mA_1S_1 = mA_1S_1$. Because mA and exposure time can be manipulated to achieve the same mAs, **it is best to think in terms of mAs when establishing technical factors.** It is important, for technical factor conversions, that the technologist be able to manipulate the mA and time to arrive at the proper mAs for a particular examination.

EXAMPLES: Given the following mA and exposure time values, calculate the mAs.

200 mA $\times$ 0.083 second = _____ mAs
100 mA $\times$ 2/5 second = _____ mAs

Answers:

200 mA $\times$ 0.083 second = 16.6 mAs
100 mA $\times$ 2/5 second = 40 mAs

EXAMPLES: Given the following mAs and mA values, calculate the exposure time.

75 mAs = 100 mA $\times$ _____ second
15 mAs = 300 mA $\times$ _____ second

Answers:

75 mAs = 100 mA $\times$ 0.75 (3/4) second
15 mAs = 300 mA $\times$ 0.05 (1/20) second

EXAMPLES: Given the following mAs and exposure time values, calculate the mA.

60 mAs = 0.3 (3/10) second $\times$ _____ mA
75 mAs = 0.15 (3/20) second $\times$ _____ mA

Answers:

60 mAs = 0.3 (3/10) second $\times$ 200 mA
75 mAs = 0.15 (3/20) second $\times$ 500 mA

Density Relationship to mAs Using Film/Screen Image Receptor Systems

Radiographic film density is the degree of blackening of an x-ray film. It is created by deposits of black metallic silver on an x-ray film that has been exposed to light or x-ray and then processed. On the radiographic image, the densities are the result of an x-ray exposure to the film and intensifying screens. Recall that as mAs is increased, x-ray exposure will increase proportionally.

While the relationship between mAs and exposure (mR) is a directly proportional one, the relationship of these two factors to film density is much more complex. Film density is determined by the amount of silver deposition in the emulsion due to the film type, exposure conditions, exposure (mR), and processing. A DlogE sensitometric curve expresses the relationship between exposure and density, with log relative exposure plotted on the x-axis and density (D) plotted on the y-axis. The relationship between exposure and density determines the shape and position of the DlogE curve for a given film under specific processing conditions. This relationship is described in detail in Chapter 21, Sensitometry.

If the exposure to a film is increased, the density to that film will increase until the point where the film reaches its maximum density (D_{max}). Since density is primarily determined by the amount of exposure a film receives, and since exposure is directly proportional to mAs, **mAs is used as the primary controller of radiographic film density.** As mAs increases, x-ray exposure increases proportionally; radiographic density also increases. The direct proportional relationship between mAs and exposure is used to calculate mAs changes necessary to maintain consistent film density when one or more technical factors are altered. By maintaining a specific exposure relative to the speed of the image receptor, consistent film density can be achieved.

The relationship of a film's reaction to exposure was described in 1875 by Bunsen and Roscoe, who studied the reaction of photographic film to light and stated that the reaction of a photographic film to light is equal to the product of the intensity of the light and the duration of the exposure. This concept is known as the **reciprocity law.** When applied to x-rays, the reciprocity law can be restated as the density on an x-ray film should remain unchanged as long as the intensity and duration of the x-ray exposure (controlled by mAs) remains unchanged. This law generally is true for x-ray films exposed using intensifying screens, because most of the film's exposure is from light and not x-rays. The reciprocity law fails for exposures made at extremely short exposure times (less than 1/100 second) or extremely long exposure times (more than a second). Under these circumstances, densities will be somewhat less than the exposures. Reciprocity law failure is not very significant in diagnostic radiology because exposure times are seldom at those extremes.

Radiographic film density should remain unchanged as long as the total exposure to the film remains unchanged. If the mAs used to create one image is the same as the mAs used to create a second image of the same structure, then both images should have the same radiographic density. As long as mAs is constant, any combination of mA and exposure time values will create the same density. The radiographs in Figures 11-1A and 11-1B illustrate this point. Remember, accurate results will depend on using equipment that is properly calibrated.

Equipment testing is an important part of a quality control program for the radiology department.

Radiographic film density will increase to D_{max} when mAs increases and will decrease to near zero when mAs decreases. Either the mA or the exposure time or both may be increased or decreased to cause an increase or decrease in the mAs. The radiographs in Figure 11-1B and Figure 11-1C illustrate this point. When mAs is increased, the radiographic density on the film is increased. The resulting film is darker than the original. If the mAs is reduced by half, the resulting film will be lighter than the original image.

Milliamperage-second (mAs) is the primary controlling factor that will affect the x-ray quantity and radiographic density. The appropriate mAs should be selected to achieve an acceptable radiograph. The technologist is usually in control of the mAs selection. However, the equipment may exert automatic control when the technologist is using an automatic exposure control system, a computerized exposure system, or falling load generators.

KILOVOLTAGE (KVP)

Kilovoltage (kVp) controls both the quantity and quality of the x-ray beam. **Increasing the kilovoltage on an x-ray control panel will cause an increase in the speed and energy of the electrons applied across the x-ray tube.** The space charge compensator corrects for the increase in speed of the electrons to maintain a constant number of electrons/second. The increased energy of the electrons results in the production of x-ray photons with greater energy. As x-ray photon energy increases, the penetrating ability of the photon increases. Kilovoltage affects the *quantity* of the x-ray beam because **more** interactions occur at the target as kVp increases, and it affects the *quality* of the x-ray beam because each electron has more energy, resulting in a beam with greater **penetrability.**

The quantity (intensity) of x-ray photons increases very quickly with increases in kVp. X-ray quantity is **approximately** directly proportional to the square of the ratio of the change in kVp. This

| 60 kVp | 3.2 mAs | 40" SID |
| No grid | 400 RS | 5.10 mR |

A

| 60 kVp | 3.2 mAs | 40" SID |
| No grid | 400 RS | 5.04 mR |

B

C

| 60 kVp | 6.4 mAs | 40" SID |
| No grid | 400 RS | 10.20 mR |

FIGURE 11-1 These three radiographs demonstrate the effect of mAs on radiographic film density. Although the mA and time may vary, if the mAs remain unchanged, then radiographic film density will be the same. A and B have the same mAs although A was exposed at 80 mA and 0.04 sec, while B was exposed at 160 mA and 0.02 sec. When the mAs is doubled, the exposure to the film doubles (C).

means that as kVp is doubled, the amount of x-ray photons increases approximately four times. Although this can be mathematically expressed, this formula would have no practical application because it does not take into account the fact that changes in kVp have a significant effect on the penetrability of the beam.

Density Relationship to kVp Using Film/Screen Image Receptor Systems

Both the quantity and quality of the x-ray beam will vary significantly with changes in the kilovoltage applied across the x-ray tube. As a result, kVp has a tremendous impact on radiographic density (Figures 11-2A and 11-2B). In addition, because changes in kilovoltage create changes in beam penetrability, kVp is the primary controller of the differences in radiographic densities. This is known as contrast. An increase in kVp causes an increase in penetrability, which will result in an image with less contrast. For the present discussion, the effect of kVp on density will be detailed. Contrast is discussed in Chapter 29.

Research was done to determine a practical formula to take into account kVp's effect on both x-ray quantity and quality. This resulted in the **15 percent rule.** The intent of this rule was to provide a guide for radiographers to maintain exposure to the image receptor. For film/screen image receptors, this will maintain radiographic film density. **The 15 percent rule states that an increase in kVp by 15 percent will cause a doubling in exposure, the same effect as doubling the mA or doubling exposure time.** The reverse is also true. If kVp is decreased by 15 percent, exposure will be reduced by one half (see Figure 11-2B and Figure 11-2C). Because both the amount and penetrability of x-ray photons increase with increases in kVp, the effect of changes in kVp will vary from low kVps to high kVps. In other words, a smaller change in kVp will have a greater impact on x-ray emission in the lower kVp ranges than in the higher kVp ranges. For example, 15 percent of 40 kVp is 6, while 15 percent of 80 kVp is 12. Exposure will nearly double when kVp is changed from 40 to 46 kVp. At 80 kVp, an increase in 12 kVp is needed to approximately double the exposure.

> **EXAMPLE:** A radiograph of the pelvis is produced using 25 mAs at 70 kVp. What kVp would be needed to double the exposure?
>
> **Answer:**
>
> 15 percent of 70 kVp = 10.5 kVp
> 70 + 10.5 = 80.5 or 81 kVp

Since kVp is expressed as a whole number, answers should be rounded to the nearest whole number.

While kVp has a tremendous impact on exposure to the image receptor and therefore on radiographic film density, **kVp adjustments should not be used to control radiographic film density.** The selection of a kVp range for specific radiographic procedures is determined by the desired contrast for the image. This is discussed in Unit IV.

DISTANCE

The intensity of x-rays varies greatly with changes in distance. Just as the intensity of light from a light bulb will decrease the further one moves from the source, so will x-ray photons spread out from their source at the x-ray tube target. As a result, the x-ray intensity will decrease as the distance from the tube is increased. The measurement of the x-ray intensity is obtained using a dosimeter. X-ray intensity (exposure) is measured in roentgens (R) or, more commonly in diagnostic radiology, in milliroentgens (mR).

From the point of origin of the x-ray beam at the tube target, the beam begins to diverge. The x-ray photons are most concentrated at the target and from there they spread out in all directions. Those photons that exit the tube port constitute the primary, useful beam. As the useful beam spreads and widens, x-ray intensity or quantity begins to diminish. The actual number of photons created remains unchanged but the distribution of the photons varies with the distance. The farther from their source, the lower will be the quantity of photons within a given area.

The relationship of x-ray quantity to distance is described in the inverse square law. **The inverse**

70 kVp	1.0 mAs	40" SID
No grid	400 RS	4.10 mR

A

60 kVp	1.0 mAs	40" SID
No grid	400 RS	2.34 mR

B

C

60 kVp	2.0 mAs	40" SID
No grid	400 RS	4.42 mR

FIGURE 11-2 These three radiographs demonstrate the effect of decreasing kVp on radiographic film density. A and B show the effect of increasing kVp on film density. In C, density and exposure are maintained by applying the 15 percent rule.

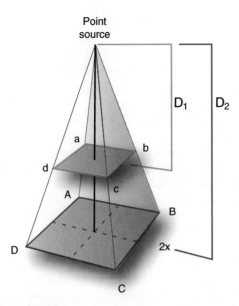

Point source

D_1 D_2

a

b

d

c

A

B

D

2x

C

FIGURE 11-3 The inverse square law states that the intensity of radiation at a given distance from a point source is inversely proportional to the square of the distance. The lower surface area (ABCD) is twice as far from the source of radiation and is four times (2^2) the surface area of the upper surface area (abcd).

square law states that the intensity of radiation at a given distance from the point source is inversely proportional to the square of the distance. The inverse square law requires an understanding of some basic rules of geometry. In Figure 11-3 the diverging lines represent the x-ray beam diverging from a collimated source. At a distance of 36 inches (D_1), the x-ray beam covers a square area (abcd). Each side has a given dimension (x) so the area of square abcd would equal x times x or x^2. If the distance is increased to 72 inches (D_2), the sides of the second square (ABCD) are now twice as long, or 2x. The area of square ABCD would be 2x times 2x or $4x^2$. A doubling of the distance has increased the area of the square by four times.

X-ray photons falling in square abcd are spread out over an area four times as large by the time it reaches square ABCD. The number of photons re-

mains the same, but they are now spread over an area four times larger. A dosimeter in square abcd would measure four times more than a dosimeter in square ABCD. For example, if a dosimeter in square abcd measures 100 mR, a dosimeter in square ABCD would measure 25 mR, or four times less.

Thus, the intensity or quantity of photons decreases with increased distance for a given area, which is an inverse relationship. More specifically, the relationship is inversely proportional to the square of the distance change. If the distance increases by a factor of three, the intensity would decrease by a factor of 3^2, or nine times.

The inverse square law can be used to calculate changes in intensity that occur as a result of changes in distance. The mathematical expression of the law is:

$$\frac{I_1}{I_2} = \frac{D_2^2}{D_1^2}$$

where: I_1 = original intensity
I_2 = new intensity
D_1 = original distance
D_2 = new distance

The formula can also be expressed as:

$$I_1 D_1^2 = I_2 D_2^2$$

In order to calculate any of the four factors, three of the four must be known. The equation can then be rearranged to place the unknown factor alone on one side of the equal sign.

EXAMPLE: An x-ray exposure of 240 mR is recorded at a distance of 20 inches. If the same technical factors are used, what will the exposure be if the distance is increased to 40 inches?

Answer:

$$\frac{240}{I_2} = \frac{40^2}{20^2}$$

$$I_2 = \frac{240 \times 20^2}{40^2}$$

$$I_2 = \frac{240 \times 400}{1,600}$$

$$I_2 = 60 \text{ mR}$$

EXAMPLE: An x-ray exposure of 400 mR is recorded at a distance of 72 inches. If the same technical factors are used, what will the exposure be if the distance is decreased to 40 inches?

Answer:

$$\frac{400}{I_2} = \frac{40^2}{72^2}$$

$$I_2 = \frac{400 \times 72^2}{40^2}$$

$$I_2 = \frac{400 \times 5,184}{1,600}$$

$$I_2 = 1,296 \text{ mR}$$

The inverse square law should be used when calculating the relationships between distance and x-ray intensity (mR).

Density Relationship to Distance Using Film/Screen Image Receptor Systems

Since distance has an effect on x-ray intensity (exposure), it will in turn affect radiographic density. **As the distance increases, intensity decreases, which causes a decrease in exposure to the image receptor** (Figures 11-4A and 11-4B). For film/screen image receptors, this will maintain radiographic film density. The reverse is also true. As the distance decreases, intensity increases, which in turn causes an increase in radiographic film density.

A practical application of the inverse square law is found in a formula which is used to compensate for the film density changes that occur when distance is changed. The formula is sometimes known as the **exposure (film density) maintenance formula** and is based on the principle of the inverse square law. This formula is a **direct square law.** A direct relationship is necessary to compensate for the changes in intensity and film density.

Since mAs is the primary controller of x-ray intensity and radiographic film density, mAs can be adjusted to compensate for changes in distance. For example, an acceptable chest film results from an exposure taken using four mAs at 100 kVp at a 72-inch distance. A second film must be taken supine at

a 36-inch distance. If the same technical factors are used, the inverse square law tells us that when the distance is decreased by a factor of 2, the intensity (exposure) will increase by a factor of 4. The second film will be too dark if the technical factors are not adjusted. The mAs can be adjusted to compensate for the distance change. The exposure (film density) maintenance formula can be used to determine the compensation necessary for any change in distance (see Figure 11-4B and Figure 11-4C). It is a direct square law because mAs should increase proportionally to the square of the change when distance increases, and mAs should decrease proportionally to the square of the change when distance is decreased. In the example above, if the distance decreases by a factor of two (72 inches to 36 inches), the mAs should be reduced by a factor of 2^2, or 4. The new mAs would be 1/4 the original, or one mAs. Four mAs at 72 inches will produce the same exposure as 1 mAs at 36 inches, provided all other factors remain the same.

The exposure (film density) maintenance formula is:

$$\frac{mAs_1}{mAS_2} = \frac{D_1^2}{D_2^2}$$

where: mAs_1 = original mAs
mAs_2 = new mAs
D_1 = original distance
D_2 = new distance

The same formula can be expressed as:

$$mAs_2 = \frac{mAs_1 \times D_2^2}{D_1^2}$$

These formulas have very direct applications to radiography because they provide the radiographer with a means for adjusting mAs to maintain film density when changes are made in distance for a given radiographic procedure.

EXAMPLE: An acceptable radiograph of the abdomen is taken using 25 mAs at 80 kVp at a distance of 40 inches. A second radiograph is requested to be taken at 56 inches. What mAs should be used to produce an acceptable radiograph if the distance is increased to 56 inches?

| 60 kVp | 2 mAs | 36" SID |
| No grid | 400 RS | 5.64 mR |

| 60 kVp | 2.0 mAs | 72" SID |
| No grid | 400 RS | 1.21 mR |

A

B

C

| 60 kVp | 8 mAs | 72" SID |
| No grid | 400 RS | 6.02 mR |

FIGURE 11-4 These three radiographs demonstrate the effect of distance on radiographic film density. A and B show the effect of increasing distance on film density. In C, density and exposure are maintained by applying the exposure (film density) maintenance direct square law.

Answer:

$$mAs_2 = \frac{25 \times 56^2}{40^2}$$

$$mAs_2 = \frac{25 \times 3,136}{1,600}$$

$$mAs_2 = 49 \text{ mAs}$$

Changes in distance will create changes in the x-ray intensity and the radiographic density. The density maintenance formula can be used to compensate for the effect that changes in distance will have on the density of the radiographic image. The radiographs of Figures 11-4A and C demonstrate the application of the direct square law for density maintenance.

DENSITY RELATIONSHIP TO mAs, kVp, AND DISTANCE USING DIGITAL IMAGE RECEPTOR SYSTEMS

With digital image detector systems, the traditional relationship between the image quality properties of density and contrast to mAs, kVp, and distance does not exist. Image density and contrast can be discussed if the digital image is printed to hardcopy film. It is possible to change the mAs, kVp, and dis-

tance and have no effect on the density (brightness) or contrast on the display monitor. This topic is covered in more detail in Unit IV that discusses image analysis. In digital image receptor systems, density and contrast are controlled primarily through post-processing parameters.

Despite the ability to control density and contrast through post-processing parameters, it is still critical to provide the digital image receptor with an appropriate exposure for a given procedure. Digital image receptors can respond to a wide range of exposures, from as low as 0.01 mR up to 100 mR. Extremely low and extremely high exposures do not produce acceptable image quality. Most acceptable images can be produced using approximately 1 mR exposure to the receptor.

Setting the appropriate mAs, kVp, and distance is the responsibility of the radiographer. These prime factors control the exposure to the image receptor. The radiographer should select the kVp based on the desired contrast, and adjust mAs to provide the appropriate total exposure to the receptor. Appropriate kVp selection is just as important with digital systems because the selected kVp will control subject contrast (signal differences to the digital detector). Distance is generally set based on the desired beam geometry. It can be used to adjust exposure but this is not generally done. Once a distance is selected based on a given procedure (e.g., chest radiography done at 72 inches and rib radiography done at 40 inches distance), mAs can be appropriately adjusted to maintain an acceptable exposure to the receptor.

SUMMARY

Prime factors are under the direct control of the radiographer and have a significant impact on x-ray photon emission from the tube. The prime factors are milliamperage-second (mAs), kilovoltage (kVp), and distance (d). X-ray emission can be described in terms of both its quantity (amount) and quality (penetrability). X-ray quantity is affected by mAs, distance, kVp, and filtration. X-ray quality is affected by kVp and filtration.

Milliamperage-second (mAs) is directly proportional to the number of x-ray photons created in the tube. Kilovoltage affects both quantity and quality, and its relationship to x-ray emission is not as easily described. Kilovoltage is approximately proportional to the square of the ratio of the change in kVp. Therefore, if kVp is doubled, the x-ray quantity would increase by a factor of four. This does not, however, take into account the increased penetrability of the beam with increasing kVp. As a result, radiographic density is more significantly affected. To maintain exposure with changes in kVp, the 15 percent rule can be applied. The 15 percent rule states that an increase in kVp by 15 percent will cause an approximate doubling of the exposure. To maintain density, if kVp is increased by 15 percent, the

mAs must be reduced to one-half its original value. The distance from the actual focal spot to the image receptor is the third prime factor. The quantity of x-ray photons is inversely proportional to the square of the distance. As distance increases, exposure will decrease in an inverse proportion to the square of the change in the distance.

REVIEW QUESTIONS

1. What are the three prime factors that affect x-ray emission?

2. What is the unit of measurement for x-ray quantity?

3. Define an ampere.

4. What is the relationship between mAs and radiographic film density?

5. What effect does increased kVp have on the speed and energy of the electrons in the x-ray tube?

6. What is the relationship between kVp and radiographic film density?

7. State the inverse square law.

8. What is the relationship between distance and radiographic film density?

REFERENCES AND RECOMMENDED READING

Ball, J. L., & Moore, A. D. (1997). *Essential physics for radiographers* (3rd ed.). Oxford: Blackwell Scientific.

Bushberg, J. T., Seibert, J. A., Leidholdt, E. M., & Boone, J. M. (2002). *The essential physics of medical imaging* (2nd ed.). Baltimore: Lippincott Williams & Wilkins.

Bushong, S. C. (2004). *Radiologic science for technologists: Physics, biology, and protection* (8th ed.). St. Louis, MO: Elsevier/Mosby.

Carroll, Q. B. (2003). *Fuchs's radiographic exposure, processing, and quality control* (7th ed.). Springfield, IL: Charles C Thomas.

Curry, T. S., Dowdey, J. E., & Murry, R. C. (1990). *Christensen's introduction to the physics of diagnostic radiology* (4th ed.). Philadelphia: Lea and Febiger.

Dendy, P. P., & Heaton, B. (1999). *Physics for diagnostic radiology* (2nd ed.). Oxford: Institute for Physics.

Fodor, J., & Malott, J. C. (1992). *The art and science of medical radiography* (7th ed.). St. Louis, MO: Catholic Health Association of the United States.

Fuchs, A. W. (1950). The rationale of radiographic exposure. *Radiologic Technology, 22*(2), 62.

Jerman, E. C. (1926). An analysis of the end-result: The radiograph. *Radiology, 6*, 59–62.

Johns, H. E., & Cunningham, J. R. (1983). *The physics of radiology* (4th ed.). Springfield, IL: Charles C Thomas.

Selman, J. (2000). *The fundamentals of x-ray physics and radiobiology for the radiologic technologist* (9th ed.). Springfield, IL: Charles C Thomas.

CHAPTER 12

X-Ray Interactions

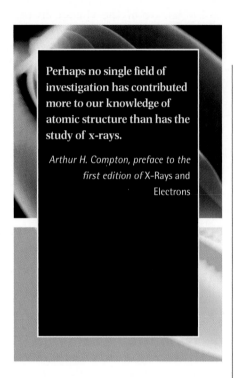

Perhaps no single field of investigation has contributed more to our knowledge of atomic structure than has the study of x-rays.

Arthur H. Compton, preface to the first edition of X-Rays and Electrons

KEY TERMS

annihilation reaction
attenuation
backscatter radiation
characteristic photon
coherent scatter
Compton effect
Compton (or recoil) electron

Compton scattered photon
Compton scattering
negatron
pair production
photoelectric absorption
photodisintegration

photoelectron
positron
radiation fog
scattering
secondary radiation

OBJECTIVES

Upon completion of this chapter, the student should be able to:

- Define attenuation.
- Explain the interactions between x-rays and matter in the following:

  photoelectric absorption

  coherent scattering

  Compton scattering

  pair production

  photodisintegration

- Describe the relationship between x-ray interactions and technical factor selections.

X-RAY INTERACTION WITH MATTER

When an x-ray beam passes through matter, it undergoes a process called **attenuation**. Attenuation is the reduction in the number of x-ray photons in the beam, and subsequent loss of energy, as the beam passes through matter (Figure 12-1).

Attenuation is the result of x-ray photons interacting with matter and losing energy through these interactions. While some photons will pass through matter and not interact, an x-ray photon can interact with the whole atom, an orbital electron, or directly with the nucleus. This will depend on the energy of the photon. Low-energy photons are most likely to interact with the whole atom, intermediate-

energy photons generally interact with orbital electrons while very high-energy photons, such as those used for radiation therapy, are capable of interacting with the nucleus. In the diagnostic x-ray range, the interactions are most commonly with orbital electrons.

To fully understand x-ray interactions with matter, it is important to recall the structure of the atom. The center of the atom is a positively charged nucleus containing protons and neutrons. The negatively charged electrons are in orbital paths around the nucleus. The energy required to remove an electron from a shell is termed the binding energy of the shell. The K-shell electrons possess the highest binding energy for a given atom and binding energies decrease progressively for successive shells. Not only is the binding energy characteristic of a given shell,

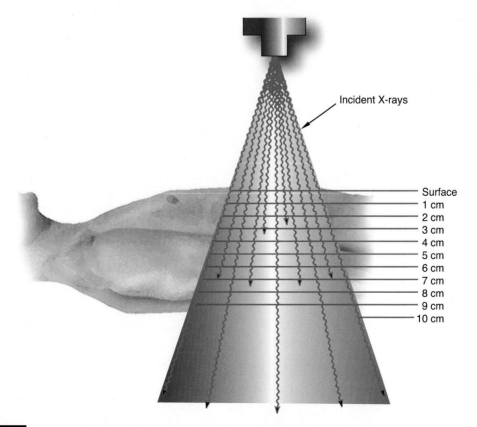

Incident X-rays

Surface
1 cm
2 cm
3 cm
4 cm
5 cm
6 cm
7 cm
8 cm
9 cm
10 cm

FIGURE 12–1   An x-ray beam undergoes attenuation as it passes through matter.

it is also specific to a given atom. K-shell electrons are more tightly bound to the nucleus in high atomic number elements. For example, the binding energy for the K-shell of tungsten (Z = 74) is approximately 70 keV while the binding energy for the K-shell of calcium (Z = 20) is only about 4 keV. The average atom in the soft tissue of the body has an approximate K-shell binding energy of only 0.5 keV. Therefore, **the higher the atomic number of an element, the more energy will be required to remove a K-shell electron from the atom.**

Because electrons that are further from the nucleus are not bound as tightly, they require less energy to remove them from their orbit. Therefore, they possess a greater total energy. Electrons that are closer to the nucleus are bound more tightly and require more energy to remove them from their position. If a free (unbound) electron is assumed to possess a total energy (ability to do work) of zero, then a bound electron would have a total energy of zero minus the binding energy. **The further an electron is from the nucleus, the higher the total energy of the electron will be.** This means that K-shell electrons possess less (more negative) total energy than outer shell electrons. As a result, when an outer shell electron moves into an inner shell, it will release energy equal to the difference between the binding energies of the two shells.

Electrons in the K-shell have the lowest energy total with the highest binding energy, and with each successive shell, **total electron energies increase and binding energies decrease.** These concepts are particularly important to the understanding of x-ray interactions with matter.

There are five basic interactions between x-rays and matter:

1. Photoelectric absorption
2. Coherent scattering
3. Compton scattering
4. Pair production
5. Photodisintegration

With each of these interactions the x-ray photons either interact and change direction, a process called **scattering,** or are absorbed by the atom. When a photon is absorbed, all of the energy of the photon is transferred to the matter and the photon

no longer exists. If a photon interacts and scatters, the photon still exists but usually possesses less energy than before the interaction. Partial energy from the photon is transferred to the matter during the interaction and the lower-energy photon then continues along its new path until again it either interacts and scatters or is absorbed. One photon may scatter several times before it is finally absorbed completely by the matter. The likelihood of one interaction occurring over another varies, depending on the incident photon's energy and the atomic number of the matter. Certain interactions, pair production and photodisintegration, for example, occur only at very high photon energy ranges, while coherent scatter is most predominant in very low photon energy ranges.

PHOTOELECTRIC ABSORPTION

Photoelectric absorption results when an x-ray photon interacts with an inner-shell electron. This interaction is most likely to occur when the incident x-ray photon possesses a slightly greater energy than the binding energy of the electrons in the inner (K or L) shells. The incident photon ejects the electron from its inner shell and is totally absorbed in the interaction (Figure 12-2). The result is an ionized atom, because of the missing inner-shell electron, and an ejected electron, called a **photoelectron.** The photoelectron travels with kinetic energy, which is equal to the difference between the incident photon and the binding energy of the inner-shell electron. This is mathematically expressed in the equation:

$$E_i = E_b + E_{ke}$$

where: E_i = energy of the incident photon
E_b = binding energy of the electron
E_{ke} = kinetic energy of the photoelctron

The incident photon needs an energy which is slightly greater than the binding energy of the electron for the interaction to occur. Since most of the atoms of the body are very low atomic number elements, the binding energies of the K-shell electrons

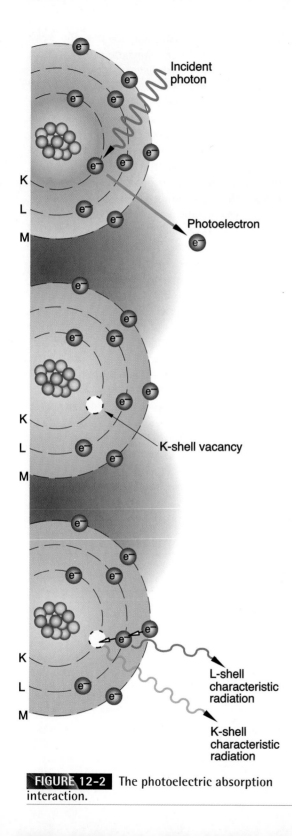

are very low. For example, the K-shell binding energy for carbon is approximately 0.28 keV and oxygen is 0.53 keV. The K-shell binding energies of elements which are important in diagnostic radiology are listed in Table 12-1. Most photoelectric interactions in the body result in the majority of the incident photon energy being given to the kinetic energy of the photoelectron. The photoelectron is matter, not just energy, and therefore will not travel far. It is usually absorbed within 1 to 2 mm in soft tissue. Despite the localized absorption, this is still a significant way in which x-ray energy can create biological changes.

The ionized atom is in an unstable state with an inner-shell electron missing. The vacancy is instantly filled by an electron from the L-shell or, less commonly, from an M-shell or free electron. In the vast majority of cases the electron transfers from an outer shell to an inner shell and, as it does, it releases energy in the form of a **characteristic photon,** known as **secondary radiation.** This secondary radiation is produced in the same manner as characteristic radiation is produced at the x-ray target—electron transfer from one shell to another. When it is created at the x-ray target it is considered primary radiation. When characteristic radiation is produced in irradiated matter outside of the x-ray target it is termed secondary radiation. Remember that outer-shell electrons possess a higher energy level than inner-shell electrons. Therefore when an outer-shell electron moves into an inner shell it has excess energy to release. This

TABLE 12-1.	K-Shell Binding Energies of Radiologically Significant Elements	
Atom	**Atomic Number**	**K-Shell Binding Energies (keV)**
Hydrogen	1	0.016
Carbon	6	0.284
Oxygen	8	0.53
Aluminum	13	1.56
Calcium	20	4.04
Molybdenum	42	20.0
Iodine	53	33.2
Barium	56	37.4
Tungsten	74	69.5
Lead	82	88.0

FIGURE 12-2   The photoelectric absorption interaction.

electron transfer process continues from shell to shell until the atom returns to a normal state and is no longer a positive ion. This process of each shell filling lower shells with a corresponding emission of photons is called a characteristic cascade. The energy of each photon of a **characteristic cascade** will be characteristic of the difference in energy in the two shells between which it dropped.

Because of the predominance of low atomic number elements comprising the human body, the secondary radiation produced is of extremely low energy. Secondary radiation energies are significantly higher for elements such as iodine and barium, which are commonly used as contrast agents in radiology.

There are three basic rules which govern the possibility of a photoelectric interaction:

1. **The incident x-ray photon energy must be greater than the binding energy of the inner-shell electron.** A 30 keV x-ray photon will not be able to remove the K-shell electron from an atom of iodine, which has a binding energy of 33.2 keV, or barium, which has a binding energy of 37.4 keV.

2. **A photoelectric interaction is more likely to occur when the x-ray photon energy and the electron binding energy are nearer to one another.** Of course, the x-ray photon energy must always be greater, but a 40 keV photon is more likely to interact by way of the photoelectric effect with an atom of iodine (K-shell E_b = 33.2 keV) or barium (K-shell E_b = 37.4 keV) than would a 100 keV x-ray photon. As photon energy increases, the chance of a photoelectric interaction decreases dramatically. The actual relationship is expressed as an inverse proportion to approximately the third power of the photon energy (photoelectric effect = $1/(energy)^3$). A significant change is therefore seen in the percentage of photoelectric interactions that will occur when using low kVp techniques versus high kVp techniques. Table 12-2 demonstrates that at 50 kVp, the percent of photon interactions that undergo photoelectric absorption is 50.45 percent with scatter interactions occurring at 49.55 percent. As the kVp increases, the percent of photon interactions by photoelectric absorption decreases. At 130 kVp, photoelectric absorption accounts for only 24.78 percent of the interactions with matter. These concepts become very important to the radiographer when establishing appropriate technical factors for specific body tissues.

TABLE 12-2. Percentage of Photon Interactions, Attenuation, and Transmission Characteristics in Soft Tissue Based on Effective Photon Energies

kVp	50	70	80	90	110	130
HVL (mm Al)	1.59	2.11	2.35	2.60	3.12	3.67
Mean Photon Energy (keV)	31.3	40.0	41.1	44.2	49.7	54.5
Effective Photon Energy (keV)	27.0	30.0	31.0	33.0	35.0	38.0
% of Photon Interactions by						
—Scattering (with coherent)	49.55%	62.70%	63.95%	66.70%	69.77%	75.22%
—Photoelectric	50.45%	37.30%	36.05%	33.30%	30.23%	24.78%
% Attenuation						
5 cm Tissue	91.45%	84.28%	83.45%	81.67%	79.70%	76.34%
10 cm Tissue	99.27%	97.53%	97.26%	96.64%	95.88%	94.40%
15 cm Tissue	99.94%	99.61%	99.55%	99.38%	99.16%	98.67%
20 cm Tissue	99.99%	99.94%	99.93%	99.89%	99.83%	99.69%
% Transmission						
5 cm Tissue	8.55%	15.72%	16.55%	18.33%	20.30%	23.66%
10 cm Tissue	0.73%	2.47%	2.74%	3.36%	4.12%	5.60%
15 cm Tissue	0.06%	0.39%	0.45%	0.62%	0.84%	1.33%
20 cm Tissue	0.01%	0.06%	0.07%	0.11%	0.17%	0.31%

Courtesy of Raymond P. Rossi, University of Colorado Health Science Center.

3. A photoelectric interaction is more likely to occur with an electron which is more tightly bound in its orbit. Binding energies of the electrons are greater in high atomic number elements than in low atomic number elements. In addition, inner-shell electrons have higher binding energies than outer-shell electrons in a given atom. With low atomic number elements, most interactions will occur with the K-shell electron. Because high atomic number elements bind their electrons more tightly, interactions will occur with the K-, L-, and M-shells. In fact, the incident x-ray photon often does not possess sufficient energy to remove a K-shell electron. For example, the K-shell binding energy for lead is 88 keV. X-ray photons below this level are incapable of removing the K-shell electrons but can be absorbed through photoelectric interactions with L- or M-shell electrons. The probability of a photoelectric interaction increases dramatically as the atomic number increases. The relationship is approximately proportional to the third power of the atomic number (photoelectric effect = (atomic number)^3). Since bone has an effective atomic number which is higher than that of soft tissue, photoelectric interactions are more likely to occur in bone than in soft tissue. **It is for this reason that radiography is so spectacularly useful in demonstrating the bones of the body.**

COHERENT SCATTERING

Coherent scatter is an interaction which occurs between very low-energy x-ray photons and matter. It is also called classical scatter or unmodified scatter. There are actually two types of coherent scattering: Thomson scattering and Rayleigh scattering. Thomson scattering involves a single electron in the interaction while Rayleigh scattering involves all of the electrons of the atom in the interaction. Both types have the same basic interaction results.

When a very low-energy photon, below approximately 10 keV, interacts with the electron(s) in an atom, it may cause the electron(s) to vibrate at the same frequency as the incident photon. The vibrating or excited atom immediately releases this excess energy by producing a secondary photon which has the same energy and wavelength as the incident photon but which travels in a direction different from the initial photon (Figure 12-3). The result is a scattered photon which possesses the same energy, frequency, and wavelength as the initial photon but which is traveling in a different direction. Since there is no energy transferred in the interaction, the atom is not ionized in the process.

Coherent scattering occurs in a very low x-ray energy range, which is generally outside the usual range for diagnostic imaging. A very small amount of the scatter radiation reaching the receptor is produced by this process and, as a result, this interaction has little significance to diagnostic imaging.

COMPTON SCATTERING

Compton scattering occurs when an incident x-ray photon interacts with a loosely bound outer-shell electron, removes the electron from its shell, and then proceeds in a different direction as a scattered photon (Figure 12-4). This interaction was described by the American Nobel laureate physicist Arthur H. Compton (1892–1962) in 1922 and is known as the **Compton effect.** Part of the energy of the incident photon is used to remove the outer-shell electron and impart kinetic energy to it. The dislodged electron is called a **Compton** or **recoil electron.** The photon which exits the atom in a different direction is called a **Compton scattered photon.** It possesses less energy than the incident photon and therefore has a lower frequency and longer wavelength.

The energy transfer in the Compton effect is mathematically expressed in the equation:

$$E_i = E_s + E_b + E_{ke}$$

where: E_i = energy of the incident photon
   E_s = energy of the Compton scattered photon
   E_b = electron binding energy of the Compton electron
   E_{ke} = kinetic energy given to the Compton electron

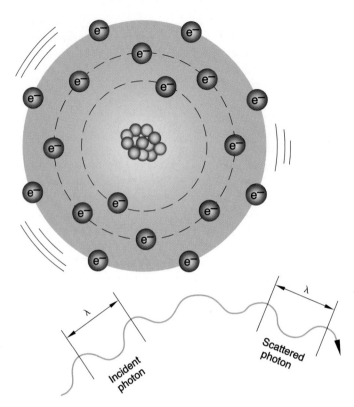

FIGURE 12-3 The coherent scatter interaction.

The incident photon energy is divided between the ejected electron and the scattered photon. The scattered photon retains most of the energy because little energy is needed to eject an outer-shell electron, due to its low binding energy. The scattered photon will continue to interact with atoms until it is eventually absorbed photoelectrically. The recoil electron is available as a free electron to fill a shell "hole" created by another ionizing interaction.

The amount of energy retained by the scattered photon is dependent on the initial energy of the photon and its angle of deflection from the recoil electron. The higher the initial energy of the photon, the greater the energy of the scattered photon. Scattered photons can be deflected at any angle from the recoil electron, just as a cue ball is deflected after it strikes a second ball in a game of billiards. At a deflection of 0°, no energy is transferred because the photon is proceeding in its original direction. As the angle of

deflection increases to 180°, more energy is imparted to the recoil electron and less energy remains with the scattered photon (Figure 12-5).

When a scattered photon is deflected back toward the source, it is traveling in the direction opposite to the incident photon. These photons are called **backscatter radiation.** Most photons will scatter in a more forward direction, especially when incident photon energy increases.

In Figure 12-5, the innermost ring represents the highest energy level and the scattered photons are all deflected in a forward direction. The third inner ring represents a typical x-ray exposure with an average effective photon energy of 50 keV. While a small number of photons are undergoing backscatter, the majority of the scatter is projected in a forward direction toward the image receptor. For this reason, scatter has a serious impact on image quality.

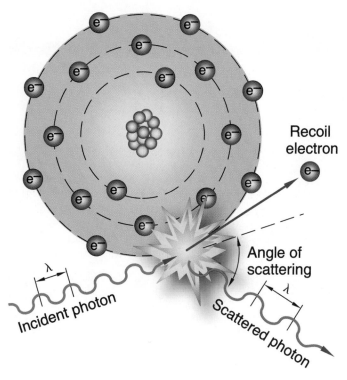

Recoil
electron

Angle of
scattering

λ

Incident photon

λ

Scattered photon

FIGURE 12-4   The Compton scatter interaction.

Scattered Compton photons possess an energy high enough to create a radiation hazard and to impair image quality. Scatter radiation emitted from the patient is the primary cause of occupational radiation exposure to the radiographer and is therefore the primary reason for wearing protective devices, such as lead aprons and gloves, and for providing protective shielding for the x-ray room. Scatter also adds unwanted exposure to the radiographic image. These unwanted esposures, caused predominantly by scattered photons and less commonly by secondary photons, are called **radiation fog.** Because scatter is coming from all directions, the scattered photons which strike the receptor places an exposure on the receptor which is unrelated to the patient's anatomy. Radiographic grids are devices designed to remove unwanted scatter and improve radiographic image quality.

PAIR PRODUCTION

In a **pair production** interaction the energy of the x-ray photon is converted to matter in the form of two electrons. For this interaction to occur, a very high-energy photon with an energy of at least 1.02 MeV is required. This is because the energy equivalent of the mass of one electron at rest is equal to 0.51 MeV. During this interaction, a high-energy incident photon comes close to the strong nuclear field and loses all its energy in the interaction. This energy is used to create a pair of electrons, one with a negative charge, a **negatron,** and the other with a positive charge, a **positron** (Figure 12-6). Since a negative electron is common in nature it is quickly absorbed by other nearby atoms. A positron, because of its unique configuration, with some of the

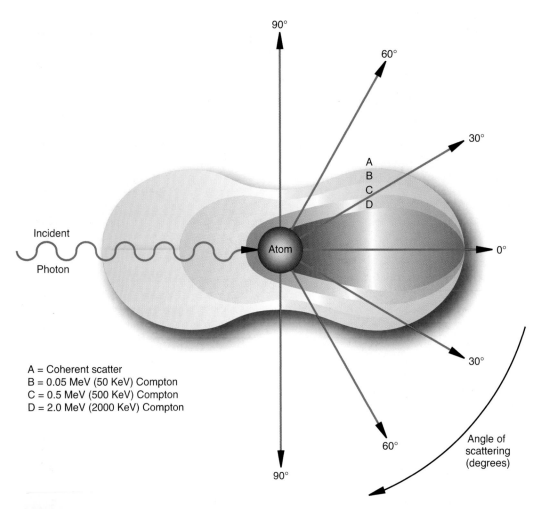

A = Coherent scatter
B = 0.05 MeV (50 KeV) Compton
C = 0.5 MeV (500 KeV) Compton
D = 2.0 MeV (2000 KeV) Compton

FIGURE 12-5 The distribution of photons in Compton scatter, along with various angles of deflection.

characteristics of a proton, is extremely volatile. It comes to rest and combines with a negative electron nearly instantaneously. When these two particles combine, they disappear and give rise to two photons moving in opposite directions and each possessing energies of 0.51 MeV. This process is called the **annihilation reaction** because matter is being converted back to energy. Pair production requires a minimum incident photon energy of 1.02 MeV but doesn't become a significant interaction until approximately 10 MeV. Therefore, it does not occur in the diagnostic x-ray imaging range.

PHOTODISINTEGRATION

Photodisintegration is an interaction between an extremely high-energy photon, above approximately 10 MeV, and the nucleus. In this interaction, the high-energy photon strikes the nucleus and all of its energy is absorbed by the nucleus, thereby exciting it. The excited nucleus responds by emitting a nuclear fragment (Figure 12-7). Because of the high-energy level needed to cause this interaction, it is not relevant to diagnostic imaging.

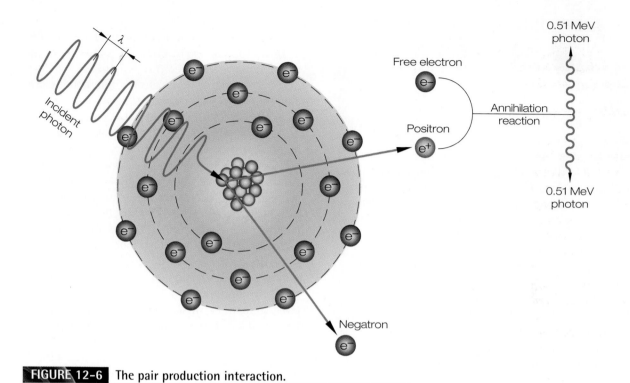

FIGURE 12-6   The pair production interaction.

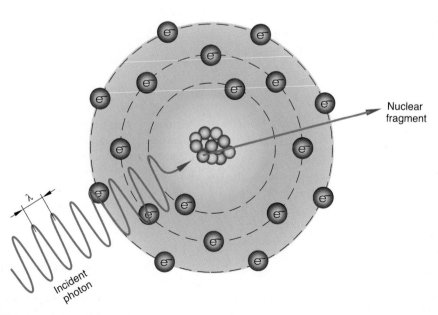

FIGURE 12-7   The photodisintegration interaction.

EFFECT ON TECHNICAL FACTOR SELECTION

Of the five interactions between x-ray and matter, only two have a significant impact on an x-ray image. These two interactions, photoelectric absorption and Compton scattering, must be considered by the radiographer when technical factors are selected.

It is important to remember that in the diagnostic x-ray range the majority of the x-ray beam is attenuated and only a small percentage of photons exit to create the image. Refer to Table 12-2. For a 10 cm tissue exposed at 50 kVp, 99.27 percent of the beam will be attenuated and 0.73 percent of the beam will be transmitted to interact with the image receptor. At 130 kVp, the same 10 cm tissue will attenuate only 94.40 percent of the beam and 5.60 percent of the beam will be transmitted. Obviously, it would be necessary to reduce the overall number of photons (mAs) when the kVp is increased, if the radiographer wants to maintain the same exit dose to the image receptor.

As kVp increases, the total number of photons which are transmitted without interaction increases. This means that the probability of photoelectric and Compton interactions decreases with increasing kVp. A shift does occur, however, in the percentages of photoelectric versus Compton interactions with increased kVp. **The percentage of photoelectric interactions decreases with increased kVp and the percentage of Compton interactions increases with increased kVp.** As a result, as kVp increases, there is an increased percentage of scatter and a decreased percentage of absorption of the attenuated beam. For example, in Table 12-2, for a 5 cm tissue exposed at 50 kVp, 91.45 percent of the beam is attenuated and 8.55 percent is transmitted. At 130 kVp, the same 5 cm tissue will attenuate only 76.34 percent of the beam and 23.66 percent will be transmitted. At 50 kVp, of the 91.45 percent that was attenuated, 50.45 percent of the interactions were photoelectric absorption and 49.55 percent were scatter. At 130 kVp, the overall percent of attenuation decreases (76.34 percent), but most of the interactions are now scatter interactions (75.22 percent) instead of photoelectric absorption (24.78 percent).

In the human body, Compton scattering is the predominant interaction through most of the diagnostic x-ray range. Photoelectric interactions predominate in two circumstances: (1) in the lower-energy ranges (25–45 keV) produced by 40–70 kVp, and (2) when high atomic number elements are introduced, such as the contrast agents iodine and barium. Iodine and barium serve as useful contrast agents because they absorb a greater percentage of the photons through photoelectric interactions. These differences in absorption between the contrast agents and the soft tissues are responsible for creating the visible radiographic image.

Figure 12-8 shows the percent attenuation by photoelectric absorption on the scale on the left and the percent attenuation by Compton scatter on the scale on the right. In the diagnostic x-ray range, for bone and soft tissue, photoelectric absorption predominates at lower energies and then Compton scatter begins to predominate. For high atomic number materials, such as sodium iodine (NaI), barium, and lead, photoelectric absorption is the predominant if not exclusive interaction. For this reason, as stated, iodine and barium serve as useful contrast agents and lead serves as a useful material for radiation protection.

When just comparing body tissues, in soft tissue (water) interactions are about 50/50 photoelectric absorption vs. Compton at approximately 26 keV. In bone, interactions are about 50/50 photoelectric absorption vs. Compton at approximately 45 keV (Figure 12-9).

When the photoelectric effect is more prevalent, the resulting radiographic image will possess high contrast. High-contrast images have great differences in densities from white to black, with fewer gray shades in between. This high contrast is the result of the complete absorption of the incident photons without the creation of undesirable scatter to fog the image. High-contrast images can be created by selecting low kVp/high mAs technical factors and through the introduction of contrast agents. In both of these instances, the photoelectric effect will be more predominant. Remember that as the

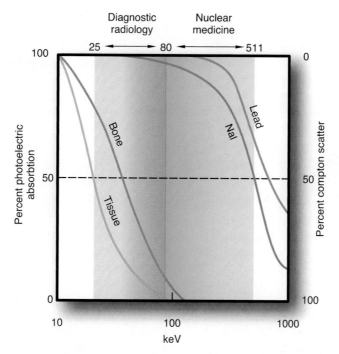

FIGURE 12-8   Percent contribution of photoelectric (left scale) and Compton (right scale) attenuation processes for various tissue as a function of energy. When diagnostic energy photons interact with low Z materials (e.g., soft tissue), the Compton process dominates. *(Reprinted with permission from Bushberg, J. T., Seibert, J. A., Leidholdt, E. M., & Boone, J. M. [2002]. The Essential Physics of Medical Imaging. [2nd ed.]. Baltimore: Lippincott Williams & Wilkins)*

FIGURE 12-9   The relative percentages of photoelectric absorption and Compton scatter in water and bone.

percentage of photoelectric interactions increases so does the absorption of radiation by the patient. This increases the likelihood of biological effects. Therefore, high-contrast, low kVp/high mAs techniques tend to result in higher patient doses.

When Compton interactions prevail, the resulting radiographic image will possess lower contrast. Low-contrast images have very small differences between densities, with more gray shades in between. Low-contrast images can be created by using high kVp/low mAs techniques because Compton interactions predominate as kVp increases. Scatter from Compton interactions is a significant cause of the lower-contrast images. However, low-contrast, high kVp/low mAs techniques tend to reduce patient dose.

SUMMARY

As an x-ray beam passes through matter it undergoes attenuation, which is the reduction in the number of x-ray photons in the beam as it passes through a given thickness of matter. Attenuation is the result of x-rays interacting with matter by way of one of five types of interactions.

The five basic interactions between x-ray and matter are photoelectric absorption, coherent scattering, Compton scattering, pair production, and photodisintegration. Only two are significant interactions within the diagnostic range of x-rays. These are photoelectric absorption and Compton scattering. Photoelectric absorption results when an x-ray photon interacts with an inner-shell electron. The incident photon is completely absorbed by the ejection of the electron, which then possesses kinetic energy and is called a photoelectron. The atom is ionized in the process and extremely unstable. The void in the inner shell is filled by the transfer of an electron from an outer shell. As the electron moves into the inner shell it releases a photon, which is characteristic for a given atom. Charac-teristic photons created in irradiated material by way of the photoelectric effect are called secondary radiation.

Compton scattering is an interaction between an x-ray photon and an outer-shell electron. The incident photon ejects the outer-shell electron (Compton or recoil electron). The incident photon loses energy and as a result changes direction or scatters. The scattered photons have sufficient energy to interact again and again. Scatter radiation is the reason for wearing radiation protection devices and for shielding x-ray rooms. Scatter also adds unwanted exposures to the receptor, which impairs image quality.

Image contrast is affected by the most predominant x-ray interaction. High-contrast images will result when the photoelectric effect is prevalent and low-contrast images will result when Compton scatter is more common. In addition, patient dose is increased when photoelectric interactions prevail. As kVp increases, more photons are transmitted without interaction and patient dose decreases as a result.

REVIEW QUESTIONS

1. Define attenuation.
2. Describe the photoelectric absorption interaction.
3. Describe the coherent scatter interaction.
4. Describe the Compton scatter interaction.

5. What is backscatter?
6. What are the two interactions which have a significant impact on the radiographic image?
7. What type of radiographic contrast will result if the prevalent interaction is photoelectric absorption?
8. What type of radiographic contrast will result if the prevalent interaction is Compton scatter?

REFERENCES AND RECOMMENDED READING

Bushberg, J. T., Seibert, J. A., Leidholdt, E. M., & Boone, J. M. (2002). *The essential physics of medical imaging* (2nd ed.). Baltimore: Lippincott Williams & Wilkins.

Bushong, S. C. (2004). *Radiologic science for technologists: Physics, biology, and protection* (8th ed.). St. Louis, MO: Elsevier/Mosby.

Compton, A. H., & Allison, H. K. (1935). *X-rays in theory and experiment* (2nd ed.). New York: Van Nostrand.

Curry, T. S., Dowdey, J. E., & Murry, R. C. (1990). *Christensen's introduction to the physics of diagnostic radiology* (4th ed.). Philadelphia: Lea and Febiger.

Dendy, P. P., & Heaton, B. (1999). *Physics for diagnostic radiology* (2nd ed.). Oxford: Institute for Physics.

Fewell, T. R., & Shuping, R. E. (1977). Photon energy distribution of some typical diagnostic x-ray beams. *Medical Physics, 4*(3), 187–197.

Glasser, O., Quimby, E. H., Taylor, L. S., Weatherwax, J. L., & Morgan, R. H. (1961). *Physical foundations of radiology* (3rd ed.). New York: Paul B. Hoeber, Division of Harper & Brothers.

Hay, G. A., & Hughes, D. (1972). *First-year physics for radiographers.* London: Bailliere Tindall.

Herman, M. W. (1980). A comparative study of scattered radiation levels from 80 kVp and 240 kVp x-rays in the surgical ICU. *Radiology, 552.*

Johns, H. E., & Cunningham, J. R. (1983). *The physics of radiology* (4th ed.). Springfield, IL: Charles C Thomas.

Meredith, W. J., & Massey, J. B. (1977). *Fundamental physics of radiology* (3rd ed.). Chicago: Yearbook Medical.

Selman, J. (2002). *The fundamentals of x-ray physics and radiobiology for the radiologic technologist* (9th ed.). Springfield, IL: Charles C Thomas.

Ter-Pogossian, M. M. (1967). *The physical aspects of diagnostic radiology.* New York: Hoeber Medical Division, Harper & Row.

van der Plaats, G. J. (1980). *Medical x-ray techniques in diagnostic radiology* (4th ed.). The Hague: Martinus Nijhoff.

Wolbarst, A. B. (1993). *Physics of radiology.* Norwalk, CT: Appleton & Lange.

Minimizing Patient Dose

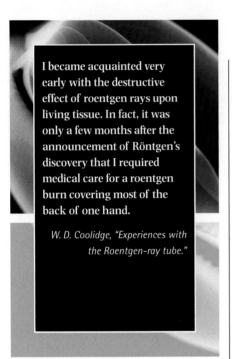

I became acquainted very early with the destructive effect of roentgen rays upon living tissue. In fact, it was only a few months after the announcement of Röntgen's discovery that I required medical care for a roentgen burn covering most of the back of one hand.

W. D. Coolidge, "Experiences with the Roentgen-ray tube."

KEY TERMS

approximate entrance
  skin exposure
entrance skin
  exposure

OBJECTIVES

Upon completion of this chapter, the student should be able to:

- Explain the relationship of entrance skin exposure to other measurement points.

- Calculate mR/mAs from a calibration exposure total.

- Calculate total entrance skin exposure when given subject part thickness, SID, kVp, mAs, and an mR/mAs chart.

- Describe typical entrance skin exposures for common radiographic procedures.

- Discuss methods of reducing patient dose through effective communication.

- Describe various methods of reducing patient dose through effective positioning.

- Explain the interrelationship of the prime factors.

- Evaluate various exposure factors for the most effective methods of reducing patient dose under various clinical conditions.

- Describe an effective method of minimizing patient dose by emphasizing radiation risk factors.
- Describe an effective method of maximizing patient diagnostic

information by emphasizing radiation benefit factors.
- Analyze various approaches to discussing radiation risk versus benefit with patients, physicians, and radiologists.

A predominant concern of radiographers is how to reduce the radiation dose to the patient. This concern is reflected in every decision made, especially when choosing technique exposure factors. The conscientious radiographer can reduce the patient dose by at least 50 percent in most examinations by choosing appropriate exposure factors.

Although exposure and dose are often used interchangeably, exposure (R) refers to radiation intensity in air, while dose (rad) is a measure of the radiation absorbed as a result of a radiation exposure. Dose is used to identify the irradiation of patients. Exposure (R) is used to calculate entrance skin exposure (ESE) in irradiated patients. Patient dose is usually estimated by conducting phantom experiments.

One of the most important characteristics of the professional is the ability to decide when it is appropriate to tip the radiation benefit versus risk issue in favor of the risk by reducing the patient dose while compromising the diagnostic quality of the image, and when to tip the issue in favor of the benefit by increasing the patient dose while maintaining the diagnostic quality of the image. There are circumstances that dictate when each choice should be made, and this chapter attempts to lay the foundation necessary to make these decisions.

ESTIMATING APPROXIMATE ENTRANCE SKIN EXPOSURE

Figure 13-1 illustrates a typical radiographic examination with the exposure indicated at various points. It is obvious that the maximum exposure

received by the patient is not at the area of interest but at the skin entrance to the body. This is known as the **entrance skin exposure** and is calculated at the minimum SOD. Note that the minimum SOD is not equal to the SOD of the area of interest and that the entrance skin receives a greater exposure. Although radiobiologists and physicists often discuss organ doses and gonadal doses, the entrance skin exposure is the most common expression to approximate patient exposure because it is safer to assume a maximum effect when attempting to minimize exposure to ionizing radiation.

Diagnostic Radiography mR/mAs Charts

Exposure to patients can be estimated by recording mR/mAs when the x-ray unit is calibrated. This is calculated by recording a reading for any average exposure and then dividing the reading in mR by the total mAs used. The expression mR/mAs represents the formula itself. The mR/mAs measurements are usually recorded for an SID of 40″ (100 cm). To estimate the entrance skin exposure, the inverse square law must be applied to determine the exposure for the source-to-entrance skin distance.

The mR/mAs readings vary according to the kVp used, with higher kVp producing greater mR/mAs. Consequently, mR/mAs readings should be recorded for each kVp range within the normal expectations of the unit. A typical mR/mAs chart is shown in Table 13-1.

A quick estimate of entrance skin exposure can be made from this chart, as shown in the following example.

Location	Exposure
Exiting collimator	1,727 mR
Entrance to skin	247 mR
Entrance to organ of interest	21.4 mR
Exit skin	9.5 mR
Exit table	6.6 mR
Exit grid	1.9 mR
Exit cassette	0.7 mR

SOD Minimum
SOD Area of interest
SID

22 cm Abdomen
14x17" Primary beam field
80kVp, 40mAs, 40" SID
8 : 1, 80 LPI Grid

FIGURE 13-1 Exposures at various locations in the imaging process.

TABLE 13-1. A Typical mR/mAs Chart

SID = 40" (100 cm)	
kVp	mR/mAs
50	0.9
60	1.7
70	2.5
80	3.5
90	4.5
100	5.6
110	6.9
120	7.9

EXAMPLE: What is the approximate entrance skin exposure for a 20 cm AP abdomen produced at 80 kVp and 20 mAs on the unit for the chart in Table 13-1?

Answer: Table 13-1 indicates that 80 kVp = 3.5 mR/mAs. The exposure required 20 mAs,

so the exposure at 100 cm = 3.5 mR/mAs $\times$ 20 mAs and the exposure at 100 cm = 70.0 mR.

$$SID = SOD + OID$$
$$100 \text{ cm} = SOD + 20 \text{ cm}$$
$$SOD = 100 \text{ cm} - 20 \text{ cm}$$
$$SOD = 80 \text{ cm}$$
$$\frac{mR_1}{mR_2} = \frac{SOD^2}{SID^2}$$
$$\frac{70 \text{ mR}}{mR_2} = \frac{80 \text{ cm}^2}{100 \text{ cm}^2}$$
$$\frac{70 \text{ mR}}{mR_2} = \frac{6,400 \text{ cm}}{10,000 \text{ cm}}$$
$$mR_2 \times 6,400 \text{ cm} = 70 \text{ mR} \times 10,000 \text{ cm}$$
$$mR_2 = \frac{70 \text{ mR} \times 10,000 \text{ cm}}{6,400 \text{ cm}}$$
$$mR_2 = \frac{700,000}{6,400}$$
$$mR_2 = 109.4$$

EXAMPLE: What is the total approximate entrance skin exposure for an intravenous pyelogram of a 24 cm abdomen if an AP preliminary scout; 5 min AP; 10 min AP, RPO, and LPO; 15 min PA; and 30 min AP radiographs of the abdomen were produced at 70 kVp and 15 mAs on the unit for the chart in Table 13-1?

Answer: Table 13-1 indicates that 70 kVp = 2.5 mR/mAs. Each exposure required 15 mAs, so the approximate entrance skin exposure = 2.5 mR/mAs × 15 mAs and the approximate entrance skin exposure = 37.5 mR per exposure; 37.5 per exposure × 7 exposures = 262.5 mR = 0.2625 R.

$$SID = SOD + OID$$
$$100 \text{ cm} = SOD + 24 \text{ cm}$$
$$SOD = 100 \text{ cm} - 24 \text{ cm}$$
$$SOD = 76 \text{ cm}$$
$$\frac{mR_1}{mR_2} = \frac{SOD^2}{SID^2}$$
$$\frac{262.5 \text{ mR}}{mR_2} = \frac{76 \text{ cm}^2}{100 \text{ cm}^2}$$
$$\frac{262.5 \text{ mR}}{mR_2} = \frac{5{,}776 \text{ cm}}{10{,}000 \text{ cm}}$$
$$mR_2 \times 5{,}776 \text{ cm} = 262.5 \text{ mR} \times 10{,}000 \text{ cm}$$
$$mR_2 = \frac{262.5 \text{ mR} \times 10{,}000 \text{ cm}}{5{,}776 \text{ cm}}$$
$$mR_2 = \frac{2{,}625{,}000}{5{,}776}$$
$$mR_2 = 454.5$$

Fluoroscopic R/min Charts

Approximate entrance skin exposure for fluoroscopic equipment is measured in R/min. Estimation of approximate entrance skin exposure is calculated in the same manner.

EXAMPLE: What is the approximate entrance skin exposure for a fluoroscopic examination of the abdomen performed for 5.5 minutes at 110 kVp at 1.7 R/min?

Answer: The exposure required 5.5 min, so the approximate entrance skin exposure = 1.7 R/min × 5.5 min and the approximate entrance skin exposure = 9.35 R = 9,350 mR.

EXAMPLE: What is the total approximate entrance skin exposure for a fluoroscopic examination of an 18 cm abdomen performed for 7 min and 45 sec at 110 kVp at 1.7 R/min and then followed by an AP at 10 mAs, left lateral at 25 mAs, and LPO projection at 20 mAs of the stomach at 120 kVp on the unit for the chart in Table 13-1?

Answer: The exposure required 7.75 min, so the approximate entrance skin exposure = 1.7 R/min × 7.75 min and the approximate entrance skin exposure = 13.175 R = 13,175 mR. The total mAs for the three projections = 10 + 25 + 20 mAs = 55 mAs. Table 13-1 indicates that 120 kVp = 7.9 mR/mAs, so the approximate entrance skin exposure = 7.9 mR/mAs × 55 mAs and the approximate entrance skin exposure = 434.5 mR; 13,175 fluoro mR + 434.5 diagnostic mR = 13,609.5 mR = 13.61 R.

$$SID = SOD + OID$$
$$100 \text{ cm} = SOD + 18 \text{ cm}$$
$$SOD = 100 \text{ cm} - 18 \text{ cm}$$
$$SOD = 82 \text{ cm}$$
$$\frac{mR_1}{mR_2} = \frac{SOD^2}{SID^2}$$
$$\frac{13{,}609.5 \text{ mR}}{mR_2} = \frac{82 \text{ cm}^2}{100 \text{ cm}^2}$$
$$\frac{13{,}609.5 \text{ mR}}{mR_2} = \frac{6{,}724 \text{ cm}}{10{,}000 \text{ cm}}$$
$$mR_2 \times 6{,}724 \text{ cm} = 13{,}609.5 \text{ mR} \times 10{,}000 \text{ cm}$$
$$mR_2 = \frac{13{,}609.5 \text{ mR} \times 10{,}000 \text{ cm}}{6{,}724 \text{ cm}}$$
$$mR_2 = \frac{136{,}095{,}000}{6{,}724}$$
$$mR_2 = 20{,}240 = 20.24 \text{ R}$$

TYPICAL ENTRANCE SKIN EXPOSURE

Numerous studies have been done regarding the exposure delivered to patients during diagnostic radiographic examinations. Diagnostic radiography is by far the greatest source of ionizing radiation exposure for the public. It is estimated that 15 percent of the radiation exposure received by the general public is a result of diagnostic radiographic examinations.

TABLE 13-2. Medical ESE Values for Selected Radiographic Exams

Projection	Patient Thickness (cm)	Grid	SID (cm)	Median ESE (mR)	3rd Quartile ESE (mR)
Chest (P/A)	23	No	183	9	13
	23	Yes	183	13	18
Pediatric Chest (P/A)	15 month old/ 11 kg infant	No		4	5
		Yes		8	10
Pediatric Chest (A/P)	15 month old/ 11 kg infant	No		5	9
		Yes		8	14
Abdomen (A/P)	23	Yes	102	271	396
Lumbar Spine (A/P)	23	Yes	102	342	477
Full Spine (A/P)	23	Yes	183	260 (200 Speed) 145 (400 Speed)	
Cervical Spine (A/P)	13	Yes	102	135 (200 Speed) 95 (400 Speed)	
Skull (Lat)	15	Yes	102	145 (200 Speed) 70 (400 Speed)	

Notes:
- Patient thickness corresponds to the dimensions of the average adult patient as clinically validated by the NEXT program.
- All measurements were made in air, without backscatter.
- The ESE values may be converted to entrance air kerma (mGy) by multiplying by 0.00876 mGy/mR.
- Chest data source: 1994 NEXT Chest Radiography Survey.
- Pediatric chest data source: 1998 NEXT Pediatric Chest Survey (preliminary data).
- Abdomen and Lumbar Spine data source: 1995 NEXT Abdomen and Lumbosacral Spine Survey (hospital data only).
- Full spine, cervical spine, and skull projections are based on data for manual mode techniques only collected by the H-7 Committee prior to the 1992 edition of this manual. ESE's are not necessarily inversely proportional to imaging system speed.
- For the full spine projection, if the facility used a wedge filter, the exposure was measured in the center of the x-ray field with the filter in the beam.

(Reprinted with permission from *Patient Exposure and Dose Guide–2003.* Conference of Radiation Control Program Directors, Inc., Frankfort, KY: CRCPD Publication E-03-2, 2003.)

Table 13-2 shows the average patient exposure guides for entrance skin exposure as published by the Conference of Radiation Control Program Directors. Within an acceptance range of ±20 percent, this guide is considered to be the standard for current practice in the United States.

Radiography of the lumbar spine, pelvis, and hip have the highest ESEs. These examinations deserve special attention from radiographers because careful consideration of the need for the examination, positioning, patient instructions, technical factors, and shielding can result in significant reduction in the total dose to the patient.

Flouroscopic systems in the United States are under a limit set by the Food and Drug Administration (FDA) for entrance exposure (kerma in the SI system) at 10 centigrays per minute (10 cGy/min), which is 11.5 R/min. High-level control mode fluo-

roscopy is limited to an entrance exposure (kerma) of 20 cGy/min, which is 23 R/min.

REDUCING PATIENT DOSE WITH COMMUNICATION

Radiographers often overlook the importance of gaining the trust and confidence of the patient. This is accomplished by a professional approach that includes technical competence, empathy for the patient and effective communication and questioning skills. When the patient has confidence in the radiographer there is a higher probability that detailed instructions will be followed, which helps to reduce motion and degradation of positioning.

REDUCING PATIENT DOSE WITH POSITIONING

An effective method of reducing patient dose is through accurate and effective positioning. Avoidance of repeated exposures far outweighs all other methods. However, once positioning skills have been developed to a degree of competence, several positioning details may further reduce the total dose.

Radiographic Projection

Some organs are especially sensitive to the effects of radiation, for example, the female breast, the kidneys, and the lens of the eye. Increased recorded detail and decreased distortion result when the area of interest is placed as close to the image receptor as possible. In most instances, a significant reduction in the total dose is achieved because this positioning also places the organ as far from the entrance exposure as possible. For example, a PA chest reduces the dose to the breast, an AP abdomen reduces dose to the kidneys, and a PA skull reduces dose to the lens of the eye. Deviation from these projections should occur only when unusual circumstances dictate an alternate projection.

Immobilization

Proper immobilization is a necessary part of achieving satisfactory recorded detail and diminishing the need for repeat exposures. Elimination of motion and decreased tissue density through compression both contribute to a reduction of patient dose.

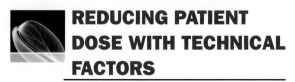

REDUCING PATIENT DOSE WITH TECHNICAL FACTORS

The radiographer can significantly reduce the approximate entrance skin exposure to the patient by judicious selection of technique exposure factors. Studies have shown that over 50 percent of repeated exposures are the result of improper technical factor selection. Table 13-3 illustrates the effect each of the major technical factors has on patient dose. In most instances when a technical factor is varied, other factors will be modified to maintain image receptor exposure. Therefore, the important information is not the direct result of the technical factor change, but the result of compensation to maintain image receptor exposure or other components of image quality.

Interrelationship of the Prime Factors

The radiation intensity from a diagnostic x-ray unit will vary in a direct relationship with mAs, directly with the square of kVp, and inversely with the square of the distance. This total relationship is often expressed as:

$$\frac{(mAs)(kVp)^2}{d^2}$$

At the image receptor the kVp is more likely to be kVp^3 or kVp^4. Although this formula includes only the three primary factors, it is useful to understand that they are interrelated and can all be used to influence the total dose.

Kilovoltage Range

When kVp is increased without compensating for other factors, patient dose is increased. Therefore, a decrease in kVp is desired when attempting to reduce patient dose. However, when an increase in kVp is compensated for by a decrease in mAs to maintain image receptor exposure, a significant reduction in patient dose is achieved. **Selection of the highest possible kilovoltage consistent with image quality is the best method of using exposure factors to reduce patient dose.** With fixed kilovoltage systems, care must be taken to achieve an optimal kVp that is within acceptance limits. Because fixed kVp technique systems tend to utilize higher optimal kVp levels, they usually reduce patient entrance skin exposures. A comparison of approximate ESE levels with the two systems is illustrated in Table 13-4.

Remember that generator phase also has an effect on kilovoltage output. Although an increase in the number of pulses from the generator would seem to increase the patient dose because of the increased average photon energy, there is actually a substantial

TABLE 13–3. Effects of Radiographic Exposure Variables on Patient Dose

Variable	Effect of Patient Dose When:		
	Variable Is Increased without Compensation	Variable Is Increased but Image Receptor Exposure Is Maintained by Compensating	
		with kVp Only	with mAs Only
Kilovoltage	+	NA	−
Milliamperage	+	+	0
Time	+	+	0
Distance SID	−	−	0
SOD	−	−	0
OID	+	+	+
Focal spot size	0	NA	NA
Filtration	−	−	+
Field Size	+	varies	varies
Gonadal shielding	−	NA	NA
Subject part density	+	+	+
Grid Ratio	0	+	+
Intensifying screens	0	−	−
Film speed	0	−	−
Film processing Developer time	0	−	−
Developer temperature	0	−	−
Developer replenishment	0	−	−

TABLE 13–4. Comparison of Approximate Entrance Skin Exposures with Fixed and Variable kVp Technique Systems

Variable—56 kVp, 5 mAs =	12.8 mR
Fixed—65 kVp, 2.5 mAs =	9.5 mR
Variable—68 kVp, 40 mAs =	175.1 mR
Fixed—80 kVp, 20 mAs =	135.4 mR
Variable—102 kVp, 20 mAs =	222.0 mR
Fixed—120 kVp, 10 mAs =	156.3 mR

These examples would produce equivalent receptor exposures.

decrease in patient ESE (from 40 to 60 percent) because of the decrease in the percentage of lower energy photons from the x-ray tube. The lower energy photons tend to be absorbed in the body instead of being transmitted to the image receptor, thus contributing to patient ESE without adding any information to the image receptor. This is clearly shown in Figure 13-2.

Milliamperage and Time

When mAs is decreased, patient dose is also decreased. When an increase in mAs is compensated by a decrease in kVp, patient dose will increase. An inverse relationship exists between mAs and kVp in maintaining image receptor exposure. To decrease patient dose, mAs should be maintained at the lowest possible level because there is a direct relationship between mAs and exposure. Because variable kVp technique systems tend to utilize lower kVp levels with higher mAs, the result can be higher average patient ESE than with fixed kVp systems.

Distance

Distance cannot be discussed alone because SID, SOD, and OID have differing relationships to patient ESE. When SID or SOD is increased, patient ESE decreases. One study found a 10 percent decrease in patient ESE between an SOD of 40 and 50 inches. When

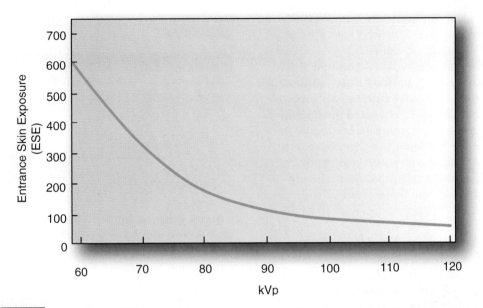

FIGURE 13-2   The effect of kVp on entrance skin exposure. This graph clearly illustrates that increased kVp causes photon energy to be carried through the object. *(Courtesy of Barry Burns, University of North Carolina)*

kVp is used to compensate for image receptor exposure, the ESE will decrease but the use of mAs for compensation will usually increase the total ESE. In most instances, when OID decreases, SOD increases and this will reduce patient ESE. This holds true regardless of whether kVp or mAs is used to compensate for the air-gap technique and exposure changes.

Focal Spot Size

Focal spot size has no appreciable effect on patient dose.

Filtration

An increase in filtration will reduce the ESE, even when kVp is compensated to maintain image receptor exposure. However, when mAs is used to compensate for lost image receptor exposure, the result is often an increase in the total ESE. This applies only to the small filtration increases used in diagnostic radiography, usually not more than 0.5 mm Al/Eq. Any significant increase in filtration (1.0 mm Al/Eq or more) would have an overall ESE reduction effect.

Field Size

When the primary-beam field size decreases, the patient dose also decreases. An increased field size will increase the total dose even when mAs or kVp is adjusted to compensate for image receptor exposure changes because a greater tissue area is irradiated. An increase in the primary technical factors is necessary to compensate for lost scatter radiation exposure when the field size is decreased. Although this appears to increase dose, the elimination of a greater percentage of tissue from the beam is a greater protective method than the increased factors.

Modern x-ray tube collimators utilize two sets of shutters or leaves to eliminate most of the off-focus radiation. When an aperture diaphragm is used instead of a collimator, off-focus radiation can increase the peripheral dose adjacent to the primary beam field.

Gonad Shielding

Gonad shielding is extremely effective in reducing dose to the gonads. There are three major types of gonad shields: flat contact, shadow contact, and shaped contact. Flat contact shields are positioned over the gonads at the skin surface. Shadow shields are positioned in the primary beam immediately below the collimator. Shaped contact shields are worn by the patient to surround the gonads. Gonadal shielding is one of the fine arts of radiography. The radiographer who is competent in the specifics of gonadal anatomy can easily satisfy the concerns of the radiologist or supervisor who has experienced suboptimal shielding that caused repeated exposure to the patient. **Properly placed gonadal shields significantly reduce patient dose while improperly placed gonadal shields can increase patient dose through repeated projections.** Consequently consistent gonadal shielding becomes a measure of the competency of the radiographer.

Gonadal shields should be used **routinely** for all patients with reproduction capabilities. The only exception to this rule should be projections that require information in the gonadal region. It is critical to locate the exact location of the ovaries or testicles prior to using gonadal shields. Most projections of the pelvic region do not permit the use of gonadal shields. This includes IVP, abdominal, colon, and bony pelvic projections. Hip projections do permit careful gonadal shielding.

Subject Part Density

A decrease in subject part density will decrease scatter production and reduce the patient dose. When compensation for lost scatter is made by increasing mAs or kVp, a reduction in total dose usually holds.

Grids

Using grids result in an increase in patient dose as opposed to non-grid procedures, in order to maintain image receptor exposure. When the grid ratio is decreased, and exposure is maintained by decreases in mAs or kVp, a significant dose reduction can be achieved. The use of a grid of unnecessarily high ratio causes routine increases in patient dose as mAs or kVp is increased to maintain exposure.

Film/Screen Image Receptor Systems

Intensifying Screens. Using intensifying screens results in a decrease in patient dose as opposed to non-screen procedures, in order to maintain radiographic density. Whenever the screen speed is increased, a significant reduction in mAs or kVp can be achieved while maintaining radiographic density. **The second most effective method of reducing**

TABLE 13-5. The Effect of Film/Screen Speed on Mean Entrance Skin Exposures

Projection	Chest	Abdomen	Lumbar
100 RS with grid	22.1 mR	553 mR	532 mR
200 RS with grid	14.9 mR	580 mR	813 mR
300 RS with grid	8.1 mR	351 mR	420 mR
400 RS with grid	7.4 mR	350 mR	383 mR

Data from 1987 NEXT survey of hospitals, U.S. Department of Health and Human Services, Food and Drug Administration, Center for Devices and Radiological Health.

patient dose is to use the highest possible film/screen combination (Table 13-5).

Film. Using higher speed film results in a decrease in patient dose as opposed to slower speed film, in order to maintain radiographic density. Base plus fog is a factor that should not be related to patient dose reductions. If base plus fog becomes too high, the detrimental effect on image quality will result in repeated exposures. However, a decrease in patient dose can be accomplished when a higher speed film is used and mAs or kVp is reduced to maintain radiographic density. Because higher contrast films also exhibit greater speed, the same effect is achieved with a higher contrast film. Film latitude becomes wider as speed and contrast decrease. Consequently, a narrow latitude film is desirable when attempting to reduce patient dose. This approach requires radiographers to be extremely accurate in selecting technical factors.

Film Processing. The compensations that are required to overcome reductions in developer time, temperature, or replenishment can result in unnecessarily high patient dose. Developer time, temperature and replenishment cannot be effectively increased to reduce patient dose. Film processing is a system that must be maintained at an optimal level to ensure satisfactory image quality. Failure to do so can result in increased dose rates, but success in maintaining the system cannot be considered a direct cause of decreased dose.

Digital Image Receptor Systems

With digital image detector systems, it is still critical to provide the digital image receptor with an appropriate exposure for a given procedure. Digital image receptors can respond to a wide range of exposures from as low as 0.01 mR up to 100 mR. Extremely low and extremely high exposures do not produce acceptable image quality. Most acceptable images can be produced using approximately 1 mR exposure to the receptor. Setting the appropriate technical factors is the responsibility of the radiographer. These prime technical factors control the exposure to the image receptor. The radiographer should select the kVp based on the desired contrast and adjust mAs to provide the appropriate total exposure to the receptor. Because of the wide exposure latitude allowed with digital systems, radiographers should be especially careful not to use higher exposure doses than necessary even though these exposures may produce an acceptable image through the post processing parameters.

DISCUSSING RADIATION RISK VERSUS BENEFIT WITH PATIENTS

The radiographer is often in the position of discussing radiation risk versus benefit with patients. To the attending physician, and sometimes even to the radiologist, the radiographer must represent the patient's interest in reducing dose. At the same time the radiographer must represent, to the patient, the physician's interest in maximizing diagnostic information. These points of view generally oppose one another. One exception is the use of higher kVp to produce a lower contrast. In this example, patient dose is decreased and the diagnostic information is increased.

Minimizing Patient Dose by Emphasizing Risk

The patient's interest in reducing the total dose must be represented even when the patient does not express such an interest. Some patients even express an opposite interest, as often occurs with minor complaints, such as lung congestion or a sprained ankle, when the patient arrives in the physician's office, a clinic or an emergency room with a request for an x-ray examination. When patients assume this attitude, the physician may prescribe an x-ray examination as a placebo. Most medical ethicists consider the prescription of a procedure for the purpose of deceiving the patient, or a procedure known to be without specific efficacy, to be unethical. This includes unnecessary radiographic examinations, which are known to be potentially detrimental.

In such a situation, the radiographer should perceive an obligation to act in such a way as to eliminate the request for the examination or at least to reduce the number of exposures. Through demonstration of professional competence, the radiographer can obtain the stature necessary to permit consultation regarding modification or elimination of examination requests.

Part of gaining this type of respect is the ability to make well considered judgments on when to advocate reductions in patient dose and when to advocate additional examinations. These judgments require all the radiographer's knowledge of anatomy, physics, radiation biology, positioning, pathology, imaging equipment, and, especially, clinical experience. For example, a radiographer should advocate an additional projection of the abdomen when an erect radiograph for an abdominal obstruction series fails to demonstrate the top of both hemidiaphragms. Conversely, the radiographer is acting professionally when advocating the elimination of separate wrist projections when both hand and wrist examinations have been requested but there is visible trauma only to the hand, the patient has no complaint of wrist pain, and the clinical history does not indicate a high probability of referred stress to the wrist joint.

For examinations that are of questionable need, the radiographer is within professional rights to inform the patient of his or her right to refuse an examination. **Under no circumstances should this be perceived by the radiographer as cause to inform the patient that an examination is not needed or to give a personal opinion regarding medical treatment or diagnosis.** The radiographer must have an introductory background in medical law in order to make judgments of this type. For example, minors, persons who have had their civil rights suspended (such as persons in the custody of law enforcement officers), mentally incompetent persons, and some other categories of patients do not have the right to refuse examinations.

The selection of patients for x-ray examinations has been the focus of considerable study, particularly when the chest, lumbar spine, and skull are involved. Patients can be divided into asymptomatic and symptomatic groups when determining which should be exposed to radiation. Asymptomatic patients should be examined only when there is significant cause, after considering the incidence and severity of the condition, the detection reliability of the examination, and the usefulness of the examination in treatment. The most common examples of asymptomatic patients are those undergoing screening procedures. Although mass chest and lumbar spine screening are now discouraged, mammography screening is encouraged for women of certain age groups. Symptomatic patients are more likely to require x-ray examination but should fit two major criteria: the examination must be capable of providing the desired information, and the information, even if negative, is expected to contribute to the management of the patient. The radiographer has a responsibility to contribute to these criteria whenever possible, primarily through history-taking. When circumstances that appear to routinely violate these principles are encountered, the radiographer should consider withdrawing from participation in the examinations.

Maximizing Diagnostic Information by Emphasizing Benefit

While advocating a reduction of patient dose, the radiographer must simultaneously impress on the patient the physician's primary concern of maximizing diagnostic information. This includes establishing credibility with the patient by demonstrating competence in answering questions, taking a medical history, manipulating the x-ray equipment, exhibiting a professional demeanor, and myriad other details. Established credibility permits the radiographer to convince the patient to follow breathing instructions, endure an additional uncomfortable projection, or permit a repeated exposure.

The benefit of radiographic procedures has been an unquestionable aspect of medicine since Röntgen's discovery in 1895. Although this is generally accepted by the public, some patients have a heightened anxiety about exposure, and there are periodic increases in publicity that cause concern over medical radiation exposures. These issues must be addressed by the radiographer as the primary professional contact with the patient. **The radiographer has a responsibility to advocate medically necessary examinations and to assure the patient that the benefit outweighs the risk.**

The primary duty of the radiographer on this issue is to provide the patient with sufficient information to permit the patient to make an informed decision regarding the examination. This can be a very sensitive topic and must be approached in a thorough and professional manner. One of the best accepted methods of providing this information to the patient is through comparison of relative radiation risks. Table 13-6 illustrates comparative risks of chest x-ray examinations to other radiation risks that are common public knowledge. Another effective method of illustrating

TABLE 13-6.	Gross Comparison of Relative Radiation Levels*	
	Scaled Relative Dose[†]	
Natural background	50–100 chest examinations/year	
Diagnostic Radiology	0.1–500 chest examinations/study[‡]	
Nuclear imaging	50–1,000 chest examinations/study[¶]	
Start of acute radiation syndrome	30,000 chest examinations in one day	
Lethal dose (LD50$_{30}$)	300,000 chest examinations in one day	
Radiation therapy (small volumes of tissue)	100,000–1,000,000 chest examinations in a few weeks	
Ultrasound	This scale does not apply	
NMR	This scale does not apply	

*Due to differential tissue distributions and sensitivities, such estimates are intended to be rough comparisons (50–100 chest examinations will have different biologic effects from that resulting from 100–200 mrads of natural background).

[†]1 PA chest examination = 5 millirad average tissue dose in thorax, which corresponds to a whole body equivalent dose of 2 millirads.

[‡]Dependent on examination types and techniques.

[¶]Does no properly account for doses received in those tissues in which the radionuclide concentrates.

(Reprinted with permission of Joseph P. Whalen and Stephen Balter, *Radiation Risks in Medical Imaging*, Chicago: Yearbook Medical Publishers, Inc., 1984.)

relative radiation risk is through a catalog of risks, such as the extract shown in Table 13-7.

When a patient requests information about the exact dose for a particular examination, the radiographer has an obligation to attempt to provide that information. However, it is important that the patient have a basic understanding that only an **approximate entrance skin exposure** can be provided. The radiographer should inform the patient that the entrance skin exposure is the maximum exposure and that the actual dose to the area of interest would be significantly less.

The Center for Devices and Radiological Health of the United States Food and Drug Administration has advocated the use of radiation record cards for patients. Proposals have been made for credit card style cards with magnetic record tapes for running totals of approximate entrance skin exposures. There are currently x-ray units available with printout capability so this information can be given to patients upon request. As the public becomes more informed about the potential risks of medical radiation exposure, additional developments in this arena can be expected.

The patient has the right to refuse radiographic examination. The radiographer is bound by professional duty to respect this right and to advocate it to physicians, including radiologists, if necessary. As long as the patient has the right to refuse treatment, proceeding with an examination under protest from the patient may place the radiographer at risk of malpractice action (usually as assault and battery).

TABLE 13-7. Estimated Loss of Life Expectancy Due to Various Causes*

Lifestyle	Estimated Loss in Days
Being unmarried—male	3,500
Cigarette smoking—male	2,250
Being unmarried—female	1,600
Cigarette smoking—female	800
Dangerous job	300
Motor vehicle accidents	207
Alcohol (U.S. average)	130
Accidents at home	95
Average job	74
Radiation job	40
Accidents to pedestrians	37
Safest job	30
Natural radiation	8
Medical x-rays	6

Individual Action	Estimated Loss in Minutes
Buying a small car	7,000
Coast to coast drive	1,000
Coast to coast flight	100
Smoking a cigarette	10
Calorie-rich dessert	50
Non–diet soft drink	15
Diet soft drink	0.15
Crossing a street	0.4
Extra driving	0.4/mile
Not fastening seat belt	0.1/mile
1 mrem of radiation	1.5

*Adapted from Cohen and Lee. Reproduced from *Health Physics* 36:707, 1979. Used by permission of the Health Physics Society.

Adapted with permission of Bernard L. Cohen and I-Sing Lee, "A catalog of risks," *Health Physics* 36, 707–722, 1979.

SUMMARY

A predominant concern of radiographers is how to reduce the radiation dose to the patient. This concern is reflected in every decision that is made, especially when choosing technique exposure factors. The conscientious radiographer can reduce the patient entrance skin exposure by at least 50 percent in most examinations by choosing appropriate exposure factors.

The maximum dose received by the patient is not at the area of interest but at the skin entrance to the body. This is known as the entrance skin exposure and is calculated at the minimum SOD. Exposure to patients can be estimated by recording mR/mAs when the x-ray unit is calibrated. This is calculated by recording a reading for any average exposure and then dividing the reading in mR by the total mAs used. The expression mR/mAs represents the formula itself. The mR/mAs measurements are usually recorded for an SID of 40″ (100 cm). To estimate the entrance skin exposure, the inverse square law must be applied to determine the exposure for the source-to-entrance skin distance. For fluoroscopy, the estimated exposure is calculated in R/min instead of mR/mAs.

Radiographers can reduce dose to the patient through their communication skills, their positioning skills, and through proper selection of technical exposure factors. Technical factors include the kilovoltage, mA, exposure time, distance, filtration, field size, gonadal shielding, subject part density, grids, and film/screen and digital image detector systems.

The radiographer is often in the position of discussing radiation risk versus benefit with patients. To the attending physician, and sometimes even to the radiologist, the radiographer must represent the patient's interest in reducing the dose. At the same time the radiographer must represent to the patient the physician's interest in maximizing diagnostic information.

REVIEW QUESTIONS

1. What is the relationship between entrance skin exposure and other measurement points?

2. What is the mR/mAs for a calibration exposure of 80 kVp at 40 mAs that produces a total exposure of 86 mR?

3. What is the total exposure for a patient measuring 26 cm when the SID is 40″ for an exposure of 70 kVp and 35 mAs and the mR/mAs at 70 kVp is 2.6 at 40″?

4. How can patient dose be reduced through effective communication?

5. How can patient dose be reduced through effective positioning?

6. What changes should be made in kVp, mA, time, and distance if each is the only factor changed to reduce patient dose?

7. What are the variables, other than the prime factors, that can be used to reduce patient dose?

8. What risk factors could be mentioned to answer a patient's inquiry about the dose for an examination?

9. What diagnostic benefits could be mentioned to answer a patient's inquiry about the need for an examination?

10. Describe an approach to discussing radiation risk versus benefit with patients, physicians, and radiologists.

REFERENCES AND RECOMMENDED READING

Anderson, P. E., Anderson, P. E., & Van-der-Kooy, P. (1982). Dose reduction in radiography of the spine for scoliosis. *Acta Radiological, 23,* 251–253.

Appleton, M. B., & Carr, S. R. (1984). Radiation protection in a neonatal intensive care unit: A practical approach. *Radiography, 50*(592), 137.

Baker, D. G. (1989). How significant are the risks from occupational exposure to ionizing radiation? *Applied Radiology, 18*(9), 19.

Ball, J. L. (1978). Does high kV reduce the dose? *Radiography, 64*(523), 163.

Barnhard, H. J. (1978). The bedside examination: A time for analysis and appropriate action. *Radiology, 129,* 539–540.

Baxter, A. (1978). Choice of kilovoltage. *Radiography, 64*(524), 196.

Beauchemin, R. (1984). Telescopic gonad protector: Analysis and experimentation of a telescopic gonad protector. *The Canadian Journal of Medical Radiation Technology, 15*(1), 39.

Bednorck, D. R., Rozenfeld, M., Lanzl, L. H., & Sabau, M. (1981). A protocol for exposure limitations in radiography. *Radiologic Technology, 53*(3), 229.

BEIR V health effects of exposure to low levels of ionizing radiation. (1990). Washington, DC: National Academy Press.

Brown, R. F., Shaver, J. W., & Lamel, D. A. (1980). *The selection of patients for x-ray examinations.* Rockville, MD: U.S. Department of Health, Education, and

Welfare, Public Health Service, Food and Drug Administration, Bureau of Radiological Health. (HEW Publication (FDFA) 80–8104)

Burkhart, R. L. (1983). *Patient radiation exposure in diagnostic radiology examinations: An overview* (HEW Publication (FDFA) 83–8217). Rockville, MD: U.S. Department of Health, Education, and Welfare, Public Health Service, Food and Drug Administration, Bureau of Radiological Health.

Bushong, S. C. (2004). *Radiation protection in Merrill's atlas of radiographic positions and radiologic procedures* (10th ed.) by Philip W. Ballinger. St. Louis, MO: Elsevier/C. V. Mosby, 39–56.

Butler, P., Thomas, A. W., Thompson, W. E., Wollerton, M. A., & Rachlin, J. A. (1986). Simple methods to reduce patient exposure during scoliosis radiography. *Radiologic Technology, 57*(5), 411.

Butler, P. F. (1985). Chest radiography: A survey of techniques and exposure levels currently used. *Radiology,* 533.

Cohen, B. L., & Lee, I. (1979). A catalog of risks. *Health Physics, 36,* 707–722.

Conference of Radiation Control Program Directors, Inc., Committee on Quality Assurance in Diagnostic Radiology. (1993). *Average patient exposure guides.* Frankfort, KY: Author.

Dowd, S. B., & Tilson, E. R. (1999). *Practical radiation protection and applied radiobiology* (2nd ed.). Philadelphia: Elsevier/W. B. Saunders.

Frank, E., Stears, J., Gray, J., Winkler, N. T, & Hoffman, A. D. (1984). Use of the P. A. projection: A method of reducing x-ray exposure to specific radiosensitive organs. *The Canadian Journal of Medical Radiation Technology, 15*(2), 63.

Frank, E. D. (1983). Use of the posteroanterior projection: A method of reducing x-ray exposure to specific radiosensitive organs. *Radiologic Technology, 54,* 343–347.

Godderidge, C. (1981). A radiology department's response to consumer concerns regarding the hazards of low-dose radiation. *Radiology Management, 4*(3), 1.

Hall, E. J. (2000). *Radiobiology for the radiologist* (5th ed.). Philadelphia: J. B. Lippincott.

Herman, M. W. (1980). A comparative study of scattered radiation levels from 80 kVp and 240 kVp x-rays in the surgical ICU. *Radiology, 134,* 552.

Jankowski, C. B. (1984). Radiation exposure of nurses in a coronary care unit. *The Journal of Critical Care, 13*(1), 55–58.

Joseph, L. P., & Wollerton, M. A. (1984). *Extremity radiography following trauma: An overview* (HEW Publication (FDFA) 84–8232). Rockville, MD: U.S. Department of Health, Education, and Welfare, Public Health Service, Food and Drug Administration, Bureau of Radiological Health.

Light, M. C., Molloi, S. Y., Yandouo, D. R., & Ranallo, F. N. (1987). Scatter radiation exposure during knee arthrography. *Radiology,* 867.

Maillie, H. D., Segal, A., & Lemkin, J. (1982). Effect of patient size on doses received by patients in diagnostic radiology. *Health Physics, 42,* 665–670.

Manny, E. F., Rudolph, H., & Wollerton, M. A. (1981). *Pre-employment low back x-rays: An overview* (HEW Publication (FDFA) 81–8173). Rockville, MD: U.S. Department of Health, Education, and Welfare, Public Health Service, Food and Drug Administration, Bureau of Radiological Health.

McClean, P. M., & Joseph, L. P. (1981). *Plain skull film radiography in the management of head trauma: An overview* (HEW Publication (FDFA) 81–8172). Rockville, MD: U.S. Department of Health, Education, and Welfare, Public Health Service, Food and Drug Administration, Bureau of Radiological Health.

McGlone, W. E. (1970). Radiation protection of the reproductive organs during radiography of the hip joints. *Radiologic Technology, 41,* 277–279.

Milner, S. C., & Naylor, E. (1989). An estimation of doses received by patients in a diagnostic x-ray department. *Radiography Today, 55*(622), 16.

National Council on Radiation Protection and Measurements (NCRP). (1987). *Ionizing radiation exposure of the population of the United States* (NCRP Report No. 93). Bethesda, MD: Author.

National Council on Radiation Protection and Measurements (NCRP). (1989). *Medical x-ray, electron beam and gamma-ray protection for energies up to 50 meV (equipment design, performance and use)* (NCRP Report No. 102). Bethesda, MD: Author.

National Council on Radiation Protection and Measurements (NCRP). (1990). *Implementation of the principle of ALARA for medical and dental personnel* (NCRP Report No. 107). Bethesda, MD: Author.

Novitch, M. (1983). Evaluation of radiation exposure in diagnostic radiology examinations. *Radiology Management, 5*(4), 33.

Noz, M. E., & Maguire, G. Q. (1985). *Radiation protection in the radiologic and health sciences* (2nd ed.). Philadelphia: Lea & Febiger.

Phillips, L. A. (1978). *A study of the effect of high yield criteria for emergency room skull radiography* (HEW Publication (FDFA) 78–8069). Rockville, MD: U.S. Department of Health, Education, and Welfare, Public Health Service, Food and Drug Administration, Bureau of Radiological Health.

Ragozzino, M. W. (1986). Average fetal depth in utero: Data for estimation of fetal absorbed radiation dose. *Radiology, 513.*

Rosenstein, M. (1988). *Handbook of selected tissue doses for projections common in diagnostic radiology* (HEW Publication (FDFA) 89–8031). Rockville, MD: U.S. Department of Health, Education, and Welfare, Public Health Service, Food and Drug Administration, Bureau of Radiological Health.

Rossi, R. P., Harnisch, B., & Hendee, W. R. (1982). Reduction of radiation exposure in radiography of the chest. *Radiology, 144,* 909–914.

Schrimpton, P. C. (1988). Monitoring the dose to patients undergoing common x-ray examinations. *Radiography Today, 54,* 619.

Seeram, E., & Travis, E. L. (1997). *Radiation protection.* Baltimore: Lippincott Williams and Wilkins.

Shleien, B., Tucker, T. T., & Johnson, D. W. (1977). *The mean active bone marrow dose to the adult population of the United States from diagnostic radiology* (HEW Publication (FDFA) 77–8013). Rockville, MD: U.S. Department of Health, Education, and Welfare, Public Health Service, Food and Drug Administration, Bureau of Radiological Health.

Sholl-Evans, B. (1989). Radiation protection training and information. *Radiography Today, 55*(620), 8.

Shrimpton, P. C. (1989). Monitoring the dose to patients undergoing common x-ray examinations. *Radiography Today, 54*(619), 38.

Skubic, S. E., & Fatouros, P. (1986). Absorbed breast dose: Dependence on radiographic modality and technique and breast thickness. *Radiology, 263.*

U.S. Department of Health, Education, and Welfare. (1975). *Gonad shielding in diagnostic radiology* (HEW Publication (FDFA) 75–8024). Rockville, MD: Author.

U.S. Department of Health, Education, and Welfare. (1976). *Specific area gonad shielding: Recommendation for use on patients during medical diagnostic x-ray procedures* (HEW Publication (FDFA) 76–8054). Rockville, MD: Author.

U.S. Department of Health, Education, and Welfare. (1980). *The selection of patients for x-ray examinations: The pelvimetry examination* (HEW Publication (FDFA) 80–8128). Rockville, MD: Author.

U.S. Department of Health, Education, and Welfare. (1981). *Procedures to minimize diagnostic x-ray exposure of the human embryo and fetus* (HEW Publication (FDFA) 81–8178). Rockville, MD: Author.

U.S. Department of Health, Education, and Welfare. (1983). *The selection of patients for x-ray examinations: Chest x-ray screening examinations* (HEW Publication (FDFA) 83–8204). Rockville, MD: Author.

U.S. Department of Health, Education, and Welfare. (1984). *Nationwide evaluation of x-ray trends (NEXT)—Eight Years of Data (1974–1981)* (HEW Publication (FDFA) 84–8229). Rockville, MD: Author.

U.S. Department of Health, Education, and Welfare. (1986). *The selection of patients for x-ray examinations: Skull x-ray examination for trauma* (HEW Publication (FDFA) 86–8263). Rockville, MD: Author.

U.S. Department of Health, Education, and Welfare. (1986). *The selection of patients for x-ray examinations: Presurgical chest x-ray screening examinations* (HEW Publication (FDFA) 86–8261). Rockville, MD: Author.

Watkins, G. L. (1988). Public health risks from low dose medical radiation. *Radiologic Technology, 59*(2), 160.

Weatherburn, G. C. (1983). Reducing radiation doses to the breast, thyroid and gonads during diagnostic radiography. *Radiography, 49,* 151–156.

Wesenberg, R. L., Blumhagen, J. D., Rossi, R. P., Hilton, S. W., Gilbert, J. M., & Nedeau, D. J. (1980). Low-dose radiography of children. *Radiologic Technology, 51*(5), 641.

Whalen, J. P., & Balter, S. (1984). *Radiation risks in medical imaging.* Chicago: Yearbook Medical.

Winkler, N. T. (1969). Minimizing radiation exposure of patients and personnel (screen-film, TFD, filters; shields; grid ratios). *Radiologic Technology, 41*(3), 142.

Yoshizumi, T. T., Drummond, K. T., Freeman, J. O., & Mullett, M. (1987). Radiation safety and protection of neonates in radiological exams. *Radiologic Technology, 58*(5), 405.

Young, A. T. (1986). SURFACE shield: A device to reduce personnel radiation exposure. *Radiology, 801.*

UNIT III Creating the Image

Creating the image that appears on the radiograph occupies the majority of the radiographer's time and requires a great deal of skill. The ability of the radiologist to make a diagnosis depends on the radiographer's ability to create a diagnostic quality image. This ability is predicated on a thorough knowledge of the scientific basis by which the image was produced as well as clinical experiences.

This unit introduces the important aspects of **vision and perception.** Understanding how the information from the radiographic image will be transmitted to the brain of the viewer is critical to understanding exactly how to manipulate the image to maximize the diagnostic information it conveys. Producing quality images requires knowledge of x-ray **beam restriction,** the concept of **the patient as a beam emitter,** the **pathology problem** inherent in many examinations, the proper use of the **grid, radiographic film,** and **film processing. Sensitometry** is necessary to evaluate films and monitor their quality, while an understanding of **intensifying screens** and **film/screen combinations** is required to permit minimum patient exposure while maximizing diagnostic information on the film. Creating the image using digital image detector systems requires an understanding of digital image processing, digital radiography, and digital image management. The diagnostic image is created only when all of these factors are applied with professional skill.

213

CHAPTER 14

Vision and Perception

She is so tall, so slender, and
her bones—
Those frail phosphates, those
carbonates of lime—
Are well produced by cathode
rays sublime,
By oscillations, amperes and
by ohms.
Her dorsal vertebrae are not
concealed
By epidermis, but are well
revealed.
Around her ribs, those
beauteous twenty-four,
Her flesh a halo makes, misty
in line,
Her noseless, eyeless face
looks into mine,
And I but whisper,
"Sweetheart, je t'adore."
Her white and gleaming teeth
at me do laugh.
Ah! Lovely, cruel, sweet
(radio)graph!

Lawrence K. Russell, Life, 1896.

KEY TERMS

cone cells
contrast perception
edge enhancement
Mach effect
rod cell
threshold detection
visual acuity

OBJECTIVES

Upon completion of this chapter, the student should be able to:

- Draw a cross-sectional image of a human eye with appropriate anatomical structures identified.

- Explain the physiological function of the eye during photopic and scotopic vision.

- Discuss the inefficiency of the medical imaging process.

- Describe the boundary effect, Mach effect, eye motion, veil glare, and the effect of viewing distance on visual perceptions.

- State why pattern recognition is the domain of the radiologist.

- Discuss the concept of controlling the radiographic image in space.

- Apply the concept of three-dimensional thinking to clinical practice.

- Identify numerous creative uses of radiography in medicine, technology, and art.

IMAGE PERCEPTION

At one time or another we have all been fooled by visual misperceptions. A common example is shown in Figure 14-1. Misperceptions of any type can be dangerous in clinical radiography. An important method of overcoming misperception is the elimination of preconceived ideas about an image. A mental erasing of these opinions is necessary to permit high-quality viewing of radiographic images. This is a skill that is cultivated by radiologists until it becomes part of their routine diagnostic procedure. Radiographers observe the diagnostic reporting of images by radiologists with amazement at first, but with increasing confidence as experience adds knowledge about the potential pathological meaning of various radiologic signs. Radiographers should strive toward developing an understanding of the perceptual problems that radiologists encounter when attempting to interpret radiographic images. Through this understanding the radiographer can work toward producing images with patterns that provide maximum assistance to the radiologist in the diagnostic process.

FIGURE 14-1   "The Lady and the Chalice" can be seen either as a pair of black faces in silhouette or as a white vase. This picture was devised by E. Rubin in 1915 and remains popular as a method of demonstrating perceptual differences.

Visual Anatomy

Because radiography depends entirely on images, it is helpful to be introduced to the complexities of visual perception. The mechanics of image perception are mostly unknown. It is little understood exactly how the eye perceives images and transmits them to the brain. Even less is known about how the brain neurologically processes the information.

The human eye is anatomically designed to gather light, focus it, convert it to nervous impulses, and transmit it to the brain for processing. The aqueous humor, cornea, iris, and lens gather and focus the light (Figure 14-2). The specialized cells of the retina, especially the fovea centralis (or macula lutea), convert the image to nervous impulses, and the optic nerve transmits the impulses to the brain for processing. With corneal malfunction, such as myopia and hyperopia, the most common problems requiring corrective lenses, a distinct loss of detail is perceived because the incoming light is not properly focused on the retina. This is easily perceived and

well-established means are available for correction. Image conversion and processing problems are not as easily perceived and these deserve some elementary study.

Visual Physiology

It is often uncertain whether conversion and processing problems are caused by the light-sensitive cells located in the retina or by mental misperceptions due to neurological processing. Sufficient research has been done at least to outline some of the factors that may cause misperceptions. Understanding that these factors exist and how they can prejudice perception can assist greatly in reducing visual problems.

An excellent example of misperception is the tendency to stare at an object that is difficult to see. Although this may be a good method of mental concentration, it does nothing to improve the visual quality of the image. In fact, it does the opposite. The length of time the human visual system can integrate (acquire information) is only 0.2 second. If the image does not provide enough information to be converted and processed in that time, the visual system will reset itself and reacquire information for the next 0.2 second. Therefore, when insufficient information is

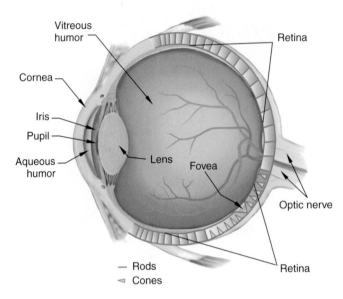

Vitreous humor

Retina

Cornea

Iris

Pupil

Aqueous humor

Lens

Fovea

Optic nerve

Rods
Cones

Retina

FIGURE 14-2 The human eye.

provided to the radiologist due to low illumination, excessive film density, or distracting reflected light, only an improvement in the quality and quantity of light photons available will improve the visual image. The radiographic film does much to resolve the integration time problem. Because the film emulsion can integrate information for a considerable length of time and then hold that information until processed, it permits the human brain to integrate much more visual information than if the image were viewed as it was acquired from the patient.

Rod and Cone Cells

Human image conversion occurs in the **rod** and **cone cells** located in the retina. Both of these types of cells contain photosensitive pigments that will respond to light by sending an electrical potential to specialized nerve cells. These bipolar cells emit neurological impulses when excited by light photons. The two types of cells are so different in their receiving and sending abilities that neurophysiologists tend to consider them as two separate visual systems. The cells are only about 1 μm in diameter and are concentrated to 100,000 per mm^2. There are approximately 7,000,000 cones, which are located

only at the fovea centralis. There are approximately 120,000,000 rods covering the remainder of the retina.

Photopic Vision

Photopic (daylight) vision is controlled by the cones. Cone cells require relatively bright light to function (a minimum of approximately 100 light photons). Cone cells contain one of three different light-sensitive pigments, each of which is sensitive to a different range of photon wavelength (color of light). The cones are most sensitive to yellow light. Color blindness is a condition that occurs when there is a lack of cones sensitive to a particular color or colors.

Because most of the cones are located at the fovea centralis in high concentration, daylight vision is sharply focused. Therefore, **visual acuity** is improved in daylight. The sparse concentration of cones in the retina outside the fovea centralis accounts for poor peripheral vision in daylight. Cones are also able to detect changes in brightness far better than rod cells. This permits much greater recognition of density differences, or contrast, and results in what is called greater **contrast perception** (Figure 14-3).

FIGURE 14-3   Human visual ability.

Scotopic Vision

Scotopic (night) vision is controlled by the rods. Rod cells are sensitive to low light levels (they may respond to as few as 15 photons) but cannot function in bright light. Rod cells cannot distinguish wavelength, although they are more sensitive to green light. As a result, humans are unable to perceive colors in extremely low light situations. Rod cells function by photosensitization of rhodopsin, also known as "visual purple," because it is most sensitive to blue-green wavelengths. When exposed to vast quantities of light photons, rhodopsin is oversensitized and becomes bleached out. The rod cells then regenerate rhodopsin at the rate of 50 percent each 7 minutes. This is the reason a bright light causes temporary blindness in both humans and animals. Because there are no rods in the fovea centralis, dim light vision is entirely peripheral and therefore difficult to bring into sharp focus. In addition, rods are not as concentrated because they are spread over a much greater area than cones. For these reasons, radiologists realize that dim objects are best viewed peripherally. Rods function better when the image information is changing. Slow scanning with an old fluoroscopic unit, night binoculars, or when walking in a dark room will increase visual acuity.

Inefficiency of the Medical Imaging Process

Few radiographers realize exactly how inefficient the entire imaging process is. An early fluoroscopic image study showed that although the x-ray tube was emitting 5,000,000 photons per second per mm^2 amplified over 5,000 times by the fluoroscopic intensification screen, only 65 photons contributed to the final impulses received by the brain. This is a conversion efficiency of 0.00005 percent (1 out of 2,000,000 photons) from the fluoroscopic screen and 0.001 percent (1 out of 100,000 photons) from the tube output.

Threshold Detection

Threshold detection is a visual phenomenon involving the perception of extremely small or faint details. This is more than an issue of the resolution, or fineness of the details, in the image. It also involves minimizing background density and other artifacts, known as visual noise.

Boundary Effect. A boundary effect occurs because the visual system has difficulty perceiving contrast differences that are distant from one another. When a distinct boundary between various densities can be achieved (this is actually contrast), adjacent differences as small as 2 percent can be perceived under high illumination (such as a radiographic view box). When the boundary is indistinct, a difference of up to 20 percent may be required. Less intense light levels also affect this perception ability.

There is a rule of thumb in radiography that density changes should be at least 25–33 percent to be visible. This is because two radiographs of differing densities are seen quite distant from one another. If a change of this magnitude formed an adjacent boundary, it would be strikingly apparent. Surrounding densities have an effect on the perception of nearby densities. This results in confusion when judging absolute and relative levels of density and contrast from one image to another.

Another aspect of the boundary effect concerns the length of the boundary line. A subtle density difference along the length of a long boundary may be perceived but when it is shortened the boundary may no longer be perceived. As yet there is no explanation for this phenomenon but radiologists can best observe extremely subtle density differences when they form a long boundary. They may fail to see diagnostic information when density differences are widely separated or form short boundaries. In these instances it is important for the radiographer to attempt to provide better perception through higher contrast.

Mach Effect. Part of the boundary effect may be explained by a phenomenon called the **Mach effect.** The retina contains neural connections that inhibit impulses under certain conditions. One of these conditions is extremely bright light; another is a dramatic change in impulse intensity. The Mach effect occurs when the eye perceives a boundary. Each time there is a change in density, there is a change in the intensity of the impulses sent to the brain. When the beginning of the new intensity

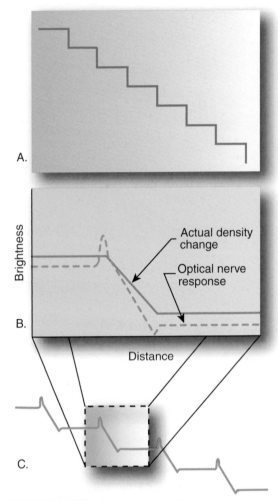

FIGURE 14-4 The Mach effect: (A) actual density differences, (B) comparison of actual density changes to optical nerve response, and (C) optical nerve response from A.

level is inhibited by the neural connectors, the impulses to the brain are transmitted as shown in the graph in Figure 14-4B. For density differences as shown in the step wedge in Figure 14-4A, the end result is a response as shown in Figure 14-4C. This creates an effect known as **edge enhancement.** Edge enhancement compresses the entire density

FIGURE 14-5 Optical step wedges. Note the prominent Mach effect through the lighter densities of the upper step wedges.

FIGURE 14-6 A continuous gray scale produced with a continuous sloping aluminum step wedge.

scale while making the boundary appear more distinct than it really is. For example, in Figure 14-5 many of the lighter density steps appear to be lighter just before the edge of the next darker step. This perceptual illusion is the Mach effect. Although this makes it easier to perceive the edges, radiologists are concerned about the possibility of a small detail being lost because its density is overwritten by edge enhancement. Figures 14-5 and 14-6 have the same light-to-dark scale. Note that the lack of a distinct boundary line causes a difference in perception of the range of visible densities.

Eye Motion. Contrast perception is dramatically increased when the eye uses a scanning motion, as when reading a book. Because the photosensitive cells in the eye can integrate a limited amount of information, eye movement maintains a constantly changing neurological signal, thus avoiding saturation of the optical nerves.

Veil Glare. Veil glare occurs when the intensely bright light from a view box floods the eye directly. This occurs in unexposed areas of the image and between images. The bright light scatters inside the eye and reduces contrast perception, much as Compton scatter does within the patient.

Viewing Distance. Data concerning threshold detection indicate that results change when the viewing distance is changed. This occurs because of the changes in intensity due to the inverse square law and because the physiological processing of the image changes when the angle of the incident light photons changes. In addition, the fovea centralis creates a blind spot at a viewing distance of about 9 inches. Therefore, radiologists often vary their viewing distances when addressing areas of perceptual difficulty.

Pattern Recognition

Pattern recognition involves perceiving combinations of details that can be defined and classified toward a diagnosis. This is the area radiologists often study the hardest. Just as it is difficult to identify a picture of a familiar face when it is shown upside down, so it is important that radiologists be presented with images in a routine manner. For example, radiographs are universally viewed as if the viewer were facing the patient (the patient's left is on the viewer's right, etc.).

Pattern recognition involves comparing mental images of patterns—anatomical, physiological, pathological, and histological—to arrive at a diagnostic opinion. Because of the complexities between the visual system and the mental capability to store and recall image patterns from memory, and because of the lack of scientific knowledge about how the brain processes information, pattern recognition is a weak area of research and no data can be provided to help the radiographer assist the radiologist. Pattern recognition is the true domain of the radiologist, who has the requisite medical knowledge to be competent in this area.

 CONTROLLING THE IMAGE IN SPACE

One of the challenges to the radiographer is to place the patient so that the area to be imaged is in a position that will enhance the quality of the image. It is helpful to visualize the object of radiographic interest (kidney, scapula, sinus, etc.) as floating in space within the body of the patient. The skill of the radiographer lies in manipulating the object to the correct position in relationship to the x-ray beam and image receptor (film). This is the art of controlling the image in space.

Thinking Three-Dimensionally

The radiographer must be capable of controlling the image in space in an artistic manner. This is one of the critical elements of professionalism. In her book, *Fundamentals of Radiology*, radiologist Lucy Frank

FIGURE 14-7 A three-dimensional effect.
(Reprinted by permission of the publisher from Squires Fundamentals of Radiology, Fifth Edition, edited by Robert A. Novelline, p. 12, Cambridge, MA: Harvard University Press, Copyright © 1975, 1982, 1988, 1997 by the President and Fellows of Harvard College)

Squire encourages us with "An Invitation to Think Three-Dimensionally." This concept is extremely valuable in forming perceptual ability. The experienced radiographer can see an incredible amount of beauty in the radiographs that are produced every day. Just as the barium-coated finger (Figure 14-7) is easily perceived in three dimensions, so are most radiographs viewed in this manner by radiographers. The magnification of structures some distance from the receptor places them further away in perspective; finely detailed structures seem to move closer, and each image assumes a three-dimensionality usually not noticed by the novice.

Radiographic positioning requires a solid knowledge of the shape and location of skeletal and soft-tissue structures and an in-depth understanding of their anatomical relationship to one another. For example, a diagnostic image of the maxillary sinuses can be obtained only after positioning the patient's head so the overlying structures of the cranium do not appear superimposed over the area of interest.

The human body is a three-dimensional object, but radiographic images possess only two dimensions—length and width. Consequently, all radiographic images are missing a critical diagnostic element—the dimension of depth. This can only be compensated for by never settling for a single radiographic view of any structure. **At least two images, as close to 90° angles to one another as possible, are required to view all three dimensions.**

The dimensional views required for all radiographic examinations are **anterior-posterior, medial-lateral, and superior-inferior.** All radiographic images will demonstrate two, but never all three, of these perspectives. For example, a posteroanterior (PA) chest radiograph demonstrates the medial-lateral dimension and the superior-inferior dimension, but not the anterior-posterior dimension. The dimension that describes the entrance and exit of the central ray, which is used to describe the projection, is the dimension not visualized. In situations where superimposition makes PA and lateral projections useless, two oblique positions at 90° angles from one another can be used to achieve the same effect.

An important skill that must be developed by the radiographer is the ability to mentally visualize the changing and moving of overlying anatomical structures from any angle in order to provide an image free of superimposition. Artistic techniques should be understood, such as making exposures while the patient is breathing, thus using patient motion to blur superimposing structures from the image (i.e., to blur ribs from the lateral projection of the thoracic vertebral column).

RADIOGRAPHY AS AN ART FORM

Radiography is an art form. In the century since its discovery it has been used to investigate an incredible variety of animals and objects. Examples of radiography as a technical and purely creative art form abound. Numerous radiographers have not only taken pride in the quality of their clinical abilities but have extended their technical skills into artistic expressions of creativity.

Radiographers can become technically artistic; innovative adaptations of routine procedures should be considered technical artistry. For example, it is technically artistic to reverse routine angles to produce a diagnostic quality acanthioparietal projection of the skull for a traumatized patient with anterior facial injuries, or to lower the tube and support a film cassette under a wheelchair patient's foot so that it is unnecessary to move a weak patient with a full leg cast onto a radiographic table.

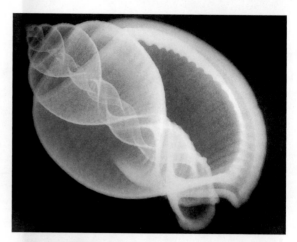

FIGURE 14-8   "Scotch Bonnet," by Willliam A. Conklin, RT FASRT. *(With permission of William A. Conklin, Inner Dimension, 1571 Marshall Avenue, Orangeburg, SC 29115)*

Artistic Radiography

William Conklin, a South Carolina radiographer artist, has achieved national acclaim for his radiography/photography of sea shells (Figure 14-8). Conklin's work has appeared in *National Geographic* and is in the permanent collection of the Smithsonian Institution. Radiography has often been used to produce a unique perspective of flowers, fruit, and other plants, as well as of shells and fish.

Nondestructive Testing

The entire industrial radiography field, known as nondestructive testing (NDT) radiography, is unknown to many medical radiographers. The intent of NDT radiography is to assist in the examination and assessment of materials such as castings, welds, and others, through noninvasive techniques.

Biological Research

Radiography has proven an invaluable tool in biological research, not only in medical studies, but also in monitoring animal functions. For example, the study of birds and bats in flight is greatly enhanced by high-speed radiography.

FIGURE 14-9 Canary with an egg. *(Courtesy of Dr. Marion Frank)*

FIGURE 14-10A A Grenz ray radiograph of a section of "Intemperance" by Hieronymus Bosch. *(Courtesy of Gerald Conlogue, Gulf Coast Community College)*

FIGURE 14-10B "Intemperance" by Hieronymus Bosch. *(Reprinted with permission from Yale University Art Gallery, The Rabinowitz Collection)*

Veterinary Radiography

Veterinary medicine and dentistry also use radiography to accomplish many diagnoses. Figure 14-9, a canary with an egg, is an example of veterinary radiography. This type of radiography is also used in zoos. Radiographers have been called on to examine all types of animals, from live venomous snakes to passive house pets.

Forensic Radiography

Forensic medicine uses radiography in a wide variety of ways. Grenz rays (5–30 kVp x-rays) are used, as are diagnostic x-rays. Grenz rays are emitted by specially designed tubes with minimal inherent filtration. They are useful for demonstrating objects as diverse as the ink on money when counterfeiting is suspected, the contents of envelopes and packages, fingerprints, and art forgery.

Art Restoration

Grenz ray radiography has also proven useful during restoration of paintings and other art objects. Radiography can detect images under existing paint, frame, and canvas construction and different types of paint and brush styles (Figure 14-10A and B).

FIGURE 14-11 A female hamadryas baboon mummy found buried with Makare, a member of an ancient Egyptian priesthood family, who was pregnant at the time of her death. *(Reprinted with permission from "X-Raying the Pharoahs," by James E. Harris and Kent R. Weeks)*

Archaeological Radiography

Radiography has become a useful archaeological tool, especially in the examination of fragile mummified remains. Numerous reports of such investigations have been published. Most notable in this area is the book, *X-Raying the Pharaohs*, in which University of Michigan researchers Harris and Weeks discuss their experiences radiographing the mummies at the National Museum in Cairo. Among their radiographic discoveries were jewelry, diseases, murders, dietary habits, and the remains of a baboon that had been assumed to be a royal child (Figure 14-11).

Poetry

Radiographic images themselves inspire many of us. The physician poet Jack Coulehan was inspired by a chest radiograph to compose this poem:

The Old Man with Stars Inside Him

I look at the X-ray,
a shadow of pneumonia
deep in this old man's chest,
and watch Antonio shake
with a cough that traveled here
from the beginning of life.
As he pulls my hand to his lips
and kisses my hand,
Antonio tells me, for a man
whose death is gnawing at his spine,
pneumonia is a welcome friend
who reaches in between his ribs
without a sound and puff!
a cloud begins to squeeze
so delicately
the great white image of his heart.
The shadow advances
every time Antonio moves—
when a nurse positions his body,

when he takes a sip of ice,
when he shakes with a cough,
moist and diminished.
I see in that delicate shadow
a cloud of gas
at the galaxy's center,
a cloud of cold stunned nuclei
beginning to spin,
spinning and shooting
a hundred thousand
embryos of stars.
I listen to Antonio's chest
where stars crackle from the past
and hear the boom
of blue giants newly caught.
I hear the snap
of white dwarves coughing, shooting.
The second time Antonio
kisses my hand
I feel his dusky lips
reach out from everywhere in space.
I look at the place
his body was
and see inside Antonio, the stars.

(*Reprinted with permission from* Midwest Poetry Review, © *Jack Coulehan 1988*)

SUMMARY

Understanding visual perception is an important aspect of clinical radiography. This understanding helps overcome misperceptions about an image.

The human eye is designed to gather light, focus it, convert it to nerve impulses, and transmit it to the brain for processing. Image conversion occurs in the rod and cone cells, which contain photosensitive pigments that will respond to light. Photopic (daylight) vision is controlled by the cones, and scotopic (night) vision is controlled by the rods.

Threshold detection is a visual phenomenon involving the perception of extremely small or faint details. The boundary effect occurs because the visual system has difficulty perceiving contrast differences that are distant from one another. When densities are adjacent, small differences can be perceived. Part of the boundary effect can be explained by the Mach effect. When the eye perceives a boundary, a change occurs in the intensity of the impulses sent to the brain. This change in intensity creates an effect known as edge enhancement, which makes the boundary appear distinct. Contrast perception is dramatically increased by eye motion or scanning the image. Veil glare occurs when bright lights, such as a view box, flood the eye. Viewing distance has an effect on threshold detection.

Pattern recognition involves perceiving combinations of details that can be defined and classified toward a diagnosis. It helps the radiologist compare mental images of patterns with medical knowledge.

Radiographers need to think three-dimensionally. Radiographic images possess two dimensions and, as a result, at least two images as close to 90° angles to one another as possible are required to view all three dimensions. It is considered technical artistry when radiographers use innovation to adapt a routine procedure.

Radiography is an art form that has been used to investigate a wide array of animals and objects. It is used in nondestructive testing; biological research and veterinary and forensic radiography; art restoration; archeological radiography; and has even been the subject of poetry.

REVIEW QUESTIONS

1. What is the human eye designed to do?
2. What is the difference between photopic and scotopic vision?
3. Explain the boundary effect.
4. What is the Mach effect?
5. How is pattern recognition used by the radiologist in making a diagnosis?
6. Why is it important for the radiographer to produce two images as close to 90° angles to one another as possible?
7. Name three examples of the use of radiography as an art form.

REFERENCES AND RECOMMENDED READING

Abildgaard, A., & Notthellen, J. A. (1992). Increasing contrast when viewing radiographic images. *Radiology, 185*(2), 475–478.

Adrian-Harris, D. (1979). Aspects of visual perception in radiography. *Radiography, 45*(539), 237–243.

Arnold, M. (1993). The importance of spatial ability in the selection of student radiographers. *Radiography Today, 59*(679), 20–22.

Bruce, V., & Green, P. R. (1985). *Visual perception physiology, psychology, and ecology.* London: Lawrence Erlbaum Associates.

Chester, M. S. (1982). Perception and evaluation of images. *Scientific Basis of Medical Imaging.* P. T. N. Wells, (Ed.). Edinburgh: Churchill Livingstone.

Cornsweet, T. N. (1970). *Visual perception.* New York: Academic Press.

Curry, T. S., Dowdey, J. E., & Murry, R. C. (1990). *Christensen's introduction to the physics of diagnostic radiology* (4th ed.). Philadelphia: Lea and Febiger.

Davson, H. (1980). *Physiology of the eye* (4th ed.). Edinburgh: Churchill Livingstone.

Fuchs, A. W. (1932). Radiography of the entire body employing one film and a single exposure. *Radiography and Clinical Photography, 10,* 9–14.

Gibbs, S. J., Price, R. R., & James, A. E. (1981). Image perception. In C. M. Coulam, J. J. Erickson, F. D. Rollo, & A. E. James (Eds.). *The physical basis of medical imaging.* (pp. 295–302). New York: Appleton-Century-Crofts.

Graham, D., & Thomson, J. (1980). *Grenz rays: An illustrated guide to the theory and practical applications of soft x-rays.* Oxford: Pergamon Press.

Gregg, E. C. (1972). Image manipulation in radiology. In D. J. Wright, (Ed.), *Physics of diagnostic radiology.* (USDHEW Publication No. (FDA) 74–8006, pp. 282–334). Rockville, MD: U.S. Department of Health, Education, and Welfare, Public Health Service, Food and Drug Administration, Bureau of Radiological Health.

Hay, G. A. (1982). Traditional x-ray imaging. *Scientific basis of medical imaging.* In P. T. N. (Ed.), Edinburgh: Churchill Livingstone.

Hendee, W. R. (1988). The human visual system and its application to perception of radiographic images. *Investigative Radiology, 24,* 25.

Hendee, W. R. (1988). Image analysis and perception. In C. E. Putnam & C. E. Ravin (Eds.), *Textbook of diagnostic imaging.* Philadelphia: W. B. Saunders.

Hendee, W. R. (1989). The perception of visual data. *American Journal of Roentgenology, 152,* 1313–1317.

Hendee, W. R., & Ritenour, R. (1993). *Medical imaging physics* (3rd ed.). St. Louis, MO: Elsevier/C. V. Mosby.

Hendee, W. R., & Wells, P. T. N. (1994). *Perception of visual information.* New York: Springer-Verlag.

Hooker, E. Z. (1981, August). The perceptual domain: A taxonomy for allied health educators. *Journal of Allied Health,* 198–206.

Jaffe, C. C. (Ed.). (1981). *Second international conference on visual psychophysics and medical imaging.* Piscataway, NJ: Institute of Electrical and Electronic Engineers (Catalog #81CH) 1676–6.

Jaffe, C. C. (1984). Medical imaging, vision, and visual psychophysics. *Medical Radiography and Photography, 60*(1), 1–48.

Manning, D., & Cooper, A. (1993). Chest x-ray image quality: Relationships between physical measurements and observer grading. *Radiography Today, 59*(678), 12–15.

Moore, H. D. (Ed.). (1981). *Materials and processes for NDT technology.* Columbus, OH: American Society for Nondestructive Testing.

Neisser, U. (1964). Visual search. *Scientific American, 210*(6), 94–102.

Randall, P. A. (1978). Mach bands in cine coronary arteriography. *Radiology, 129,* 65–66.

Richardson, H. D. (1968). *NDT radiography manual.* Washington, DC: U.S. Government Printing Office, U.S. Department of Health, Education, and Welfare.

Rose, A. (1948). The sensitivity performance of the human eye on an absolute scale. *Journal of the Optical Society of America, 38*(2), 196–208.

Schnitzler, A. D. (1973). Image-detector model and parameters of the human visual system. *Journal of the Optical Society of America, 63*(11), 1357–1368.

Squire, L. F. (1982). *Fundamentals of radiology* (3rd ed.). Cambridge, MA: Harvard University Press.

Tuddenham, W. J. (1957). The visual physiology of Roentgen diagnosis. *American Journal of Roentgenology, 78*(1), 116–123.

CHAPTER 15

Beam Restriction

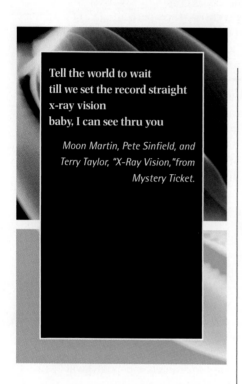

Tell the world to wait
till we set the record straight
x-ray vision
baby, I can see thru you

*Moon Martin, Pete Sinfield, and
Terry Taylor, "X-Ray Vision," from
Mystery Ticket.*

KEY TERMS

aperture diaphragm
collimator
cone/cylinder
penumbra
positive beam
  limitation (PBL)
  device

OBJECTIVES

Upon completion of this chapter, the student should be able to:

- Identify the factors that affect the amount of scatter radiation produced.

- Discuss the primary methods used by radiographers to control the amount of scatter radiation reaching the image receptor.

- Explain the purpose and construction of beam-restricting devices.

- Compare the advantages and disadvantages of the various beam-restricting devices.

- Describe the effect of beam restriction on image quality and patient dose.

CONTROLLING SCATTER

Scatter radiation is produced during a Compton interaction. In this interaction, a primary photon interacts with an outer-shell electron and changes direction, thereby becoming a scattered photon. Scattered photons are not a part of the useful beam and will impair image quality by placing exposures on the image receptor that are unrelated to patient anatomy. In order to provide the best possible image, the radiographer must try to minimize the amount of scatter radiation reaching the image receptor. **This can best be accomplished by restricting the x-ray beam and by using a grid.** Proper beam restriction will keep the total amount of tissue irradiation to a minimum and has great importance in both improving image quality and reducing patient dose.

As the beam is restricted, fewer primary photons are emitted from the tube and collimator and fewer scattered photons are created. Additionally, the decrease in the number of primary photons results in a decrease in the dose to the patient. The only way to improve image quality once scattered photons have been created is to try to decrease the number that are allowed to interact with the image receptor. Grids are devices that are placed between the patient and the image receptor to absorb scatter radiation.

The principal factors that affect the amount of scatter produced are (1) kilovoltage and (2) the irradiated material. In order to control the amount of scatter produced, it is important to understand how kilovoltage and the irradiated material affect scatter production.

Kilovoltage

Kilovoltage affects the penetrability of the beam. As kVp increases, fewer photons undergo interaction with matter and more pass through the patient to interact with the image receptor. For the photons that undergo an interaction, photoelectric absorption and Compton interactions are predominant in the diagnostic x-ray range. Although the total number of photons that undergo interaction decreases with increased kVp, a shift is seen in the percentage of photoelectric versus Compton interactions as kVp increases. As the kilovoltage increases, the percentage of x-rays that undergo a Compton interaction increases and the percentage of photons that undergo photoelectric absorption decreases. Because Compton interactions create scatter, as kilovoltage increases the percentage of primary photons that will undergo scattering also increases. At the same time, the percentage of primary photons that are absorbed photoelectrically decreases, resulting in a reduction in patient dose.

If kilovoltage is increased with no other change in the technical factors selected for a given exposure, the end result will be an increase in the transmission of photons and therefore an increase in the exit dose from the patient. More radiation will reach the image receptor. This increase in kilovoltage will also result in an increase in the percent and amount of scatter radiation produced. Table 12-2 illustrates this point. At 50 kVp with a 10 cm tissue, for every 1000 photons, 990 photons (approximately 99 percent) will be attenuated and 10 photons (approximately 1 percent) will be transmitted. Of the 990 attenuated photons, approximately one-half interact by photoelectric absorption and one-half by Compton scatter (495 interactions each). At 130 kVp with a 10 cm tissue, for every 1000 photons, 940 photons (approximately 94 percent) will be attenuated and 60 photons (approximately 6 percent) will be transmitted. Of the 940 attenuated photons, approximately 25 percent (235 photons) interact photoelectric absorption and 75 percent (705 photons) by Compton scatter.

In radiography, the kilovoltage level is selected based predominantly on the size of the part being examined and the radiographic contrast desired for the image. When kilovoltage is increased without any other changes in technical factors, more scatter will result. If, however, the increase in kilovoltage is accompanied by a reduction in mAs to maintain the same exit dose, the overall result will be a decrease in the amount of scatter produced. Overall less photons are needed to create an acceptable image.

An x-ray image is created when some photons pass through the patient unaffected and others are absorbed photoelectrically. This difference is the basis for varying shades of radiographic density. When more photons pass through unaffected, the result is greater image receptor exposure. When more photons are absorbed photoelectrically, the result is less image receptor exposure. Scattered photons from Compton interactions are of no use in demonstrating the structures of interest. They merely add unwanted exposure to the image receptor that does not correspond to any particular structure. Much of the overall image receptor exposure is created by scattered photons. Image quality is improved when the amount of scatter reaching the image receptor is reduced.

Irradiated Material

The amount of scatter created during an interaction is affected by the volume and atomic number of the material being irradiated. The volume of irradiated material is controlled by field size and patient thickness (Figure 15-1).

As the volume of irradiated tissue increases, the amount of scatter increases. Volume increases as the field size increases or as the patient thickness increases. Larger field sizes, such as with 14″ × 17″ (35 × 43 cm) film, allow for more photons to interact with tissue, thereby creating more scatter. Larger body parts have more tissue to interact with the photons, resulting in greater scatter production. In order to decrease scatter, the smallest possible field size should be used. It is for this reason that beam restriction is an important part of scatter reduction and, of course, of patient protection. Patient thickness cannot be significantly altered by the radiographer, but certain techniques, such as the use of compression bands, can be useful in slightly reducing patient thickness.

The atomic number of the irradiated material also has an impact on the amount of scatter produced because higher atomic number materials have a greater number of electrons within each atom and photons have a greater chance of striking an electron, creating an absorption interaction. Therefore, the higher the atomic number of a material, the greater will be the number of photoelectric absorption interactions and the less scatter. Bone absorbs more radiation and scatters less than soft tissue. For this same reason, high atomic number materials, such as iodine, barium and lead, absorb

FIGURE 15-1   The amount of scatter increases with increased field size and patient thickness.

more radiation through the photoelectric interaction than low atomic number materials do. These photoelectric absorption interactions create the high contrast seen when contrast media are used.

Of the factors affecting the amount of scatter produced, the kilovoltage and the field size are under the direct control of the radiographer. Kilovoltage levels must be selected based on the area being radiographed, and the smallest possible field size should always be used. Beam restriction is, therefore, important to image quality. Remember, however, that **when the beam is restricted, less scatter radiation will reach the image receptor and, as a result, technical factors may need to be increased to compensate for the reduction in the overall image receptor exposure.** For example, the technical factors used for an AP projection of the abdomen using a 14″ × 17″ (35 × 43 cm) film would be insufficient to produce a good image of the same patient's bladder imaged on an 8″ × 10″ (18 × 24 cm) receptor. Technical factors would typically need to be increased 25 to 50 percent to compensate for this type of reduction in the field size.

BEAM RESTRICTORS

There are three basic types of beam-restricting devices used to control scatter and reduce patient dose: **aperture diaphragms, cones/cylinders,** and **collimators.** Each of these devices has advantages and disadvantages which determine how and when they are used in radiography.

Aperture Diaphragm

The aperture diaphragm is a flat sheet of metal, usually lead, with a hole cut in the center and attached to the x-ray tube port. This is the simplest of all beam-restricting devices both in design and in application. Different diaphragms are needed to accommodate different receptor sizes and different distances. The opening can be made in any size or shape but most are rectangular, square or round. Rectangular diaphragms are most common, to correspond to image receptor sizes. The size of the opening depends on the desired exposure field, the source to image receptor distance (SID), and the distance from the aperture to the focal spot.

The main advantages in using an aperture diaphragm are its simple design, low cost, and ease of use. The principal disadvantage is the increase in **penumbra,** a geometric unsharpness around the periphery of the image. This is the result of the diaphragm's close proximity to the tube port. Penumbra is reduced when the beam restrictor is at an increased distance from the port.

Penumbra is the result of x-ray photons being created in all areas of the focal spot rather than at just a single point. Primary photons diverge from the tube port at varying angles and intersect with the structures of interest at varying angles when creating the image. Reducing penumbra will improve the sharpness of the recorded image edges (Figure 15-2). While the use of different types of restrictors does not alter the sharpness of the internal image details, the farther the beam restrictor is from the port, the sharper the edges of the exposed area will be.

Another problem when using an aperture diaphragm is the increase in *off-focus (stem) radiation* reaching the image receptor. This occurs because of the aperture's close proximity to the tube port. Off-focus radiation originates within the x-ray tube but not at the focal spot. Off-focus radiation can result in images, similar to shadows of the patient, beyond the exposed field of radiation (see Figure 6-23). These shadows are often believed to be caused by scatter radiation. However, scatter will never create an image of a specific anatomical structure.

The aperture diaphragm was the original type of beam restrictor, but its use is somewhat limited today. Since it is merely a flat sheet of metal with a hole cut in it, no light field is available for use as an aid in positioning. Its primary application is in dedicated equipment, such as for chest radiography, where the field size and the SID do not vary.

Determining the Diaphragm Field Size. When using an aperture diaphragm it may be necessary for the radiographer to determine the size of the projected image on the image receptor. Aperture diaphragms, when used alone, do not provide the radiographer with a light field for viewing the projected image size. To avoid exposing an area larger than necessary, selection of the correct diaphragm and proper SID is critical. The following formula is used to determine the size of the projected image when using a specific aperture diaphragm. This formula is especially useful when a given diaphragm is used at varying distances.

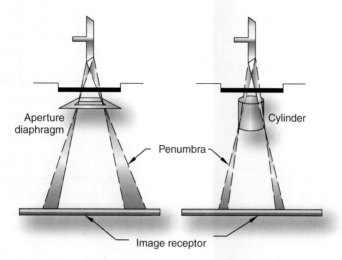

FIGURE 15-2 Penumbra increases as the beam restrictor moves closer to the port. Use of an aperture diaphragm results in greater penumbra than does use of a cylinder.

projected image size =

$$\frac{\text{SID} \times \text{diameter of diaphragm}}{\text{distance from focal spot to diaphragm}}$$

> **EXAMPLE:** A diaphragm is placed 5 inches from the focal spot. The diameter of the opening in the aperture is a 2-inch circle. What would be the projected image size if the SID is 40 inches?
>
> **Answer:** projected image size =
>
> $$\frac{40 \times 2}{5} = \frac{80}{5} = 16\text{- inch circle}$$

This same formula can be applied to a rectangular or square diaphragm by substituting length or width for the diameter of the diaphragm.

Cones/Cylinders

Cones and cylinders are essentially circular aperture diaphragms with metal extensions (Figure 15-3). A cone has an extension which flares or diverges, with the upper diameter smaller than the bottom flared end. A cylinder does not flare. Instead, it has the same diameter at the bottom of the extension as it has at the top. A cylinder may be equipped with an extension sleeve which can expand or collapse to vary the degree of beam restriction.

FIGURE 15-3 Cones and cylinders.

Cones and cylinders are also relatively inexpensive and simple to use. They are most commonly employed in radiography of the skull, spine, gallbladder, and breast. The physical weight of a cone sometimes makes it difficult to handle and, when used with a horizontal beam, the weight of the cone may cause the tube to angle slightly, causing cone cutting if the central ray is not checked carefully just prior to the exposure.

Cones, like aperture diaphragms, have the disadvantage of a fixed field size unless they are equipped with an extension sleeve. In addition, flared cones are no better at reducing penumbra along the edges than are aperture diaphragms.

Cylinders, however, do reduce penumbra and off-focus radiation because they provide better beam restriction at a greater distance from the focal spot (see Figure 15-2). This is especially true when they are used in conjunction with a collimator, as is most often the case.

Determining the Cone Field Size. Determining the field size for a cone/cylinder involves a method similar to that used with an aperture diaphragm. The following formula can be used to calculate the size of the projected image when using a cone/cylinder.

$$\text{projected image size} = \frac{\text{SID} \times \text{lower diameter of cone}}{\text{distance from focal spot to bottom of cone}}$$

> **EXAMPLE:** The diameter of the lower rim of a cone is 3 inches. The bottom of the cone is placed at a distance 16 inches from the focal spot. What will be the size of the projected image at a 40–inch SID?
>
> **Answer:** projected image size =
>
> $\dfrac{40 \times 3}{16} = \dfrac{120}{16} = 7.5\text{-inch circle}$

Collimator

The collimator is the most commonly employed beam restrictor in radiography. Although it is more complex and expensive, the collimator permits an infinite number of field sizes using only one device

(Figure 15-4). It also has the advantage of providing a light source for the radiographer as an aid in properly placing the tube and central ray.

A collimator consists of sets of lead shutters at right angles to one another which move in opposing pairs. Each set moves symmetrically from the center of the field. These lead shutters can be adjusted to correspond to an infinite number of square or rectangular field sizes.

The shutters serve to regulate the field size and, in addition, have two other purposes. The bottom shutters reduce penumbra along the periphery of the beam because of their greater distance from the focal spot. The upper shutters help in reducing the amount of off-focus (stem) radiation reaching the image receptor by absorbing this radiation before it exits the tube.

The collimator offers the radiographer a light field which outlines the exposure field and provides a crosshair to identify the center of the beam. Some units also provide an outline of the automatic exposure control (AEC) chambers' size and location. The light field is provided by mounting a mirror in the path of the x-ray beam at a 45° angle. A light source is then placed opposite the mirror and the light is projected through the collimator. The light source and the x-ray source must be equidistant from one another to ensure that the light field and the x-ray field are the same size. Improper positioning of the mirror or the light can result in improper alignment of the light field to the exposure field. Collimator accuracy should be checked on a regular basis as a part of the department's quality control program.

In the United States it was required by law from 1974 to 1993 for all fixed radiographic equipment to be equipped with automatic collimators. These devices are known as **positive beam limitation (PBL) devices.** When a cassette is placed in the Bucky tray and secured in position, sensing devices determine the size and placement of the cassette. The sensing devices activate an electric motor which drives the collimator lead shutters into proper position. When operating properly, automatic collimators should leave a small unexposed border on all four sides of the exposed image. However, it is possible to override the PBL devices so that the field size can be controlled by the radiographer.

Stators
Rotating anode
Cathode
Tube housing
Rotor
Filters
Glass envelope
Mirror
Collimators
Light source
X-ray beam

FIGURE 15-4 **Schematic drawing of an x-ray tube and collimator.** *(Courtesy of Siemens Medical Systems, Inc., Iselin, NJ)*

The use of a collimator results in some filtration of the x-ray beam because the primary beam is passing through the mirror in the collimator. The added filtration is equivalent to approximately 1 mm of aluminum. Because collimators result in increased filtration of the x-ray beam, their use during low-kVp radiography (such as mammography) is restricted.

Proper collimation is the responsibility of the radiographer. Under no circumstances should the exposure field exceed the size of the image receptor. Automatic collimation helps to ensure that the exposure field does not exceed the size of the image receptor, but the radiographer should always limit the field to the part being examined. By so doing,

image quality can be improved and patient dose can be minimized.

 ANCILLARY DEVICES

Beam restrictors may be made for a very specific purpose. Ancillary devices are generally designed with a special need in mind. Examples include lead blockers and lead masks. These devices are tailored for a specific use during a given procedure. They are designed to restrict the beam to a specific shape for a particular examination.

A lead blocker is simply a sheet of lead-impregnated rubber that can be cut to any size or shape. Placement

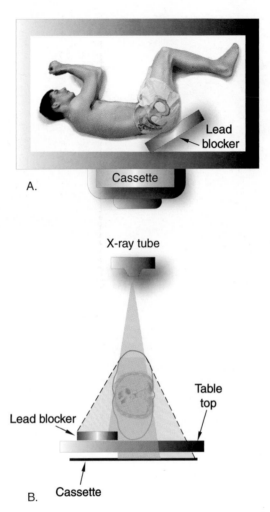

A.

Cassette

X-ray tube

Lead blocker

Table top

B. Cassette

FIGURE 15-5 The use of a lead blocker for radiography of the lower spine (A), and cutaway view of absorption of scatter (B).

of a lead blocker on the radiographic table during radiography of the lower spine in the lateral position will help to absorb the scatter that is produced in the soft tissue of the patient's back (Figure 15-5). A lead blocker may also be helpful when placed on the radiographic table above the level of the shoulder during positioning for AP projections of the shoulder joint. Lead blockers are most helpful when examining large patients, because the amount of scatter increases with increases in the size of the patient.

A lead mask is usually cut to correspond to the particular field size desired and is then secured to the end of the collimator. The most common use of a lead mask is during cerebral angiography. The lead mask helps improve image quality by reducing scatter (Figure 15-6 A and B).

FIGURE 15-6 Two radiographs of an AP cerebral angiogram, with and without a lead mask. *(Courtesy of Dr. Marion Frank)*

SUMMARY

In order to provide the best possible image, the radiographer must try to control the amount of scatter radiation reaching the image receptor. The principle factors that affect the amount of scatter produced are: (1) kilovoltage and (2) the irradiated material. As kilovoltage increases, the percentage of primary photons that will undergo scattering also increases. As the volume of irradiated tissue increases, the amount of scatter produced is increased. Volume will increase as the field size increases or as the patient thickness increases. The atomic number of the irradiated material also has an impact on the amount of scatter produced. Higher atomic number materials have a greater number of electrons within each atom. Photons have a greater chance of being absorbed by these materials.

There are three basic types of beam-restricting devices that are used to control scatter and reduce patient dose: aperture diaphragms, cones/cylinders, and collimators. Each of these devices has advantages and disadvantages which determine how and when they are used in radiography. The collimator is the most commonly employed beam restrictor in radiography because it permits an infinite number of field sizes using only one device. It also has the advantage of providing a light source for the radiographer as an aid in properly placing the tube.

Proper collimation is the responsibility of the radiographer. Under no circumstances should the exposure field ever exceed the size of the image receptor. In addition, the radiographer should always limit the field to the part being examined. By so doing, image quality will be improved and patient dose will be minimized.

REVIEW QUESTIONS

1. Why does beam restriction reduce scatter radiation production?

2. What are the two principal factors that affect the amount of scatter produced?

3. How does the atomic number of a material affect the amount of scatter produced?

4. What are the three basic types of beam-restricting devices?

5. What is penumbra and how can it be minimized?

6. What is the formula for determining the size of the projected image when using a cone?

7. How is a collimator constructed?

8. What is PBL?

9. How does beam restriction affect patient dose?

REFERENCES AND RECOMMENDED READING

Bushberg, J. T., Seibert, J. A., Leidholdt, E. M., & Boone, J. M. (2002). *The essential physics of medical imaging* (2nd ed.). Baltimore: Lippincott, Williams & Wilkins.

Carroll, Q. B. (2003). *Fuchs's radiographic exposure, processing, and quality control* (7th ed.). Springfield, IL: Charles C Thomas.

Crooks, H. E., & Ardran, G. M. (1976). Checking x-ray beam field size. *Radiography, 42(503),* 239.

Cullinan, A., & Cullinan, J. (1994). *Producing quality radiographs* (2nd ed.). Philadelphia: J. B. Lippincott.

Curry, T. S., Dowdey, J. E., & Murry, R. C. (1990). *Christensen's introduction to the physics of diagnostic radiology* (4th ed.). Philadelphia: Lea and Febiger.

Mattsson, O. (1955). Practical photographic problems in radiography with special reference to high-voltage technique. *Acta Radiologica Supplementum, 120,* 1–206.

Mitchell, F. (1991). Scattered radiation and the lateral lumbar spine part 1: Initial research. *Radiography Today, 57(644),* 18–20.

Mitchell, F., Leung, C., Ahuja, A., & Metreweli, C. (1991). Scattered radiation and the lateral lumbar spine part 2: Clinical research. *Radiography Today, 57(645),* 12–14.

Rogers, K. D., & Matthers, I. P. (1986). X-ray field collimation in diagnostic radiology. *Radiography, 52(604),* 161.

Seeram, E., & Travis, E. L. (1997). *Radiation protection.* Baltimore: Lippincott, Williams & Wilkins.

Thomas, S. R., Freshcorn, J. E., Krugh, K. B., Henry, G. C., Kereiakes, J. G., & Kaufman, R. A. (1983). Characteristics of extrafocal radiation and its potential significance in pediatric radiology. *Radiology, 146,* 793–799.

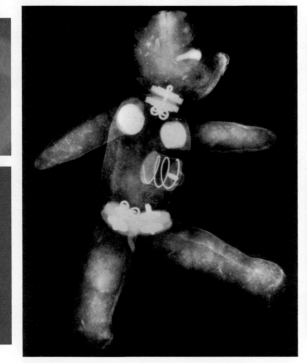

(Courtesy of Dr. Marion Frank)

The Case of Lumpy

What is this lumpy object's name?

Answers to the case studies can be found in Appendix E.

CHAPTER 16

The Patient as a Beam Emitter

. . . the patient . . . would shape up into something that called for attention, his peculiarities, her reticences or candors. And though I might be attracted or repelled, the professional attitude . . . would steady me and dictate the terms on which I was to proceed.

By William Carlos Williams, from The Autobiography of William Carlos Williams, copyright © 1951 by William Carlos Williams. Reprinted with permission of New Directions Publishing Corp.

KEY TERMS

subject contrast
subject density
subject detail
subject distortion

OBJECTIVES

Upon completion of this chapter, the student should be able to:

- Explain the process of attenuation.

- Describe the basic composition of the human body.

- Describe the effect of the human body on the attenuation of the x-ray beam.

- Explain the relationship of the subject (patient) to the density, contrast, recorded detail, and distortion of the recorded image.

ATTENUATION

Attenuation is the reduction in the total number of x-ray photons remaining in the beam after passing through a given thickness of material (see Figure 12-1). It is the result of x-rays interacting with matter and being absorbed or scattered. The amount of attenuation is determined by the amount and type of irradiated material. X-rays are attenuated exponentially. This means that they are reduced by a certain percentage for each given thickness of material they pass through. Theoretically, then, the number of x-rays passing through an absorber will never reach zero. This is because each succeeding thickness of material reduces the number of photons by only a fraction of the previous amount.

As an x-ray beam passes through a patient, the beam is attenuated. The thicker the body part being radiographed, the greater the attenuation. In order to provide a sufficient number of x-ray photons for interaction with the image receptor, the original quantity and quality of the photons must be increased with increased body part thickness. The incident beam is significantly altered as it passes through the patient. **The beam emitted from the patient contains the radiologically significant information needed by the radiologist to make a diagnosis.**

Attenuation is also affected by the type of absorber. **Higher atomic number materials** (such as lead and barium) **attenuate a greater percentage of the beam than low atomic number materials** (such as hydrogen, carbon, and oxygen). This is due to the presence of a greater number of electrons with which photons may interact. Bone produces less image receptor exposure because it attenuates the x-ray beam more than soft tissue. This is predominantly because of the presence of calcium in bone, which has a higher atomic number than the majority of the elements found in the human body. The effective atomic number of the important materials comprising the human body are listed in Table 16-1.

The density of the absorbing material also has an impact on attenuation. **Density is the quantity of matter per unit of volume measured in kilo-**

TABLE 16-1.	Basic Substances Comprising the Human Body	
Substance	Effective Atomic Number	Density (kg/m³)
Air	7.78	1.29
Fat	6.46	916
Water	7.51	1000
Muscle	7.64	1040
Bone	12.31	1650

grams per cubic meter. It describes how tightly the atoms of a given substance are packed together. For example, the molecules in an ice cube are more tightly packed than the same molecules when they are in their liquid state. Bone tissue is a denser substance than lung tissue. Table 16-1 lists the densities of the important materials comprising the human body. Because density and atomic number affect attenuation, it is important to understand the basic composition of the human body, particularly in terms of the average atomic number and density of the major substances.

THE HUMAN BODY AS AN ATTENUATOR

The patient is the greatest variable the radiographer faces when performing a radiographic procedure. The human body is comprised of a variety of organic and inorganic substances. At the atomic level, the body consists primarily of hydrogen, carbon, nitrogen, and oxygen. These elements have atomic numbers of 1, 6, 7, and 8, respectively. Calcium, found in concentrated amounts in bones and teeth, has an atomic number of 20.

The composition of the human body determines its radiographic appearance (Figure 16-1). Although human anatomy and physiology are quite complex, when studying the absorption characteristics of the body, four major substances account for most of the variations in x-ray absorption: air, fat, muscle, and bone (Figure 16-2).

FIGURE 16-1 An antique full-body radiograph.
(Reprinted with permission of the International Society of Radiographers and Radiological Technicians from the K. C. Clark Archives, Middlesex Hospital, London, England)

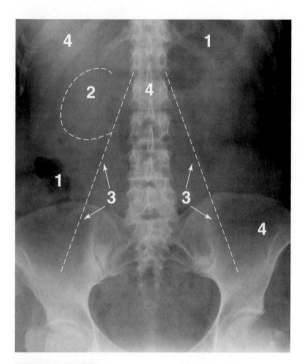

FIGURE 16-2 A radiograph of the abdomen demonstrating (1) air in the stomach and colon; (2) fat around the kidneys; (3) muscle to the right and left of the spine (psoas muscle); and (4) ribs, spine, and pelvis.

Air

Air has an effective atomic number of 7.78, which is greater than either fat or muscle. Despite the slightly higher effective atomic number, air has a significantly lower tissue density. As a result, air will absorb fewer photons as they pass through it. Because air absorbs fewer photons than other body substances, more photons reach the image receptor, thus producing a greater image receptor exposure.

Air is naturally present in the lungs, the sinuses and, in small amounts, in the gastrointestinal tract. On a typical radiograph of the abdomen, air can usually be seen in the stomach and colon.

Fat

Fat is similar to muscle in that they are both among the soft-tissue structures in the body. The soft-tissue structures have effective atomic numbers and tissue densities which are very similar to water's. For this reason, water is sometimes used to simulate soft tissue for experimental purposes. Fat has an effective atomic number which is slightly less than muscle's. In addition, fat has less tissue density than muscle. Muscle cells are more closely packed than fat cells. The amount of fatty tissue varies considerably between patients. While this is also true of muscle tissue, the variations are generally less pronounced and therefore have less effect on the overall attenuation of the beam. On a radiograph of the abdomen, the kidneys can often be outlined because of the perirenal fat capsule that surrounds them.

Muscle

Like fat, muscle is a soft tissue. Muscle, however, has a slightly higher effective atomic number and a greater tissue density than fat. As a result, muscle is a greater attenuator of the beam. On a radiograph of the abdomen, it is often easy to distinguish the psoas muscle on each side of the spine because of the increased absorption of radiation by these muscles.

Bone

The skeletal anatomy is easily seen radiographically because of the calcium content of bone. Calcium has a higher atomic number than most of the elements found in the human body. As a result, bone has the highest effective atomic number of the four basic substances. It also has the greatest tissue density and, as a result, absorbs radiation at a greater rate than any of the soft tissues or air-filled structures. This absorption means that fewer photons will reach the image receptor and less image receptor exposure will be produced. On a radiograph of the abdomen, the lower ribs, spine and pelvis are all very easily distinguished because of the increased x-ray absorption that occurs in bone.

THE PATIENT'S RELATIONSHIP TO IMAGE QUALITY

The patient has an impact on all properties affecting radiographic quality: density, contrast, recorded detail, and distortion. These are described in detail in Chapters 28–31. The relationships between these factors and the patient (subject) are termed **subject density, subject contrast, subject detail,** and **subject distortion.**

Subject Density

The various tissues in the human body are responsible for the differing exposures to the image receptor. Subject density refers to the impact the subject (patient) has on the resultant radiographic density. **Image receptor exposure will be altered by changes in the amount or type of tissue being irradiated.** In other words, thicker and denser body parts absorb more radiation, thus producing less image receptor exposure and vice versa.

Subject Contrast

Radiographic contrast is the difference in densities of a recorded image. The differences in density are the result of differences in the absorption of the x-ray beam as it passes through the patient. **Subject contrast is the degree of differential absorption resulting from the differing absorption characteristics of the tissues in the body.** Subject contrast is dependent on the specific characteristics of an individual patient's tissues.

When there is little difference in the absorption characteristic of the given body tissues within a part being examined, as in mammography, subject contrast will be low. When there is a greater difference in the absorption characteristics of the body tissues within a part being examined, as in the chest with the lungs, heart, and spine, subject contrast is high.

Subject Detail

One of the primary factors that affects the sharpness or detail of an image is the distance between the structure of interest and the image receptor. Because anatomical structures are located at varying distances from the image receptor, **the recorded detail of the structures is dependent on their position within the body and also on the body's placement in relationship to the receptor**. The overall size and placement of the patient has a great impact on the recorded detail. The larger the patient, the greater the distance between the anatomical structures and the image receptor. This results in less sharpness in the recorded details. Conversely, greater sharpness will result when the anatomical part is closer to the image receptor, as is the case with thinner patients.

Specific positions have been established to place the anatomical structures of interest in as close proximity to the image receptor as possible. For example, chest radiography is typically performed in the PA projection and in the left lateral position to place the heart closer to the image receptor.

Subject Distortion

Distortion is the misrepresentation of the size or shape of the structure of interest. Because of the way in which certain structures lie within the body, **unless the patient is positioned specifically to demonstrate a particular structure, it may not be accurately represented on the image receptor.** For example, to properly demonstrate the apophyseal joints of the lumbar spine, the patient should be in the oblique position. In the AP projection of the lumbar spine, these joints will be distorted. Distortion, in the form of magnification, also occurs because various anatomical structures sit at varying levels.

SUMMARY

Attenuation is the reduction in the total number of x-ray photons remaining in the beam after passing through a given thickness of material. It is the result of x-rays interacting with matter and being absorbed or scattered. The amount of attenuation will be determined by the amount and type of irradiated material.

The patient is the greatest variable that the radiographer faces when performing a radiographic procedure. The composition of the human body determines its radiographic appearance. When studying the absorption characteristics of the body, four major substances account for most of the variations in x-ray absorption: air, fat, muscle, and bone.

The patient has an impact on all the properties that affect radiographic quality: density, contrast, recorded detail, and distortion. The relationships between these factors and the patient (subject) are termed subject density, subject contrast, subject detail, and subject distortion.

REVIEW QUESTIONS

1. How does atomic number affect attenuation?
2. How does tissue density affect attenuation?
3. What elements comprise the majority of those found in the human body?
4. What are the differences between air, fat, muscle, and bone with respect to their attenuation and the resultant radiographic film density?
5. How does the patient affect each of the factors of image quality?

REFERENCES AND RECOMMENDED READING

Bower, R. (1989). Stripes in the abdomen. *Radiologic Technology, 60*(6), 511.

Bushberg, J. T., Seibert, J. A., Leidholdt, E. M., & Boone, J. M. (2002). *The essential physics of medical imaging* (2nd ed.). Baltimore: Lippincott Williams & Wilkins.

Carroll, Q. B. (2003). *Fuchs's radiographic exposure, processing, and quality control* (7th ed.). Springfield, IL: Charles C Thomas.

Cohen, M. (1971). Attenuation of x-rays in the human body. *Radiography, 37*(436), 88–90.

Curry, T. S., Dowdey, J. E., & Murry, R. C. (1990). *Christensen's introduction to the physics of diagnostic radiology* (4th ed.). Philadelphia: Lea and Febiger.

Fuchs, A. W. (1948). Relationship of tissue thickness to kilovoltage. *Radiologic Technology, 19*(6), 287.

Handbook of chemistry and physics. (1998). (78th ed.). Boca Raton, FL: C. R. C. Press.

Lindsay, R., & Anderson, J. B. (1978). Radiological determination of changes in bone mineral content. *Radiography, 44*(517), 21–26.

Seeram, E., Travis, E. L. (1997). *Radiation protection.* Baltimore: Lippincott Williams & Wilkins.

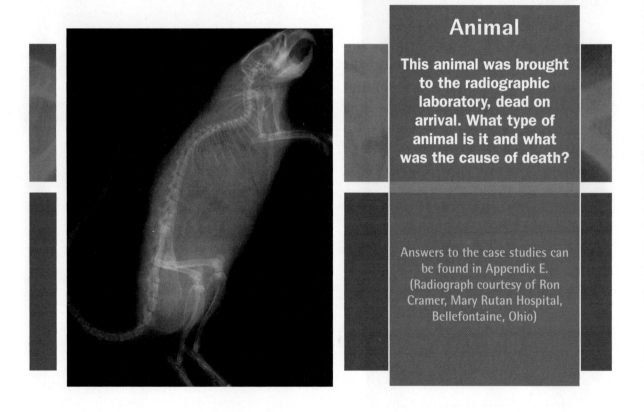

Animal

This animal was brought to the radiographic laboratory, dead on arrival. What type of animal is it and what was the cause of death?

Answers to the case studies can be found in Appendix E. (Radiograph courtesy of Ron Cramer, Mary Rutan Hospital, Bellefontaine, Ohio)

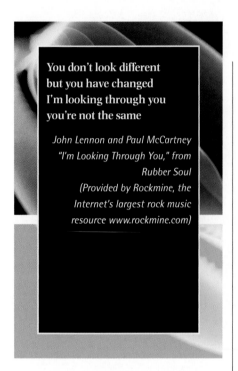

CHAPTER 17   # The Pathology Problem

You don't look different
but you have changed
I'm looking through you
you're not the same

John Lennon and Paul McCartney
"I'm Looking Through You," from
Rubber Soul
(Provided by Rockmine, the
Internet's largest rock music
resource www.rockmine.com)

KEY TERMS

abscess	congestive heart	osteochondroma
acromegaly	failure	osteolytic metastases
active osteomyelitis	degenerative arthritis	osteomalacia
additive condition	destructive condition	osteoporosis
aerophagia	edema	Paget's Disease
anorexia nervosa	emaciation	pathology
aortic aneurysm	emphysema	pleural effusions
ascites	empyema	pneumoconiosis
aseptic necrosis	fibrosarcoma	pneumonectomy
atelectasis	gout	pneumonia
atrophy	hemothorax	pneumonitis
bowel obstruction	hydrocephalus	pneumothorax
bronchiectasis	hydrothorax	pulmonary edema
calcified stones	hyperparathyroidism	sclerosis
carcinoma	multiple myeloma	tuberculosis
cardiomegaly	osteitis deformans	tumor
chronic osteomyelitis	osteoblastic	
cirrhosis	metastases	

OBJECTIVES

Upon completion of this chapter, the student should be able to:

- Explain the effect that a pathological condition can have on radiation absorption.

- Describe the effect of pathology on the radiographic image.

- Differentiate between pathological conditions that result in increased attenuation versus those that result in decreased attenuation of the x-ray beam.

- Identify pathological conditions that result in an increased attenuation of the x-ray beam.

- Identify pathological conditions that result in a decreased attenuation of the x-ray beam.

PATHOLOGY AND RADIATION ABSORPTION

As radiation passes through the patient it undergoes attenuation or absorption of the x-ray photons. The patient is the greatest variable the radiographer faces when trying to select adequate exposure factors for a specific procedure. Attenuation will vary, depending on the thickness and the composition of the patient's tissues. As an added dilemma, the radiographer must also realize that pathological conditions can affect the overall thickness and composition of the patient's tissues. The radiographer must first be aware of the variations between normal body tissues and then be concerned about possible additional variations as a result of a specific disease process.

Pathology is the medical science that is concerned with all aspects of disease, including the structural and functional changes caused by a disease process. Disease will often bring about changes in body tissues that can be viewed radiographically and interpreted by the radiologist. If this were not true, radiography would be of no use in diagnosing disease. These changes may be structural and/or functional in nature and they may or may not have an impact on the degree of radiation absorbed by the patient. Certain diseases can increase or decrease tissue thickness or alter tissue composition (change the effective atomic number or density). When this occurs, the disease will affect the degree of radiation absorption for that specific body tissue. Two common pathologies of the chest demonstrate the differences in radiation absorption (Figure 17-1A and B). In Figure 17-1A, the patient has pneumonia, which causes air-filled lung tissue to fill with fluid. Fluid will absorb more radiation than air. In Figure 17-1B, the patient has emphysema. With emphysema, normal lung tissue is destroyed and the air sacs become enlarged. A greater amount of air is then present in the lungs, which results in less attenuation of radiation.

Radiographers must have an understanding of pathology in order to properly select the technical factors for a procedure. Properly reading the x-ray requisition, taking an adequate patient history and close observation of the patient are the essential responsibilities of the radiographer. Fulfilling these responsibilities reduces the need to repeat an image, due to the patient's condition. For example, it may be necessary to adjust the technical factors if a chest x-ray is requested for a patient with emphysema. By taking a good history, the radiographer can determine how long the patient has had the condition and what signs and symptoms the patient has exhibited. By observing signs, such as shortness of breath or prolonged exhalation, the radiographer can assess the extent of the disease. Of course, disease conditions are not always known prior to performing the examination. This is one of the primary reasons a repeat exposure may be necessary, even though there was no error in judgment on the part of the radiographer. As an individual gains clinical experience, his assessment skills improve and he is able to make better judgments concerning the presence and extent of disease.

If a disease causes the affected body tissue to increase in thickness, effective atomic number, and/or density, there will be a greater attenuation of the x-ray beam. As more photons are absorbed by the body tissues, fewer will be available to reach the image receptor to create an adequate exposure. These diseases are harder to penetrate and are called **additive conditions** because they require increasing technical factors to achieve the proper image receptor exposure. There is an inverse relationship between additive conditions and image receptor exposure. This means that when additive conditions are present, image receptor exposure will decrease as the extent of the disease increases.

If a disease causes the affected body tissue to decrease in thickness, effective atomic number, and/or density, there will be less attenuation of the x-ray beam. As more photons are able to pass through the body tissues, more will be available to reach the image receptor. These diseases are easier to penetrate and are called **destructive conditions.** They require decreasing the exposure to achieve the proper image receptor exposure. There is a direct relationship between destructive conditions and image receptor exposure. This means that when destructive conditions are present, the image receptor exposure will increase as the extent of the disease increases.

A

B

FIGURE 17-1 (A) The patient has bilateral pneumonia, resulting in an increase in radiation absorption. (B) The patient has severe emphysema, resulting in a decrease in radiation absorption.

A disease influences radiation absorption when it alters the overall number or types of atoms comprising the affected tissue. For example, if a person sprains an ankle, one of the body's responses to the injury is swelling or edema at the site. The ankle becomes enlarged because there is an increase in blood and serous fluid around the ankle joint. The body tissue increases in thickness, but, in this example, the opacity of the tissue is generally the same. Blood and serous fluid have approximately the same opacity as the soft tissue around the ankle. What is occurring at the molecular and atomic level is an increase, primarily in the number of water molecules (hydrogen and oxygen atoms), which comprise most of blood and serous fluid. If there are more water molecules present around the ankle, a greater number of x-ray photons will interact with that tissue, resulting in increased radiation absorption and decreased exposure to the image receptor. Technical factors must be increased to compensate for an increase in the thickness of the part. Proper

measurement of the body part and the use of technique charts will ensure that the correct technical factors are selected.

The extent to which a body part is affected by disease will determine if technical factors must be adjusted. For example, no change in technical factors is necessary to visualize a small, localized tumor in the lung or a small kidney stone. If, however, the tumor is large and diffuse, or the kidney stone causes severe hydronephrosis, adjustments in the technical factors may be required to adequately visualize the pathology (Figure 17-2A and B). It is important to remember that the degree or extent of the pathology is critical in determining the technical factor adjustments. If the technical factors must be adjusted, the change must be enough to make a noticeable difference in image receptor exposure. **To produce a visible difference requires a minimal change of 25–50 percent in the overall exposure to the image receptor for film/screen radiography.** This issue is more complex with digital image

A

B

FIGURE 17-2 (A) When a tumor is smaller and more localized, there is less need for technical factor adjustments. (B) Tumors that are larger and more diffuse throughout both lungs require greater technical factor adjustments.

detector systems, where the traditional relationship between density and mAs, kVp, and distance no longer exist. It is possible to change the mAs, kVp, and the distance and have no effect on the density or brightness on the display monitor. A wider range of patient exposures can all produce acceptable images, and it is the technologist's responsibility to keep the patient dose for a given exam as low as possible without compromising image quality.

Many diseases do not affect the thickness or opacity of body tissues but can be diagnosed by way of radiography simply because of the structural or functional changes that they produce. These diseases generally do not require an adjustment in the selected technical factors. Examples include ulcers, diverticula, and simple fractures (provided there is minimal swelling). There are many diseases that do not affect the thickness or alter the composition of the body tissues and therefore cause no radiographically evident structural or functional changes.

These conditions generally do not require radiography; they are usually diagnosed through laboratory testing. Diseases such as diabetes mellitus, anemia, and meningitis are examples.

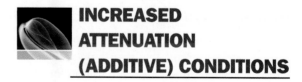 **INCREASED ATTENUATION (ADDITIVE) CONDITIONS**

Many disease processes will result in an increase in thickness, effective atomic number, and/or density of the body tissue. Recall that the body tissues vary in thickness (the femur is thicker than the humerus) and in composition (bone has a higher effective atomic number and greater tissue density than muscle). These diseases absorb more radiation and require the radiographer to increase technical factors to compensate for the changes in the body tissues.

The extent of the disease also plays an important role in technical factor adjustment. The technical factor adjustments will vary, depending on the degree to which the body tissues are affected. Because of this, each patient will be different and must be examined individually.

No magic formula exists to adjust technical factors to compensate for a pathologic problem. The radiographer must carefully review the requisition, obtain a patient history, and then examine the patient. By following these steps, the radiographer can make a judgment concerning the necessary technical adjustment to be made. Experience is particularly valuable in determining the proper changes to be made. As a general rule, additive conditions will require an increase in kilovoltage to adequately penetrate the thicker, more opaque body parts. Remember that an increase of 15 percent in kVp will approximately double the exposure to the image receptor. An increase of 5–15 percent in kilovoltage will compensate for most additive pathologic conditions. Automatic exposure control (AEC) systems will compensate for most pathological changes by adjusting the exposure automatically. However, the compensation will be the result of increased mAs rather than increased kVp.

Some of the common conditions that cause an increase in attenuation and may therefore require an increase in technical factors are outlined. A summary of the conditions is provided in Table 17-1.

Conditions Affecting Multiple Systems

Certain diseases can occur in a wide variety of body systems and, as a result, they may be present in various sites. Whenever an x-ray requisition indicates the presence of any of the following conditions, it may be necessary to increase technical factors for the procedure.

Abscess—an encapsulated infection increases tissue thickness and may alter composition, particularly in the lungs.

Edema—swelling causes an increase in tissue thickness and may alter composition if it occurs in the lungs.

TABLE 17-1. Summary of Pathology Problems

Increased Attenuation Conditions	Decreased Attenuation Conditions
Multiple Sites	**Multiple Sites**
Abscess	Anorexia Nervosa
Edema	Atrophy
Tumors	Emaciation
The Chest	**The Chest**
Atelectasis	Emphysema
Bronchiectasis	Pneumothorax
Cardiomegaly	
Congestive Heart Failure	
Empyema	
Pleural Effusions	
Pneumoconiosis	
Pneumonia	
Pneumonectomy	
Pulmonary Edema	
Tuberculosis (advanced/miliary)	
The Abdomen	**The Abdomen**
Aortic Aneurysm	Aerophagia
Ascites	Bowel Obstruction
Cirrhosis	
Calcified Stones	
The Extremities and Skull	**The Extremities and Skull**
Acromegaly	Active Osteomyelitis
Chronic Osteomyelitis	Aseptic Necrosis
Hydrocephalus	Carcinoma
Osteoblastic Metastases	Degenerative Arthritis
Osteochondroma	Fibrosarcoma
Paget's Disease	Gout
Sclerosis	Hyperparathyroidism
	Multiple Myeloma
	Osteolytic Metastases
	Osteomalacia
	Osteoporosis

Tumor—an abnormal new growth in tissue results in an increase in tissue thickness and may alter composition, particularly in the lungs or bones or when calcification results.

Conditions of the Chest

The chest is a common site for pathologic conditions, and chest radiography is a common diagnostic procedure. It may be necessary to increase technical factors for a procedure whenever an x-ray requisition indicates the presence of any of the following conditions.

Atelectasis—a collapse of the lung results in airlessness of all or part of the lung tissue. This causes lung tissue density to increase.

Bronchiectasis—the chronic dilatation of the bronchi can result in peribronchial thickening and small areas of atelectasis. This causes an increase in lung tissue density.

Cardiomegaly—an enlargement of the heart causes an increase in thickness of the part.

Congestive Heart Failure—when the heart is in failure, the cardiac output is diminished. This results in backward failure, or increased venous congestion in the lungs. Lung tissue density is increased and the heart is enlarged as well.

Empyema—pus in the thoracic cavity causes an increase in tissue density.

Pleural Effusions (Hemothorax, Hydrothorax)—when the pleural cavity fills with either blood or serous fluid, it displaces normal lung tissue. This results in an increased tissue density within the thoracic cavity.

Pneumoconiosis—the inhalation of dust particles can cause fibrotic (scarring) changes. When healthy lung tissue becomes fibrotic, density of the tissue increases.

Pneumonectomy—the removal of a lung will cause the affected side to demonstrate an increase in density since normal air-filled lung tissue is removed.

Pneumonia (pneumonitis)—inflammation of the lung tissues causes fluid to fill in the alveolar spaces. Fluid has much greater tissue density than the air normally present.

Pulmonary Edema—when fluid fills the interstitial lung tissues and the alveoli, tissue density increases. This is a typical complication of congestive heart failure.

FIGURE 17-3   This patient has miliary tuberculosis with bronchopneumonia. These are both additive conditions, resulting in increased radiation absorption.

Tuberculosis (advanced and miliary)—an infection by a mycobacteria causes the inflammatory response, which results in an increase in fluid in the lungs. If the mycobacteria were inhaled, it generally begins as a localized lesion (usually upper lobes), which can spread to a more advanced stage. If the infection reaches the lungs by the bloodstream, it has a more diffuse spread (miliary TB). Increased tissue density results in both advanced and miliary TB (Figure 17-3).

Conditions of the Abdomen

Abdominal conditions usually cause the abdomen to distend. It may be necessary to increase technical factors for a procedure when an x-ray requisition indicates the presence of any of the following conditions. Most technical factor changes, however, will be the natural result of the noted increase in abdominal size when measuring patient thickness.

Aortic Aneurysm—a large dilatation of the aorta will result in increased thickness of the affected part.

Ascites—fluid accumulation within the peritoneal cavity causes an increase in tissue thickness. The free fluid has a unique "ground glass" appearance radiographically.

Calcified stones—stones are most commonly found throughout the abdomen in such organs as the gallbladder and the kidney. Calcium may be deposited, which causes an increase in the effective atomic number of the tissue.

Cirrhosis—fibrotic changes in the liver cause the liver to enlarge and ascites can result. The result is an increase in the thickness of the liver and the entire abdomen.

Conditions of the Extremities and Skull

Conditions that result in new bone growth are termed osteoblastic. These conditions generally require an increase in technical factors. It may be necessary to increase technical factors for a procedure whenever an x-ray requisition indicates the presence of any of the following conditions.

Acromegaly—an overgrowth of the hands, feet, face, and jaw as a result of hypersecretion of growth hormones in the adult will result in an increase in bone mass.

Chronic Osteomyelitis—a chronic bone infection results in new bone growth at the infected site.

Hydrocephalus—a dilatation of the fluid-filled cerebral ventricles causes an enlargement of the head, resulting in an increased thickness.

Osteoblastic Metastases—the spread of cancer to bone can result in uncontrolled new bone growth.

Osteochondroma—a tumor arising in the bone and cartilage will result in an increased thickness of the bone.

Paget's Disease (osteitis deformans)—an increase occurs in bone cell activity which leads to new bone growth. The result is increased bone

FIGURE 17-4 Paget's disease is an additive condition, resulting in increased radiation absorption.

thickness, with the pelvis, spine, and skull most often affected (Figure 17-4).

Sclerosis—an increase in hardening as a result of a chronic inflammation in bone. This increases the density of the bone tissue.

DECREASED ATTENUATION (DESTRUCTIVE) CONDITIONS

Various disease processes can result in a decrease in thickness, effective atomic number and/or density of the body tissue. These conditions cause the absorption of less radiation and require the radiographer to decrease technical factors to compensate for the changes in the body tissues. Recall also that the extent of the disease plays an important role in technical factor adjustment. As a general rule, compensations for destructive conditions can be made by decreasing the mAs. Remember that a decrease of 50 percent in mAs will reduce the exposure to the image receptor by half. A decrease of 25–50 percent in mAs will compensate for most of these pathologic conditions. Automatic exposure control (AEC) systems will compensate for most pathological changes by adjusting the exposure automatically.

Some of the common conditions that cause a decrease in attenuation and may therefore require a decrease in technical factors are outlined. A summary of the conditions is provided in Table 17-1.

Conditions Affecting Multiple Sites

Certain diseases can occur in a wide variety of body systems and, as a result, they may be present in various sites. Whenever an x-ray requisition indicates the presence of any of the following conditions, it may be necessary to decrease technical factors for the procedure.

Anorexia Nervosa—a psychological eating disorder which results in an extreme weight loss. Overall body thickness is reduced.

Atrophy—a wasting away of body tissue with diminished cell proliferation, resulting in reduced thickness of a specific part or the entire body.

Emaciation—a generalized wasting away of body tissue, resulting in reduced thickness of the body.

Conditions of the Chest

The chest is a common site for pathologic conditions and chest radiography is a common diagnostic procedure. It may be necessary to decrease technical factors for a procedure when an x-ray requisition indicates the presence of the following conditions.

Emphysema—the overdistention of the lung tissues by air will result in a decrease in lung tissue density.

FIGURE 17-5 A large, right-sided pneumothorax is a destructive condition, resulting in decreased radiation absorption.

Pneumothorax—free air in the pleural cavity displaces normal lung tissue and results in decreased density within the thoracic cavity (Figure 17-5).

Conditions of the Abdomen

Abdominal conditions usually cause the abdomen to distend. This distention may be the result of the accumulation of fluid (in which case technical factors need to be increased) or air. Distention of the abdomen from air will require a decrease in technical factors. Whenever an x-ray requisition indicates the presence of the following conditions, it may be necessary to decrease technical factors for the procedure because of the presence of air.

Aerophagia—a psychological disorder resulting in abnormal swallowing of air. The stomach becomes dilated from the air and overall tissue density decreases.

FIGURE 17-6 An obstruction of the large bowel is a destructive condition, resulting in decreased radiation absorption.

Bowel Obstruction—an obstruction in the bowel results in the abnormal accumulation of air and fluid. If a large amount of air is trapped in the bowel, the overall density of the tissues is decreased (Figure 17-6).

Conditions of the Extremities and Skull

Conditions that result in the destruction of bone tissue are termed osteolytic. These conditions result in a loss of bone mass or calcium within the bone. They alter the composition of the bone by decreasing the effective atomic number and/or the tissue density. The result is areas of radiolucency, which are easier to penetrate than normal bone. Approximately 50 percent of the bone substance must be lost before changes can be seen radiographically. As a result, these conditions must generally be extensive before technical factor changes are necessary.

Active Osteomyelitis—with a bone infection, there is initially a loss of bone tissue (containing calcium), resulting in a decrease in the thickness and composition of the part.

Aseptic Necrosis—death of bone tissue results in a decrease in composition and thickness of the part.

Carcinoma—malignancies in bone can cause an osteolytic process, resulting in decreased thickness and composition of the part.

Degenerative Arthritis—inflammation of the joints results in a destruction of adjoining bone tissue, which decreases the composition of the part.

Fibrosarcoma—this malignant tumor of the metaphysis of bone causes an osteolytic lesion with a "moth-eaten" appearance. The result is reduced bone composition.

Gout—during the chronic stages of this metabolic disease, areas of bone destruction result in punched-out lesions that reduce the bone composition.

Hyperparathyroidism—oversecretion of the parathyroid hormone causes calcium to leave bone and enter the bloodstream. The bone becomes demineralized and composition is decreased.

Multiple Myeloma—this malignant tumor arises from plasma cells of bone marrow and causes punched-out osteolytic areas on the bone. Often many sites are affected and reduced bone tissue composition results.

Osteolytic Metastases—when some malignancies spread to bone they produce destruction of the bone, resulting in reduced composition.

Osteomalacia—a defect in bone mineralization results in decreased composition of the affected bone.

Osteoporosis—a defect in bone production due to the failure of osteoblasts to lay down bone matrix results in decreased composition of the affected bone (Figure 17-7).

FIGURE 17-7 This patient has a severe bone deformity from a fracture that resulted in chronic osteomyelitis and diffuse osteoporosis. The chronic osteomyelitis is an additive condition (seen around the fracture site) and the osteoporosis is a destructive condition, resulting in a decrease in radiation absorption throughout the remaining bone.

SUMMARY

The presence of a pathologic condition can greatly affect the degree of radiation absorption. Radiographers must have an understanding of pathology in order to properly select the technical factors for a procedure. Properly reading the x-ray requisition and taking an adequate patient history are essential responsibilities of the radiographer. Fulfilling these responsibilities reduces the need to repeat an image, due to the patient's condition.

If a disease causes the affected body tissue to increase in thickness, effective atomic number, and/or density, that disease will result in a greater attenuation of the x-ray beam. As more photons are absorbed by the body tissues, fewer will be available to reach the image receptor to create adequate exposure. These diseases are harder to penetrate and are called additive conditions because they require adding to the exposure to achieve the proper image receptor exposure.

If a disease causes the affected body tissue to decrease in thickness, effective atomic number, and/or density, that disease will result in less attenuation of the x-ray beam. As more photons are able to pass through the body tissues, more will be available to reach the image receptor to create the required exposure. These diseases are easier to penetrate and are called destructive conditions. They require decreasing the technical factors to achieve the proper image receptor exposure.

REVIEW QUESTIONS

1. Why do some pathological conditions affect the attenuation of the x-ray beam?

2. Why is it important that radiographers have an understanding of pathological conditions?

3. What is the relationship between additive conditions and attenuation? Destructive conditions and attenuation?

4. Why should the radiographer take a good clinical history and closely observe the patient?

5. Describe how the following additive conditions may affect the radiographic image:
   a. edema
   b. congestive heart failure
   c. pneumonia
   d. ascites
   e. Paget's disease

6. Describe how the following destructive conditions may affect the radiographic image:

   a. atrophy
   b. emphysema
   c. pneumothorax
   d. degenerative arthritis
   e. osteoporosis

REFERENCES AND RECOMMENDED READING

Eisenberg, R. L., & Dennis, C. A. (2003). *Comprehensive radiographic pathology* (3rd ed.). St. Louis, MO: Elsevier/Mosby.

Hiss, S. S. (2003). *Understanding radiography* (4th ed.). Springfield, IL: Charles C Thomas.

Mace, J. D., Kowalczyk, N. M., Evans, K. D. (Contributor), McCarthy, B. (Contributor), and Pfeiffer, B. (Contributor) (2004). *Radiographic pathology for technologists* (4th ed.). St. Louis, MO: Elsevier/Mosby.

Sheldon, H. (1992). *Boyd's introduction to the study of disease* (11th ed.). Lippincott, Williams & Wilkins.

The Case of the White Snakes

What is the most likely cause of these white, snakelike structures circling the upper corner of the patient's abdomen?

Answers to the case studies can be found in Appendix E.

CHAPTER 18

The Grid

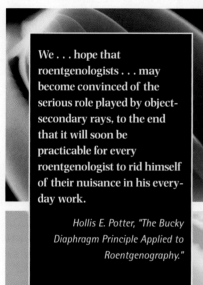

We . . . hope that roentgenologists . . . may become convinced of the serious role played by object-secondary rays, to the end that it will soon be practicable for every roentgenologist to rid himself of their nuisance in his every-day work.

Hollis E. Potter, "The Bucky Diaphragm Principle Applied to Roentgenography."

KEY TERMS

criss-cross grid
cross-hatched grid
focused grid
grid
grid cut-off
grid frequency
grid ratio
linear grid
parallel grid

OBJECTIVES

Upon completion of this chapter, the student should be able to:

- Describe the purpose of the grid.
- Explain the construction of a grid, including grid materials, grid ratio, grid frequency, and lead content.
- Describe the various grid patterns.
- Differentiate between parallel and focused grids.
- Differentiate between the uses of a stationary and a moving grid.
- Explain the process of grid selection for specific radiographic procedures.
- Explain the relationship of grid selection to patient dose and image receptor exposure.
- Calculate changes in technical factors to compensate for changes in grid selection.
- Describe methods for evaluating the performance of a grid.
- Discuss common errors that are made when using a grid and the effects of these errors on the radiographic image.
- Describe other scatter reduction methods.

PURPOSE OF THE GRID

A **grid** is a device used to improve the contrast of the radiographic image. It does this by absorbing scatter radiation before it can reach the image receptor. When an x-ray beam passes through the body, one of three things will occur with the primary photons that originated at the target. They will: (1) pass through the body unaffected; (2) be absorbed by the body; or (3) interact and change direction (Figure 18-1).

The photons that pass through the body unaffected will interact with the image receptor to create the image. These are the photons responsible for creating the contrast (differences in the densities) on the image. These differences exist because some photons pass through the body while others are absorbed. Absorption of photons occurs as the result of photoelectric interaction. This interaction results in the complete absorption of the primary photon and the production of a secondary photon. The secondary radiation created by this interaction is, with few exceptions, very weak and is quickly absorbed in the surrounding tissues.

Primary radiation that interacts and, as a result of this interaction, changes direction is known as scatter radiation. The interaction that produces scatter radiation is known as a Compton interaction. These interactions can result in photons which are strong enough to be emitted by the patient and interact with the image receptor. Since these photons have changed direction, they are no longer able to record exposures on the image receptor that relate to the patient's anatomy. The exposures that they add to the image receptor are of no diagnostic value. Scattered photons add an overall density to the receptor and, as a result of this overall graying of the image, contrast is lowered. An important point to remember is that the percentage of Compton interactions increases with increased kVp. Therefore, **scatter increases and contrast is further impaired as kVp increases.**

Since the patient is the source of the scatter that is degrading the image, it is logical to assume that the patient will also control the quantity of scatter produced. Scatter increases with increases in the volume of the tissue irradiated and decreases with increased atomic number of the tissue. The volume of tissue that is irradiated is controlled by the thickness of the patient and the exposure field size. While thickness of the patient is predetermined (although it can sometimes be reduced by compression), the field size can be kept to a minimum by collimation. The atomic number of the tissue will also affect the quantity of scatter. The greater the atomic number of the tissue, the less will be the quantity of scatter created. For example, less scatter is produced in bone than in soft tissue, because bone absorbs more photons photoelectrically. This is the result of changes in the number and types of atoms that are present for interaction. In summary, **the amount of scatter radiation increases with (1) increases in patient thickness; (2) larger field sizes; and (3) decreases in atomic number of the tissue.** (This is discussed in further detail in Chapter 15.)

Since a grid is designed to absorb the unwanted scatter radiation, it is necessary to use a grid with thicker, larger body parts and with procedures that require higher kVp techniques. As a general rule, a grid is employed when:

FIGURE 18-1 When x-rays interact with the patient, they will either **(1) pass through unaffected; (2) be absorbed; or (3) interact and change direction (scatter).**

1. body part thickness exceeds 10 cm

2. kVp is above 60

A grid is a thin, flat, rectangular device made by placing a series of radiopaque lead strips side by side and separating the strips by an interspace material which is radiolucent. The lead strips are of very thin foil and the interspace material is thicker and usually made of aluminum. These strips are then encased in an aluminum cover to protect them from damage.

The very first grid was made in 1913 by the American radiologist Gustav Bucky (1880–1963). Dr. Bucky's first grid consisted of wide strips of lead spaced 2 cm apart and running in two directions, along the length of the image and across the image (Figure 18-2). This crude design created an image of the grid that was superimposed on the patient's image. Despite having to view the anatomy through this checkerboard pattern, the original grid did remove scatter and improve contrast.

In 1920 Hollis Potter (1880–1963), a Chicago radiologist, improved Dr. Bucky's grid design. Dr. Potter realigned the lead strips so they would run in only one direction, made the lead strips thinner and therefore less obvious on the image, and then designed a device (now known as the Potter-Bucky diaphragm) which allowed the grid to move during the exposure. By moving the grid, the lead strips became

FIGURE 18-2 **Dr. Bucky's original grid.** *(Courtesy of Smithsonian Institution's Division of Science, Medicine, & Society)*

blurred and were no longer visible on the image. All these improvements resulted in a practical grid device, which significantly improved contrast without impairing the view of the patient's anatomy.

GRID CONSTRUCTION

A wide variety of grids are available today (Table 18-1). The choice of the proper grid for a particular clinical procedure requires an understanding of a grid's function. Grid construction involves the selection of materials, grid ratio, and grid frequency.

Grid Materials

A grid is a series of radiopaque strips which alternate with radiolucent interspace strips. These strips are bonded firmly together and then sliced into flat sheets. The radiopaque strips are needed to absorb the scatter radiation and must therefore be made of a dense material with a high atomic number. Lead is the material of choice because it is relatively inexpensive and is easy to shape into very thin foil.

The interspace material must be radiolucent. In other words, it allows radiation to pass easily through it. Several organic and inorganic materials have been tried but only two are commercially available—aluminum and fiber. Ideally, this material should not absorb any radiation. However, in reality, it does absorb a small amount. Aluminum is more commonly used than fiber because it is easier to use in manufacturing and is more durable. Also, because it has a higher atomic number than fiber, it can provide additional absorption of low-energy scatter. With its higher atomic number, aluminum also increases the absorption of primary photons. This can be a disadvantage, especially with low kVp techniques where this absorption would be greater. Fiber interspace grids are preferred when using low kVp techniques where their application can contribute to lower patient dose, such as in pediatric radiography.

Grid Ratio

Grid ratio has a major influence on the ability of the grid to improve contrast. It is defined as the ratio of the height of the lead strips to the distance

TABLE 18-1. Typical Grid Specifications

Ratio	Linear/ Crosshatch	Focused/ Parallel	Interspace	Lines/Inch	Weight (g/cm²)	Thickness (mm)
15:1	L	F	Al	103	1.74	3.7
15:1	L	F	Al	85	1.64	4.4
12:1	L	F	FIBER	80	1.45	4.4
12:1	L	F	Al	152		1.86
12:1	L	F	Al	103	1.21	3.2
12:1	L	F	Al	85	1.35	3.8
8:1	L	F	FIBER	80	0.96	3.4
8:1	L	F	Al	152		1.34
8:1	L	F	Al	103	0.87	2.3
8:1	L	F	Al	85	0.96	2.8
6:1	L	F	Al	103	0.67	1.9
6:1	L	F	Al	85	0.77	2.3
6:1	L	P	Al	85	0.77	2.3
6:1	C	F	Al	85	1.40	3.8
			Specialty Mammography Grid			
5:1	L	F	FIBER	80		

between the strips (Figure 18-3). This is expressed in the formula:

$$\text{Grid ratio} = \frac{h}{D}$$

where: h = lead strip height
        D = interspace width

> **EXAMPLE:** If the lead strips are 3 mm high and are separated by an interspace of 0.25 mm, what is the grid ratio?
>
> **Answer:**
>
> $$\text{grid ratio} = \frac{3.0}{0.25}$$
> $$\text{grid ratio} = 12{:}1$$

If the height of the grid is a constant, decreasing the distance between the lead strips would result in an increase in the grid ratio. Conversely, if the height of the grid is a constant, increasing the distance be-

FIGURE 18-3 Grid ratio is the height of the lead strips divided by the width of the interspace.

8 : 1 Grid

Maximum angle

16 : 1 Grid

Maximum angle

FIGURE 18-4   Grid ratio affects the amount of scatter absorbed by determining the maximum angle of a scattered ray that can get through the grid. The smaller the angle, the less scatter reaches the image receptor.

1 inch

A.   10 : 1 Grid
     10 Line/inch

B.   10 : 1 Grid
     8 Line/inch

FIGURE 18-5   Grid frequency is the number of grid lines per inch or centimeter. Grids A and B have the same grid ratio, but A has a higher grid frequency than B.

mary photons in order to reach the image receptor. This means that higher grid ratios are more effective at removing scatter. For the same reason, higher-ratio grids require greater accuracy in their positioning and are more prone to grid errors.

Grid Frequency

Grid frequency is defined as the number of grid lines per inch or centimeter. Grids are made with a range in frequency from 60–200 lines/inch (25–80 lines/cm). Most commonly used grids have a frequency of 85–103 lines/inch (33–41 lines/cm). In general, grids with higher grid frequencies have thinner lead strips (Figure 18-5). Very high-frequency grids of approximately 103 to 200 lines/inch (41–80 lines/cm) are recommended for stationary grids used with digital image receptor systems to minimize the possibility of seeing the grid lines on the image.

By combining information about grid ratio and frequency, one can determine the total quantity of lead in the grid. It is the grid's lead content that is most important in determining the grid's efficiency at cleaning up scatter. Lead content is measured in mass per unit area, or grams per square centimeter. In general, the lead content is greater in a grid that has a higher grid ratio and lower grid frequency. **As the lead content of a grid increases, the ability of the grid to remove scatter and improve contrast increases.**

tween the lead strips would result in a decrease in grid ratio. **An inverse relationship exists between the distance between the lead strips and grid ratio when the height of the grid strips remains the same.**

Higher grid ratios allow less scatter radiation to pass through their interspace material to reach the image receptor. Figure 18-4 demonstrates the effect of grid ratio on the maximum angle possible for a scattered photon to pass through the grid. The higher the grid ratio, the straighter the scattered photon has to be in order to pass through the interspace material. Scattered photons, therefore, have to be more closely aligned to the direction of the pri-

Linear
Grid Pattern

Criss-Cross
Grid Pattern

FIGURE 18-6 A linear vs. a criss-cross grid pattern.

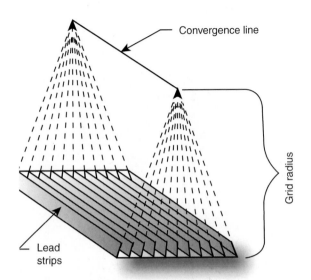

FIGURE 18-7 A focused grid is designed to match the divergence of the x-ray beam. The grid radius is the distance from the face of the grid to the points of convergence of the lead strips.

 GRID PATTERNS

Grid strips can be made to run in one or two directions. Grids with lead strips running in only one direction are called linear grids. Grids are also made by placing two linear grids on top of one another so the grid lines are running at right angles. These grids are termed **criss-cross** or **cross-hatched** (Figure 18-6). Dr. Bucky's original grid was made using this pattern.

Linear grids are more commonly used in clinical practice because they can be used when performing procedures that require tube angulation. Linear grids allow the technologist to angle the tube only *along* the long axis of the grid. Angulation *across* the long axis would result in the primary beam being directed into the lead strips. If the primary beam is angled into the lead, the lead will absorb an undesirable amount of primary radiation, resulting in a problem known as **grid cut-off**. When criss-cross grids are used, no tube tilt is permitted, since any angulation would result in grid cut-off because lead strips are running in both directions.

 GRID TYPES

Grids are manufactured with either a parallel or a focused design. **Parallel grids** are made with the lead and interspace strips running parallel to one another. This means that if the grid lines were extended into space they would never intersect. **Focused grids** are designed so that the central grid strips are parallel and as the strips move away from the central axis they become more and more inclined (Figure 18-7).

The focused design results in a grid with lead strips designed to match the divergence of the x-ray beam. If these lead strips were extended, the strips would intersect along a line in space known as the convergence line. The distance from the face of the grid to the points of convergence of the lead strips is called the grid radius. **For the grid to be properly focused, the x-ray tube must be located along the convergence line.** Each focused grid will identify the focal range within which the tube should be located. For example, grids are made with short, medium, or long focal ranges, depending on the distance for which they are designed. Short focal range grids (14–18 inches or 36–46 cm) are made for use in mammography; long focal range grids (60–72 inches or 152–183 cm) are used for chest radiography. Focused grids with lower grid ratios allow for greater latitude in the alignment of the tube with the grid. With higher grid ratios, proper alignment of the grid with the tube is more critical.

Parallel grids are less commonly employed than focused grids. Because the strips do not try to coincide with the divergence of the x-ray beam, some grid cut-off will occur along the lateral edges, especially when the grid is employed at short SIDs. The

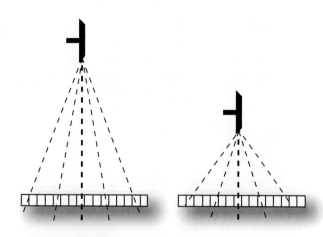

FIGURE 18-8   Parallel grids function best at long, as opposed to short, SID.

parallel grid is best employed at long SIDs because the beam will be a straighter, more perpendicular one (Figure 18-8).

GRID USES

A grid is used either in a stationary position or mounted in a Potter-Bucky diaphragm to move it during exposure. Most radiology departments have a supply of stationary grids, in various sizes, which can be mounted to the front of a cassette. These are generally made approximately one inch larger than the image receptor size they are intended to cover. Stationary grids are used primarily in portable procedures or for upright or horizontal beam views. Some departments may also purchase a special cassette with a grid built into it. This design, called a grid cassette, requires reloading between exposures using the grid. This may be an inconvenience in situations where multiple images are needed. When grids are used in a stationary fashion, grid lines on the image will usually be noticed on close inspection. This is especially true with low-frequency grids. High-frequency grids, like those used for digital imaging, have a minimal visual effect.

The most common use of the grid is for procedures using the Potter-Bucky diaphragm (usually called the bucky). This device is mounted below the tabletop of radiographic and radiographic/fluoroscopic tables and holds the cassette in place below the grid. It can move the grid during the exposure so that grid lines

will be blurred and therefore not evident on the image. These grids are approximately $17'' \times 19''$ (43×48 cm), large enough to cover a $14'' \times 17''$ (35×43 cm) cassette placed either lengthwise or crosswise in the cassette tray. Only moving grids are used for film/screen mammography studies.

The direction in which the grid moves is important if it is to accomplish the job of blurring the grid lines. The lead strips of the grid run along the long axis of the table. To blur the lead lines, the grid must move at a right angle to the direction of the lines. This means that it will be moving back and forth across the table and not from top to bottom.

There are two movement mechanisms used today. The movements are described as reciprocating and oscillating. With the reciprocating grid, a motor drives the grid back and forth during the exposure for a total distance of no more than 2–3 cm. With the oscillating grid, an electromagnet pulls the grid to one side and then releases it during exposure. The grid oscillates in a circular motion within the grid frame.

GRID SELECTION/ CONVERSIONS

Selecting the best grid to use for a specific radiographic procedure is a complex process. Most procedures which are done with a grid use a moving grid mounted in a table or upright holder. Grid choice must be made in the equipment purchase phase of quality control. Once a grid is selected and mounted in the Potter-Bucky diaphragm, it is not easily changed. Purchase decisions are generally made by the department administrator in collaboration with the radiologist.

Grids absorb scatter and scatter adds exposure to the image receptor. The more efficient a grid is at absorbing scatter, the less exposure will be received by the image receptor. Therefore, compensations must be made to increase this exposure. This is generally accomplished by increasing mAs, which, in turn, results in greater patient dose. The better the grid cleans up scatter, the greater will be the dose given to the patient to achieve an adequate exposure. The amount of mAs needed can be calculated using the following formula:

$$\text{Grid Conversion Factor (GCF)} = \frac{\text{mAs with the grid}}{\text{mAs without the grid}}$$

TABLE 18-2. Grid Conversion Factors

Grid Ratio	60 kVp	85 kVp	110 kVp
No grid	1	1	1
5:1	3	3	3
8:1	3.75	4	4.25
12:1	4.75	5.5	6.25
16:1	5.75	6.75	8

Adapted with permission from *Characteristics and Applications of X-Ray Grids*, Liebel-Flarsheim division of Sybron Corporation, Cincinnati, Ohio.
Approximate values based on clinical tests of pelvis and skull.

This formula is referred to as the Bucky factor as well as the grid conversion factor. **Grid-conversion factors (GCF) increase with higher grid ratios and increasing kVp.** Since grids vary in respect to their ratio, frequency and lead content, it would be useful to check the grid conversion factor for each of the common grids used in a department. Table 18-2 offers a guide of grid conversion factors for commonly purchased grids.

> **EXAMPLE:** A satisfactory chest radiograph is produced using 5 mAs at 85 kVp without a grid. A second image is requested using a 12:1 grid. Using Table 18-2, what mAs is needed to produce a second satisfactory image?
>
> **Answer:**
>
> $$GCF = \frac{mAs \text{ with the grid}}{mAs \text{ without the grid}}$$
>
> $$5.5 = \frac{X}{5} \text{ mAs}$$
> $$X = 5.5 \times 5 \text{ mAs}$$
> $$X = 27.5 \text{ mAs}$$

When converting from one grid ratio to another, the following formula is used:

$$\frac{mAs_1}{mAs_2} = \frac{GCF_1}{GCF_2}$$

where: mAs_1 = original mAs
mAs_2 = new mAs
GCF_1 = original grid conversion factor
GCF_2 = new grid conversion factor

> **EXAMPLE:** A satisfactory abdominal image is produced using an 8:1 grid, 35 mAs, and 85 kVp. A second image is requested using a 12:1 grid. Using Table 18-2, what mAs is needed to produce a second satisfactory image?
>
> **Answer:**
>
> $$\frac{mAs_1}{mAs_2} = \frac{GCF_1}{GCF_2}$$
>
> $$\frac{35}{X} = \frac{4}{5.5}$$
> $$4X = 192.5$$
> $$X = 48 \text{ mAs}$$

GRID PERFORMANCE EVALUATION

The efficiency of a grid in cleaning up or removing scatter can be quantitatively measured. The International Commission on Radiologic Units and Measurements (ICRU) Handbook 89 defines two criteria for measuring a grid's performance: selectivity and contrast improvement ability.

Selectivity

Although grids are designed to absorb scatter, they also absorb some primary radiation. Grids that absorb a greater percentage of scatter than primary radiation are described as having a greater degree of selectivity. Selectivity is identified by the Greek sigma (Σ) and is measured by using the following formula:

$$\text{Selectivity} = \frac{\% \text{ primary radiation transmitted}}{\% \text{ scatter radiation transmitted}}$$

The better a grid is at removing scatter, the greater will be the selectivity of the grid. **This means that a grid with a higher lead content would have a greater selectivity.**

Contrast Improvement Ability

The best measure of how well a grid functions is its ability to improve contrast in the clinical setting. The contrast improvement factor is dependent on the amount of scatter produced, which is controlled by the kVp and volume of irradiated tissue (see Chapter 29). As the amount of scatter radiation increases, the lower will be the contrast and the lower the contrast improvement factor. The contrast improvement factor (K) can be measured using the following formula:

$$K = \frac{\text{Radiographic contrast with the grid}}{\text{Radiographic contrast without the grid}}$$

If K = 1, then no improvement in contrast has occurred. Most grids have contrast improvement factors between 1.5 and 3.5. This means that contrast is 1.5–3.5 times better when using the grid. **The higher the K factor, the greater the contrast improvement.**

GRID ERRORS

Poor images can result from improper use of the grid. Errors in the use of the grid occur mainly with grids that have a focused design. This is because fo-

cused grids are made to coincide with the divergence of the x-ray beam. The tube must be centered to the focused grid and aligned at the correct distance. Additionally, a focused grid has a tube side and a receptor side based on the angulation of the grid strips. Proper tube/grid alignment is essential to prevent the undesirable absorption of primary radiation known as grid cut-off.

Off-Level

An off-level grid error occurs when the tube is angled across the long axis of the grid strips. This can be the result of improper tube or grid positioning (Figure 18-9). Improper tube positioning results if the central ray is directed across the long axis of the radiographic table. Recall that it is only possible to angle along the long axis of the table with a linear grid and it is not possible to angle at all with a criss-cross grid. Improper grid positioning most commonly occurs with stationary grids being used for mobile procedures or decubitus views. If, for example, a patient is lying on a grid for a mobile abdominal procedure and

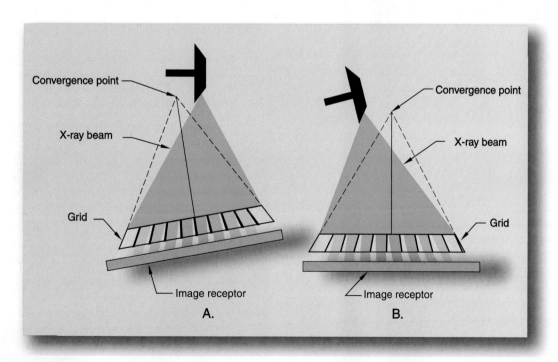

FIGURE 18-9 An off-level grid error can occur with a parallel or focused grid. A linear grid can be off-level in one direction while a criss-cross grid can be off-level in both directions (across and along the grid).

| 75 kVp | 15 mAs | 40" SID |
| 15:1 grid | 400 RS | 63.4 mR |

FIGURE 18-10 A radiograph illustrating an off-level grid error.

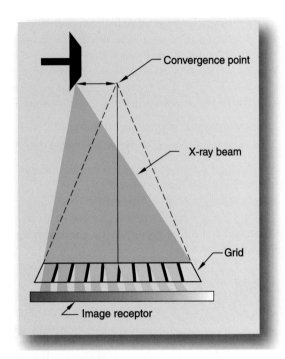

FIGURE 18-11 An off-center grid error.

the patient's weight is unevenly distributed on the grid, the grid may not be properly aligned to the tube.

An off-level grid error can occur with a focused grid and it is the only positioning error possible with a parallel grid. Care must always be taken when aligning the tube to the grid, especially when using stationary grids, to avoid this error. When this error occurs, there is an undesirable absorption of primary radiation, which results in a radiograph with a decrease in exposure across the entire image (Figure 18-10).

Off-Center

The x-ray tube must be centered along the central axis of a focused grid to prevent an off-center (off-axis or lateral decentering) grid error (Figure 18-11). The center grid strips are perpendicular and become more and more inclined away from the center. This design coincides with the divergence of the x-ray beam from the tube. If the central ray is off-center, the most perpendicular portion of the x-ray beam will not correspond to the most perpendicular portion of the grid. The result is a decrease in exposure across the entire image (Figure 18-12).

The greater the degree of lateral decentering, the greater the grid cut-off.

| 75 kVp | 15 mAs | 40" SID |
| 15:1 grid | 400 RS | 66.1 mR |

FIGURE 18-12 A radiograph illustrating an off-center grid error.

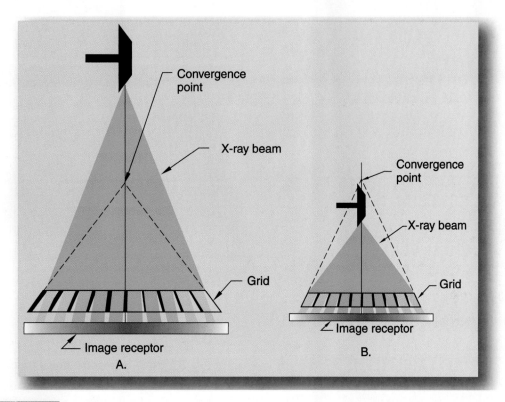

FIGURE 18-13 An off-focus grid error occurs when the grid is used at distances less than or greater than the focal range.

Off-Focus

A focused grid is made to be used at very specific distances identified as the focal range labeled on the front of the grid. When a grid is used at a distance other than that specified as the focal range, an off-focus error results (Figure 18-13). For example, if a grid has a focal range of 36–44 inches (91–112 cm) and it is used at 72 inches, severe grid cut-off will occur. Off-focus errors result in grid cut-off along the peripheral edges of the image (Figure 18-14). Higher grid ratios require greater positioning accuracy to prevent grid cut-off.

Upside-Down

A focused grid has an identified tube side based on the way the grid strips are angled. If the grid is used upside-down, severe peripheral grid cut-off will

75 kVp	15 mAs	40" SID
15:1 grid	400 RS	69.3 mR

FIGURE 18-14 A radiograph illustrating an off-focus grid error taken at less than the recommended focal range distance.

FIGURE 18-15 An upside-down grid error.

75 kVp	15 mAs	40" SID
15:1 grid	400 RS	64.2 mR

FIGURE 18-16 A radiograph illustrating an upside-down grid error.

occur (Figure 18-15). Radiation will pass through the grid along the central axis where the grid strips are most perpendicular and radiation will be increasingly absorbed away from the center (Figure 18-16). It is important that the technologist check the tube side prior to using a focused grid.

The Moire Effect

The Moire effect is a grid error that occurs with digital image receptor systems when the grid lines are captured and scanned parallel to the scan lines in the imaging plate readers. This error occurs with grids used in a stationary fashion for examinations such as portable radiography or translateral hip images. In order for the Moire pattern to demonstrate on the image, the grid lines must be running in the same direction as the movement of the laser beam that is scanning the imaging plate (Figure 18-17). Most imaging plates are scanned

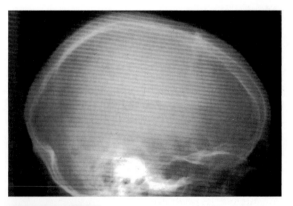

FIGURE 18-17 The Moire effect. *(Courtesy of Barry Burns, MS.R (R), DABR, UNC, Division of Radiographic Science)*

across the short axis of the plate, and, most often, grid lines run parallel to the long axis of the imaging plate. In these instances, the Moire pattern will not demonstrate. To prevent this grid error, it is recommended that high-frequency grids of 103 lines per inch or greater be used for digital image receptor systems when a stationary grid is needed.

AN ALTERNATE SCATTER REDUCTION METHOD—THE AIR-GAP TECHNIQUE

In addition to the use of a grid, there are a number of other methods that can be employed to reduce the amount of scatter reaching the image receptor. Remember, the most important way to improve image quality is to decrease the amount of scatter initially being created. This is best done by restricting the primary beam. Collimating to the size of the area being examined is critical to image quality. Even with the use of close collimation, it is still necessary to reduce scatter reaching the image receptor when radiographing larger body parts or when using higher kVps. The grid is the primary device employed to reduce scatter. The body part may also be compressed to decrease the amount of scatter created.

The air-gap technique is an alternative to the use of a grid. It has primary applications in magnification radiography and, to a lesser extent, in chest radiography. The technique involves placing the patient at a greater object image receptor distance (OID), thus creating an air gap between the patient and the image receptor. By moving the patient away from the image receptor, the amount of scatter reaching the image receptor will be reduced. As stated earlier, the patient is the source of the majority of scatter. While the same amount of scatter will be created during the exposure, less of the scatter will reach the image receptor if the pa-

FIGURE 18-18   The air-gap technique reduces the amount of scatter reaching the image receptor.

tient is moved farther away (Figure 18-18). The result is improved contrast without the use of the grid. The primary disadvantage of the air-gap technique is the loss of sharpness that results from increased OID.

Gould and Hale evaluated contrast improvement between the use of a grid and the air-gap technique, showing that a 10-inch (25-cm) air gap has the same degree of clean-up of scatter as a 15:1 grid for a 10 cm body part. This same grid was shown to be more effective at eliminating scatter than the air gap with a thicker (20 cm) body part.

SUMMARY

A grid is a tool used by the radiographer to improve image contrast. Grids are made of lead strips alternating with an interspace material, which is usually made of aluminum. Grids are constructed with a specific grid ratio and frequency. The grid ratio and frequency are important in determining the total lead content of the grid. Generally, grids with higher grid ratios and lead content are more efficient at removing scatter. This can be quantitatively studied by measuring the selectivity and contrast improvement ability of the grid.

Grids absorb scatter and scatter adds exposure to the image receptor. The more efficient a grid is at absorbing scatter, the less image receptor exposure. Therefore, compensation must be made to increase exposure. This is generally accomplished by increasing the mAs, which, in turn, results in greater patient dose. The better the grid is at cleaning up scatter, the greater is the dose given to the patient to achieve adequate exposure.

Grids are manufactured in either a linear or criss-cross pattern, with either a parallel or focused design. They can be used in either a stationary manner or may be placed in a device that moves the grid and thereby blurs the grid lines.

An alternative to the use of a grid is the air-gap technique.

REVIEW QUESTIONS

1. Why does a grid improve contrast?

2. As a general rule, when should a grid be used?

3. How is a grid constructed?

4. Define grid ratio.

5. What type of grid pattern has lead strips running in only one direction?

6. How is a focused grid designed?

7. As the ability of a grid to clean up scatter increases, what is the effect on patient dose and image receptor exposure?

8. How is the contrast improvement of a grid measured?

9. How does an off-level grid error occur?

10. How does the air-gap technique improve contrast?

REFERENCES AND RECOMMENDED READING

Bednarek, D. P., Rudin, S., & Wong, R. (1983, April). Artifacts produced by moving grids. *Radiology, 255.*

Bushberg, J. T., Seibert, J. A., Leidholdt, E. M., & Boone, J. M. (2002). *The essential physics of medical imaging* (2nd ed.). Baltimore: Williams & Wilkins.

Chan, H. P. (1985, March). Ultra-high-strip-density radiographic grids: A new antiscatter technique for mammography. *Radiology, 807.*

Cullinan, A., & Cullinan, J. (1994). *Producing quality radiographs* (2nd ed.). Philadelphia: J. B. Lippincott.

Curry, T. S., Dowdey, J. E., & Murry, R. C. (1990). *Christensen's introduction to the physics of diagnostic radiology* (4th ed.). Philadelphia: Lea and Febiger.

Doi, K., Frank, P. H., Chan, H. P., Vyborny, C. J., Makino, S., Iida, N., et al. (1983). Physical and clinical evaluation of new high-strip-density radiographic grids. *Radiology, 147*(2), 575–582.

Egan, R. L. (1983, February). Grids in mammography. *Radiology, 359.*

Fry, O. E., & Cesare, G. (1960). Bedside radiography reduction of patient exposure and orientation of grid cassettes. *Radiologic Technology, 31*(4), 387.

Gould, R. G., & Hale, J. (1974). Control of scattered radiation by air gap techniques: Applications to chest radiography. *American Journal of Roentgenology, 122,* 109–118.

Harlow, C. (1993). Off-centering secondary radiation grids. *Radiography Today, 59*(674), 11–13.

Heriand, J., & Varma, D. G. K. (1986). A lung opacity caused by grid artifact. *Radiologic Technology, 58*(2), 147.

Hufton, A. P., Crosthwaite, C. M., Davies, J. M., & Robinson, L. A. (1987). Low attenuation material for table tops, cassettes, and grids: A review. *Radiography, 53*(607), 17.

Jensen, G., & Scheid, C. (1980). The performance of radiographic grids. *Optimization of chest radiography* (HHS Publication (FDA) 80–8124). Rockville, MD: U.S. Department of Health and Human Services.

Potter, H. E. (1920). The Bucky diaphragm principle applied to roentgenology. *The American Journal of Roentgenology, 7*, 292.

Potter, H. E. (1931). History of diaphragming roentgen rays by the use of the Bucky principle. *The American Journal of Roentgenology, 25*, 396.

Seeman, H. E., & Splettstosser, H. R. (1954). The physical characteristics of Potter-Bucky diaphragms. *Radiology, 62*, 575–583.

Seeman, H. E., & Splettstosser, H. R. (1955). The effect of kilovoltage and grid ratio on subject contrast in radiography. *Radiology, 64*, 572–580.

Stanford, R. W., Moore, R. D., & Hills, T. H. (1959). Comparative performance of grids in relation to their stated ratio. *British Journal of Radiology, 32*(374), 106–113.

Stears, J. G., Gray, J. E., & Frank, E. D. (1986). Grids are not created equal. *Radiologic Technology, 57*(4), 345.

Stober, E. V. (1947). Off-distance cut-off. *Radiologic Technology, 19*(3), 111.

Stober, E. V. (1951). The term 'ratio' as applied to an x-ray grid. *Radiologic Technology, 23*(3), 180.

Switzer, D. (1981). The use of grids in diagnostic radiography. *The Canadian Journal of Medical Radiation Technology, 12*(2), 60.

Trout, E. D., Kelley, J. P., & Cathey, G. A. (1952). The use of filters to control radiation exposure to the patient in diagnostic roentgenology. *American Journal of Roentgenology, 67*(6), 946–963.

CHAPTER 19

Radiographic Film

> Any discussion relating to the rationale of radiographic exposure should begin with the understanding that the characteristics and the exposure response of x-ray film are the foundations of an exposure system.
>
> *Arthur W. Fuchs, from the Jerman Memorial Lecture at the 1950 Annual Meeting of the American Society of X-Ray Technicians*

KEY TERMS

adhesive
antihalation coating
base
cathode ray tube (CRT) imaging
coating
contact surgical radiography
crossover effect
crystal production

detail extremity radiography
duplication film
duplitized
emulsion with crystals
fluoroscopic spot filming
halation
laser film
mammography

mixing
orthochromatic
panchromatic
ripening
sensitivity speck
silver bromide
silver chloride
silver iodide
silver iodobromide
supercoat

OBJECTIVES

Upon completion of this chapter, the student should be able to:

- Describe the components of radiographic film.

- Explain the production of silver halide crystals.

- State the purpose of various additives to radiographic film.

- Describe latent image formation.

- Discuss the differences between direct exposure film, screen film, and films for various special applications, such as duplication.

- Explain the fundamentals of proper film storage and handling.

- Identify common radiographic film artifacts.

- Discuss automated and film systems.

- Explain the responsibilities involved in proper radiograph identification.

Photosensitive film remains the most common radiographic image receptor, although modern imaging technology has developed many other receptors (e.g., fluoroscopic screens and computer-linked detectors). Film was the first image receptor chosen by Röntgen, and it has remained the primary means of recording radiographic images to the present day, although some computer images are now being read for diagnosis without being recorded on film.

Radiographic and photographic film are very similar in nature and both derive from early experiments in recording light images. The discovery of photography cannot be assigned to one person. A permanent photographic process was discovered about 1816 by the French inventor Joseph Nièpce (1765–1833). Nièpce eventually collaborated with the French artist Louis Daguerre (1787–1851), who improved the process and sold it to the French government, which released it to the public in 1839. Simultaneously, between 1835 and 1840, the English photographer William Fox Talbot (1800–1877) developed the now common negative-to-positive process that was given the name photography. Many photographers contributed to the scientific understanding of the process, and by the 1850s the process was similar to, although more primitive than, that used today.

Photographic materials are photosensitive, or capable of responding to exposure by photons. Both are sensitive to the wavelengths and energies that comprise most of the electromagnetic spectrum of both light and x-rays (see Figure 2–12), although it is possible to manufacture film that is insensitive to portions of the spectrum. Proper use of photosensitive materials requires an understanding of how film is constructed and how the image is formed.

 ## CONSTRUCTION

Diagnostic radiographic film is manufactured by coating both sides of a base material with an emulsion containing photosensitive crystals. Several other materials are also used to improve the performance and permanence of the film. The complete construction of diagnostic radiographic film includes the **base, adhesive, emulsion with crystals** and **supercoat** (Figure 19-1). The total thickness of the film varies with the manufacturer, from 175 to 300 μm (0.007″ to 0.012″).

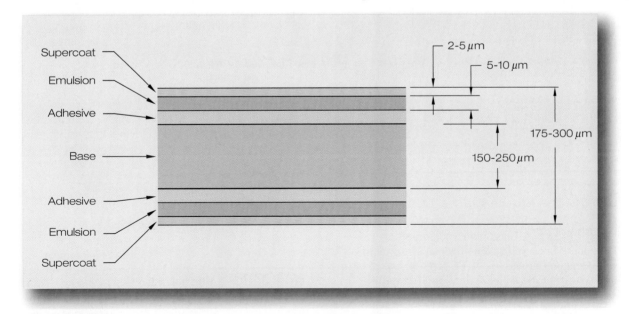

FIGURE 19-1   Cross-sectional view of diagnostic radiographic film.

Base

The film base was originally composed of a glass plate. Glass plates coated with emulsion were used in photography from soon after its discovery until World War I (circa 1914) (Figure 19-2). Modern radiography has retained in the professional jargon an old-fashioned term, *flat plate of the abdomen,* from this period. Of course, the physician requesting such an image intends the film base to be of polyester plastic, not a glass plate. Modern plastic bases solved problems such as cut fingers from broken films and strained backs from carrying and filing stacks of heavy radiographs.

During World War I a shortage of the good, optical quality glass needed for the film base caused film manufacturers to switch to cellulose nitrate. Because of its flammable nature (which caused several tragic hospital fires), nonflammable cellulose triacetate was introduced in the 1920s. Modern radiographic film base is polyester, which was introduced in the 1960s by DuPont. It is usually 150–200 μm (0.006″–0.008″) thick.

The film base must be flexible yet tough, stable, rigid, and uniformly lucent. It must be flexible to permit easy handling in the darkroom and to make good contact with the cassette pressure pads. It must be stable so that it does not change its dimensions during the heating and immersion in chemicals required for processing. It must be rigid enough to be conveniently placed onto a view box (radiographic illuminator). Most important, it must be uniformly lucent so that it permits the transmission of light without adding artifacts to the diagnostic image.

The film base usually includes a blue dye to tint the film and reduce eyestrain for the interpreting radiologist, thereby increasing the diagnostic accuracy available from the image. The film base is also often coated with a special substance to prevent light from one screen crossing over to the other, causing blurring of the image. This reflection of light is called the **crossover effect.** Some manufacturers use an ultraviolet emission from the intensifying screen to reduce the crossover effect. **Halation** is a different effect caused by light being reflected from the air interface on the back of the base material (Figure 19-3). An **antihalation coating** may be applied to the back of single-emulsion

FIGURE 19-2   Glass plate radiograph of Theodore Roosevelt taken at Mercy Hospital in Chicago on October 15, 1912, after he was shot in the chest during an assassination attempt in Milwaukee. *(Reprinted with permission from the American College of Surgeons, Chicago, IL)*

Light beam

Primary image

Secondary image by reflection

Film emulsion

Film base

Reflection at film base-air interface

FIGURE 19-3   The halation effect. *(Reprinted with permission of David Jenkins from Radiographic Photography and Imaging Processes, MTP Press, Lancaster, England)*

film. This coating is designed to absorb the light coming from the emulsion and prevent backscatter, visible light, or reflected light from degrading the image. The coating is removed by the processing chemicals to permit light to be transmitted through the film for viewing. Antihalation layers contribute to patient dose and are often used only in extremity systems.

If a single emulsion film is loaded into a cassette with the antihalation coating toward the intensifying screen (the source of the light photons), most of the light will be absorbed. **Single-emulsion film must be loaded with the emulsion toward the intensifying screen.** The emulsion side of the film always appears dull, the nonemulsion side shiny. In addition, single emulsion films have an identifying notch cut in the lower left corner. The mnemonic double L (LL) for the lower left corner makes this easy to remember.

Adhesive

A thin coating of adhesive is applied to the base material before it is coated with the emulsion. This substratum coating is designed to glue the emulsion to the base and prevent bubbles or other distortion when the film is bent during processing or handling, or when it is wet and heated during development.

Emulsion

The emulsion is composed of gelatin in which photosensitive silver halide crystals are suspended. It is spread in an extremely even coating that, depending on the manufacturer, ranges from 5–10 μm (0.0002″–0.0004″) of thickness on each side of the base. The purpose of the gelatin is to act as a neutral lucent suspension medium for the silver halide crystals that must be separated from one another to permit processing chemicals to reach them. Gelatin serves as a nonreactive medium through which chemicals can diffuse to reach the silver halides. The gelatin also distributes the crystals evenly over the surface of the film, thus preventing clumping of silver halides that would make one area of the film more photosensitive than another. Additionally, the gelatin must be clear, to per-

mit light to travel through it uniformly, and flexible enough to permit bending without distorting the recorded image. The gelatin that is used for film is of extremely high quality.

The photosensitive agents suspended in the emulsion are silver halide crystals (or grains). The silver halides used in radiographic film are **silver bromide, silver iodide,** and **silver chloride.** Although the exact formula of each company is a closely guarded trade secret, film manufacturers agree that modern silver halides are 95–98 percent silver bromide, with the remainder usually consisting of silver iodide. This has led to the term **silver iodobromide** as a generic specification of the silver halide crystals.

Because photographic film normally has emulsion on a single side, diagnostic radiographic film is sometimes called **duplitized,** double emulsion, or double-coated film. Not all radiographic film is duplitized though. There are special radiographic films (such as duplication, mammography, and fine-detail extremity films) that are coated on a single side.

Supercoat

The supercoat is a layer of hard, protective gelatin designed to prevent the soft emulsion underneath from being physically or chemically abused by scratches, abrasions from stacking, and skin oils from handling. It is usually designed to be antistatic as well. The supercoat is extremely strong and, when combined with the tough base material, makes it nearly impossible to tear a radiograph. A Chicago phone book would be easier to tear in half than a radiograph unless an edge is cut first.

The only items routinely used during film handling that are capable of permanently damaging the surface of a radiograph are a paper clip and a staple. For this reason, plastic holders or paper film envelopes should always be used to keep radiographs together. Radiographs should not be paper-clipped to reports or requisition orders, and stapled medical records should not be filed in the same envelope with radiographs. To avoid this problem, a properly designed radiograph envelope has a separate compartment for the consultation report.

Manufacturing

Radiographic film is manufactured in four stages: **crystal production, ripening, mixing,** and **coating.**

Crystal Production. Silver-bromide crystal production is accomplished, in total darkness, by combining silver nitrate and potassium bromide in the presence of gelatin. The silver bromide will precipitate out and the potassium nitrate can be washed away as a waste product. The gelatin must be present as a medium to permit the crystals to form. The gelatin functions to limit oxidation and reduce crystal surface energy tension, as well as to facilitate other chemical reactions. This process is described by the formula:

$$AgNO_3 + KBr \rightarrow AgBR \downarrow + KNO_3$$

| silver nitrate | + | potassium bromide | $\rightarrow$ | silver bromide (precipitate) | + | potassium nitrate |

The silver halide crystals are flat and roughly triangular in shape (Figure 19-4). Although different types of film emulsions require different size crystals, they are all very small, about 1 μm (0.00004") on each side. A cubic millimeter contains over half a billion ($> 500,000,000$) crystals.

The tabular grain process develops flat, tabular crystals two to four times larger that can be more evenly dispersed throughout the emulsion. The advantages of tabular grains include the absorption of a

T-grain

A

conventional grain

B

FIGURE 19-4 Photomicrographs of silver halide crystal. (A) Flat, triangular tabular crystals (T-grain). **(B) Conventional crystals.** *(Used with permission of Eastman Kodak Company, Rochester, NY)*

FIGURE 19-5   Cubic lattice arrangement of ions in a silver halide crystal. The surfaces are primarily negative bromine and iodine halides, while the interior is primarily positive silver. Note the free silver atom and the sensitivity speck.

TABLE 19-1.	Relationship of Film Crystal and Emulsion to Film Factors			
	Crystal Size		Emulsion Layer	
	Small	Large	Thin	Thick
Resolution	high	low	high	low
Speed	slow	fast	slow	fast

The silver halide crystals must have an impurity added, usually gold-silver sulfide, to form **sensitivity specks**. The gold-silver sulfide may adhere to the surface of the crystal or even be partially incorporated into its structure. There can be a few or many specks, but they must be present to provide film sensitivity. During latent image formation the sensitivity specks serve as electrodes to attract the free silver ions. During development, the bromide concentrations will serve as ion pumps to assist in the deposition of silver, thus amplifying the image.

Ripening.   Ripening is the period during which silver halides are allowed to grow. The size of the crystals determines their total photosensitivity, so the longer the ripening period, the larger the crystals (or grains) and the more sensitive the emulsion. The relationship of crystal size and emulsion thickness to various film factors is shown in Table 19-1. At the proper time, the emulsion is cooled, shredded, and washed to remove the potassium nitrate.

Mixing.   The mixing process follows ripening. The shredded emulsion is melted at a precise temperature to properly sensitize the crystals. A number of additives are then mixed into the emulsion. Usually included among these are:

colored dyes that improve the sensitivity of the silver halides to match the wavelengths of photons that will be striking the emulsion during exposure,

hardeners to prevent physical trauma,

bactericides and fungicides to inhibit the growth of these organisms (especially in warmer climates or where water supplies are not chemically treated), and

antifogging agents to decrease sensitivity to environmental factors, such as heat.

greater portion of the exposing photons, reduced light crossover from one emulsion to the other, and reduced silver coating requirements. Tabular grains may also permit 45-second processing but are very sensitive to fluctuations in the developer replenishment rate.

Each crystal is a cubic lattice (or matrix) of silver, bromide, and iodine atoms (Figure 19-5). A conventional crystal contains approximately 10^{10} (10,000,000,000) atoms. They are bound together by moderately strong ionic bonds with the silver positive (Ag^+) and the bromine or iodine negative (Br^- or I^-). The crystal structure permits both free silver atoms and free electrons to drift through the lattice. This ability is the key to the formation of the latent image.

It is thought that the halide ions (bromine and iodine) tend to cluster on or near the surface of the crystal while the silver ions form the center. This results in silver halide crystals having negatively charged surfaces and positively charged interiors.

Films are often classified as **panchromatic** or **orthochromatic,** according to their sensitivity to the color of light. Panchromatic films are sensitive to all colors, while orthochromatic films are not sensitive to the red spectrum. This sensitivity is controlled by the dyes that are added during this stage.

Coating. The coating process requires extremely precise and expensive coating equipment. There are only a few factories in the world that can coat emulsions. First, the adhesive layer is applied to the base, then the emulsion, and, finally, the supercoat. The emulsion is applied to 40-inch-wide (102 cm) sheets of film, which are stored on rolls, cut to size, and packaged for the consumer. Standard film sizes are shown in Table 19-2. All film manufacturing, packaging, transport, exposure, and processing must be accomplished in total darkness.

LATENT IMAGE FORMATION

The photons that reach the emulsion are primarily light photons from the intensifying screens that are in contact with the film. However, x-ray photons are also involved in the production of the image. This deposits energy from the photon within the lattice of the silver halide crystals.

The latent image is the unseen change in the atomic structure of the crystal lattice that results in the production of a visible image. Although there is still much that is unknown about the exact mechanisms that control the formation of the latent image, the theory proposed by Gurney and Mott in 1938 remains almost unchallenged. Their theory accounts for sensitivity specks being essential to the image formation process.

The arrangement of the silver and halide ions, free silver ions, and sensitivity specks (see Figure 19-5) has been simplified to illustrate the Gurney-Mott theory (Figure 19-6) of latent image formation. The process begins when an incident photon (light or x-ray) interacts with one of the halides (bromine or iodine). The ejected electron is freed to

TABLE 19-2.	Standard Radiographic Film Sizes
SI	U.S. Customary
35 × 91 cm	14 × 36 inches
40 × 40 cm	
35 × 43 cm	14 × 17 inches
35 × 35 cm	14 × 14 inches
30 × 40 cm	
30 × 35 cm	
28 × 35 cm	11 × 14 inches
25 × 30 cm	10 × 12 inches
24 × 30 cm	
24 × 24 cm	9.5 × 9.5 inches
20 × 40 cm	
20 × 25 cm	8 × 10 inches
18 × 24 cm	
18 × 43 cm	7 × 17 inches
	5 × 12 inches
15 × 30 cm	6 × 12 inches
	6.5 × 8.5 inches

Bold sizes are in routine use at most institutions.

NOTE: In most cases the metric and English sizes are not equivalent; they are similar but not exactly interchangeable.

wander and may eventually be attracted and trapped by a sensitivity speck, giving the speck a negative charge. The negatively charged sensitivity speck attracts a free silver ion. The silver ion neutralizes the sensitivity speck (thus resetting the "trap"). This process is known as the ionic stage and is repeated several times until a clump of silver atoms rests at the sensitivity speck. A single incident photon may free thousands of electrons for deposition at sensitivity specks. However, not all freed silver is deposited at sensitivity specks. At least three silver atoms must be deposited for a visible clump of black metallic silver to be formed by chemical development of the image.

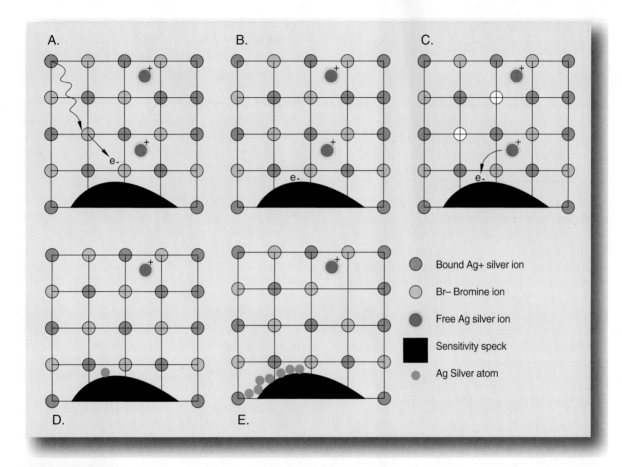

FIGURE 19-6   Latent image formation according to the Gurney-Mott theory.

A—A bromine ion absorbs an incident photon and ejects an electron.

B—The ejected electron is trapped at the sensitivity speck, giving it a negative charge.

C—The negatively charged sensitivity speck attracts a free silver ion.

D—The silver ion neutralizes at the sensitivity speck.

E—Repetition of the process deposits several silver atoms at the sensitivity speck.

TYPES OF FILM

The first radiographs were exposed to x-ray photons only. Film is still manufactured for direct exposure, but because it requires a much greater radiation dose, its use is severely limited for medical applications. Once the technology had been developed to use the x-rays to produce light at the intensifying screen, the dose reduction resulted in intensifying screen film (usually called screen film) becoming predominant in medical radiography. In addition, numerous special application films have been developed, such as mammography, detail extremity, contact surgical, computer-driven cathode ray tube (CRT), laser exposed, duplication, and fluoroscopic films.

Direct Exposure or Nonscreen Film

Although used primarily for industrial nondestructive testing (NDT) radiography, occasional use of direct exposure film can be justified when extremely fine detail is critical to the diagnostic quality of the image. Because of the extremely high radiation exposure that results from the use of nonscreen film, it is unusual to justify its use on living patients. Dental radiography, reconstructive surgery of the hands, biopsy specimen radiography, and forensics are examples of appropriate applications. Direct exposure film has a single emulsion, extremely fine grain silver halide crystals, and a much greater silver content. It also requires a much thicker emulsion layer (two or three times that of medical screen film) in order to achieve sufficient sensitivity and still maintain a fine grain. Because of the emulsion thickness, many brands of direct exposure film cannot be processed in automatic radiographic processors and require manual processing.

Intensifying Screen Film

Commonly called screen film, this type of film is available in a wide variety of speeds, contrast ranges, latitudes, and resolutions. Each manufacturer has developed specific characteristics for its particular films.

The primary differences are in speed (sensitivity of the silver halides), which is controlled by the size of the crystals and the thickness of the emulsion layer. Contrast, latitude, and resolution tend to be linked to speed. Larger crystals and thicker emulsions usually provide lower contrast, wider latitude, and less resolution. Screen films are made faster through their double emulsion, while a reduction in the silver content has been achieved through more efficient distribution of the silver.

Special Application Films

Most special applications require single-emulsion films, although some have a pure gelatin coating on one side to avoid shrinking and curling during pro-

cessing. **Mammography** and **detail extremity radiography** films have developed as fine-grain films sensitive to a single screen. **Contact surgical radiography** is accomplished with nonscreen film in sterilized plastic packages. **Cathode ray tube (CRT) imaging,** also called video imaging, requires a film that is sensitive to the light emitted by the CRT. Films for CRT are available in blue and green sensitivities as well as orthochromatic for either. They are usually fine grain because patient dose is not a factor when recording CRT images. **Laser films** are directly exposed by the laser used in the imaging camera. Consequently, the film must be sensitive to the color (frequency) of light emitted by the particular camera. The laser light is extremely accurate and because it operates with parallel instead of divergent photons, it produces a near distortion-free image. Fine-grained films are used for this purpose because their exposure is usually not related to the level of patient exposure to radiation, and because the accuracy of the laser image demands a film that can record fine detail.

Duplication film is designed to provide an exact image of the original film. Diagnostic radiographs are actually negatives because they reverse the blacks and whites of the subject (white-bone). Fluoroscopy produces a positive image (black-bone). If an unexposed diagnostic film is laid under a processed film with a good image, a light is turned on for a brief moment and the exposed film is processed, the duplicate film will have densities opposite from the original (i.e., the white-bone image will be converted to black-bone). Duplicating film is pre-exposed to permit it to duplicate the original image (i.e., a white-bone image is recorded as a white-bone image). It is sensitive to the ultraviolet light used in duplicating machines.

Fluoroscopic spot filming can be accomplished with screen film but is often done with 70 mm roll film or 105 mm film chips. These films are similar to cineradiography film in that they are sensitive to the green light from the fluoroscope.

Special minimum sensitivity films have been developed for verifying the radiation field during MeV radiation therapy treatments. These films are exposed to massive amounts of radiation.

THE DUPLICATION PROCESS

Duplication is the process by which a nearly exact copy, the same size or miniaturized, is made of a radiographic image. Duplicates arose from the need to share visual information with other institutions, with other hospital departments for educational purposes, and for volume storage and medical legal purposes. Film manufacturers have made duplication relatively easy by producing ready-to-use duplicating film that is processed in automatic processors and devices for exposing it (Figure 19-7).

Solarization Effect

The solarization effect is a technique from the early days of photography that produces prints by exposure to sunlight. If an ordinary silver halide emulsion is exposed long enough, it will reach the reversal phase and actually lose density.

Duplicating Film

Modern duplicating film has a single emulsion and is presolarized; it is chemically fogged to D-Max by the manufacturer. Therefore, further exposure decreases optical density (OD).

Duplicating film has an average gradient of OD 1.0 to 1.5 and is sensitized to about 359 nm, which is in the ultraviolet range. It is possible to post a simple technique chart by a duplicating unit after a brief trial with duplicating film and a control radiograph.

Various authors have written of techniques used to save overexposure radiographs in order to avoid having to repeat the examination. Diagnostic information from images that are overexposed as much as 75 percent can often be saved via duplication with long exposure times. This technique is limited to original radiographs with a density of OD 3.1 or less.

With some of the faster emulsions now available, the exposure requirements may be so low that the copying unit cannot accurately time them. In these instances, the duplicating system can be slowed down to match the emulsion by blocking part of the

unit's ultraviolet tube with blackened film, black electrical tape, or by an orange/yellow filter.

Very large institutions and other mass users of radiographic images, such as the military and survey units, often need to reduce the size of images because of limited storage facilities. In these situations a copy-stand device with a roll-film camera can be used. These units use 16 mm to 100 mm photographic roll-film.

FILM STORAGE AND HANDLING

Although often overlooked, the proper storage and handling of film is an important part of radiography. It is not uncommon for a hospital diagnostic radiography department to have an annual film budget of over $1,000,000, and any unit performing radiography quickly discovers that film cost is a considerable budget item. Improper storage and handling of film can be very expensive. More importantly, it can produce film artifacts that compromise image quality. Appendix B (AGFA's Troubleshooting the Radiographic System) details film artifacts and their causes.

Basic Storage and Handling

Attention must be given to the **age** of the film, heat, **humidity, light,** radiation, and **handling.** All film is sold with an expiration date stamped on the box. Photosensitive materials are constantly absorbing photons of both heat and background radiation and, over time, this exposure can reach a level where the fog on the film interferes with image quality. Rotation of new stock must be established to observe expiration dates.

Film should be stored at a temperature of 20°C (68°F) or lower at all times. Professional photographers refrigerate all film, and radiography departments should follow this recommendation. Most radiography departments avoid the problem by arranging film shipments to keep film in storage for only 45 to 60 days. Special application films that

FIGURE 19-7 A radiographic duplication unit. A radiograph is duplicated by the following steps:

1. A clean radiograph requiring duplication is placed on the glass plate and centered using the view light control.
2. The view light is switched off. Under safelight, a duplicating film of appropriate size is placed emulsion down on the original radiograph to be duplicated. (Notch in lower left [LL] means the emulsion is facing the operator.)
3. The lid is attached tightly to achieve good film-to-film contact.
4. The timer is set and an exposure is made in the duplicating mode.
5. Both films are removed from the glass plate; the duplicating film is processed, and the original is returned to storage.

Exposure adjustments are made by comparing the duplicate to the original. Because duplicating film is a positive emulsion, exposure adjustments are the opposite of those used for radiographic film. For example, a darker duplicate is produced by decreasing exposure time.

The duplicate image will be slightly less sharp than the original because of the divergence of light as it travels through the two emulsions of the original onto the single emulsion of the duplicate. In addition, the duplicate image will have significantly higher contrast because the slope of the solarized D log E curve is always steeper than with radiographic films. *(Courtesy of Roger Smith, British Columbia Institute of Technology, Vancouver, BC)*

must be stored for long periods of time should be frozen. All refrigeration and freezing must be done with the film sealed in moisture-proof containers, as sold by the manufacturer. This essentially arrests the aging process. **Film must be brought to room temperature in advance of use** and before breaking the moisture-proof seal. Failure to do this will destroy the film when atmospheric moisture condenses on the cool film surface, creating waterspot artifacts.

The humidity must be maintained between 30 and 60 percent. Static discharge artifacts are a danger at low humidity, and high humidity causes condensation. A basement area that contains steam, cold water or other fluid pipes and is not included in the building's heating and cooling system is a poor choice for film storage.

All photosensitive materials must be protected from unfiltered light. Because film is sold in light- and moisture-proof packaging, this becomes a problem only with damaged or opened packages. Darkroom safelighting permits film handling with the convenience of limited visibility. All film must be protected from exposure to ionizing radiation. Lead lining of film storage areas will eliminate this problem. Handling of film is often overlooked as a source of problems. **Film should be stored on end,** not flat. Film boxes should be opened carefully, and under no circumstances should a film, paper interleaf, or cardboard insert be removed quickly. Abrasion artifacts can occur from quick movement over film and under pressure. Even at the proper humidity, quick movement can cause static discharge with artifact exposure from the resulting light (see Figure 3-5). Chemical fumes can also cause film fog. Film should not be stored near cleaning solutions, formaldehyde, or other strong chemicals.

Automated Systems

Automatic film handling systems involve a transport mechanism that feeds a single film from a storage unit, transports it into position for exposure between a pair of intensifying screens, and then transports it into a processor after exposure. Automatic feed diagnostic units have been marketed successfully. However, in spite of the fact that they save the expense of cassettes, they have not been extremely popular, but automatic feed dedicated chest units are a more common fixture in high-volume departments.

FILM IDENTIFICATION

All radiographs should be permanently identified with medical record information. This includes the date of the exposure, the full name of the patient, the institution where the exposure was made, the referring physician, the patient identification number, the examination ordered, and any other important information. The identification information is usually added to the film by a light exposure after the radiographic exposure and can be accomplished with a special daylight identification camera and cassette system. It can also be done in the darkroom after the film has been removed from the cassette but before it is processed. Most radiographic cassettes have a lead blocker space in one corner to prevent the film from being exposed to x-rays in that small area. This reserves the space for identification information to be "flashed" by light. This information, like the radiograph, becomes part of the legal medical record and should be treated as such. Additionally, a method of identifying right and left sides of the patient should be required. Many institutions use lead markers, although film punches and blocker placement systems can also be used. The radiographer performing the examination is usually identified through some means; initials or number on a lead marker and signature of accompanying paperwork are common.

Depending on institutional policy, it may or may not be acceptable to change the identification information if it is recorded incorrectly. Some institutions permit changes to be made with wax pencil, stickers, or punches, while others require that the radiograph be repeated. The radiographer is nearly always held responsible for recording the identification information correctly.

SUMMARY

Photographic materials are photosensitive, or capable of responding to exposure by photons. Diagnostic radiographic film is duplitized; in other words, the base is coated on both sides with an adhesive, an emulsion with crystals, and a supercoat.

The film base is polyester, the adhesive glues the emulsion to the base to prevent distortion during processing or handling, the emulsion is gelatin in which photosensitive silver halide crystals are suspended, and the supercoat is a protective layer. An antihalation coating is used to decrease light reflections within the base itself.

Radiographic film is manufactured in four stages: crystal production, ripening, mixing, and coating. The silver halides used are silver bromide, silver iodide, and silver chloride. The term silver iodobromide best describes the silver halides used in radiographic film. They are produced in total darkness by combining silver nitrate and potassium bromide in the presence of gelatin. The silver halide crystals that are produced are flat and roughly triangular in shape. Each crystal is a cubic lattice of silver, bromide, and iodine atoms with sensitivity specks. Ripening time determines crystal size and sensitivity. During mixing, additives are included in the emulsion. Panchromatic films are sensitive to all colors, while orthochromatic films are not sensitive to red. Coating is the final stage before the film is cut and packaged.

The latent image is the unseen change in the atomic structure of the crystal lattice that results in the production of a visible image. At least three silver atoms must be deposited to form a visible clump of black metallic silver.

Direct exposure or nonscreen film can be used when extremely fine detail is critical, although the extremely high radiation exposure requires a careful justification. Intensifying screen film is the most common radiographic film. Films vary in speed, contrast, latitude, and resolution. Special application films have been developed for mammography, detail extremity, contact surgical, cathode ray tube (CRT), laser-exposed, duplication, and fluoroscopic films.

Duplication produces a nearly exact copy of a radiographic image.

Care must be taken in storing and handling film because it is affected by age, heat, humidity, light, radiation, and handling. Some of the handling is avoided by automated systems. All radiographs should be permanently identified with the appropriate medical record information.

REVIEW QUESTIONS

1. What are the primary components of radiographic film?

2. Explain the production of silver halide crystals.

3. What is the purpose of various additives to radiographic film?

4. How is the latent image produced?

5. What are the primary differences between direct exposure film and screen film?

6. Describe the duplication process.

7. Describe common problems due to improper film storage and handling.

8. What are the radiographer's responsibilities concerning proper radiograph identification?

REFERENCES AND RECOMMENDED READING

Arnold, B., Eisenberg, H., & Bjarngard, B. (1978). Measurements of reciprocity law failure in green-sensitive x-ray films. *Radiology, 126,* 493.

Bruce, G. (1980). Tests to compare two film-materials for use in chest radiography. *Radiography, 46*(547), 170.

Busching, L. W. (1978). Implementing a new x-ray film management system. *Radiologic Technology, 49*(5), 603.

Chow, M. F. (1988). The effect of a film's sensitivity to its speed, contrast, and latitude. *The Canadian Journal of Medical Radiation Technology, 19*(4), 147.

Cullinan, A., & Cullinan, J. (1994). *Producing quality radiographs* (2nd ed.). Philadelphia: J. B. Lippincott.

Curry, T. S., Dowdey, J. E., & Murry, R. C. (1990). *Christensen's introduction to the physics of diagnostic radiology* (4th ed.). Philadelphia: Lea and Febiger.

Daniels, C., & Halloway, A. F. (1983, January). Comparison and variations of the speed of radiographic film. *Radiology,* 203.

Doi, K. (1981, June). Effect of crossover exposure on radiographic image quality of screen-film systems. *Radiology,* 707.

Egyed, M., & Shearer, D. R. (1981). A comparative physical evaluation of four x-ray films. *Radiology Management, 3*(4), 11–20.

Frantzell, A. (1950). The practical roentgenographic importance of reciprocity law failure. *Acta Radiologica, 34,* 6–16.

Fuchs, A. (1956). Evolution of Roentgen film. *American Journal of Roentgenology, 75,* 30–48.

Jaffke, R. C. (1957). That versatile non-screen film. *Radiologic Technology, 29*(1), 14.

James, T. H. (1977). *The theory of the photographic process* (4th ed.). New York: Macmillan.

Jenkins, D., & Latham, S. M. (1979). The duplication of chest radiographs. *Radiography, 45*(539), 244–248.

Kelsey, C. A. (1983, January). Anticrossover emulsions evaluated by observer performance tests. *Radiology, 209.*

Kim, O., Ahn, M., & Bahk, Y. (1992). Use of film duplicator to lighten dark radiographs. *Radiology, 184*(2), 573.

Kofler, J., & Gray, J. (1991). Sensitometric responses of selected medical radiographic films. *Radiology, 181*(3), 879–883.

Mathias, J. L., & Marquis, J. R. (1976). Radiographic duplication: A simple method of minimizing radiation dosage to the patient. *Radiologic Technology, 48*(3), 293.

McKinney, W. (1988). *Radiographic processing and quality control.* Philadelphia: J. B. Lippincott.

Morgan, R. H. (1944). Reciprocity law failure in x-ray films. *Radiology, 42,* 471–479.

Morgan, R. H. (1946). An analysis of the physical factors controlling the diagnostic quality of roentgen images: Part IV. Contrast and the film contrast factor. *American Journal of Roentgenology and Radiation Therapy, 55*(5), 627–633.

Newhall, B. (1964). *The history of photography.* New York: The Museum of Modern Art.

Ramsey, L. J. (1978). Notes on x-ray film speeds. *Radiography, 44*(524), 200.

Rao, G. U. V., Witt, W., Beachley, M. C., Bosch, H. A., Fatouros, P. P., & Kan, P. T. (1981). Radiographic films and screen-film systems. In C. M. Coulam, J. J. Erickson, F. D. Rollo, & A. E. James, (Eds.), *The physical basis of medical imaging.* New York: Appleton-Century-Crofts.

Rossi, R. P., Hendee, W. R., & Aherns, C. R. (1976). An evaluation of rare-earth screen-film combinations. *Radiology, 121,* 465.

Sanford, L. (1992). The continuing story of film technology. *Radiography Today, 58*(661), 27–29.

Sturge, J., Walworth, V., & Shepp, A. (1989). Imaging processes and materials: Neblette's 8th edition. New Jersey: Wiley.

Sweeney, R. J. (1983). *Radiographic artifacts: Their cause and control.* Philadelphia: J. B. Lippincott.

Wilson, P. (1976). Principles of formation of the latent and developed images. *Canadian Journal of Radiography, Radiotherapy, and Nuclear Medicine, 7*(6), 268–278.

CHAPTER 20

Film Processing

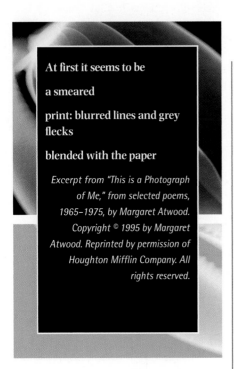

At first it seems to be

a smeared

print: blurred lines and grey flecks

blended with the paper

Excerpt from "This is a Photograph of Me," from selected poems, 1965–1975, by Margaret Atwood. Copyright © 1995 by Margaret Atwood. Reprinted by permission of Houghton Mifflin Company. All rights reserved.

KEY TERMS

activator
agitation
chemical fog
chemical
    precipitation
circulation system
clearing agent
clearing time
crossover network
developing
drive system
dryer system
drying
dwell time
electrolytic

entrance rollers
fixing
flood replenishment
hardener
heat exchanger
hydroquinone
metallic replacement
pass box
phenidone
preservative
reducing agent
replenishment system
resin
restrainer
solvent

standby
    replenishment
standby switch
starter solution
superadditivity
tailing
temperature control
    system
timed replenishment
transport racks
transport system
volume
    replenishment
washing

OBJECTIVES

Upon completion of this chapter, the student should be able to:

- Explain the process of film development.

- Describe the synergistic properties of automatic processor reducing agents.

- Identify the primary chemical and its function for each of the developer and fixer agents.

- Explain the process of film fixation.

- Explain the washing and drying processes of film archiving.

- Describe the functions of the subsystems of an automatic processor.

- Discuss the design of a radiographic darkroom, including entrances, pass boxes, centralized and decentralized plans, and ventilation.

- Explain the rationale for the use of silver recovery systems.

- Compare the advantages and disadvantages of metallic replacement, electrolytic, chemical precipitation, and resin silver recovery units.

The primary purpose of radiographic processing is to deposit enough black metallic silver at the latent image sites to permit a permanent visible image to form. The development of the latent image can be accomplished manually or with automatic processing equipment. Due to the predominance of automatic processors in radiography, manual processing will not be discussed. The process is very similar to automatic processing and any radiographer can apply his or her knowledge of automatic processing to manual processing with the modifications provided by the manufacturer's information inserts that are packed with the chemicals.

Quality control experts agree that the radiographic film processor is the most sensitive and variable factor in the production of a radiograph. A high percentage of radiographic quality problems can be traced to processor variations or malfunctions. It is the role of the radiographer to monitor the performance of the processor, troubleshoot problems, and repair minor malfunctions.

Automatic processing of a radiograph involves four primary steps: **developing, fixing** and two archiving steps—**washing** and **drying.** Developing and fixing are accomplished in solutions of numerous chemicals. Archiving involves a two-step process of washing and drying the radiograph for use as a medical record.

 DEVELOPING

Developing is the first step in processing the film. At this stage silver is deposited at the latent image sites and an image becomes visible. The deposition of silver amplifies the density of the image. Modern x-ray developers are capable of amplifying the image by a factor of 10^8–10^9 within 3 to 4.5 minutes. The silver ions of the latent image are stabilized and more silver is added to the site until a visible silver clump is formed. The primary agents of the developer are two **reducing agents,** although automatic radiographic developer solutions also include an **activator, restrainer, preservative, hardener** and water as a **solvent** (Table 20-1). The action of the developer is controlled by the immersion time, solution temperature and chemical activity.

Reducing Agents

Reducing agents provide electrons to the silver ions attached to the sensitivity specks of the silver halide crystals (the latent image). Silver halides have negative exteriors (where bromine and iodine ions are located) and positive interiors (where silver ions are located). This arrangement effectively prohibits the reducing agent from supplying electrons to the silver ions because the bromine and iodine repel electrons. However, when a sensitivity speck has attracted silver ions, a gate exists through which the interior of the crystal can be supplied with electrons. When a silver ion obtains an extra electron, it is converted to a stable black metallic silver atom. Reduction is actually the process of the reducing agents giving up electrons to neutralize the positive silver ions. This reduction process is illustrated in Figure 20-1.

The secret to the production of the various densities is that the sensitivity speck gate will be larger when more silver ions are deposited at the speck during exposure. A larger gate permits faster reduction of the internal silver atoms. When the reduction process is stopped at the appropriate time, the silver halides have accumulated black metallic silver in proportion to the size of the sensitivity speck gate. This produces a film with varying degrees of blackness. Of course, all silver halides with gates will become totally reduced, and the entire film will appear black if the reducing agents are permitted to work for too long a time, if they work too fast due to high temperature, or if the solution has too high a concentration. The term **chemical fog** is used to describe development when these factors cause unexposed silver halides to be reduced.

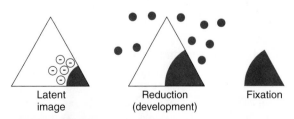

Latent image | Reduction (development) | Fixation

FIGURE 20-1 The reduction of a silver halide crystal through a sensitivity speck gate.

TABLE 20-1. Automatic Radiographic Processing Chemicals and Their Functions

Solution	Time in 90-second Processor	Chemical	Function
Developer	20–25 sec		reduces latent image to visible black metallic silver
reducing agent		phenidone	rapidly produces fine detail shades of gray
reducing agent		hydroquinone	slowly produces heavy densities
activator		sodium carbonate	produces alkaline pH, swells gelatin
restrainer		potassium bromide	decreases reducing agent activity, antifogging agent
preservative		sodium sulfite	controls oxidation, buffer agent
hardener		glutaraldehyde	hardens emulsion, reduces gelatin swelling
solvent		water	dissolves chemicals
Fixer	20 sec		stops reduction and removes undeveloped silver halides from emulsion
clearing agent		ammonium thiosulfate	removes undeveloped silver halides from emulsion
activator		acetic acid	provides acidic pH, stops reduction
hardener		potassium alum	hardens emulsion
preservative		sodium sulfite	maintains pH
solvent		water	dissolves chemicals
Wash	20 sec		removes developing and fixing chemicals
solvent		water	removes excess chemicals
Dry	25–30 sec		removes water and seals emulsion
		hot air	evaporates water and hardens emulsion

Those silver halide crystals that have fewer than three silver atoms on their sensitivity specks are unable to open a gate and remain unreduced (undeveloped). Each reduced silver atom is accompanied by a liberated bromine ion with a negative charge. A bromide ion barrier is created when too many liberated bromine ions are permitted to accumulate. They may produce sufficient charge to repel reducing agents and effectively stop silver halide development. This is the same effect that is achieved by using potassium bromide as a "starter" solution to slow down the hyperactivity of newly mixed developer replenisher solutions. The problem is overcome by replenishment of the developer strength at regular intervals. A freshly cleaned processor may require seasoning by running for 20 to 30 minutes to thoroughly mix the starter solution.

The reducing agents used in automatic radiographic processors are **phenidone** (known as P developer) and **hydroquinone** (known as Q developer). **Phenidone quickly reduces silver, enhancing fine detail and subtle shades of gray and works only in areas of light exposure.** It cannot reduce heavily exposed areas. Phenidone replaces the function of metol (often known by the Kodak brand name Elon) in manual processing. **Hydroquinone slowly reduces silver and produces heavy density.** Hydroquinone is ineffective

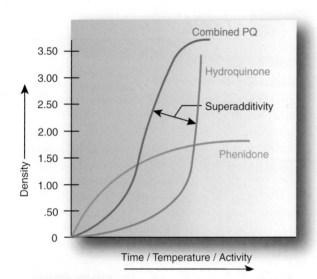

Density

3.50
3.00
2.50
2.00
1.50
1.00
.50
0

Combined PQ

Hydroquinone

Superadditivity

Phenidone

Time / Temperature / Activity

FIGURE 20-2 The superadditivity or synergistic effect of phenidone and hydroquinone combined, as compared to their independent reducing abilities.

at first but then rapidly increases in action. When the two reducing agents are combined, forming a PQ developer, their reducing ability is greater than the sum of their independent abilities. This is a synergistic phenomenon known as **superadditivity** (Figure 20-2). As can be seen from the graph, phenidone controls the lower part of the curve (the toe), while hydroquinone controls the upper portion (the shoulder).

Oxidation and reduction are opposite processes. When the reducing agent is oxidized, it gives up electrons. Reduction occurs when a silver halide crystal takes one of the electrons and is changed to black metallic silver. The oxidation/reduction process reduces the strength of the developer solution. As developer oxidizes, it changes color, first to a deep amber, then to brown, and, finally, to a thick, rust red.

Activator

The action of the reducing agents is enhanced by maintaining the developer solution in an alkaline state (around pH 10.0 to 10.5) by using an activator, usually sodium carbonate. Potassium carbonate, sodium hydroxide, and potassium hydroxide may also be used. The activator also assists the reducers in reaching the silver halides by causing the gelatin to swell and become more permeable. The activator is caustic, and, therefore, rubber gloves and an apron should be worn when handling developer solutions. Developer solution that is splashed onto clothing and walls is corrosive and should be neutralized with fixer solution or diluted with water.

Restrainer

A restrainer, usually potassium bromide, is also added to the developer to restrict the reducing action to those crystals with sensitivity speck gates. It does this by permitting overactive reducers to attack it, instead of unexposed silver halides.

Preservative

Sodium sulfite is used as a preservative agent to help decrease the oxidation of the reducing agents when they are combined with air. The attraction of air for the reducers is so strong that developer solutions remain effective for only a few weeks after mixing. Common techniques to assist with this problem include floating plastic lids and styrofoam balls to reduce the air-developer interface. This is also a consideration when buying developer solution tanks. Tall, narrow tanks reduce the surface and the oxidation effect. They are more desirable than low, wide tanks. A floating plastic cover or balls (e.g., ping-pong balls) will also reduce the surface area. The tank should not hold more than a 2-week supply of solution.

Hardener

Glutaraldehyde is the most common developer solution hardener. It controls the swelling of the gelatin to prevent scratches and abrasions to the emulsion during processing. It also maintains uniform film thickness to assist in transport through an automatic processor. Insufficient hardener will cause films to deposit gelatin on processor rollers, which may cause transport and artifact problems for subsequent films. Insufficient hardener may also cause films to exit the processor with moist, softened surfaces. Hot-air drying alone cannot seal the emulsion. Excessive hardener may cause the emulsion to harden prematurely, preventing chemical interactions with the silver halides and trapping moisture in the gelatin.

Solvent

The chemicals are suspended in water as a solvent. The water used for mixing chemistry should be filtered to remove impurities (a 5–10 μm filter is recommended). In tropical climates, it should be treated to eliminate bacteria and fungus that may find the gelatin emulsion an attractive meal.

Contamination

The developer is the only solution that is dramatically affected by contamination. Only 0.1 percent fixer in a developer tank will destroy the ability of the reducing agents (10 ml in a 2.5 gallon [10 liter] tank). Films processed in contaminated developer appear extremely gray (they exhibit extremely low contrast). Because the fixer tank is adjacent to the developer, it is easy for splashing to occur during quality control and repair procedures. The most common cause of contamination is splashing, which occurs during lifting or replacing the fixer transport rack. Special splash guards are supplied with automatic processors, and they should always be used. Developer contamination requires total dumping, washing, refilling and seasoning of the developer tank. Not only is this difficult and time consuming but it also wastes money. When cleaning a processor, the fixer tank should always be filled first. If splashing occurs, it is a simple matter to re-clean the developer tank before it is filled.

Evaporation of solutions can also cause contamination. Due to the heat necessary for processing, solutions evaporate and condense on the processor lid. Contamination can occur if fixer condensation drips into the developer tank. Individual evaporation covers for both developer and fixer tanks should be in place at all times. When a processor is shut down, excessive condensation can occur as it cools. To prevent contamination, the processor lid should be propped open whenever the processor is not in use. Splashing or evaporation of developer into the fixer tank does not cause contamination. Developer is regularly carried into the fixer by the films being processed.

 ## FIXING

If a film is exposed to light after development, the unreduced silver halides will open gates and be converted to black metallic silver. This is seen as a slow blackening of the film, which obscures the image. Undeveloped silver halides must be removed from the emulsion to permanently fix the image before exposure to light for viewing. (This was the last reaction to be discovered and delayed development of the photographic process by nearly 25 years.) This important step is accomplished by using a clearing agent that bonds with the unexposed silver halides and removes them from the emulsion. The primary agent of the fixer is the **clearing agent,** although automatic radiographic fixer solutions also include an activator, preservative, hardener, and water as a solvent (see Table 20-1).

Clearing Agent

Nearly all fixer solutions use ammonium thiosulfate as the clearing (fixing) agent (also known by the old-fashioned term "hypo"). Ammonium thiosulfate uses silver in the emulsion to form ammonium thiosilversulfate. Within 5–10 seconds after the clearing agent has begun to function, the film can be exposed to full room light for inspection without damage to the image. If the fixer has not completely cleared the film of unexposed silver halides, the film will have a milky appearance. The **clearing time** is defined as twice the time necessary for the milky appearance to disappear. In a 90-second automatic processor, the clearing time is usually 15–20 seconds.

Activator

Acetic acid is used as the activator in the fixer. It maintains an acidic pH (4.0–4.5) to enhance the functioning of the clearing agent. It also serves as a stop bath to keep the reducing agents from continuing to function when the film is immersed in the fixer. Recall that reducing agents function in an alkaline solution. An acidic solution will neutralize and thereby stop the alkaline developing solution from continuing its reduction of the silver halides.

Preservative

The fixer uses the same preservative as the developer—sodium sulfite. It dissolves silver from the ammonium thiosilversulfate, thus permitting it to continue to remove silver from the emulsion.

Hardener

The hardener in the fixer must function in an acidic environment. Glutaraldehyde is effective only in an alkaline solution, so fixer hardeners are aluminum chloride, chromium alum, or potassium alum. The hardener serves the same purpose as glutaraldehyde in the developer—prevention of scratches and abrasions to the emulsion during processing and maintenance of a uniform thickness of the film during transport. Insufficient hardener will cause films to exit the processor with moist, softened surfaces.

Solvent

Water (which should be filtered and treated) is used as the solvent.

Depletion

After a time, the fixer solution will become saturated with silver ions from the emulsion. The solution slowly becomes unable to accept additional silver and requires a longer clearing time. Automatic processors constantly replenish the fixer solution to eliminate this problem. The silver ions in the fixer can be reclaimed through various silver recovery processes.

 ARCHIVING

The archiving process is composed of two steps: washing and drying. Archiving prepares the film for long-term storage as a medical record by protecting it from deterioration by chemicals, fading, and physical forces.

Washing

The washing process uses water to remove as much of the fixer and developer solutions as possible. The water temperature should be slightly lower than the other solutions (about 5°F or 3°C lower) because some processors use the water to help control temperature fluctuations in the developer and fixer. The emulsion may reticulate (crack into many pieces) if the temperature is changed too dramatically.

Both fixer and developer solutions contain chemicals that, even in weak concentrations, can damage the image over time. Because most of the developer action is stopped by the acidic pH of the fixer, the main concern is removing the fixer from the emulsion. Failure to provide sufficient agitation or wash time to clear fixer from the film may result in silver stains or a yellowing of the emulsion after a few years.

Warm water will increase the efficiency of the wash. Wash tanks, especially those not made of stainless steel, are susceptible to algae and bacteria growth during periods when the processor is turned off. To eliminate this problem, the wash tank should be drained whenever the processor is shut down.

Drying

Drying is done by forcing hot air over both sides of the film as it begins its exit from the processor. The air temperature ranges from 120–150°F (43–65°C). The hot air sets a final hardening to the emulsion and seals the supercoat. Table 20-1 illustrates all of the automatic processing steps, the processing times, and the functions of the component chemicals.

Storage

Proper storage is a critical part of the archiving process. The length of time an original radiograph is stored is usually 5–7 years, depending on institutional policies and applicable laws. Films taken of minors and cases involved in litigation may be retained much longer (sometimes permanently). Processed radiographs should be stored at about 70°F (23°C) and 60 percent humidity.

 AUTOMATIC PROCESSING

Radiographic films were manually processed until Eastman Kodak introduced the first continuous roller automatic processor in 1957. This unit processed a film in 15 minutes and was so large that an overhead winch was required to lift the racks of rollers from the chemical tanks for cleaning. It was a

FIGURE 20-3 (A) A modern automatic x-ray film processor. (B) A transport rack and crossover networks in a single tank.

great improvement over manual processing, which required an hour to process and dry a film, and often produced erratic results. Modern processors are much more compact (their racks can easily be lifted by hand) and they process a film in 45–120 seconds (Figure 20-3A).

Automatic processors are complex and utilize several subsystems to completely process a radiograph: the **transport system, dryer system, replenishment system, circulation system,** and **temperature control system.** Table 20-2 illustrates the processor systems and subsystems and their functions. The radiographer should understand the functions of automatic processing systems well enough to diagnose

problems that affect image quality. The radiographer should also be capable of basic disassembly of a processor for cleaning or removal of lost or stuck films.

Transport System

The transport system is designed to move a film through the developer, fixer, wash and dryer sections of the processor. As it does this, it controls the length of time the radiograph is immersed in each of the solutions and agitates the chemistry to ensure maximum reaction. The transport system consists of three subsystems: **transport racks, crossover networks,** and a **drive system.**

TABLE 20-2.	Automatic Radiographic Processor Systems and Subsystems	
System	**Subsystem**	**Function**
Transport		Move the film through the processor, control immersion time, agitate solutions
	Transport rack	Move the film down in and up out of solution tanks
	Crossover network	Turn the film down into the next tank
	Drive system	Turn rollers
Dryer system		Remove excess water, shrink and seal emulsion
Replenishment system		Replace depleted chemicals in the developer and fixer
Circulation system		Stabilize solution temperatures, agitate solutions, mix replenishment chemistry into the tank
Temperature control		Maintain solution temperatures

Transport Racks. The transport racks consist of three series of rollers designed to move a film through a processing tank (see Figure 20-3B). The offset of the three series of rollers provides constant tension to propel the film down into and up out of the processing tank. Note that the center series of rollers may handle films traveling down and up at the same time. The original processors had difficulty handling films due to shrinking and expansion of the emulsion. The solution temperature, quantity of hardeners and expandability of the emulsion are all designed specifically for automatic processing. Films without these characteristics may not transport through the processor and may even leave artifact causing emulsion deposits on rollers. Single-emulsion films are especially difficult because the single emulsion tends to cause the film to curl as it expands and contracts.

Special turnaround equipment is needed to bend and turn a film at the bottom and top of the transport racks. This is accomplished at the bottom of the rack by a combination of master roller, planetary rollers, and guide shoes (deflectors) (see Figure 20-3B). The master roller pushes the leading edge of the film against the guide shoes. The guide shoes then force the edge around the master roller with the help of the planetary rollers until it is pointed upward and can be pulled by the offset rollers. Guide shoes are ribbed to prevent wet films from sticking to

a smooth metallic surface. Each transport rack can be lifted from its tank for easy cleaning. The final set of rollers in a transport rack are special squeegee rollers that remove excess solution from the film as it is pulled from each tank.

Crossover Networks. A crossover network is used to bend and turn the film when it reaches the top of the transport rack and must be directed down into the next tank or section (see Figure 20-3B). Each crossover network operates with a master roller and guide shoes system similar to that in the transport rack. Misaligned guide shoes will scratch the film emulsion as it is driven past. The most common cause of guide shoe misalignment is improper seating of transport racks and crossover networks.

The **entrance rollers** are a special crossover network designed to start the film traveling from the feed tray down into the developer section. These rollers are specially designed with ribs to grip the film and feed it evenly into the first rack. It is important that the entrance rollers grip the film so that it will feed straight through the entire processor. A film that is fed at a slight angle will be driven into the transport gears by the time it travels a distance into the processor.

Always use the guides at each side of the feed tray to align each film as it is fed into the entrance rollers. Films should be fed from alternate sides of

A.

CORRECT: Short side of film against feed tray guide

B.

WRONG: Long side of film and not against feed tray guide

FIGURE 20-4 (A) Proper film feeding. (B) Improper film feeding.

the feed tray to avoid excess wear to one side of the transport rollers (i.e., first film right side, second film left side, etc.). **Films should always be fed with the short axis along the feed tray side guide** (Figure 20-4). In some processors, the entrance rollers also open a microswitch that activates the replenishment system.

Drive System. The drive system consists of a series of mechanical devices designed to turn the numerous rollers in the processor from power supplied by a single motor. The speed of the drive system is usually set to move a film from the entrance rollers to the feed tray (dry to dry) in 45–120 seconds. This speed controls the time the film is immersed in each chemical solution, and slowing or speeding by as little as 2 percent can dramatically affect image quality.

Dryer System

The final stage of processing is drying the film with the dryer system. The emulsion of a wet film is sticky and may adhere permanently if brought into contact with another film. The dryer system begins with a series of squeegee crossover rollers removing excess wash water from the surface of the film. The film is then driven between a double row of slotted, hot forced-air tubes (see Figure 20-3A). A high-speed fan draws room air past electric heating coils, producing air at 120–150°F (50–65°C). The film emulsion

shrinks and seals dry in a single pass and the film is ready for viewing and storing when it exits the processor. The excess air is returned to the room. This is the primary cause for uncomfortable temperatures in processing areas during hot weather. When damp films exit the processor, the cause is more likely to be in the fixer (depletion or lack of hardener) or wash tank (saturation or insufficient fresh water) than in the dryer section.

Replenishment System

The replenishment system replaces chemicals that are depleted through the chemical reactions of processing, oxidation, and evaporation. The developer replenisher solution has a different composition than the solution in the processing tank. Because bromides build up in functioning developer, they tend to restrain the activity of the reducing agents on the silver halides. For this reason, developer replenisher lacks sufficient restrainer. A special **starter solution** of acetic acid and potassium bromide (the restrainer) must be added to the replenisher solution when starting a fresh tank of developer. Potassium bromide is needed to develop films properly. Potassium bromide gets into the developer solution from the bromide in the emulsion of the film. However, when new developer is mixed and put into the developer tank, no bromide is present because no films have been processed. This is why

FIGURE 20-5 A typical processor replenishment and circulation system. *(Adapted with permission of David Jenkins from Radiographic Processing and Imaging Processes, MTP Press, Lancaster, England)*

starter solution needs to be added to fresh developer chemistry. If starter solution is not added to the fresh developer, images will be dark and the sensitometry will be out of control. The tank of fresh solution must then be seasoned by running the processor for 15 to 20 minutes to permit adequate mixing of the solutions.

Volume replenishment is used for high-volume and **flood replenishment** for low-volume units. A volume replenishment system is activated when films enter the processor. The entrance rollers may activate a microswitch or an infrared sensor. In this manner, replenishment of chemical solution strength begins when a film enters the processor and ends when it passes the entrance rollers. This permits replenishment according to the amount of film entering the processor. (A 14″ film would replenish solutions more than a 10″ film. This is appropriate since it would require more chemistry to process the longer film.) Infrared sensors provide more accurate replenishment as they are capable of sensing not only the length but also the width of the film. A microprocessor can then activate the replenishment pumps for an appropriate length of time. Flood replenishment (also called **timed** or **standby replenishment**) is designed for low-volume units, in which films enter the processor at irregular intervals. The replenishment unit is controlled by a timer that automatically floods the developer and fixer

tanks with replenisher solution at a regular interval regardless of the number of films processed.

Although not a replenishment system, a **standby switch** is supplied on many processors. These processors are programmed to shut down some systems when 2 minutes pass without a film entering the unit. The standby switch usually must be manually activated to bring the entire unit to processing readiness. The standby mode inactivates the entrance rollers so films cannot be fed until the unit is activated.

The replenishment rate can be adjusted so that more fixer is replenished than developer. Although they must be adjusted for specific conditions, procedures, and manufacturers' recommendations, developer replenishment rates often range from 4–5 ml per inch (1.5–2.0 ml per cm) of film feed. This is about 55–70 ml per 14-inch (36 cm) length of film. Fixer rates range from 6–8 ml per inch (2.5–3.0 ml per cm). This is about 85–110 ml per 14-inch (36 cm) length of film. Some processors provide a digital display of this information on the front panel.

A replenishment system is designed to pump replenisher solutions from separate storage tanks for the developer and fixer (Figure 20-5). Replenisher tubing usually includes a filter at the exit of the supply tank to collect dirt and sediment. Processors often use dual pumps operated by a single motor. The motor rotates a magnet, which, in turn, causes magnets in vanes inside the plastic pump bodies to rotate. This system isolates the solutions from each other and the pump motor and makes replacement of pump bodies easy and inexpensive. The replenishment system uses a metering pump, which is more complicated but operates on the same principle.

The storage tanks may be under or adjacent to the processor or, in the case of some large institutions, replenisher may be pumped great distances from a central mixing station. The tanks must be located at a site convenient for the mixing of chemical solutions. A clean area with a drain and corrosive-resistant floor and wall coverings is required.

All mixing should be done strictly according to the manufacturer's recommendations regarding temperature and the proper sequence of additives (for example, solution A, then B, then C, etc.). Always mix additives to water. Adding water to additives will cause splashing of corrosives and a decrease in solution strength. There are occasions when the chemicals react in undesirable ways with one another, the water, and air. For example, if hardener is added to fixer replenisher too rapidly, it may precipitate sulfur and aluminum, leaving the solution with insufficient hardener.

Processing solutions are hazardous materials and are covered by several federal agencies in the United States. Since 1986 the Occupational Health and Safety Administration (OSHA), the Environmental Protection Agency (EPA), and the Department of Transportation have all implemented regulations affecting processing chemicals. Users of the chemicals are required to have material safety data sheets (MSDS) on hand, policies regarding handling, a teaching program, and safety equipment, particularly an eyewash station.

Radiographic solutions are not available to the general public in the United States. When developer solution is mixed on-site, the concentrated solution containing hydroquinone and the preservative and activator (usually the first part mixed) has a pH of about 12.0, which is extremely destructive to the eyes if splashed. For this reason, protective eyeglasses should always be worn when mixing solutions. Additionally, hydroquinone can be absorbed through the skin, and glutaraldehyde is a tanning agent that will work on human skin just as it works in leathermaking.

Circulation System

The circulation system is designed to **stabilize temperatures, agitate solutions, mix the chemistry, and filter the solutions.** Temperatures are maintained in conjunction with the temperature control system. Constant mild agitation of the developer and fixer solutions is required so the chemicals will enter and exit the emulsion. The fresh chemistry added by the replenishment system must be constantly mixed throughout the tanks to avoid overdevelopment, underdevelopment, and underfixation. Separate developer, fixer, and wash tank circulation systems are required, although a single motor may drive all of the pumps.

Most circulation systems draw chemistry from the bottom ends of the developer and fixer tanks and pump it to the upper ends. Because old chemistry tends to rise in the tank, the excess solution is permitted to overflow from the top of the tank into a drain. In addition, the replenishment pumps usually add fresh chemistry to the upper or middle end of a tank. Some wash systems are made more efficient by the addition of a circulation pump (see Figure 20-5). The fixer circulation lines are usually fitted with a 100 μm wire mesh filter to trap dirt or bits of gelatin that have been washed from films.

The fixer tank overflow has sufficient accumulated silver content to make it financially feasible to attempt to recover as much as possible. **Fixer overflow should be considered toxic and under no circumstances should it be dumped directly into an open drain.**

The wash tank uses a discard circulation system. Constantly recirculated water would quickly become saturated with fixer, which would set up an ionic barrier against additional fixer leaving the emulsion. To prevent this problem from occurring, the wash tank uses a constant flow of fresh water, which is pumped in at the bottom ends of the tank and overflows from the top to a drain. Most manufacturers recommend 4 to 8 liters per minute (1–2 gallons [U.S.] per minute). **It is environmentally unsound to drain wash tank water into sewer lines.** Increasing concern over heavy metal pollution may place liability on persons or institutions responsible for dumping processing chemicals, especially silver. Although expensive, storage of processing overflow and disposal by hazardous materials professionals is advisable.

Temperature Control System

The temperature control system maintains all three solutions at compatible temperatures. This is accomplished in conjunction with the circulation system by various methods, depending on the model and manufacturer. A **heat exchanger** is the most common system. It uses a thermostat to heat the developer, since its temperature is the most critical. The developer is then routed through a circulation coil in the bottom of the fixer or wash tank to permit exchange of heat to the fixer by conduction. Developer in a circulation coil does not mix with the fixer or wash water. A 90-second automatic processor will usually require a developer temperature of 92–96°F (33–35°C), while a 2-minute processor will operate at 83–86°F (28–30°C).

Cold water processors accept incoming water at cold line temperatures and divert it to the wash tank, where it is heated and stabilized. Some systems require mixing of incoming hot and cold water within a set temperature range. The incoming water is then added to the wash tank, where the temperature stabilizes. Wash tank overflow is diverted to surround the developer and fixer tanks where heat can be conducted through the metal tank wall to maintain solution temperatures. These systems may also use circulation or heater coils in the developer and fixer tanks.

The developer temperature is especially critical. A difference is visible with a fluctuation of only 0.5° (F or C). Some processors provide a digital display of this information on the front panel. The optimal reducing agent temperature is 68°F (20°C) for an immersion time of 4–8 minutes. Much research has been devoted to the formulation of special developer solutions that will produce quality images at temperatures of 92–96°F (33–35°C). These high-temperature developers reduce immersion time to 20–22 seconds, thus permitting 90-second or less processing. Specific developing temperatures vary with manufacturer and can be adjusted with a thermostat. The thermostat is often not easily accessible (sometimes requiring a screwdriver or set screw) to remove the temptation for casual adjustment.

Periodic maintenance of an automatic processor is essential to obtain dependable performance. Since the processor affects the final image produced by nearly all radiographic equipment, and because the unit is often expected to operate 24 hours a day, nonstop, it should have a top maintenance priority.

DARKROOM

The darkroom is the light-proof laboratory used for loading and unloading cassettes and feeding film into the automatic processor. Film is twice as sensitive after exposure and must be handled carefully to preserve a diagnostic quality image. An exposed film should be handled in the darkroom with the understanding that mishandling will require a double radiation dose to the patient.

Safelights

Radiographic film is designed to be insensitive to specific wavelengths of orange-red light. This permits the use of low level illumination within this wavelength to make work in the darkroom easier. The amount of light is controlled by the type of filter, wattage of the light source, and distance from the working surface. Not all films are insensitive to the same wavelengths. For example, some films designed for rare-earth intensifying screen phosphors require shorter wavelengths (dark red), and some cathode ray tube (CRT) films are sensitive to all light and require total darkness.

Sodium vapor safelights emit an orange-yellow light but their intensity is too high for direct illumination. These safelights must be installed to indirectly illuminate the working area. Installation near the ceiling facing up makes certain that the light loses intensity as it reflects from the ceiling to the working area.

Direct illumination for most radiographic films is possible with a Kodak GBX filter (dark red) over a low intensity (7–15-watt) bulb that is 4 feet (1.25 meters) from the working area. Films that are sensitive only to blue emitting phosphor light (blue-violet) may be handled with a Kodak Wratten Series 6B filter (orange-brown) at the same intensity and distance. Light-emitting diode (LED) safelights are also available. They emit light in the 660 nm range, use very low power, and last 10 to 15 years. Although they are more expensive, their long life makes them more cost effective.

Too many safelights may result in too great an intensity. A safelight test calculates how long a film may be handled before fogging becomes a problem. Darkroom walls and floor should be light colored to increase the amount of light in the darkroom. If light is safe at its first reflection, it loses intensity and remains safe on additional reflections. When benches and flooring are light colored, it is much easier to locate films and other objects.

Entrance

The darkroom entrance may be of several types. A single door, double interlocking doors, revolving door, or light-proof maze may be used. The disadvantage of the single door is that all film must be protected from light, film storage bins must be closed, processor feed tray must be empty, and so on, each time the door is opened. The advantage is in space and cost savings. Single-door darkrooms should be equipped with an electric lock on the door that will not open when the film bin is open. This eliminates costly accidental exposure of the entire film bin. The electric lock must open automatically in the event of a power failure. Otherwise, another emergency entrance must be provided for the darkroom. Radiographers and darkroom aides should make it a habit to **always check all film bins before opening a single-door entrance.** Double interlocking doors, revolving doors, and light-proof mazes permit persons to enter and leave the darkroom without disrupting work in progress.

Pass Box

Film cassettes are passed into the darkroom through a **pass box,** or cassette hatch, which is a light-proof container set in the darkroom wall. Most pass boxes have two sides, one labeled "exposed," the other "unexposed," and both have interlocking light-proof doors. The interlocking doors are designed to prevent both doors from being opened at once, allowing light into the darkroom. A film cassette is taken from the "unexposed" side and the

door is closed. The film is then exposed in a radiographic room and returned to the "exposed" side of the pass box. When the door is closed, the darkroom aide may remove the exposed cassette from the pass box, remove and process the film, refill the cassette, and return it to the "unexposed" side of the pass box again. This system is very popular because of its speed and convenience.

Plan

A typical darkroom plan is shown in Figure 20-6. This plan has the automatic processor set in the wall between the darkroom and the viewing area. Only the feed tray of the processor extends into the darkroom. The processor is actually located in the viewing area to facilitate periodic maintenance.

When planning a darkroom, one should ensure that the pass boxes and film bins are located where the darkroom aide (who may often be the radiographer) does not have to take steps to reach the processor feed tray. A grounded loading bench should be located directly under each pass box. Grounding of the bench by connecting a wire between the bench top and a well-grounded object (such as a water pipe) reduces the possibility of electrostatic discharge. The film bin should be located under the loading bench.

Darkrooms should be small enough so the darkroom aide does not have to move more than 1–2 steps to perform any operation. A large darkroom is poorly designed and serves no purpose unless other light-proof procedures are routinely performed there (e.g., manual subtraction or duplication, loading specialized cassettes or film holders, etc.).

The darkroom plan should also include a communication system, such as a light-proof speaking grill installed in the door or an intercom. Lighting should be controlled by two separate switches removed from one another. Both full white light illumination (for maintenance and repairs) and safelight illumination (for normal work) should be controlled by a switch. To avoid accidental exposure, the white-light switch should be located higher than the safelight switch (5–6 feet [1.5–1.75 meters] from the floor).

Darkroom ventilation should be a primary concern. Chemical fumes must be vented directly to the

FIGURE 20-6 A typical darkroom plan.

outside of the building. Failure to do so can result in toxic fumes being picked up by ventilation systems and delivered to critical areas within a hospital. Most automatic processors have special connections to assist in venting. Good circulation of air from outside the darkroom should also be maintained. Darkrooms in colder climates may also require humidifiers to ensure humidity of 40–60 percent during winter months so electrostatic discharge conditions are reduced.

Floor drains are required both inside the darkroom and near the automatic processor outside the darkroom to facilitate maintenance, repairs, and daily clean-up. Drains are also a safety precaution against leaks and overflow. They must not be made of copper because processing chemicals will react with copper.

Large departments may use a central processing plan where all films are routed through one or more central darkrooms. These darkrooms are often equipped with two processors. In a compact, well-designed darkroom, an experienced, full-time dark-

room aide can feed a steady stream of films faster than a single 90-second processor can handle them. Dual processors also permit the darkroom to function even if one is inoperable or undergoing maintenance. Central processing saves the cost of numerous processors and economizes space usage, staffing, etc.

Because of the time required in carrying exposed films to a central darkroom, many large departments utilize a satellite darkroom plan, where single processor darkrooms are placed throughout the department and institution. If a processor is inoperable or undergoing maintenance, the radiographer uses the next nearest darkroom. Satellite processing saves time but is more expensive in equipment, maintenance, facilities, and staffing.

Regardless of the plan selected, the area where the processors deposit the finished radiographs should be equipped with benches for handling films and illumination view boxes for viewing them. This area becomes the natural gathering point for the entire radiology department and it is often equipped with computers, telephones, log books, seats, and so on, to make it a convenient place to do paperwork and data entry while waiting for radiographs to be processed.

SILVER RECOVERY SYSTEMS

As mentioned in the fixer and circulation system sections, sufficient silver is dissolved in the fixer solution to make recovery before discarding feasible from a financial standpoint and to prevent toxic heavy metal pollution of the environment. In the United States, the Water Control Act of 1972, Resources Conservation-Hazardous Waste Act of 1976, Clean Water Act of 1984, and Resource Conservation and Recovery Act of 1986 all affect the disposal of heavy metals into the public environment. In essence, these laws require that the best available methods be used to clear silver from fixer overflow solutions prior to disposal. In addition, they limit liquid waste to a toxic level of 5 parts per million (ppm). A permit is required for dumping more than 27 gallons (U.S.) per month into a public sewer and any amount into the ground. Even shipping the waste to a treatment plant requires a permit. Compliance with these regulations is the reason commercial firms are usually employed to handle silver recovery.

The fixer may accumulate silver at the rate of as much as 100 mg/m^2 of film processed. This is well above the dumping limits allowed by law in the United States. In fact, **the fixer is as valuable, if not more valuable, after processing than before.**

About half of the silver in the film remains in the emulsion after processing. The other half is dissolved into the fixer solution. Much of this silver may be removed from the fixer by diverting the overflow through a silver recovery system before discarding. About 5 percent of the silver is carried into the wash tank, which, in extremely high-volume circumstances, may also be worth recovery. It is estimated that about 10 percent of the purchase price of film may be recovered, depending on the type of recovery system used and the market price for silver. The cost of recovery will almost always pay for the processing and handling and usually provides a modest financial return to help offset film costs. Silver mining and refining is expensive, and as a result, about half of all silver on the market worldwide comes from recycling.

There are several types of silver recovery units. The most common fixer recovery units are **metallic replacement, electrolytic, chemical precipitation** and **resin.** All of these units operate by providing electrons that can be used by the silver in the fixer solution to form black metallic silver. They differ in the method by which the electrons are provided and by the process used to refine the metallic silver.

All silver recovery methods require that the fixer sit within the unit for some time to permit the chemical interactions to occur. This **dwell time** is the single most important factor in unit effectiveness. **Agitation** of the fixer solution during this time is also important because it enhances the ability of electrons and silver to contact each other. Finally, the surface area controls the region from which electrons are available or where silver can be deposited.

Metallic Replacement

Metallic replacement units are also called metallic displacement because in these units the fixer acid breaks down the iron in a steel screen or in steel wool and displaces or replaces it with silver. The iron oxides give up electrons for the silver. The metallic silver is precipitated onto the steel. These units are sometimes called silver buckets or cartridges (Figure 20-7). They operate by having the fixer drain into the top, filter through the steel wool or screen, and overflow through a tube connected to the bottom of the container. Metallic replacement buckets are designed for low-volume situations only. They are inefficient as they age and processing is expensive. Fixer overflow from metallic replacement buckets should not be sent to the same drain as the developer overflow. As the steel wool or screen reacts with the fixer, it produces iron oxide, which can form drain-clogging fibers when it reacts with developer.

Electrolytic

Electrolytic units pass a current from a cathode to an anode through the fixer. The ionized silver in the fixer solution is attracted to the negatively charged cathode. It then plates onto the cathode as

FIGURE 20-7   A metallic replacement silver recovery unit. *(Reprinted courtesy of Eastman Kodak Company)*

Bypass

Line from processor

Connection to drain

Space for flow of solution

Iron filter

Plastic spacer

Space for flow of solution

metallic silver (Figure 20-8). These units are sometimes called cells because they function like a cell in a battery. They are rated according to their recovery capacity (i.e., troy ounces per gallon). They are also classified by their method of agitation, rotating anode, rotating cathode, and pumped solution. Electrolytic units are available that will recirculate the fixer for reuse in the processor. Electrolytically processed fixer is deficient in sodium sulfite (the preservative) and this can lead to incomplete fixing. A method of replenishing sodium sulfite must be added when a recirculating fixer system is used. If no silver is present in the fixer, the current will cause the thiosulfate to form sulfur, a smelly process that degrades the quality of the silver plating. This problem can be avoided by using an automatic electrolytic unit that is programmed to increase the current during high-volume operation and to reduce it during other periods. **Electrolytic units should not be run when the processor has not been used for a long period of time (such as overnight).** Electrolytic units are designed for moderate- and high-volume situations and produce easily processed silver flakes (which are chipped from the coated cathode). Most units require regular maintenance because they are an electrical hazard. Their electrical components are exposed to moisture, they are prone to short-circuiting, and their failure, overuse, or underuse may cause hazardous fumes.

Chemical Precipitation

Chemical precipitation units use chemicals (such as zinc chloride and sodium sulfite) that break down in the fixer and release electrons. The metallic silver is heavy enough to precipitate out and fall to the bottom of the tank, where it forms silver sludge. The chemical reactions produce hazardous gasses that are both toxic and explosive. New reagents are available for precipitating extremely large volumes of fixer. Because of the complexity of the process, they are currently used only by commercial silver dealers.

Resin

Resin units use acid to form resin ions. The silver in the solution is attracted to the resin and forms black metallic silver. The resin is then processed to remove the silver.

Monitoring

All silver recovery units must be properly sized for the amount of silver in the fixer. If undersizing is suspected, a second (**tailing**) unit may be added to process the solution exiting from the first unit. Various types of test strips are available to determine the silver content remaining in the solution as it exits the silver recovery unit. A copper test can be done by dropping a copper penny into the exiting solution. A very light gray coating after 10 seconds is acceptable. A heavy coating indicates too much silver is not being recovered. Correction should begin by checking the function of the existing recovery unit. If it is functioning within acceptable limits, either a larger-capacity recovery unit is needed or a tailing unit should be installed.

Used fixer from processor

Anodes

Rotating cathode plating disk

Motor

Drain

Pump

FIGURE 20-8 An electrolytic silver recovery unit.

Film

The film itself retains half the silver (about 0.1 troy ounce per pound [0.45 kg]) and this can also be recovered. Unexposed (green) film has twice the amount of silver as processed film. However, recycling firms will not pay more for unexposed film. To reclaim the silver, it is recommended that unexposed film be run through a processor to permit the fixer to reclaim half the silver. All scrap film should be saved for recycling, as should all original film when medical files are purged. Because of the weight, space required, and value of the silver in radiographs, storage is expensive in hospitals, clinics, and physician's offices. When original films are discarded, recycling is a very profitable undertaking.

SUMMARY

The primary purpose of radiographic processing is to deposit enough black metallic silver at the latent image sites to permit a permanent visible image to form. Quality control experts agree that the radiographic film processor is the most sensitive and variable factor in the production of a radiograph. Automatic processing of a radiograph involves developing, fixing, washing, and drying.

During development, silver is deposited at the latent image sites and an image becomes visible. The primary agents of the developer are the two reducing agents, phenidone and hydroquinone;

an activator, sodium carbonate; a restrainer, potassium bromide; a preservative, sodium sulfite; a hardener, glutaraldehyde; and water as the solvent. The action of the developer is controlled by immersion time, solution temperature, and chemical activity.

Fixing removes the undeveloped silver halides from the emulsion. This is necessary before exposure to light for viewing. The primary agent is the clearing agent, ammonium thiosulfate. Fixer solutions also include an activator, acetic acid; a preservative, sodium sulfite; a hardener, aluminum chloride; and water as the solvent.

The archiving process prepares the film for long-term storage as a medical record. Archiving involves washing the film with water to remove the processing chemicals and drying to harden and seal the radiograph.

Automatic processors utilize several subsystems to completely process a radiograph: (1) the transport system to move a film through the developer, fixer, wash, and dryer at a controlled speed; (2) the dryer system to force hot air across the film for drying; (3) the replenishment system to replace chemicals which are depleted through the chemical reactions of processing, oxidation, and evaporation; (4) the circulation system to stabilize temperature, agitate solutions, mix the chemistry, and filter the solutions; and (5) the temperature control system to maintain all three solutions at compatible temperatures.

The darkroom is the light-proof laboratory used for loading and unloading cassettes and feeding them into the automatic processor. Radiographic film is designed to be insensitive to specific wavelengths of orange-red light. Safelights use low-level illumination within this wavelength to make work in the darkroom easier.

Sufficient silver is dissolved into the fixer solution to make recovery before discarding feasible from a financial standpoint and desirable for environmental reasons. The most common types of silver recovery units are metallic replacement, electrolytic, chemical precipitation, and resin.

REVIEW QUESTIONS

1. What are the four primary steps in automatic processing?

2. How do the reducing agents phenidone and hydroquinone differ in their functions?

3. What is the chemical name and function of the hardener in the developer?

4. What is the purpose of fixing?

5. What are the two steps of the archiving process?

6. How should a film be fed into the automatic processor?

7. Differentiate between volume replenishment and flood replenishment.

8. What is the function of the circulation system in an automatic processor?

9. Under what conditions is direct illumination of a radiographic film safe?

10. How does an electrolytic silver recovery unit operate?

REFERENCES AND RECOMMENDED READING

Anslow, L. (1991). Silver recovery—an evaluation of existing disposal methods in a district general hospital. *Radiography Today, 57*(653), 24–28.

Ball, J., & Price, T. (1995). *Chesneys' radiographic imaging* (6th ed.) Oxford: Blackwell Scientific.

Bruce, G. (1980). Darkroom safelighting and its effects. *Radiography, 46*(542), 45.

Carroll, Q. B. (2003). *Fuchs's radiographic exposure, processing, and quality control* (7th ed.). Springfield, IL: Charles C Thomas.

Chesney, D. N. (1973). Building materials and film fogging. *Radiography, 39*(466), 262.

Curry, T. S., Dowdey, J. E., & Murry, R. C. (1990). *Christensen's introduction to the physics of diagnostic radiology* (4th ed.). Philadelphia: Lea and Febiger.

Dohms, J. (1992). OSHA safety requirements for hazardous chemicals in the workplace. *Radiology Management, 14*(4), 76–80.

Eastman Kodak Company. (1980). Recovering silver from photographic materials (Publication No. J–10). Rochester, NY: Author.

Electrifying artifacts. (1984). *Radiologic Technology, 56*(2), 99.

Fodor, J., Malott, J. C., & Sweeny, R. J. (1989). A common artifact. *Radiologic Technology, 60*(4), 325.

Gordon, M. (1988). Chemical hazards in film processing. *International Society of Radiographers and Radiological Technicians Newsletter, 24*(1), 9–12.

Griffiths, R. (1994). The presence of sulphur dioxide and other toxic fumes within processing environments, and associated health problems. *Radiography Today, 60*(690), 13–16.

Haus, A. G. (Ed.) (1993). *Film processing in medical imaging.* Madison, WI: Medical Physics.

Jenkins, D. (1980). *Radiographic photography and imaging processes.* Lancaster, England: MTP Press Limited.

McKinney, W. (1988). *Radiographic processing and quality control.* Philadelphia: J. B. Lippincott.

Newhall, B. (1982). *History of photography: 1839 to the present.* New York: Bulfinch Publishers.

Sturge, J., Walworth, V., Shepp, A., (1989). *Imaging Processes and Materials: Neblette's eighth edition.* New Jersey: Wiley.

Sweeney, R. J. (1983). *Radiographic artifacts: Their cause and control.* Philadelphia: J. B. Lippincott.

Wilson, P. (1978). Principles of formation of the latent and developed images. *Canadian Journal of Radiography, Radiotherapy, and Nuclear Medicine, 7*(6), 268–278.

Wolbarst, A. B. (1993). *Physics of radiology.* Norwalk, CT: Appleton & Lange.

The Case of the Colon in the Spider's Web

This radiograph of a barium-filled colon has strange vertical lines that seem to enclose the lower GI tract in a web. What is the cause of these lines?

Answers to the case studies can be found in Appendix E.

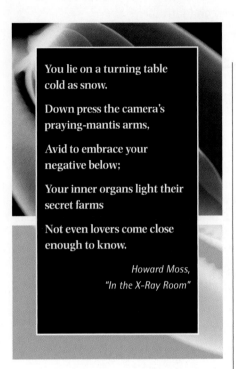

CHAPTER 21

Film Sensitometry

You lie on a turning table
cold as snow.

Down press the camera's
praying-mantis arms,

Avid to embrace your
negative below;

Your inner organs light their
secret farms

Not even lovers come close
enough to know.

Howard Moss,
"In the X-Ray Room"

KEY TERMS

average gradient
base plus fog
calibrate
characteristic curve
contrast
D log E curve
definition
densitometer
detail
D_{max}
gamma

gradient point
Hurter and Driffield
  (H&D) curve
latitude
opacity
optical density
  numbers
penetrometer
resolution
resolving power
reversal

sensitometer
sensitometric curve
sensitometry
sharpness
solarization
speed exposure point
speed point
step wedge
straight line portion

OBJECTIVES

Upon completion of this chapter, the student should be able to:

- Define *sensitometry* as it is applied to radiography.

- Describe the production of a step wedge on radiographic film through the use of a penetrometer and a sensitometer.

- Explain the function of a densitometer.

- Estimate the percentage of light transmitted by a radiograph according to optical density logarithms.

- Construct a D log E curve from sensitometric data.

- State acceptable base-plus-fog and diagnostic range optical density numbers.

- Describe the effect of automatic-processor reducing agents on the shape of a D log E curve, especially with relation to speed and contrast.

- Define resolution, speed, contrast, and latitude.

- Explain the effect of silver halide crystal size on image resolution.

- Discuss the physical and processing factors that affect film speed.

- Calculate speed points, speed exposure points, and relative speeds from D log E curves.

- Calculate gamma, gradient point, average gradient, and latitude from D log E curves.

- Analyze D log E curves to determine speed, contrast, and latitude relationships.

- Discuss the relationships between speed, contrast, and latitude.

Sensitometry is the measurement of the characteristic responses of film to exposure and processing and is accomplished by exposing and processing a film and then measuring and evaluating the resulting densities. It is primarily the responsibility of the radiographer to use sensitometric methods to evaluate technical factor exposure systems, films, intensifying screens, and processing equipment. In addition, sensitometric methods are useful in establishing, evaluating, and maintaining technical exposure factor charts and systems, a duty that can be done only by a qualified radiographer.

SENSITOMETRIC EQUIPMENT

A variety of equipment is necessary to carry out sensitometric procedures. Either a **penetrometer** or a **sensitometer** is required to produce a uniform range of densities on a film. A **densitometer** is required to provide an accurate reading of the amount of light transmitted through the film.

Penetrometer

A penetrometer is a series of increasingly thick, uniform absorbers. They are usually made of aluminum steps, although tissue-equivalent plastic is sometimes used (Figure 21-1). A penetrometer is referred to as a **step wedge** because of its shape. It is used to produce a step wedge on radiographic film by exposure to x-rays (Figure 21-2). Because of the vast number of variables in x-ray-generating equipment, the use of a penetrometer is not recommended for quality control monitoring of film processors. However, it is an excellent method for monitoring both x-ray equipment and film/intensifying screen combinations because it reproduces the variables associated with a clinical situation.

Sensitometer

A sensitometer is designed to expose a reproducible, uniform, optical step wedge onto a film (Figure 21-3). It contains a controlled intensity light source (a pulsed stroboscopic light is best) and a piece of film with a standardized optical step wedge image (a step tablet).

FIGURE 21-1   Two basic types of penetrometers or step wedges: (A) aluminum and (B) tissue equivalent plastic. *(Courtesy of Fluke Biomedical)*

FIGURE 21-2 **FIGURE 21-2**   A density curve produced from graphing the exposures of a penetrometer exposure. (A) The exposure. (B) The graph.

FIGURE 21-3   A sensitometer.

The controlled light source reproduces the same amount of light each time it is triggered. Voltage fluctuations and other factors that might cause the intensity to vary are controlled by circuits that supply an exact quantity of power to a capacitor that discharges to the stroboscopic light when triggered. The optical step wedge absorbs a calibrated amount of this light, leaving a uniform and reproducible "light penetrometer" to expose any film placed in the sensitometer over the optical step wedge. The optical step wedge should not be touched because hands leave a film of oil that interferes with the light intensity.

Optical step wedges (step tablets) are available in 11- and 21-step versions. The 11-step wedges usually increase density 100 percent (by a factor of two) per step. The 21-step wedges usually increase density 41 percent (by a factor of 1.41 times [which is $\sqrt{2}$]) per step. Because the rigid control of the densities produced on the film eliminates other variables, sensitometer-produced step wedges are perfect for processor quality control monitoring. Very slight density differences can be detected by sensitometric equipment. When a film is processed, there is a tendency for exhausted reducing agents and bromine ions to be carried backward on the emulsion as it is driven through the rollers of an automatic processor. For this reason, sensitometric film strips should be fed into automatic processors with either the long axis of the step wedge parallel to the entrance rollers or with the light edge entering the processor first.

Densitometer

A densitometer is an instrument that provides a readout of the amount of blackening (density) on a film. A densitometer consists of a calibrated uniform light source, a stage for placing the film to be measured, a light aperture to control the amount of light from the source, a sensor arm with an optical sensor, a readout display, and a calibration control (Figure 21-4). Density readings are accomplished by comparing the amount of light emitted by the light source with the amount of light transmitted through the film. To do this, the densitometer must be calibrated before each reading by recording the amount of light the light source is emitting. This is done by pushing the sensor arm so that the sensor is in contact with the light source (this eliminates the inverse square law factor) and by using the calibration control to set the readout display at zero. This **calibrates** or zeroes the densitometer and prepares it for a reading. When a film is placed on the stage and the sensor arm is pushed down into contact with the film, the densitometer can calculate the difference between the calibration intensity and the intensity of light the film is transmitting. Some densitometers include a filter to negate the blue tint in the film base.

Because films are sensitive to a wide range of exposures, their densities are best visualized if the range is compressed into a logarithmic scale. When using a logarithmic scale with a base of 10, an increment of 0.3 represents a doubling of exposure. This is because the log of 2 is 0.3. The numbers that are displayed by a densitometer are known as **optical density numbers.** They can be expressed with the term *OD* in front of the number (e.g., OD 1.5). They are calculated using the following formula:

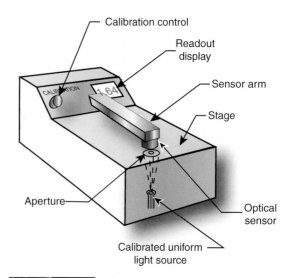

FIGURE 21-4 A densitometer.

$$OD = \log_{10}\frac{I_o}{I_t}$$

where: OD = optical density number
I_o = intensity of the incident light
I_t = intensity of the transmitted light

This formula can be stated as the log of the intensity of the incident light divided by the intensity of the light transmitted through the film. Radiographic film densities range from OD 0.0 to 4.0.

The ability of a film to stop light is termed **opacity.** Opacity is calculated using the following formula:

$$opacity = \frac{I_o}{I_t}$$

where: I_o = intensity of the incident light
I_t = intensity of the transmitted light

Note that density is the $\log_{10}$ of opacity (density = $\log_{10}$ of opacity). Table 21-1 shows both the opacity and optical density numbers for various percentages of light transmitted within the radiographic film density range of 0.0 to 4.0. For example, if a region of a radiograph has an OD of 1.0, this means only 10 percent or 1/10 of the incident light is transmitted through the radiograph in this region. The opacity of the region would be 10. If the OD

TABLE 21-1.	Example Opacities, Optical Density Numbers, and Light Transmission Percentages		

Opacity	OD Number	Percentage of Light Transmitted through Film
1	0.0	100
2	0.3	50
4	0.6	25
8	0.9	12.5
10	1.0	10
20	1.3	5
40	1.6	2.5
80	1.9	1.25
100	2.0	1
200	2.3	0.5
400	2.6	0.25
800	2.9	0.125
1,000	3.0	0.1
2,000	3.3	0.05
4,000	3.6	0.025
8,000	3.9	0.0125
10,000	4.0	0.01

number is increased to 1.3, the opacity is doubled (to 20) and the percentage of light transmitted through the film is halved (to 5 percent or 1/20). Increments of 0.3 changes in OD numbers represent a doubling or halving of opacity.

THE D LOG E CURVE

Sensitometry is normally shown as a graphic relationship between the amount of exposure and the resultant density on the film (Figure 21-5). The horizontal exposure axis (x axis) is compressed into a logarithmic scale (because of the wide range of densities possible) and the vertical density axis (y axis) is shown as a linear scale. Consequently, the curves

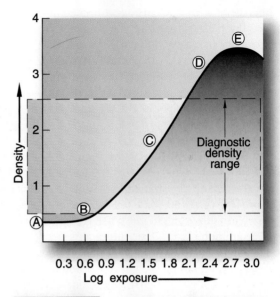

FIGURE 21-5 A typical D log E (characteristic, sensitometric, or H&D curve). (A) Base plus fog; (B) toe; (C) straight line portion; (D) shoulder; (E) D_{max}.

are known as density log exposure, or **D log E curves.** They are also called **characteristic, sensitometric,** and **Hurter and Driffield (H&D) curves** after the two photographers who first described the relationships in 1890. The important elements of a typical D log E curve are the base plus fog, toe, straight line portion (gamma), shoulder, and maximum density (D_{max}).

The **base plus fog** (b+f) (see Figure 21-5A) is the density at no exposure, or the density that is inherent in the film. It includes the density of the film base, including its tints and dyes, plus any fog the film has experienced. Radiographic film base density ranges around OD 0.05–0.10. Processing the film usually adds about OD 0.05–0.10 in fog density. The total base plus fog is seldom below OD 0.10 but should not exceed OD 0.22. Fog may be caused by heat, chemical fumes, light, and x-radiation. Over time, the natural amounts of these radiations will produce a slight density that is sometimes called age fog. Most of the fog level will be produced by the processing system. This includes the hyperactivity of the developer solution, primarily caused by the high temperature at which automatic processors operate.

Phenidone is the reducing agent that controls the subtle gray tones early in the development process. This region of the curve is known as the toe (see Figure 21-5B) and is predominantly controlled by phenidone.

The **straight line portion** of the curve is that portion between the toe and shoulder (see Figure 21-5C). It is usually fairly straight because the film is reacting in a linear fashion to exposure in the range of its primary sensitivity, which is in this region. The range of diagnostic densities varies from a low of OD 0.25–0.50 to a high of OD 2.0–3.0. The majority of diagnostic quality information on a radiograph will measure between OD 0.5 and OD 1.25. These densities are within the straight line portion of the curve.

Hydroquinone is the reducing agent that controls the heavy black tone later in the development process. This region of the curve is known as the shoulder (see Figure 21-5D) and is entirely controlled by hydroquinone.

D_{max} is the maximum density the film is capable of recording (see Figure 21-5E). It is the highest point on the D log E curve. It represents the point where all the silver halides have a full complement of silver atoms and cannot accept more. Additional exposure beyond D_{max} will result in less density because silver atoms attached to sensitivity specks will be ionized again, reversing their charge and causing them to be repelled from the speck. This process of **reversal,** or **solarization,** reduces the intensity of the latent image and will produce less density. The true D log E curve is bell-shaped (Figure 21-6). Duplication film is actually film that is preexposed to D_{max} so that additional exposure will cause a reversed, duplicated image instead of a negative one.

Modern film manufacturing techniques permit photochemical engineering of the exact shape of the D log E curve. For example, a film can be engineered for chest radiography that will increase the density of the mediastinal region by enhancing the densities produced for those exposures to the film typical of that region.

FILM CHARACTERISTICS

The primary characteristics of film are classified as **resolution,** speed, **contrast,** and **latitude.** Sensitometry permits analysis of speed, contrast, and lati-

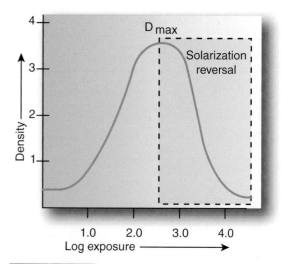

FIGURE 21-6 Solarization or reversal of duplicating film.

tude within the normal exposure ranges of the film. Extremely long or high-intensity exposure can overload the silver halide crystals and cause a phenomenon known as reciprocity failure. Although films are designed to handle a wide range of exposures, when unusual circumstances require large exposures, films may deviate from their expected performance.

Resolution

Resolution is the ability to accurately image an object. It is also called **detail, sharpness, definition,** and **resolving power.** Resolution is measured by the ability to see pairs of lines. The unit of resolution is line pairs per millimeter, expressed as lp/mm.

Film resolution is determined by the **size of the silver halide crystals.** Smaller crystals will darken a smaller area of the film, while larger ones will darken larger areas. Information that is smaller than an individual silver halide crystal cannot be visualized. **An inverse relationship exists between film resolution and crystal size** (the smaller the crystals, the higher the resolution; the larger the crystals, the lower the resolution). Silver halide crystals are sometimes called grains, thus the term *graininess* for poor resolution. Although film graininess can sometimes be seen, radiographic film/screen system resolution is generally controlled by the size of the intensifying screen phosphors, not the size of the silver halide crystals in the film emulsion.

FIGURE 21-7 The effect of film speed on D log E curves.

Speed

The amount of density (degree of blackening) a film produces for a given amount of exposure is the film speed. It is determined by the film's sensitivity to exposure. Speed is controlled by the activity of the phenidone because it affects the toe of the D log E curve. The position of the toe determines how soon the straight line portion will begin, and this indicates the overall speed of the film. Figure 21-7 illustrates the effect of the toe and shoulder on the overall position of the curve.

Film sensitivity is determined primarily by the **size of the silver halide crystals**. However, **the number of sensitivity specks and the thickness of the emulsion layer** also have an effect. Larger crystals will receive more photons because of the greater area they cover. They will also produce more photons than smaller crystals for the same reason. Larger crystals will darken a greater area of the film than smaller crystals with the same exposure. Therefore, **film speed and crystal size are directly related** (the larger the crystals, the faster the film speed; the smaller the crystals, the slower the film speed). **Film speed and the number of sensitivity specks are also directly related** for the same reason.

A thicker emulsion layer will place more crystals in a given area. Each incoming photon may interact with more than one crystal, so when more crystals are stacked on top of one another in the same area, the same number of photons will produce more film density. Therefore, **film speed and thickness of emulsion layer are directly related** (the thicker the emulsion, the faster the film speed; the thinner the emulsion, the slower the film speed).

Screen films are capable of responding to (producing visible densities for) exposures as low as 1 mR and as high as 1,000 mR. In Figure 21-7, film A produces all density levels with less exposure than film B requires for the same density. This demonstrates that film A is more sensitive to exposure, or faster. Film B is less sensitive, or slower.

The **speed point** of a film is that point on the D log E curve where a density of OD 1.0 + b+f is achieved. The American National Standards Institute (ANSI) specifies x-ray film speed as the exposure required to reach OD 1.00. However, many users add base plus fog to this standard. The **speed exposure point** is the log exposure that will produce the speed point for a given film. Film A in Figure 21-7 has a speed exposure point of 1.5, while film B has a speed exposure point of 2.0.

In clinical radiography it is important to be able to adjust technical factors from one film to another. The radiographer must be able to calculate the difference in exposure that will produce a diagnostic quality image on a new film when the proper factors are known for a previous one. In Figure 21-7, film B would require a log exposure of 2.0 to produce OD 1.0. Film A would require a log exposure of 1.5 to produce the same density. The difference in film speed is calculated as:

$$\text{antilog } (\log E_1 - \log E_2)$$

where: $\log E_1$ = log exposure of 1st film
$\log E_2$ = log exposure of 2nd film

Note: The antilog of a number is found by using an antilog table or by entering the number into a scientific calculator and then pressing the INV (inverse) key followed by the LOG key. For calculators without an INV key, review instructions for computing antilogs.

EXAMPLE: What is the difference in speed between film A and film B in Figure 21-7?

Answer:

$$\text{antilog}(\log E_1 - \log E_2) =$$
$$\text{antilog}(2.0 - 1.5) =$$
$$\text{antilog}(0.5) = 3.16$$

Film A is 316 percent faster than film B.

Relative speeds have been assigned by film manufacturers to assist radiographers in relating films to one another as they are used in film and intensifying screen combinations (film/screen combinations). Relative film/screen speed can be determined by using the reciprocal of the exposure required to produce a given density:

$$\text{relative speed} = \frac{1}{\text{exposure in R needed to produce speed point density (OD 1.0 + b+f)}}$$

EXAMPLE: What is the relative speed for a film that requires an exposure of 5 mR to produce the speed point density?

Answer:

$$\text{relative speed} = \frac{1}{\text{exposure in R needed to produce speed point density (OD 1.0 + b+f)}}$$

$$\text{Relative speed} = \frac{1}{5 \text{ mR}}$$

$$\text{Relative speed} = \frac{1}{0.005 \text{ R}} = 200$$

Film speed is affected by immersion time, solution temperature and chemical activity. The immersion time in a high-speed automatic processor may be as short as 20–25 seconds. The longer the film is subjected to the chemical action of the developer solution, the greater is the amount of black metallic silver deposited on the latent image sites through the reduction process (Figure 21-8). Film speed is most affected by developer solution temperature (Figure 21-9). Only 0.5° will cause a visible change in film density. Higher temperature increases the activity level of the reducing agents in the developer and this produces greater density on the film. High-speed automatic processors use high temperatures to permit sufficient development to occur in the 20–25 seconds the film is immersed in the devel-

FIGURE 21-8 The effect of developer solution immersion time on film speed.

oper. The chemical activity of the developer solution will also increase the development of density. Film speed is affected when the bromide ion barrier has not formed properly (due to insufficient restrainer or overreplenishment) or when it is too strong (due to excess restrainer or underreplenishment). Determination of the proper time, temperature, and activity for a particular developer and film is done by graphing speed, contrast, and base plus fog levels for various activity concentrations (Figure 21-10). This is how the manufacturer arrives at the recommended time and temperature for optimal results.

Contrast

Contrast is the difference between adjacent densities. This concept can be confusing when one tries to understand the difference between density and con-

FIGURE 21-9 The effect of developer solution temperature on film speed.

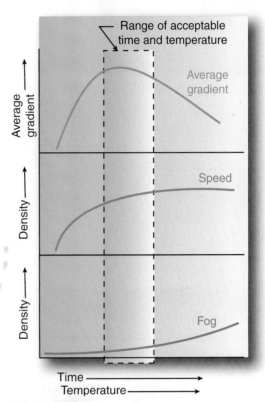

FIGURE 21-10 Determination of optimal development time and temperature for a particular film by comparison of contrast, speed, and base plus fog for a particular developer solution concentration.

trast. There is a relationship between contrast and density because contrast consists of the difference between adjacent densities. For the same film type, **a change in density will affect contrast only when above or below the straight line portion of the D log E curve**.

Contrast is controlled by the level of activity of the hydroquinone. Hydroquinone establishes the shoulder of the D log E curve and the position of the shoulder affects the slope of the straight line portion of the curve (Figure 21–11).

Contrast is defined by the slope of the straight-line portion of the D log E curve, but, because the straight line portion is actually a curve, it is important to define the point at which the slope is measured. **Gamma** is simply a measure of the slope of the straight line portion of the curve at the speed point (OD 1.0). In practice, a gamma may be read with the

speed point in the center, top end or bottom end, as long as all comparative readings are done from the same reference point. Contrast differences cannot be appreciated unless they are measured from identical reference points.

The slope can be read as "rise over run" (Figure 21-12). More sophisticated measurements, such as the trigonometric tangent of the slope, are also used. The slope of any portion of the D log E curve can be calculated, and this is known as a **gradient point**. Gradient points must have their OD values stated, for example, a gradient of 1.75 at OD 0.80. Gradient points are sometimes known by their location: toe gradient, middle gradient, and upper gradient. The toe gradient is calculated between OD 0.25 and OD 1.00. The middle gradient is calculated

FIGURE 21-11 Comparison of film contrast.

FIGURE 21-12 Average gradient from a D log E curve.

between OD 1.00 and OD 2.00. The upper gradient is calculated between OD 2.00 and OD 2.50. Overall radiographic film contrast is more commonly defined by the **average gradient** of the straight line portion of the D log E curve between OD 0.25 + b+f and OD 2.50 + b+f. Opinions differ on whether b+f should be added to average gradient calculations. The average gradient is calculated as:

$$\text{average gradient} = \frac{\Delta D}{\Delta E} \text{ or}$$

$$\text{average gradient} = \frac{D_2 - D_1}{E_2 - E_1}$$

where: $D_1 = \text{OD } 0.25 + \text{b+f},$
$D_2 = \text{OD } 2.50 + \text{b+f},$

$E_1 = \text{exposure that produces } D_1$
$E_2 = \text{exposure that produces } D_2$

Note: ΔD is a constant of OD 2.25 (OD 2.50 − 0.25).

Figure 21-13 illustrates the difference between various gradient points and the average gradient. Most radiographic film average gradients are between 2.5 and 3.5.

The important part of the D log E curve is that portion between the toe and the shoulder (the diagnostic range of the film). In this central straight line portion, the density is approximately proportional to the log relative exposure. This is because a straight line will always have a constant ratio. If the slope of the straight line portion is at a 45° angle, the average gradient will measure 1.0. In this example, a doubling of exposure will result in a doubling of the opacity. (Note that the term *doubling of density* is not used because density is a log number. A change of 0.3 in density reflects a doubling or halving of opacity.) **A common misnomer in radiography is that doubling the exposure will double the density.** This is not true for typical radiographic film/screen systems.

Radiographic films have a slope steeper than 45°. In these films, when exposure is doubled, opacity is increased by more than a factor of 2. Because of the steepness of the slope (and the average gradient above 1.0), radiographic films amplify exposure by producing a greater proportion of density per exposure increase. **Doubling the radiographic expo-**

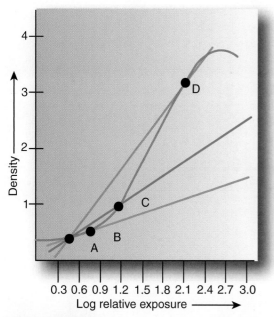

FIGURE 21-13 Average gradient and gradient point calculations from a D log E curve. The slopes of points A-B, A-C, and A-D are quite different.

sure will produce more than a doubling of radiographic opacity.

Toe and shoulder gradients are less than a 45° angle (<1.0) and therefore not only fail to amplify the contrast but actually decrease it. This is one reason why extremely light or dark areas on radiographs are not acceptable for diagnosis.

A contrast index is often used in quality control to indicate contrast. Because the definition of average gradient depends on comparable densities, when the density itself shifts, a different measure must be established. A contrast index is simply two density points that are subtracted from each other. It gives a measure of the difference between set densities, which represents the contrast. (Contrast is defined as the difference between densities.)

The relationship between density and contrast is complex. To understand how density affects contrast, it is important to realize that the changes in average gradient between the toe and shoulder of

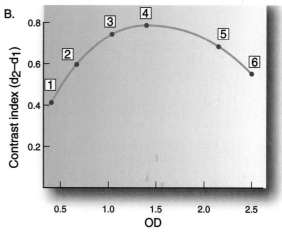

FIGURE 21-14 (A) Density ranges (1–6) from D log E curve of film measured for contrast index. (B) Contrast index for the density ranges (1–6) measured from Figure A. Note that the maximum contrast (range 4) is essentially the straight line portion of the curve. Contrast is decreased for toe and shoulder measurements but is maximized for the straight line portion of the D log E curve (OD 1.2–1.5). (Also note that this range corresponds to the speed point [OD 1.2].) *(Courtesy of Barry Burns, UNC Division of Radiologic Science)*

the D log E curve are actually changes in contrast. When insufficient or excessive density causes the range of visible densities on the radiograph to change, contrast is affected. For example, the film used for the data in Figure 21-14 achieved a maximum optimal contrast with an OD of 1.2–1.5. For OD measurements above or below this range, contrast is decreased. For radiographic films under most conditions, contrast is maximized when the density range is within the range of diagnostic densities (low of OD 0.12–0.50 and a high of OD 2.0–3.0). When the diagnostic densities are below or above this range, the contrast will be decreased. This occurs because the slope of the range of diagnostic densities has moved into the toe or shoulder of the D log E curve.

The contrast must exist within the diagnostic range of the film if it is to be visualized; in other words, within the straight line portion of the curve.

Latitude

For clinical radiographic purposes, latitude is the range of exposures that will produce densities within the diagnostic range (Figure 21–15). Latitude can be recorded as the width of the range of exposures that will produce diagnostic range densities according to the following formula:

$$latitude = E_h - E_l$$

where E_h = OD 2.50 exposure point
E_l = OD 0.25 exposure point

when E_h = high exposure point
E_l = low exposure point

EXAMPLE: What is the latitude for film A in Figure 21-15?

Answer:

latitude = $E_h - E_l$
latitude = 1.8 − 1.1
latitude = 0.7

The latitude for film B can be calculated to be 1.0. Film A has a narrow latitude while film B has a wider latitude. Because a wide latitude film permits considerable variation in the exposure while still exhibiting densities within the diagnostic range, it is

FIGURE 21-15 Comparison of film latitude. The range of relative exposure is indicated for each film.

sometimes called a forgiving film. The use of a narrow latitude film for routine radiography requires greater exposure accuracy.

Latitude and contrast are inversely related. As contrast increases, latitude tends to decrease. This affects the overall shape of the D log E curve. Latitude changes whenever there is a change in the average gradient of the D log E curve. Speed could change without altering the average gradient and latitude. A difference in film speed usually results in different contrast and latitude because it is rare for the entire D log E curve to shift the same degree. Usually the toe and shoulder will not shift exactly the same amount and this causes a change in the slope of the straight line portion of the curve (which changes contrast and latitude). The relationships of speed, contrast and latitude to patient dose are listed in Tables 21-2 and 21-3.

TABLE 21-2.	Relationship between Contrast, Latitude, and Patient Dose	
Contrast	Latitude	Patient Dose
high	narrow	high
low	wide	low

TABLE 21-3.	Relationship between Speed and Patient Dose
Speed	Patient Dose
slow	high
fast	low

SUMMARY

Sensitometry is the measurement of the characteristic responses of a film to exposure and processing. It is accomplished by exposing and processing a film and then measuring and evaluating the resulting densities. Either a penetrometer or a sensitometer is required to produce a uniform range of densities on the film. A densitometer is required to provide an accurate reading of the amount of light transmitted through the film.

Because films are sensitive to a wide range of exposures, their densities are best visualized if the range is compressed into a logarithmic scale. When using a logarithmic scale with a base of 10, an increment of 0.3 represents a doubling of exposure. This is because the log of 2 is 0.3.

Sensitometry is normally shown as a graphic relationship between the amount of exposure and the resultant density on the film. The horizontal axis (exposure) of the graph is compressed into a logarithmic scale and the vertical axis (density) is a linear scale. Consequently, the curves are known as density log exposure, or D log E, curves. They are also called characteristic, sensitometric and Hurter and Driffield (H&D) curves. The important elements of the D log E curve are the base plus fog, toe, straight-line portion (gamma), shoulder, and maximum density (D max).

The primary characteristics of film are resolution, speed, contrast and latitude. Resolution is the ability to accurately image an object and is measured by the ability to see line pairs. The amount of density a film produces for a given amount of exposure is the film speed. The film speed is determined by the size of the silver halide crystals, the number of sensitivity specks, and the thickness of the emulsion. Relative speeds have been assigned by film manufacturers to assist radiographers in relating films to one another as they are used in film/screen combinations. Contrast is the difference between adjacent densities. It is defined as the slope of the straight line portion of the D log E curve. Latitude is the range of exposures that will produce densities within the diagnostic range. As contrast increases, latitude tends to decrease.

REVIEW QUESTIONS

1. What is the purpose of sensitometry?

2. Explain the design of a penetrometer.

3. Why is a logarithmic scale used for describing optical densities?

4. Describe the five important elements of the D log E curve.

5. What is the relationship between film resolution and the size of the silver halide crystals?

6. What is the relationship between film speed and emulsion layer thickness?

7. State the formula for relative speed.

8. How is the average gradient calculated?

9. What is the relationship between contrast and latitude?

REFERENCES AND RECOMMENDED READING

Carroll, Q. B. (2003). *Fuchs's radiographic exposure, processing, and quality control* (7th ed.). Springfield, IL: Charles C Thomas.

Chow, M. F. (1988). The effect of a film's sensitivity to its speed, contrast, and latitude. *The Canadian Journal of Medical Radiation Technology, 19*(4), 147.

Eastman Kodak Co. *Sensitometric properties of x-ray films.* Rochester, NY: Eastman Kodak Company Radiography Markets Division.

Fuji. *X-ray sensitometry.* Tokyo: Fuji Photo Film Co., Ltd., Medical X-Ray Products Technical Handbook.

Haus, A. G. (Ed.) (1993). *Film processing in medical imaging.* Madison, WI: Medical Physics.

Kofler, J., & Gray, J. (1991). Sensitometric responses of selected medical radiographic films. *Radiology, 181*(3), 879–883.

McKinney, W. (1988). *Radiographic processing and quality control.* Philadelphia: J. B. Lippincott.

Thompson, M. A., Hattaway, M. P., Hall, J. D., & Dowd, S. B. (1994). *Principles of imaging science and protection.* Philadelphia: W. B. Saunders.

Wolbarst, A. B. (1993). *Physics of radiology.* Norwalk, CT: Appleton & Lange.

CHAPTER 22

Intensifying Screens

> I decided to try a combination of Edison's fluorescent screen and the photographic plate. . . . The combination succeeded even better than I had expected. A beautiful photograph was obtained with an exposure of a few seconds. That was the first x-ray picture obtained by that process during the first part of February 1896.
>
> *Autobiography of M. Pupin, From Immigrant to Inventor*

KEY TERMS

afterglow	K-shell absorbtion	reflective layer
base	edge	relative speed
conversion efficiency	luminescence	screen lag
fluorescence	phosphorescence	spectral emission
intensification factor	phosphor layer	
intensifying screen	protective coat	

OBJECTIVES

Upon completion of this chapter, the student should be able to:

- Explain the purpose of radiographic intensifying screens.
- Describe the function of each layer of an intensifying screen.
- Evaluate the desirability of phosphor materials according to atomic number, conversion efficiency, spectral emission, and fluorescence.
- Describe luminescence.
- Analyze the effect of phosphor crystal size, layer thickness, and concentration on intensifying screen resolution.
- Explain the effect of film/screen contact on resolution.
- Describe how to remedy quantum mottle.
- Classify intensifying screens according to intensification factor, descriptive rating, and relative speed number.

- Describe the effect of K-shell absorption edges on intensifying screen efficiency.

- Describe the components of a radiographic cassette.

- Describe the proper cleaning and care of radiographic cassettes and screens.

- Evaluate film/screen combinations for specific clinical uses.

Intensifying screens are used to amplify the incoming x-ray beam and reduce patient radiation dose. Introduced in 1896 by the American inventor Thomas Edison (1847–1931), intensifying screens produce large quantities of light photons when struck by x-rays. In this manner they intensify the latent imaging power of the beam, even though less than 33 percent of the x-ray photons that strike the cassette interact with the intensifying screen. Over 99 percent of the latent image is formed by this light, with less than 1 percent contributed by x-ray photons. This permits a great reduction in the amount of radiation necessary to produce a diagnostic quality image. Intensifying screens are normally used in pairs with duplitized film, although there are specialized cassettes that are designed for a single screen with single emulsion film.

CONSTRUCTION

Intensifying screens are composed of radiolucent plastic, coated with phosphors that will emit light when struck by x-ray photons. They are designed to be mounted in pairs inside the top and bottom of a light proof cassette so that a sheet of radiographic film can be sandwiched tightly between them. A screen consists of a **base**, a **reflective layer**, a **phosphor layer**, and a **protective coat** (Figure 22-1).

Base

The base is usually made of polyester plastic 1 mm thick, although cardboard and metal have been used. Its requirements are similar to those for a film base. It must be flexible yet tough, rigid, chemically inert, and uniformly radiolucent. It must be flexible to permit it to achieve good contact with the film. It must be rigid enough to stay in place in the top and bottom of a cassette. It must be chemically inert so that it does not react with the phosphor and interfere with the conversion of x-ray photons to light. It also must not react with air or chemicals in a manner that would cause discoloration. Discoloration filters and changes the wavelengths of the light emitted by the screen by absorbing wavelengths that could be used to create the radiographic image. Because films are designed to be most sensitive to

FIGURE 22-1 Cross-sectional view of a typical radiographic intensifying screen.

the particular wavelength of light emitted by the screen, discoloration may require more light, and consequently more patient radiation dose, to form the latent image. Most important, base material must be uniformly radiolucent so that it permits the transmission of x-ray photons without adding artifacts to the diagnostic image.

Reflective Layer

The base material is not transparent to light. In fact, a special layer of reflective material, such as magnesium oxide or titanium dioxide, about 25 μm thick, is used to reflect light toward the film. When a phosphor is struck by an x-ray photon, it will emit light isotropically (in all directions) (Figure 22-2A). When a reflective layer is added (Figure 22-2B), nearly twice as much light is reflected toward the film. This increase in light striking the film assists in creating the latent image and decreases the radiation dose to the patient.

Light that is emitted at a large angle from the direction of the incident x-ray photon will have a slightly longer wavelength. Some intensifying screens use dyes in the reflective layer to selectively absorb this longer-wavelength light. This assists in reducing the scattering of light that would decrease the resolving ability of the screen. Scattered light of this type causes a large area of penumbra, which reduces the sharpness of the image.

Phosphor Layer

The active layer of the intensifying screen is the phosphor layer. Phosphors are materials that are capable of absorbing the energy of an incident x-ray photon and then emitting light photons. Röntgen discovered x-rays when he observed the luminescence of the phosphor barium platinocyanide from a piece of cardboard in his laboratory. This phosphor layer varies from 150 to 300 μm, depending on the speed and resolving power of the screen.

Protective Coat

A coating of protective plastic about 25 μm thick is applied on top of the phosphor layer. The coating protects the phosphor layer from abrasions and stains during the loading and unloading of films. Fingernails and jewelry are the prime trauma to screens in the darkroom. Although the protective coating will prevent scratching of the phosphor layer during normal handling, repeated trauma can remove the coating. When intensifying screens are scratched, phosphor crystals may be removed, creating unexposed white line artifacts on the radiographic image.

PHOSPHORS

Phosphors must have a high atomic number, high **conversion efficiency**, appropriate **spectral emission**, and minimal **phosphorescence.**

Atomic Number

A high atomic number is desirable to increase the probability of an incident x-ray photon interaction. Because x-ray photons are of high energy, a high atomic number is required to permit photoelectric and Compton interactions.

Conversion Efficiency

The ability of the phosphor to emit as much light per x-ray photon interaction as possible is a measurement of the screen speed. As this conversion efficiency increases, the radiation dose to the patient decreases. A typical conversion efficiency would produce 1×10^3 light photons per incident 50 keV x-ray photon for a rare-earth screen.

FIGURE 22-2 Intensifying screen reflective layer redirection of isotropic light emission to film.

Spectral Emission

The spectral emission is an indication of the precise wavelength of light emitted by the phosphor. It is important that the spectral emission match the sensitivity of the film to ensure maximum latent image formation.

Luminescence

Luminescence is the ability of a material to emit light in response to excitation (usually by increased outer-electron-shell energy levels). Because of the narrow energy band within which these interactions occur, luminescent materials emit light with wavelengths that are characteristic of the particular luminescent material. This results in light emissions of a characteristic color. **Fluorescence and phosphorescence are the two types of luminescence.** Fluorescence occurs when the light is emitted within the time it takes an electron to complete one orbit of the affected shell electrons (within 1 nanosecond). Phosphorescence occurs when the light is emitted for a period longer than that necessary for one orbit of the affected shell electrons. In other words, **fluorescence is instantaneous emission while phosphorescence is delayed emission,** sometimes considerably delayed. Phosphorescence occurs when the phosphor continues to emit light after the incident x-ray photon energy has dissipated. Maximum fluorescence and minimal phosphorescence are desirable because delayed emission of light may permit the film to be removed from the cassette before the maximum latent image formation has occurred. Additionally, if another film is loaded into the cassette it may be faintly exposed to a previous image.

Delayed phosphorescent emission is called **screen lag** or **afterglow** and is common in older intensifying screens with exhausted phosphors. The normal life of intensifying screen phosphors is 5 to 7 years. All intensifying screens must be replaced routinely. As screens age, their phosphors decrease in activity. Because of this, it is highly recommended that all screens in a particular working area be replaced simultaneously. For example, all radiographic rooms serviced by a single darkroom should have the screens replaced at the same time. This assures the radiographer that all cassettes contain intensifying screens of approximately the same activity level.

A simple demonstration of phosphor activity is achieved by darkening an x-ray room and observing the light emitted by intensifying screen phosphors when an exposure is made. Observations of this type can be made through leaded glass and from behind leaded walls. The light emissions can be varied by using screens of different phosphors, different ages, and exposures of different mAs and kVp levels. Roughly 50,000 photons per mm^2 must exit the object being examined to produce a radiographic image. The intensifying screens must produce enough light from these photons to create the latent image in the film emulsion.

Several phosphors have been used in radiography since Röntgen's discovery: zinc sulfide, barium lead sulfate, calcium tungstate ($CaWO_4$), and a family of hybrid rare earths, including gadolinium, lanthanum, and yttrium. Calcium tungstate was used by Edison and it predominated as the best phosphor until the late 1970s, when the rare earths were introduced. Rare earths now predominate.

Rare Earths

Rare earths are the preferred phosphor materials because they have greater absorption abilities, intensification factors, and conversion efficiency. The older calcium tungstate screens have an x-ray-to-light conversion efficiency of about 5 percent, as compared to rare-earth conversion efficiencies of 15–20 percent. The rare-earth screens use phosphors with atomic numbers of 57–71. These elements are known as rare earths because they are difficult to isolate, although more common than cobalt in nature. Gadolinium and lanthanum are being used in compounds with activators and other chemicals (Table 22-1). The primary reason rare-earth phosphors are preferred is because they offer increased speed while maintaining resolution, when compared to similar speed calcium tungstate screens. Phosphor technology has outstripped advancements in other radiographic equipment. Some rare earths are so fast, tubes have insufficient time to produce enough mAs to prevent quantum mottle, automatic exposure control minimum reaction times are too long to avoid erratic exposures, and reciprocating grids are not

TABLE 22-1. Rare-Earth Intensifying Screen Phosphors with Manufacturer and Trade Name

Rare Earth	Primary Emission Color	Manufacturer	Trade Name
gadolinium oxysulfide	green	Kodak	Lanex
gadolinium oxysulfide	green	Fuji	
gadolinium oxysulfide	green	Agfa	Curix
lanthanum oxybromide	blue	Agfa	Quanta III

fast enough to prevent grid lines from being imaged. These factors must be considered when using extremely fast rare-earth screens (film/screen combinations above RS 500).

 CHARACTERISTICS

Intensifying screens exhibit the same types of characteristics as films. Consideration must be given to screen **resolution, speed, contrast** and **latitude.**

Resolution

Resolution is the ability to accurately image an object. Intensifying-screen resolution is controlled by the size of the phosphor crystals, the thickness of the layer, and the concentration (packing density) of the crystals, exactly as silver halide size and distribution affect film resolution (Figure 22-3). Smaller crystals

60 kVp
5 mAs
40" SID
No **grid**
100 RS
10.7 mR

60 kVp
0.8 mAs
40" SID
No **grid**
600 RS
1.74 mR

FIGURE 22-3   The effect of intensifying screen resolution on image quality: (A) fine-detail intensifying screens; (B) high-speed intensifying screen.

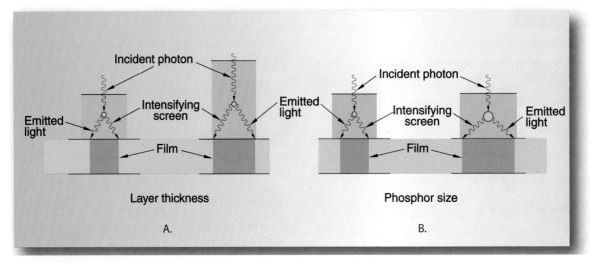

FIGURE 22-4 The effect of intensifying screen phosphor layer thickness and crystal size on film resolution.

and a thinner layer increase resolution but decrease screen speed. Larger crystals and a thicker layer decrease resolution but increase screen speed (Figure 22-4). **Phosphor crystal size and layer thickness are both inversely related to resolution and directly related to screen speed.** A greater concentration of crystals will increase both resolution and screen speed. Phosphor concentration is directly related to resolution and screen speed. Intensifying screen phosphor crystals are much larger than the silver-halide crystals in the film emulsion. In radiographic film and intensifying screen combinations, **the screen resolution always predominates over the film resolution.**

Measurement. Under ideal conditions, the naked eye can resolve approximately 10–20 lp/mm. Direct exposure nonscreen radiographic film can resolve up to 100 lp/mm, detail-speed screens about 15 lp/mm, par-speed screens about 10 lp/mm, and high-speed screens about 7 lp/mm.

Film/Screen Contact. One of the most common screen resolution problems is caused by poor contact between the film and the intensifying screen in the cassette (Figure 22-5). Poor film/screen contact also decreases the image density. There are numerous possible causes of poor film/screen contact, including foreign objects in the cassette and warped or damaged cassettes.

Quantum Mottle. Each phosphor crystal emits light that exposes a corresponding area of silver-halide crystals in the film emulsion. When insufficient phosphor crystals emit light to expose a coherent expanse of film, the resulting image will appear grainy (Figure 22-6). Quantum mottle is caused by an insufficient quantity of photons striking the intensifying screen. Although film graininess may appear mottled, radiographic mottle is nearly always a result of intensifying screen quantum mottle. The radiographer controls the quantity of photons with the mAs setting, so an increase in this factor will eliminate quantum mottle. Fluoroscopic tubes normally operate at very low mA levels. For this reason, quantum mottle is more commonly seen in fluoroscopy.

Speed

The speed or sensitivity of the intensifying screen is determined by the same factors that control resolution. Increasing phosphor size and layer thickness increase speed. An increase in phosphor concentration also increases speed. In addition, there are factors that affect speed but not resolution. As kVp

FIGURE 22-5   Poor resolution and increased image density due to loss of film/screen contact.

FIGURE 22-6   Quantum mottle.

is increased, the efficiency of the intensifying screen will also increase. **An increase in kVp will cause an increase in screen speed.** Intensifying screen phosphors have relatively high atomic numbers, so higher kVp will increase the probability of light-producing interactions within the phosphors. **Temperature** increases (over 100°F [38°C]) will decrease screen speed significantly. This is usually of concern only in extremely hot climates or during outdoor radiography.

Screen Speed Classifications. Three casual systems of classifying intensifying-screen speed have developed: the intensification factor, descriptive rating, and relative-speed number.

The most accurate factor that measures the speed or sensitivity of an intensifying screen is the **intensification factor.** It is a measurement of the amplification of the image that occurs due to the screen's ability to convert x-ray photons to light. It is directly related to the conversion efficiency of the phosphor. It is calculated as:

$$\text{intensification factor} = \frac{D_n}{D_s}$$

where: D_n = exposure in mR nonscreen
D_2 = exposure in mR with screens

Most radiographic intensifying screens are also classified with a descriptive rating of either high speed, par speed (also called universal or medium speed), and fine detail (high resolution). Some manufacturers use their own descriptive terms and many of these are trademarks.

The most useful rating of intensifying screens is the **relative speed.** Relative speed is expressed with par-speed screens, and, film, being arbitrarily assigned a relative speed (RS) number of 100, as a control point. High-speed screens are usually rated RS 200–1,200 while fine-detail screens are usually rated RS 20–80.

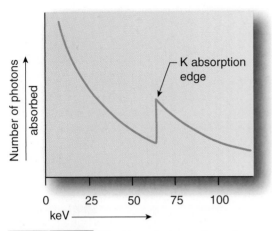

FIGURE 22-7 The K-shell absorption edge effect for calcium tungstate phosphors.

K-shell Absorption Edge. Calcium tungstate screens will absorb about 20–40 percent and rare-earth screens will absorb about 50–60 percent of the incident beam. These percentages vary depending upon the keV level of the incident photons. Nearly 100 percent of the absorption occurs through photoelectric interactions. Because photoelectric interactions produce characteristic photons, when the incident x-ray photons match the K-shell binding energy of the phosphor, there is a dramatic increase in characteristic production within the screen. This is the **K-shell absorption edge** (Figure 22-7). The K-shell edges for screen phosphors can result in a dramatic increase in light emission. This causes problems for the radiographer who uses a variable kVp technical factor system. If the kVp selected happens to be on or slightly above the K-shell edge, a slight decrease in kVp can cause a tremendous decrease in light emission, greatly reducing film density, instead of the slight decrease intended. In the reverse situation, if the original kVp happens to be slightly below the K-shell edge and a slight increase is desired, if the increase activated the K-shell peak, the resulting increase in density might be excessive. On a repeated examination, these situations could require third exposures. Table 22-2 provides the K-shell edges for the most common phosphors. **The kVp level should not be varied around screen-phosphor K-shell edges.** Note that the K-shell

TABLE 22-2. K-Shell Edges for Intensifying Screen Phosphors

Phosphor	K-Shell Edge	Atomic Number
lanthanum	39 keV	57
gadolinium	50 keV	64
tungsten	70 keV	74

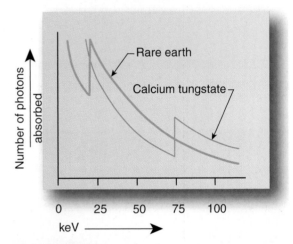

FIGURE 22-8 The increased efficiency range of rare-earth phosphors due to the K-shell edge effect.

edges are stated in keV levels. About 5–6 percent higher kVp levels would be required to produce the maximum number of K-shell edge-level photons for single-phase generators.

The reason rare-earth phosphors are more efficient is because they take advantage of the increased absorption of x-ray photons after the K-shell edge. Figure 22-8 compares the absorption of both calcium tungstate and rare-earth phosphors. The range of increased efficiency due to the K-shell edge is highlighted. This increased efficiency range is approximately 35–70 keV (roughly equivalent to 40–75 kVp). However, there is not a linear relationship when comparing the speed of calcium-tungstate and rare-earth phosphors (Figure 22-9). Therefore, it is important not to assume that one set of intensifying screens is twice or half as fast as another **across the entire kVp range.** This relationship may not hold true, especially at lower kVps.

FIGURE 22-9 The approximate kVp dependence of the relative speed of calcium tungstate and gadolinium–oxysulfide intensifying screens. *(By permission of John Stears, Joel Gray, and Eugene Frank, Mayo Foundation, Rochester, MN)*

Asymmetrical Screens. Extremely efficient intensifying screens may require that they be used as matched pairs. When the conversion efficiency is very high, significantly more light is emitted by the top screen than the bottom one. To compensate for the top side of the film being overexposed and the bottom underexposed, the top screen may be thinner to equalize the light emission between the screens. These types of screens are provided with labels for top and bottom. If they are installed improperly, a significant loss of screen speed results.

Contrast and Latitude

Intensifying-screen contrast and latitude are insignificant factors because most phosphors have a relatively linear conversion efficiency except for their K-shell edges. Film contrast and latitude are much more critical because of the nonlinear shape of the D log E curve. A slight improvement in screen contrast is achieved by the use of antihalation crossover dyes in the screens, but their use remains primarily with film base and emulsion. However, the effect of intensifying screens on image contrast is so slight as to be negligible.

CASSETTES AND HOLDERS

Cassettes and holders are designed to create a portable, lightproof case for film to utilize the intensifying screens to best advantage and to attenuate the residual x-ray beam as much as possible (Figure 22-10). A wide variety of sizes and types of cassettes are available. Originally, direct exposure film was exposed in a cardboard holder, which is simply a lightproof container. Today there are numerous specialty cassettes available, such as curved cassettes and cassettes designed for specialty equipment, such as panoramic facial units.

Characteristics

The front of the cassette must be uniformly radiolucent to eliminate artifacts, rigid to provide good support for body parts, and lightweight. The intensifying screens are attached to the inside of the front and back of the cassette. At least one must be mounted on a foam pressure pad to provide good contact between the screens and the film. The back must be rigid and lightweight and may also include a sheet of lead foil to reduce the residual beam and absorb backscatter. Backscatter is a significant problem with large body parts, especially in hypersthenic chest and abdomen examinations. It is caused when the incident beam is of such magnitude that enough backscatter is produced from behind the cassette to form a second image (Figure 22-11). The lead sheet must be minimal in cassettes designed to be used with automatic exposure controls (AECs).

Extremely low-attenuation graphite carbon fiber materials are sometimes used for cassettes, grid interspaces, and tables when low-energy photons may be carrying critical information. Computed tomography and angiography tables, grids, and cassettes are examples. Although expensive, graphite can reduce attenuation by up to 50 percent and permits a corresponding reduction in patient dose.

Cross section of a typical radiographic cassette.

Eastman Kodak introduced the X-Omatic™ cassette (Figure 22-12) in the 1970s. This cassette was a significant improvement in film-screen contact, beam attenuation, and weight. X-Omatic™ cassettes are manufactured with a slight curve, thus causing squeegeeing of air as they are closed and eliminating the air pockets that cause poor film/screen contact. The cassettes are made of lightweight plastic with excellent radiolucent qualities. A thin sheet of lead foil in the back of the cassette is designed to eliminate residual scatter. The lead foil absorbs sufficient scatter to permit the cassette to be used backwards as a no-line grid. Specialized mammography cassettes are available with polystyrene fronts for low attenuation and thin sides to permit film edges to demonstrate chest wall tissues.

CARE

Loading and Storage

When loading cassettes, the tops should never be fully open in order to prevent dust and condensation from accumulating and to prevent the formation of the artifacts they cause on the radiograph. The cassette top should be opened slightly; 2–3 inches, or 6–8 cm, is enough for the experienced darkroom technician to unload and load any cassette.

Cassettes should be stored on end like a book and empty of film. Because of the frequency of cassette use, nearly all radiography departments observe the first recommendation but not the second.

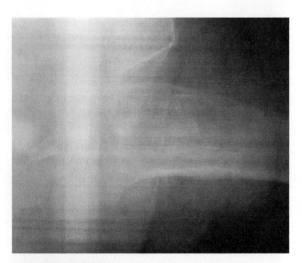

FIGURE 22-11 Backscatter forming an image of a cassette hinge. This resulted from lack of collimation, which permitted the remnant beam to strike a wall and backscatter through the back of the cassette onto the film. *(By permission of Mayo Foundation for Medical Education and Research. All rights reserved.)*

FIGURE 22-12 The Eastman Kodak X-Omatic™ cassette.

Cleaning

Intensifying screens and cassettes should be cleaned regularly. They must not be cleaned with tap water or any cleaning solution not specifically designed for intensifying screens. Most commercial firms offer an electrostatic cleaning solution that will not leave mineral stains, will not become sticky (resulting in damage when screens stick to film or to one another after cleaning), and discourages static electricity that could discharge and expose film.

The proper procedure for cleaning intensifying screens is to unload the cassette in the darkroom and then use unsterile 1″ × 1″ or 2″ × 2″ gauze sponges to apply an electrostatic cleaning solution liberally to the screen, working in strokes from side to side across the cassette. The procedure should then be repeated at right angles to the first series of strokes and followed by using dry sponges to remove excess liquid. **Never close a wet cassette** because the screens may adhere to one another, permanently damaging their surfaces. Set the damp cassettes in a clean location until they dry thoroughly (an x-ray table top is ideal). The cassettes may be reloaded in the darkroom and returned to use.

Artifacts

A loaded cassette that is stored near heat, bright sunlight, or in an ionizing radiation area may fog the film as the heat, light, or ionizing radiation activates the screen phosphor slightly. Always store cassettes away from any type of radiation.

A white spot (low density) represents an area where an artifact blocked the transmission of light between the screen and film or prohibited the ionizing radiation from activating the intensifying screen. Pitted screens or dust on the film or screen in the cassette are common causes of white spots. Cleaning the screens will often remove the artifacts.

Poor contact between the film and screens can produce lack of detail. A screen contact quality control test may be performed to verify the artifact diagnosis, but often the cassette and screens must be discarded.

SUMMARY

Intensifying screens produce large quantities of light photons when struck by x-rays, thereby amplifying the incoming x-ray beam and reducing patient radiation dose. Over 99 percent of the latent image is formed by light from the screens, with less than 1 percent being contributed by x-ray photons.

An intensifying screen consists of a base, reflective layer, phosphor layer, and protective coat. The base is usually made of polyester plastic and serves to hold the phosphor layer. The reflective layer is added to increase the amount of light reaching the film. The phosphor layer is the active, light-emitting layer of the screen, and the protective coat protects the phosphor layer from abrasions.

The phosphors used in intensifying screens must have a high atomic number, high conversion efficiency, appropriate spectral emission, and minimal phosphorescence. Luminescence is the ability of a material to emit light in response to excitation. The two types of luminescence are fluorescence and phosphorescence.

A variety of phosphor materials have been used in radiography. The most popular of the phosphors are the rare earths.

Intensifying screens exhibit the same characteristics as film: resolution, speed, contrast, and latitude. Resolution and speed are affected by phosphor crystal size, layer thickness, and the concentration of the crystals. Contrast and latitude are relatively insignificant factors.

Cassettes and holders are designed to create a portable, lightproof case for the film, to utilize the intensifying screens to best advantage, and to attenuate the residual x-ray beam as much as possible. Cassettes should never be fully open when loading and unloading film. Both cassettes and intensifying screens should be cleaned regularly.

REVIEW QUESTIONS

1. How do intensifying screens reduce patient dose?

2. What are the four basic components of an intensifying screen?

3. What characteristics should an intensifying screen phosphor possess?

4. What is the difference between fluorescence and phosphorescence?

5. What is the relationship between resolution and phosphor crystal size, layer thickness, and phosphor concentration?

6. What is quantum mottle?

7. What is the difference between calcium tungstate screens and rare-earth screens in terms of x-ray beam absorption?

8. What is the purpose of a cassette?

REFERENCES AND RECOMMENDED READING

Ardran, G. M., Crooks, H. E., & James, V. (1969). Testing x-ray cassettes for film-intensifying screen contact. *Radiography, 35*(414), 143.

Burgess, A. E., & Hicken, P. (1982, May). Comparative performance of x-ray intensifying screens. *Radiology, 55.*

Bushberg, J. T., Seibert, J. A., Leidholdt, E. M., & Boone, J. M. (2003). *The essential physics of medical imaging* (2nd ed.). Baltimore: Lippincott, Williams & Wilkins.

Carroll, Q. B. (2003). *Fuchs's radiographic exposure, processing, and quality control* (7th ed.). Springfield, IL: Charles C Thomas.

Cullinan, A., & Cullinan, J. (1994). *Producing quality radiographs* (2nd ed.). Philadelphia: J. B. Lippincott.

Curry, T. S., Dowdey, J. E., & Murry, R. C. (1990). *Christensen's introduction to the physics of diagnostic radiology* (4th ed.). Philadelphia: Lea and Febiger.

Doi, K., Loo, L., Anderson, T. M., & Frank, P. H. (1981). Effect of crossover exposure on radiographic image quality of screen-film systems. *Radiology, 139,* 707–714.

Fuchs, A. W. (1947). Edison and roentgenology. *The American Journal of Roentgenology and Radium Therapy, 57*(2), 145–156.

Fuchs, A. W. (1956). Evolution of Roentgen film. The *American Journal of Roentgenology and Radium Therapy, 75*(1), 30–48.

Hollis, K. D. (1975). Rare-earth phosphor intensifying screens. *Radiography, 41*(491), 249.

Hufton, A. P., Crosthwaite, C. M., Davies, J. M., & Robinson, L. A. (1987). Low attenuation material for table tops, cassettes, and grids: A review. *Radiography, 53*(607), 17.

Jenkins, D. (1980). *Radiographic photography and imaging processes.* Lancaster, England: MTP Press Limited.

Keefe, D. D., & De Brusk, D. (1980). A systematic approach toward rare-earth imaging. *Applied Radiology, 9*(6), 105.

Kodera, Y., Doi, K., & Chan, H. (1984). Absolute speeds of screen-film systems and their absorbed-energy constants. *Radiology, 151,* 229–236.

McKinney, W. (1988). *Radiographic processing and quality control.* Philadelphia: J. B. Lippincott.

Morgan, R. H. (1953). Roentgenoscopic screen intensification. *Radiologic Technology, 25*(2), 80.

Olson, A., & High, M. (1981, August). Performance of automatic exposure controls when used with rare-earth intensifying screens. *Radiology,* 491.

Roberts, D. P., & Smith, N. L. (1988). *Radiographic imaging: A practical approach.* Edinburgh: Churchill Livingstone.

Sackett, M. H. (1977). Caution: Speed ahead—rare earth imaging systems. *Radiologic Technology, 48*(5), 537.

Schmidt, R. A. (1983, March). Evaluation of cassette performance: Physical factors affecting patient exposure and image contrast. *Radiology,* 801.

Shearer, D. R., & Moore, M. M. (1986). Lag in radiographic imaging systems: Simple methods for evaluation. *Radiology, 159*(1), 259–263.

Sklensky, A. F., Buchanan, R. A., Maple, T. G., & Bailey, H. N. (1974). Quantum utilization in x-ray intensifying screens. *The Institute of Electrical and Electronics Engineers Transactions on Nuclear Science, 21,* 685–691.

Skucas, J., & Gorski, J. (1980). Application of modern intensifying screens in diagnostic radiology. *Medical Radiography and Photography, 56*(2), 25–36.

Sprawls, P. (1987). *Physical principles of medical imaging.* Rockville, MD: Aspen.

Sprawls, P. (1990). *Principles of radiography for technologists.* Rockville, MD: Aspen.

Sturm, R. E., & Morgan, R. H. (1949). Screen intensification systems and their limitations. *The American Journal of Roentgenology and Radium Therapy, 62*(5), 617–634.

Sweeney, R. J. (1983). *Radiographic artifacts: Their cause and control.* Philadelphia: J. B. Lippincott.

Thompson, M. A., Hattaway, M. P., Hall, J. D., & Dowd, S. B. (1994). *Principles of imaging science and protection.* Philadelphia: W. B. Saunders.

Trout, E. D., & Kelley, J. P. (1973). The effect of the temperature of intensifying screens on radiographic exposure. *Radiologic Technology, 45*(2), 70–72.

van der Plaats, G. J. (1980). *Medical x-ray techniques in diagnostic radiology* (4th ed.). The Hague: Martinus Nijhoff.

Venema, H. W. (1979). X-ray absorption, speed, and luminescent efficiency of rare earth and other intensifying screens. *Radiology, 130,* 765–771.

Vyborny, C. J. (1980, August). Relative efficiencies of energy to photographic density conversions in typical screen-film systems. *Radiology,* 465.

Wilson, P. (1977). Principles of intensifying screens in image formation. *Canadian Journal of Radiography, Radiotherapy, and Nuclear Medicine, 8*(3), 134–140.

Wolbarst, A. B. (1993). *Physics of radiology.* Norwalk, CT: Appleton & Lange.

The Case of the Line in the Stomach

Although barium has been used to coat this stomach for the air contrast study, an odd line appears at its midpoint. What is causing the line?

Answers to the case studies can be found in Appendix E.

CHAPTER 23

Film/Screen Combinations

Mr. Edison has discovered . . .
tungstate of calcium . . .
[with which] you can see
other people's bones with the
naked eye . . . . On the
revolting indecency of this
there is no need to dwell. But
what we seriously put before
the attention of the
Government is that the
moment tungstate of calcium
comes into anything like
general use, it will call for
legislative restriction of the
severest kind.

Pall Mall Gazette, March 1896

KEY TERMS

line pairs per
   millimeter (lp/mm)
line spread
   function (LSF)
modulation transfer
   function (MTF)

OBJECTIVES

Upon completion of this chapter, the student should be able to:

- Relate the emission spectra of various intensifying screens to specific types of radiographic film.

- Explain radiographic film/screen combination relative speed numbering systems.

- Calculate relative speed conversions from one film/screen combination to another.

- Describe various methods of measuring resolution, including a basic description of line pairs per millimeter, line spread function, and modulation transfer function.

- Relate film/screen contrast to latitude.

- Determine appropriate film/screen combinations for various clinical situations.

Radiographic film and intensifying screens are designed to complement each other and to produce the highest quality image with the lowest patient radiation dose. Film and screens must be matched to each other to achieve diagnostic quality images. If the screens have been designed to emit a specific wavelength, then the film must be designed to have enhanced sensitivity to the same wavelength. **Mismatching of film and screens often increases patient dose.**

 EMISSION SPECTRA

The spectral emissions of intensifying screen phosphors and radiographic films are shown in Figure 23-1. Note that blue sensitive film will not respond to most of the wavelengths emitted by the rare-earth phosphors. However, green sensitive film is more sensitive to the entire range of phosphor emissions, including the yellow-green wavelengths. Note also that green sensitive film is not quite as sensitive to the blue-violet wavelengths as the blue sensitive film. The spectral emission colors for various brands of intensifying screens are shown in Table 22-1.

The appropriate film/screen combination for a specific clinical situation must be selected based on the combined qualities of the film and the screen. Clinical selection cannot be accomplished by evaluating film and intensifying screens separately. The qualities that must be considered are **speed, resolution, contrast,** and **latitude.** Film/screen combination relationships are the same as the interrelationships of these factors for film (see Tables 21-2 and 21-3). The most common decision that must be made when selecting film/screen combinations is image resolution versus patient dose.

 CHARACTERISTICS

The important characteristics of film/screen combinations are **speed, resolution, contrast, and latitude.**

Speed

The speed of an imaging system depends on the **thickness of the layer** of phosphor or silver halide, the **crystal/phosphor** size, and the **efficiency** of the crystal/phosphor in emitting (in the case of intensifying screens) or capturing (in the case of silver halides) photons.

Commercial firms use relative speed (RS) numbers to rate film/screen combinations. The numbers are not quantitative and represent no units. They are based on a relative value of 100 for calcium tungstate intensifying screens used with a medium contrast and latitude blue sensitive film. This was the standard film/screen combination known as par or medium speed before the advent of rare-earth screens (Table 23-1). Each manufacturer tends to calibrate film/screen combinations to its own brands. However, it has been suggested that the base RS 100 be calibrated equal to 1.28 mR to produce the film speed point (OD 1.00 + base + fog). **Rela-**

FIGURE 23-1 Light sensitivity of various films and intensifying screens. Note that blue sensitive screens are not sensitive to the major rare-earth light emissions. *Note.* from "An Improved X-Ray Intensifying Screen," by Robert A. Buchanan, New York, New York. 1971, *IEEE Transactions on Nuclear Science.* Copyright 1971 by the IEEE. Reprinted with permission.

TABLE 23-1.   Typical Radiographic Intensifying Screen Comparisons

Intensifying Screen	Typical Relative Speed When Combined with Appropriate Film	Approximate lp/mm	Minimum Receptor Activation Dose
rare-earth detail	100	8	1 mR
rare-earth par regular speed	200	5.5	0.4 mR
rare-earth high speed	400	4.5	0.2 mR

TABLE 23-2.   Relationship between Relative Speed Number and Exposure Sensitivity

RS Number	Exposure Sensitivity in mR
1200	0.10
800	0.16
400	0.32
200	0.64
100	1.28
50	2.56
25	5.00
12	10.00

Note. From *Physical Principles of Medical Imaging*, by P. Sprawls, 1987, Rockville, MD: Aspen. Reprinted with perΜission.

tive speed numbers are usually established at 70–80 kVp, with 80 kVp preferred. When kVp values below 70 or above 100 are used, RS numbers may be less consistent. Therefore, the relationship between the RS number and the sensitivity of the film/screen combination is established by the following formula:

$$\text{Sensitivity in mR} = \frac{128}{RS}$$

Table 23-2 shows the relationship of RS number to the sensitivity in mR to produce the film speed point.

Relative speed (RS) numbers are accurate enough to be used by radiographers to convert exposure technique settings from one situation to an-

other. The formula for converting mAs from one relative speed to another is:

$$\frac{mAs_1}{mAs_2} = \frac{RS_2}{RS_1}$$

where: mAs_1 = old mAs
mAs_2 = new mAs
RS_1 = old relative speed
RS_2 = new relative speed

The most common problem is to determine a new mAs for use with a relative speed that is different from the one for which an acceptable technique is known. To determine a new mAs, the following version is used:

$$mAs_2 = \frac{RS_1 \times mAs_1}{RS_2}$$

EXAMPLE: What is the proper mAs for use with a 400 RS system when technical factors of 80 kVp and 50 mAs produce an acceptable image with a 200 RS system?

Answer:

$$\frac{mAs_1}{mAs_2} = \frac{RS_2}{RS_1}$$

$$\frac{50}{mAs_2} = \frac{400}{200}$$

$$mAs_2 \times 400 = 50 \text{ mAs} \times 200$$

$$mAs_2 \times 400 = 10,000 \text{ mAs}$$

$$mAs_2 = \frac{10,000 \text{ mAs}}{400}$$

$$mAs_2 = 25 \text{ mAs}$$

TABLE 23-3. Manufacturer's Relative Speed/Film Combinations

Agfa Relative Speed Film/Screen Combination Chart (Green Systems)

Film sensitivity/speed/contrast/latitude	Screen				
	Curix® Ortho Fine	Curix® Ortho Medium	Curix® Ortho Regular	Curix® Ortho Fast	Curix ® Opthos H
Curix® Ortho HT-G green/low/high/narrow	100	250	400	600	not recommended
Curix® Ortho HT-L Plus green/low/low/wide	100	250	400	600	not recommended
Curix® Opthos H green/low/low/wide	not recommended	not recommended	not recommended	not recommended	400
Curix® Ortho HT-C green/low/high/narrow	100	250	400	600	not recommended

Agfa Relative Speed Film/Screen Combination Chart (Ultra Violet (Blue) Systems)

Film sensitivity/speed/contrast/latitude	Screen			
	Quanta Detail Extremity	Quanta Fast Detail Medium Speed	Quanta Rapid Fast Speed	Quanta Super Rapid Ultra Fast Speed
Cronex® 10T ultraviolet/low/high/narrow	80	250	400	600
Cronex® 10TL ultraviolet/low/low/wide	80	250	400	600
Cronex® 4/5 ultraviolet/fast/high/narrow	100	400	800	1200

EXAMPLE: What is the proper mAs for use with a 250 RS system when technical factors of 80 kVp and 50 mAs produce an acceptable image with an 800 RS system?

Answer:

$$\frac{mAs_1}{mAs_2} = \frac{RS_2}{RS_1}$$

$$\frac{50}{mAs_2} = \frac{250}{800}$$

$$mAs_2 \times 250 = 50 \text{ mAs} \times 800$$

$$mAs_2 \times 250 = 40,000 \text{ mAs}$$

$$mAs_2 = \frac{40,000 \text{ mAs}}{250}$$

$$mAs_2 = 160 \text{ mAs}$$

Film/screen combinations are available from RS 20 to RS 1,200 (Table 23-3). An RS combination of 400 is the most common compromise between patient dose and resolution in hospital settings. Although not an absolute relationship, for the most part higher RS numbers reduce patient dose, decrease latitude, and decrease resolution. Film/screen combinations to RS 1,800 have been produced but are not available due to unacceptable image quality.

Resolution

Recorded detail, sharpness, and resolution are measured as **line pairs per millimeter (lp/mm,** or cycles per mm), **line spread function (LSF),** and **modulation transfer function (MTF).**

Line Pairs per Millimeter. Line pairs per millimeter, or cycles per millimeter, measures the minimum size and space between objects that can be visualized on the final image.

Line Spread Function. The line spread function (LSF) measures the ability of a film/screen system to

Fuji Relative Speed Film/Screen Combination Chart (Green Systems)

Film sensitivity/speed/control/latitude	Screen			
	HR Fine	HR Medium	HR Regular	HR Fast
S HR–G green/low/high/narrow	100	200	400	600
S HR–L green/low/low/wide	100	200	400	600
S HR–C green/low/low/very wide	100	200	400	600
S HR–H green/high/high/narrow	not recommended	300–400	600	900

Kodak Relative Speed Film/Screen Combination Chart (Green Systems)

Film sensitivity/speed/contrast/latitude	Screen			
	Lanex® Fine	Lanex® Medium	Lanex® Regular	Lanex® /Fast
T–Mat G/RA green/low/high/narrow	100	300	400	600
T–Mat L/RA green/low/low/wide	100	300	400	600
T–Mat S/RA green/low/high/narrow	100	300	400	600
T–Mat H/RA green/high/high/narrow	not recommended	400	600	900

This table illustrates only the combinations available when both film and screen are ordered from the same manufacturer. There are other manufacturers of film and intensifying screens and some manufacturers listed in this table make additional films. Film manufacturers should always be consulted prior to attempting to create a film/screen combination for clinical use to ensure that current information is considered. Film and screen names change with advancements in manufacturing technologies. These charts are provided as examples based on information available at the time of publication. Film manufacturers' technical information with laboratory verification by the authors were used to establish comparable classifications in this table. The authors are aware that manufacturers and other radiologic researchers' data may differ slightly due to laboratory conditions.

accurately measure the boundaries of an image. It is calculated by using a microdensitometer to measure the ability of the image receptor to record a line from a 10 µm wide beam of radiation. A typical film/screen system might display densities from a 10 µm line over 600–800 µm.

Modulation Transfer Function. The modulation transfer function (MTF) provides the best measurement of the resolving ability of a film/screen combination. It measures the information lost between the subject and the image receptor. There are no units of MTF. The MTF is determined primarily by the amount of light diffusion that occurs between the screens and the film. The MTF is primarily controlled by the chemical composition of the screen, phosphor size, thickness of the phosphor layer, absorbing dye, and, most important, by film/screen contact. Therefore, MTF is a function of the screens because the resolving power of film is far superior to that of the intensifying screens. The intensifying screens impose the resolution limitations on the film/screen system.

FIGURE 23-2 MTF versus lp/mm for several different film/screen combinations. *(Note. Reprinted from MTF's and Wiener Spectra of Radiographic Screen-Film Systems (HHS Publication FDA 82-8187), by Doi Kunio, G. Holje, L. Loo, and H. Chan, 1982, FDA 82-0187, Rockville, MD: U.S. Department of Health and Human Services, Public Health Service, Food and Drug Administration, Bureau of Radiological Health)*

The MTF is sometimes presented as a formula:

$$MTF = \frac{Recorded\ Detail\ (Resolution)}{Available\ Detail\ (Resolution)}$$

A perfect MTF would be 1.0. Therefore, MTFs are less than 1.0 because more information cannot be recorded than what is available. An MTF curve plots MTF against resolution (lp/mm) (Figure 23-2). Faster film/screen combinations exhibit an obvious decrease in resolution when compared to the detail combinations.

Contrast

Contrast is primarily the contrast of the film, although intensifying screens, especially the rare earths, also exhibit contrast. The effect of higher contrast that is achieved when lower kVp can be used due to higher speed screens is often overlooked. In addition, the rare-earth phosphors often exhibit slightly higher contrast.

Latitude

The film/screen system latitude is primarily dependent upon the latitude of the film, which is directly related to the contrast. Narrow latitude film/screen systems

exhibit high contrast. High-speed film/speed systems tend to have lower resolution (decreased detail).

SELECTING FILM/SCREEN COMBINATIONS

The selection of appropriate film/screen combinations requires consideration of the various film and screen characteristics. For example, Figure 23-3 illustrates the differences between two types of screens and three types of film. The radiographs on the left were produced with detail screens, while those on the right were produced with high-speed screens. Radiographs A and B were produced with a general-purpose film, C and D with a wide-latitude film, and E and F with a high-contrast film. The exposure factors were adjusted to maintain a consistent density. Variations in resolution can be seen by comparing the resolution tools from the right column with those from the left. Variations in contrast can be seen by comparing the number of steps visible on the penetrometer from the different types of film used.

60 kVp	5 mAs	40" SID
No grid	100 RS	10.7 mR

60 kVp	5 mAs	40" SID
No grid	100 RS	10.0 mR

60 kVp	2.5 mAs	40" SID
No grid	200 RS	4.88 mR

A   C   E

B   D   F

60 kVp	0.8 mAs	40" SID
No grid	600 RS	1.74 mR

60 kVp	0.8 mAs	40" SID
No grid	600 RS	1.66 mR

60 kVp	0.4 mAs	40" SID
No grid	1200 RS	0.88 mR

FIGURE 23-3
Differences between two types of screens and three types of film. The radiographs on the top were produced with detail screens, while those on the bottom were produced with high-speed screens. Radiographs A and B were produced with a general-purpose film; C and D with a wide-latitude film; and E and F with a high-contrast film.

CLINICAL CHOICES

Film and intensifying-screen manufacturers publish film/screen combination charts that compare all possible combinations of their films and intensifying screens. These charts often highlight the RS numbers and provide commentary on appropriate clinical uses and the image quality factors (speed, resolution, contrast, and latitude).

Various types of intensifying-screen phosphors are more efficient at various kVp levels (Figure 23-4). These factors must be considered when selecting combinations for various clinical situations. The primary advantages and disadvantages of rare-earth film/screen combinations are shown in Table 23-4.

The objectives of high-quality images and reduced patient dose are well within the focus of modern film/screen combination technology. However, this depends considerably on the appropriate choice of film/screen combination for specific clinical situations.

Angiography

Rare-earth film/screen combinations were immediately recognized for their value in angiographic studies. The advantage of decreased patient dose while maintaining image resolution is obvious

TABLE 23-4.	Advantages and Disadvantages of Rare-Earth Film/Screen Combinations

Advantages	Disadvantages
Reduced patient dose	Increased quantum mottle noise
Reduced staff dose	
Increased tube life	Increased cost
Use of lower power generators	kVp influences efficiency
Reduced patient motion	
Reduced kVp (while maintaining contrast)	
Reduced mA (while maintaining focal spot size)	

FIGURE 23-4 Absorption efficiency of various intensifying-screen phosphors. Note that although rare earths are significantly more efficient between 40 and 70 keV, calcium tungstate is slightly more efficient above 70 keV. *(Note. "Quantum utilization in x-ray intensifying screens," by A. F. Sklensky, R. A. Buchanan, I. G. Maple, and H. N. Bailey, 1974, IEEE Transactions on Nuclear Science. Copyright 1974 by the IEEE. Reprinted with permission. New York, New York)*

when short exposure times are critical at the same time that numerous exposures are required, resulting in high total exposure. Because angiography produces high subject contrast between injected vessels and surrounding tissues, quantum mottle noise is less of a problem than in other studies.

Gastrointestinal and Urologic Radiography

Both gastrointestinal and urologic examinations are procedures in which high subject contrast permits the use of high-speed rare-earth film/screen combinations. High subject contrast often permits higher quantum mottle noise ratios without objectionable interference with the diagnostic information of the image.

Abdominal Radiography

Faster calcium tungstate or slower rare-earth systems have been suggested for abdominal radiography because of low subject contrast, which requires reducing quantum mottle noise.

Skeletal Radiography

Skeletal examinations are usually divided into extremity examinations, in which detail film/screen combinations are very desirable due to the subtle differences that provide clues to some pathologies. Pelvic and lumbar examinations present totally different problems because of large subject thickness and the less subtle nature of regional pathologies.

Chest Radiography

High kVp chest radiography ($> 100\,kVp$) is achieved more efficiently with calcium tungstate film/screen combinations than with rare earths.

Pediatric Radiography

Pediatric examinations are also prime candidates for higher-speed film/screen combinations because large portions of the body are often included within the primary-beam field, effects of the radiation exposure will be carried longer, and motion is the primary imaging problem for the radiographer.

SUMMARY

Radiographic film and intensifying screens are designed to complement each other and to produce the highest quality image with the lowest patient radiation dose. To accomplish this, film and screens must be matched to each other, especially with regard to their emission spectra. Mismatching of film and screens increases patient dose.

The qualities that must be considered in a film/screen combination are speed, resolution, contrast, and latitude. The most frequent decision that must be made when selecting film/screen combinations is image resolution versus patient dose.

Commercial firms use relative speed (RS) numbers to rate film/screen combinations. The formula for converting mAs from one relative speed to another is:

$$\frac{mAs_1}{mAs_2} = \frac{RS_2}{RS_1}$$

Recorded detail, sharpness, and resolution are measured as line pairs per millimeter (lp/mm, or cycles per mm), line spread function (LSF), and modulation transfer function (MTF). Contrast is primarily the contrast of the film, although intensifying screens, especially the rare earths, also affect contrast. The film/screen system latitude is primarily dependent upon the latitude of the film. The selection of appropriate film/screen combinations requires consideration of the various film and screen characteristics and of the clinical situation for which they are to be used.

REVIEW QUESTIONS

1. What are the emission spectra of calcium tungstate and rare-earth intensifying screens?

2. What is the formula used to calculate a relative speed conversion from one film/screen combination to another?

3. What are the three methods of measuring resolution?

4. How is film/screen contrast related to latitude?

5. What clinical situation(s) would justify the use of a detail-speed film/screen combination?

6. What clinical situation(s) would justify the use of a high-speed film/screen combination?

REFERENCES AND RECOMMENDED READING

Braun, M., & Wilson, B. C. (1982). Comparative evaluation of several rare-earth film-screen systems. *Radiology, 144,* 915.

Buchanan, R. A. (1971). An improved x-ray intensifying screen. *IEEE Transactions on Nuclear Science,* New York, New York.

Burgess, A. E., & Hicken, P. (1982, May). Comparative performance of x-ray intensifying screens. *Radiology,* 55.

Bushberg, J. T., Seibert, J. A., Leidholdt, E. M., & Boone, J. M. (2003). *The essential physics of medical imaging* (2nd ed.). Baltimore: Lippincott Williams & Wilkins.

Bushong, S. C. (2004). *Radiologic science for technologists: Physics, biology, and protection* (8th ed.). St. Louis: C. V. Mosby.

Carroll, Q. B. (2003). *Fuchs's radiographic exposure, processing, and quality control* (7th ed.). Springfield, IL: Charles C Thomas.

Cullinan, A., & Cullinan, J. (1994). *Producing quality radiographs* (2nd ed.). Philadelphia: J. B. Lippincott.

Curry, T. S., Dowdey, J. E., & Murry, R. C. (1990). *Christensen's introduction to the physics of diagnostic radiology* (4th ed.). Philadelphia: Lea and Febiger.

DeSmet, A. A. (1982). An evaluation of screen-film combinations for detail skeletal radiography. *Radiology, 143,* 259.

Doi, K., Holje, G., Loo, L., & Chan, H. (1982). *MTF's and Wiener spectra of radiographic screen-film systems* HHS Publication FDA 82-8187. Rockville, MD. United States Department of Health and Human Services, Public Health Service, Food and Drug Administration, Bureau of Radiological Health.

Doi, K., Loo, L., Anderson, T. M., & Frank, P. H. (1981). Effect of crossover exposure on radiographic image quality of screen-film systems. *Radiology, 139,* 707–714.

Haus, A. G., & Cullinan, J. E. (1989). Screen film processing systems for medical radiography: A historical review. *Radiographics, 9*(6), 1203–1224.

Higashida, Y., Frank, P. H., & Doi, K. (1983, November). High-speed, single-screen/single-emulsion film systems: Basic imaging properties and preliminary clinical applications. *Radiology,* 571.

Jenkins, D. (1980). *Radiographic photography and imaging processes.* Lancaster, England: MTP Press Limited.

Kodera, Y., Doi, K., & Chan, H. (1984). Absolute speeds of screen-film systems and their absorbed-energy constants. *Radiology, 151,* 229–236.

McKinney, W. (1988). *Radiographic processing and quality control.* Philadelphia: J. B. Lippincott.

Rao, G. U. V., & Fatouros, P. P. (1978). The relationship between resolution and speed of x-ray intensifying screens. *Medical Physics, 5,* 205–208.

Rao, G. U. V., Fatouros, P. P., & James, A. E. (1978). Physical characteristics of modern radiographic screen-film systems. *Investigative Radiology, 13,* 460.

Rossi, R. P., Hendee, W. R., & Aherns, C. R. (1976). An evaluation of rare-earth screen-film combinations. *Radiology, 121,* 465.

Sackett, M. H. (1977). Caution: Speed ahead—rare earth imaging systems. *Radiologic Technology, 48*(5), 537.

Shearer, D. R., & Moore, M. M. (1986). Lag in radiographic imaging systems: Simple methods for evaluation. *Radiology, 159*(1), 259–263.

Sklensky, A. F., Buchanan, R. A., Maple, I. G., Bailey, H. N. (1974). Quantum utilization in x-ray intensifying screens. *IEEE Transactions on Nuclear Science.* New York, New York.

Sprawls, P. (1987). *Physical principles of medical imaging.* Rockville, MD: Aspen.

Taylor, K. W., McLeich, B. P., Hobbs, B. B., & Hughes, T. J. (1980). Selection of screen-film combinations. *The Canadian Journal of Medical Radiation Technology, 11*(3), 154.

Thompson, M. A., Hattaway, M. P., Hall, J. D., & Dowd, S. B. (1994). *Principles of imaging science and protection.* Philadelphia: W. B. Saunders.

Thompson, T. T. (1974). Selecting medical x-ray film. *Applied Radiology, 3,* 47–51.

Thompson, T. T. (1985). *A practical approach to modern imaging equipment* (2nd ed.). Boston: Little, Brown.

U.S. Department of Health, Education, and Welfare, Food and Drug Administration. (1976). Bureau of Radiological Health. *First Image Receptor Conference: Film/screen combinations.* (HEW Publication [FDA] 77-8003). Washington, DC: Authors.

Venema, H. W. (1979). X-ray absorption, speed, and luminescent efficiency of rare earth and other intensifying screens. *Radiology, 130,* 765–771.

Vyborny, C. J. (1980, August). Relative efficiencies of energy to photographic density conversions in typical screen-film systems. *Radiology,* 465.

Wolbarst, A. B. (1993). *Physics of radiology.* Norwalk, CT: Appleton & Lange.

The Case of the Missing Lower Pelvis

For some unexplained reason, this patient's lower hips and pelvis disappeared. Why?

Answers to the case studies can be found in Appendix E.

CHAPTER 24

Digital Image Processing

> . . . the digital computer has revolutionized virtually every element of diagnostic imaging . . . diagnostic imaging is one of the most exciting and rapidly evolving fields of medicine, and without question is leading all of medicine into the computer-electronic era.
>
> *William R. Hendee, Preface to Christopher C. Kuni's Introduction to Computers and Digital Processing in Medical Imaging*

KEY TERMS

analog computer	edge enhancement	read-only memory
array detection	hardware	(ROM)
bandwidth	high-pass filtering	scanning
band-pass filtering	low-pass filtering	sharpening
binary machine	masking	signal-to-noise ratio
language	matrix	slow scanning
bit	pixel	smoothing
byte	program	software
central processing	progressive scanning	voxel
unit (CPU)	random-access	
data	memory (RAM)	
digital computer		

OBJECTIVES

Upon completion of this chapter, the student should be able to:

- Describe the differences between analog and digital computers.

- Describe the differences between programs and data.

- State reasons why binary machine code is used in place of other languages.

- Describe the basic function of a central processing unit, read-only memory, and random-access memory.

- Describe the basic function of various memory storage and input and output devices.

- Explain the basic function of an array processor.

- Describe the process of digital image data acquisition.

- Describe the effects of frequency, contrast, and noise on digital image quality.

- Explain the function of digital image window level and width controls.

- Describe various factors that directly affect digital image resolution.

- Explain the digital subtraction process and various filtering techniques.

The future of medical imaging continues to be driven by computerized applications of the numerous modalities that currently exist, as well as in the integration of those now on the horizon. The explosion of the imaging sciences that took place between the early 1970s and the 1990s was caused by the first wave of digital computerization in computed tomography (CT) and ultrasound. Computed tomography captured the imagination of the public; digital processing has now been successfully applied to nuclear medicine, cardiovascular imaging and magnetic resonance imaging (MRI) and now predominates in diagnostic imaging and mammography as well.

The method by which these imaging modalities handle digital processing of imaging information requires radiographers to understand anatomy from transverse, sagittal, and coronal perspectives. Those who work in the radiologic and imaging sciences must often visualize anatomy as a dynamic three-dimensional tilting, rotating, and tumbling process due to computer manipulation of imaging data in four dimensions.

THE COMPUTER

Computers are devices that process information. The earliest computer device, the abacus, dates to around 3,000 B.C., and calculating machines were developed in the 1600s. The modern electronic computer, ENIAC, was developed in 1945 at the University of Pennsylvania. The addition of the mathematical theories of Baron Jean Fourier (1768–1830) and George Boole (1815–1864), solid-state electronics in the 1940s, and microchip technology in the 1960s were all required prior to the first digital computer applications in medical imaging.

Analog and Digital Computers

Analog computers handle data composed of continuously varying electrical currents. **Digital computers** handle data composed of definite quantities of current (i.e., current on versus current off). For example, an analog watch displays time with hands while a digital watch uses a numerical readout. All medical imaging is achieved with digital computers, often from information that has been processed by an analog-to-digital converter (ADC). Digitization of analog information, such as the vast number of incident photons that comprise a radiographic image, always reduces the quantity and quality of the remaining information. Figure 24-1 illustrates the digitization process. Digital-to-analog converters (DAC) are sometimes used to permit faster transmission of data. After transmission, an ADC is used to convert the data for digital display or processing.

Programs and Data

Computers use two types of information: operating instructions, called the **program** and collected facts, called **data.** Programs provide specific instructions for calculations and sequential steps to be followed. Special computer languages are used for programming. Programs are called **software** while computer

FIGURE 24-1 Analog-to-digital conversion of imaging information. The line represents the input data; the blocks represent the digitization of the data.

equipment is called **hardware.** One of the most useful programming techniques is the ability to program a computer to do problem solving, such as an if-then statement in which a computer can determine if a condition has been met, and then perform various operations depending on the exact conditions.

1	read memory 1
2	if memory 1 is less than 5 then go to line 5
3	if memory 1 equals 5 then go to line 6
4	if memory 1 is greater than 5 then go to line 7

For example, this program provides three alternative actions depending on the value of the information stored in memory 1. Complex programs have many alternative functions that can be performed as variables are processed by the computer.

Binary Machine Language

Computers operate from a **binary machine language.** Just as English has a 26-letter symbol alphabet, the binary system operates with a two-symbol alphabet. Because electrical currents are most easily understood as being either on or off, the binary system consists of information recorded as either a 0 for off or a 1 for on. Each binary number is called a **bit,** for binary digits. Nominal numbers function on a base 10 system instead of base 2. Table 24-1 illustrates how the numbers 1 through 10 are written in binary code. An 8-bit word is required to form the 26 letters of the English alphabet. As a convenience, an 8-bit word is called a **byte.** Computer memory is often rated in terms of the total byte memory (rounded off). For example, a 10 megabyte magnetic hard disk will store over 10,000,000 bytes (80,000,000 bits) of information.

Central Processing Unit (CPU)

The **central processing unit (CPU)** is the heart of every computer. It directs information to and from the various components that make up the computer system. For example, when a computer is turned on, the CPU may extract information from a permanent memory that loads an operating system program into

TABLE 24-1. Binary Code Numbers

Arabic	Binary
1	1
2	10
3	11
4	100
5	101
6	110
7	111
8	1000
9	1001
10	1010
.	.
.	.
.	.
.	.
16	10000
.	.
.	.
.	.
32	100000
.	.
.	.
.	.

the working memory. This operating system may then display instructions on the monitor. When a keyboard is used to input information, the CPU may then extract a program from memory and begin to carry out its instructions to operate imaging equipment.

The electrical connections between the CPU and the components run along a system of parallel or series conductors called a bus. Parallel connections permit simultaneous transmission of information, but they are expensive because a separate conductor must exist for each channel of information. Serial connectors are less expensive but require significantly more transmission time because information must be transmitted sequentially instead of simultaneously. Peripheral devices, such as memory storage units, printers, modems, and imaging systems, also use parallel and serial connectors.

TABLE 24-2. Typical Memory Requirements for Various Imaging Modalities

Imaging Modality	Typical Image Matrix	Grayscale Bit Depth	Images Per Typical Exam	Approximate Storage Requirements
Mammography	2,000 × 2500	32	4	80 Mb
Computed Radiography	2500 × 2500	16	4	50 Mb
Digital Fluoroscopy	1024 × 1024	8	24 sec × 5 min	7.5 Gb
Computed Tomography	512 × 512	16	120	60 Mb
Computed Tomography—MSCT	512 × 512	16	2,000	1 Gb
Ultrasound	512 × 512	32	50	50 Mb
Magnetic Resonance Imaging	512 × 512	16	2,000	1 Gb
Nuclear Medicine	512 × 512	8	100	25 Mb

Memory

Information can be stored in a computer's memory as magnetic variations and can be transferred as voltage. Magnetic field direction or greater and lesser voltage represent "on," or 1, and "off," or 0 indications. Memory is also classified as read memory or write memory. Read memory simply extracts information without alteration. Write memory replaces (deletes) old memory with new information.

ROM and RAM. Memory is classified as **read-only memory (ROM)** or **random-access memory (RAM).** Both standard ROM and programmable ROM (PROM) usually contain basic operating instructions that are rarely, if ever, changed. The RAM usually functions as temporary storage for programming and operating instructions during their use and is constantly changed. When the main power to the computer is turned off, RAM is erased while ROM is maintained.

Bus

A bus is the system of conductors that connects the various components of a computer system. It functions in a manner similar to a city bus route in that it permits the computer processing system to accept inputs from any point along the conductor as if it were a bus picking up jobs to do instead of people to carry. The bus speed is critical to how fast the computer system can function. For example, a 2 GHz system is significantly more efficient than an old 120 MHz system.

Peripherals

Peripheral devices permit input and output of information to or from the CPU. Some peripherals may appear to be a physical part of the computer, such as an input memory disk drive, while others may appear to be separate devices, such as a paper printer.

Memory Storage Devices. A number of memory storage devices for data have become popular. These include magnetic and optical tapes and disks. Information can be stored by optical (laser) recording and reading as well as by electronic and magnetic fields. Magnetic tape is often called "mag tape" and, although inexpensive, is difficult to access because data is stored serially. Consequently, it is seldom used today. Magnetic disks have evolved from large (8″) to small (5¼″) floppy disks and even smaller (3½″) diskettes. For large amounts of data a hard disk CD or DVD storage is required. Optical tape and disks permit the storage of significantly more data. Medical imaging modalities have used all of these devices for storing images and their associated data. Table 24-2 illustrates typical memory requirements for various imaging modalities.

Input Devices. The most familiar computer input device is a keyboard with a monitor for visualization of information before it is sent into the CPU. For example, a CT unit may wait for an entire examination protocol to be entered before it is sent to the CPU. In addition to keyboards, some units provide a visual marker known as a cursor on the monitor.

The cursor can be moved by keyboard arrows, a joystick, track ball, pad and pen, light or ultrasonic pen, or a specialized sliding control unit called a mouse. Most vendors offer touch screen monitors for input, and voice-activated units are becoming feasible. Input via these devices can be remarkably simple. For example, ultrasound units will place a centimeter ruler through the anatomical image from a cursor location and CT units will provide radiation attenuation coefficient numbers (CT numbers) for the tissue at the cursor location. Image receptors, such as television cameras, ultrasonic transducers, CT ion detectors, and MRI radiofrequency detectors also input information signals to CPUs for processing into visual images.

Output Devices. The most familiar output devices are monitors and printers. Computerized imaging systems often send output information directly to a monitor or hardcopy display for the production of visual images. Most computerized imaging systems incorporate both input and output CRTs into their control consoles. Some systems use a single monitor for both input and output information.

Array Processors. An array processor is a specialized computer that functions as a peripheral. It uses its CPU memory to perform simultaneous mathematical operations in a parallel fashion at extremely high speed instead of performing them sequentially. Array processors are useful when vast numbers of repetitive calculations are required, as in the processing of image detector data from CT or MRI equipment.

DIGITAL IMAGE ACQUISITION

A digital image is one that has been converted into numerical values for transmission or processing. A detector of some type must be used to acquire the image information. There are many types of detectors for various types of input information—ionizing radiation, ultrasonic waves, radiofrequencies, etc. Detectors acquire information either by **scanning** an area for information or by area or **array detection,** in which information is received from an entire area

at once. For example, a fluoroscopic image is digitized by the plumbicon™ camera for transmission to the display monitor. Although the monitor image is of significantly less resolution than the original image, it is simply a matter of numbers. The monitor is limited to 525 or 1,050 lines of resolution, while the primary photon beam has millions of incident photons. If the monitor could display millions of lines of data, the image would exhibit comparable resolution. Most monitors are capable of only 1–2 lp/mm. Specialized high-resolution monitors up to 5,000 × 5,000 lines of resolution are available.

Although digital images currently have diagnostic limits due to resolution, as display capabilities increase diagnostic confidence will also increase. Computerized digital images are described in terms of the number of values displayed per image side. A **matrix** is a square series of boxes that gives form to the image (Figure 24-2A). Each box of an image matrix will display a numerical value which can be transformed into a visual brightness or density level (Figure 24-2B and C). The individual matrix boxes are known as picture elements or **pixels.** The greater the matrix size, the better the resolution because a larger matrix provides smaller pixels. Pixel size determines resolution (Figure 24-3). Each pixel location is determined by its address. (For example, in Figure 24-2A the address of the labeled pixel is 4-4.) In medical imaging, each pixel value corresponds to a three-dimensional volume of tissue known as a **voxel** (see Figure 24-2A).

Each pixel in the matrix is capable of representing a wide range of different shades of gray from pure white through total black. The number of shades of gray is determined by the gray scale bit depth. Imaging modalities differ in the bit depth that is available depending on the capabilities of the image receptor. For example, digital radiography may have a bit depth of 16 whereas nuclear medicine may only require an 8 bit depth. A byte is equal to 8 bits, so byte size is the bit depth divided by 8. A gray scale bit depth of 8-16 represents a range of 1-2 bytes of storage that would be required per pixel in the image matrix. A gray scale bit depth of 12 produces 2^{12} or 4,096 gray levels that are available for diagnosis.

The radiologic community has promulgated a digital standard for imaging known as the Digital Imaging and Communication in Medicine (DICOM) standard. It is designed to ensure that all

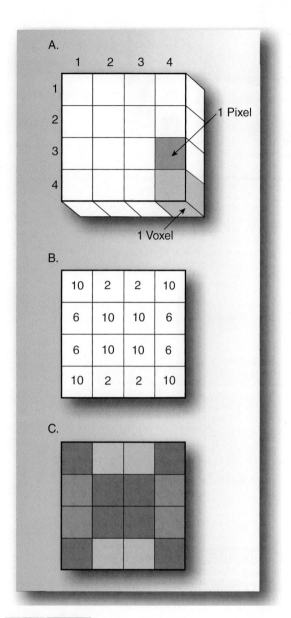

FIGURE 24-2 Digital image matrix expressions: (A) a matrix; (B) a matrix with numerical values; and (C) a matrix with visual density values corresponding to the numerical values in B.

equipment from all manufacturers who choose to adhere to the standard are speaking the same computer language that can be understood across manufacturer and device lines. For example, a central display or printing unit needs to be able to understand how to handle a CT image from one

manufacturer's scanner as well as a digital fluoroscopy image from a different manufacturer and be able to send both to a teleradiology system if necessary. The original DICOM standard was for output devices, while subsequent standards require that both input and output data meet the same compatibility standards. DICOM imaging now includes compatibility via a database system known as Health Level 7 (HL7). This standard includes linkage of the patient images with the patient's electronic medical record (EMR).

 DIGITAL IMAGE QUALITY

Data Characteristics

The quality of the data acquired from the image receptor is measured by its frequency, contrast, and noise.

Frequency. The frequency data is the raw data to which a Fourier transformation is applied to create the digital image. The acquired frequency is a measure of the total amount of contrast within the image. A high-contrast image has high frequency, while a low contrast image has low frequency.

Contrast. As with any image contrast, the acquired contrast is a measure of the differences between the data values. A **direct** relationship exists between subject contrast and acquired data contrast. When the subject contrast is high, the acquired data contrast will be high.

Noise. Image noise is random background information that is detected but does not contribute to image quality. It is congruent with audio noise, such as the static "white noise" heard on frequencies between radio stations. White noise is visualized as "snow" on frequencies between television stations. It is measured as the **signal-to-noise ratio** (S/N). A high S/N indicates little noise in the image. Most fluoroscopic image noise is from electronic sources (e.g., the television chain). Background noise can be seen when the unit is used without a subject, although static digital images also contain visual noise. The noisiest component of most digital systems is the television camera. Commercial systems often have an S/N of 200 but the high-resolution

FIGURE 24-3 **The effect of matrix size on resolution.** *(Photographs courtesy of Doug Raver, James A. Rhodes State College)*

systems used in digital fluoroscopy have an S/N between 500 and 1,000.

Although noise looks like quantum mottle, the effect of the noise level on the digital image is more like the effect of base plus fog on radiographic film. Image noise has an **inverse** relationship to contrast. Increased noise decreases image contrast. Conversely, increased image contrast tends to obscure or decrease noise. The effect of image noise on density is irrelevant in digital imaging, because the computer can easily compensate for lack of density as long as sufficient contrast exists to differentiate diagnostic data from noise.

Display Qualities

The density and contrast of the digital image are controlled by varying the numerical values of each pixel. The human visual range encompasses 32 or fewer shades of gray, while the photon beam that exits the patient encompasses over 1,000 shades. Most digital image detectors are sensitive to the majority of these 1,000 differences. Because the range of stored densities is so much wider than the visual range, any digital image is only a small part of the total data obtained by the computer. Each image is only a "window" on the total range of data (Figure 24-4). The computer can easily change the level and width of the display window by mathematical recalculations.

The quantity of information stored for each pixel varies depending on the gray scale imaging abilities of the system. For example, if a black and white image is desired with no intermediate shades of gray, each pixel will require a single bit. Each pixel will either be turned on for white or off for black. When shades of gray are required, as for all diagnostic images, as many as 32 bits may be required per pixel.

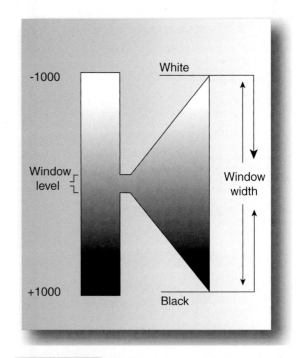

FIGURE 24-4 Digital image windows. The window level can be moved up and down the density scale. The window width can be expanded and contracted.

A 512 × 512 CT image at a 12-bit depth requires 3,145,728 bits (393,216 bytes or 394 Kb).

The radiographer usually controls which portion of this vast amount of information will be seen by controlling the display image density and contrast recorded on the hardcopy from which many radiologists diagnose, although more and more radiologists are reading from monitors. This practice makes the radiographer responsible for choosing the appropriate density and contrast ranges to be dis-

FIGURE 24-5   A clinical example of window level and width changes. Computed tomography of the chest requires two images to demonstrate the entire range of diagnostic densities. **(A)** High window level and narrow window width demonstrate the mediastinum and chest wall. **(B)** Low window level and wide window width demonstrate the lung fields. *(Courtesy of Van Wert County Hospital, Van Wert, OH)*

played. It is critical that radiographers who are required to produce digital images be familiar with the manner in which the computer determines what portion of the image information will be displayed. Careful image processing is critical to avoid obscuring diagnostically critical information.

Window Level.   When the values of each pixel are changed by addition or subtraction, the total value of the entire image changes. Because a computer can express a vast range of values, it can "see" image densities far below and beyond the range of human vision. One of the most important values of digital imaging is the ability of the computer to mathematically bring density differences into the visual range from extremely low-input doses that would produce densities far below the normal range of vision.

The **window level controls image density.** There is a **direct** relationship between window level and image density (see Figure 24-4). When the window level is increased, image density increases. The window level must be adjusted to the proper level to display diagnostically relevant information. Information outside the chosen window level is lost from diagnosis. In some instances, two images may have to be produced to visualize an appropriate range of densities. For example, in routine chest CT an image

with appropriate densities for the mediastinum and chest wall must be recorded in addition to a second image with appropriate densities for the lung fields (Figure 24-5).

Window Width.   When the values of each pixel are changed by multiplication or division, the value range of the entire image changes. A computer can expand or compress image densities to fill the range of human vision. Window width changes are sometimes called gray scale expansion or compression. Another important value of digital imaging is the ability of the computer to mathematically expand the visual density differences from similar input doses that would produce contrast far below the normal range of vision.

The **window width controls image contrast.** There is an **inverse** relationship between window width and image contrast (see Figure 24-4). When the window width is increased, image contrast decreases. An extremely wide window width requires the computer to ignore fine contrast differences in order to display the entire range of data. An extremely narrow window width requires the computer to ignore a large amount of data outside the chosen range. For this reason, **window width can be said to control visibility of detail.** Extremely narrow window widths may cause an objectionable

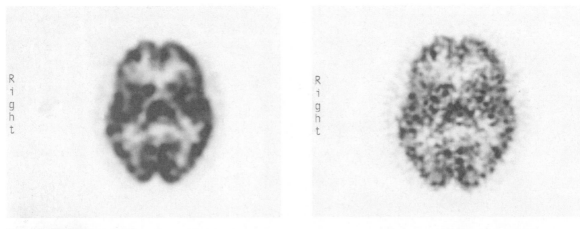

FIGURE 24-6 Low-pass filtering or smoothing. Transverse brain sections from a nuclear medicine study: (A) smoothed, and (B) noisier filter. *(Courtesy of Mike Ballistrea, Department of Nuclear Medicine, Meridia Hillcrest Hospital, Mayfield Heights, OH)*

increase in the image noise level. Information outside the chosen window width is lost from diagnosis. The window width must be adjusted to display a maximum amount of diagnostically relevant contrast.

Resolution. Resolution is controlled by the matrix size, as discussed above. There is a direct relationship between matrix size and image resolution (see Figure 24-2). When matrix size is increased, image resolution increases. Matrix size is not variable within a system. It is controlled by the quantity of image detectors and the accompanying electronics built into the system.

As discussed in Chapter 40, the primary limitation on digital images is the raster scan pattern of the display CRT. Commercial units achieve only 525 lines of interlaced scanning in which only 262.5 lines are scanned in one pass. This produces only 1–2 lp/mm for diagnostic imaging. The frequency response of the incoming signal is termed the **bandwidth.** The bandwidth also affects the resolution. In the United States, commercial television is broadcast at 4 MHz, which produces about 320 lines of resolution.

Progressive scanning increases resolution slightly by scanning all 525 lines in order. **Slow scanning** also increases resolution but cannot be used in real-time dynamic studies with digital fluoroscopy. High-resolution video is now available commercially and has been used in radiological ap-

plications for some time. The raster pattern is increased to 1,050 lines (often called a 1,000-line system) and the bandwidth is increased to 20 MHz, which produces about 800 lines of resolution. The result is a resolving ability of about 5–7 lp/mm.

Filtering. Digital filtering of images utilizes the computer to extract more diagnostic information. It is usually accomplished by transforming the image into frequencies, mathematically altering the frequency by convolution and then using deconvolution and an inverse Fourier transformation to reproduce the image. The computer either accentuates or suppresses selected frequencies during the filtering process. Digitized image filters are classified as low-pass, band-pass, or high-pass, although various equipment manufacturers have developed trade names and added unique modifications to many of them. The term **masking** is sometimes applied to the filtering process to indicate which frequencies have been suppressed. Masking of high frequencies produces low-pass filtering and vice versa.

Low-pass filtering either amplifies or deletes all but the low frequencies. It frequently appears to reduce image contrast and is often used to remove high-frequency noise, especially when very little data is available (Figure 24-6). Low-pass filtering can also be accomplished by averaging each pixel's value

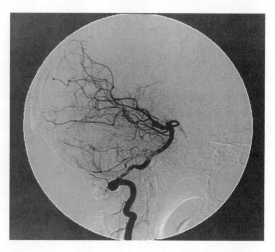

FIGURE 24-7 High-pass filtering or sharpening. Edge enhancement is demonstrated on these digital subtraction angiograms: (A) normal image, and (B) with high-pass filtering. *(Courtesy of Rick Halker, Lima Memorial Hospital, Lima, OH)*

with that of adjacent pixels. This type of low-pass filtering is sometimes called **smoothing.** Nine-point smoothing averages each pixel with the 8 adjacent pixels to accomplish a 9-pixel average. Low-radiation count nuclear medicine studies often use smoothing techniques.

Band-pass filtering either amplifies or deletes all but a selected range or band of frequencies. It is useful in the elimination of characteristic emission peaks, or in nuclear medicine, when a particular characteristic emission permits the localization of an injected radioisotope.

High-pass filtering either amplifies or deletes all **but** the high frequencies. It often appears to increase

image contrast and is sometimes called **edge enhancement** filtering or **sharpening** (Figure 24-7). When the frequencies that represent structures of interest can be identified, as in contrast medium filled vessels, amplification of their frequencies can produce an edge enhancement effect while other frequencies are actually suppressed. The result is an image with edge enhancement and greatly increased contrast. This type of high-pass filtering is useful in digital vascular imaging and in digital mammography. However, extremely small structures can sometimes be buried in an edge, and undesirable edges are usually enhanced as well as those that are of diagnostic value.

SUMMARY

The future of medical imaging lies in computerized applications of the numerous modalities. The method by which these imaging modalities have been computerized is digital processing of imaging information.

Computers are devices that process information. Analog computers handle data composed of continuously varying electrical currents. Digital

computers handle data composed of definite quantities of current (for example, current on versus current off). All medical imaging is achieved with digital computers, often from information that has been processed by an analog-to-digital converter (ADC). Computers use two types of information: operating instructions, called the program, and collected facts, called data. Programs are called software, while computer equipment is called hardware.

Computers operate from a binary machine language with a two-symbol alphabet. Because electrical currents are most easily understood as being either on or off, the binary system consists of information recorded as either a 0 for off or a 1 for on. Each binary number is called a bit, for binary digits. An 8-bit word is called a byte. Computer memory is often rated in terms of the total byte memory.

The CPU directs information to and from the various components that make up the computer system. Information is stored in a computer's memory and is classified as read-only memory (ROM) or random-access memory (RAM). Peripheral devices permit input or output of information to and from the CPU and include memory storage devices, along with a variety of input and output devices.

A digital image is one that has been converted into numerical values for transmission or processing. A detector of some type must be used to acquire the image information. A matrix is a square series of boxes that gives form to the image. The individual matrix boxes are known as picture elements or pixels. Pixel size determines resolution. In medical imaging each pixel value corresponds to a three-dimensional volume of tissue, known as a voxel.

The quality of the data acquired from the image receptor is measured by its frequency, contrast, and noise. The density and contrast of the digital image are controlled by varying the numerical values of each pixel. The window level controls image density. Window width changes the gray scale expansion or compression and therefore controls contrast. Resolution is controlled by the matrix size.

Digital filtering of images is usually accomplished by transforming the image into frequencies, mathematically altering the frequency by convolution and then using deconvolution and an inverse Fourier transformation to reproduce the image. The computer either accentuates or suppresses selected frequencies during the filtering process. Digitized image filters are classified as low-pass, band-pass, or high-pass.

REVIEW QUESTIONS

1. What is the difference between analog and digital computers?

2. Why do computers operate from a binary machine language?

3. What is the function of the central processing unit?

4. What is the most common input device?

5. How is a digital image acquired?

6. What is image noise?

7. How do the window level and the window width affect the digital image display?

8. What are the three types of digital image filtering methods?

REFERENCES AND RECOMMENDED READING

Bedard, L., & Delisle, C. (1992). Image digitizing in conventional radiology. *Canadian Journal of Medical Radiation Technology, 23*(2), 67–70.

Berland, L. L. (1987). *Practical CT technology and techniques.* New York: Raven Press.

Brody, W. R. (1984). *Digital radiography.* New York: Raven Press.

Brody, W. R., & Macovski, A. (1981). Dual-energy digital radiography. *Diagnostic Imaging, 3,* 18–25.

Burns, C. (1993). Using computed digital radiography effectively. *Seminars in Radiologic Technology, 1*(1), 24–35.

Bushberg, J. T., Seibert, J. A., Leidholdt, E. M., & Boone, J. M. (2003). *The essential physics of medical imaging* (2nd ed.) Baltimore: Williams & Wilkins.

Bushong, S. C. (2004). *Radiologic science for technologists: Physics, biology, and protection* (8th ed.). St. Louis, MO: Elsevier/C. V. Mosby.

Curry, T. S., Dowdey, J. E., & Murry, R. C. (1990). *Christensen's introduction to the physics of diagnostic radiology* (4th ed.). Philadelphia: Lea and Febiger.

De Brusk, P. D. (1983). Digital x-ray imaging: The basics. *Radiologic Technology, 54*(4), 280.

Dobbins, J. T., & Powell, A. O. (1989). Variable compensation technique for digital radiography of the chest. *Radiology, 157,* 451.

Dreyer, K., Mehta, A., & Thrall, J. (2002). *PACS: A guide to the digital revolution.* New York: Springer Verlag.

Forster, E. (1985). *Equipment for diagnostic radiography.* Lancaster: MTP Press.

Glazer, H. S., Muka, E., Sagel, S. S., & Jost, R. G. (1994). New techniques in chest radiography. *Radiologic Clinics of North America, 32*(4), 711–729.

Gould, R. G. (1984). Digital hardware in radiography and fluoroscopy. *Applied Radiology, 13,* 137–140.

Hindel, R. (1983). Digital imaging: The technology of the future. *The Canadian Journal of Medical Radiation Technology, 14*(4), 128.

Hedrick, W. R. (1993). Digital image acquisition and processing in computed radiography. *Seminars in Radiologic Technology, 1*(1), 6–15.

Hruby, W. (2001). *Digital revolution in radiology.* New York: Springer Wein.

Huda, W., & Szeverenyi, N. M. (1999, February). The filmless radiology department: A primer. *Applied Radiology,* 30–34.

Kuni, C. C. (1988). *Introduction to computers and digital processing in medical imaging.* Chicago: Year Book Medical.

Kushner, D. C. (1986). Radiation dose reduction in the evaluation of scoliosis: An application of digital radiography. *Radiology, 154,* 175.

Long, B. W. (1989). Computed radiography: Photostimulable phosphor image plate technology. *Radiologic Technology, 61*(2), 107–112.

Malott, J. C., & Fodor, J. (1982). Digital video angiography. *Radiologic Technology, 54*(2), 83–89.

Marjois, J. D. (1985). Minimizing dose associated with digital subtraction angiography. *The Canadian Journal of Medical Radiation Technology, 16*(4), 141.

Mistretta, C. A., & Crummy, A. B. (1981). Digital fluoroscopy. In C. M. Coulam, J. J. Erickson, F. D. Rollo, & A. E. James, *The physical basis of medical imaging.* New York: Appleton-Century-Crofts.

Mistretta, C. A., Crummy, A. B., Strother, C. M., & Sackett, J. F. (1982). *Digital subtraction arteriography: An application of computerized fluoroscopy.* Chicago: Year Book.

Nishitami, H. (1986). Dual energy projection radiography using a condenser x-ray generator and digital radiography apparatus. *Radiology, 154,* 533.

Schaefer, C. (1989). Improved control of image optical density with low-dose digital and conventional radiography in bedside imaging. *Radiology, 153,* 713.

Sherrier, R., & McAdams, H. P. (1986, July). Digital processing of portable films can reduce need for repeat studies. *Diagnostic Imaging,* 117.

Siegel, E., & Kolodner, R. (2001). *Filmless radiology.* New York: Springer.

Smith, C. B. (1984). Physical principles of digital radiography. *Radiography, 50*(590), 41–44.

Toth, B., Edmonds, E. W., Rowlands, J. A., Porter, A. J., & Hynes, D. M. (1985). The 'digital' compromise. *The Canadian Journal of Medical Radiation Technology, 16*(2), 28.

Wiederhold, G., Shortliffe, E., Fagan, L., & Perreault, L. (2000). *Medical informatics: Computer applications in health care and biomedicine (health informatics)* (2nd ed.) New York: Springer.

Wilson, P. (1984). Digital imaging: An introduction. *Radiography, 50*(590), 449.

(Reprinted by permission of the International Society of
Radiographers and Radiological Technicians from K. C. Clark
Archives, Middlesex Hospital, London, England, Courtesy of Dr.
Marion Frank)

The Case of the Deep Sea Rodeo

This creature was radiographed after a sojourn in the deep. What is it?

Answers to the case studies can
be found in Appendix E.

CHAPTER 25

Digital Radiography

Barbara Smith, Richard R. Carlton

> My body is the frame wherein 'tis held,
>
> And perspective it is the painter's art.
>
> For through the painter must you see his skill,
>
> To find where your true image pictured lies;
>
> *Shakespeare, Sonnet XXIV*

KEY TERMS

computed radiography (CR)
direct acquisition
direct digital radiography (DR)
flat field detector
flat panel detector
histogram
indirect acquisition

OBJECTIVES

Upon completion of this chapter, the student should be able to:

- Describe various digital radiography image receptor and detector systems.

- Explain critical elements used in the different digital radiography systems.

- Discuss limitations inherent in each of the currently available digital radiography systems.

- Describe the process by which the digital radiography histogram is acquired and the display algorithm is applied to the collected data.

- Explain why digital radiography systems have significantly greater latitude than conventional film-screen radiography systems.

- Analyze elements of digital radiography systems that make them prone to violation of ALARA radiation protection concepts.

- Explain the causes of several digital radiography artifact problems.

INTRODUCTION

Digital radiography systems replace traditional film with a reusable detector. These systems can be divided into two groups, either "cassette based" or "cassette-less." The cassette-based system uses a **photostimulable storage phosphor imaging plate** (PSP or IP) inside a cassette. This cassette can be used in a bucky or for portable exams, similar to traditional film screen. Once the PSP is exposed, it is taken to a reader to process the plate and create the image. The term used for this system is **computed radiography (CR),** and it is considered "indirect digital" because the radiographer must move the detector between image acquisition and display. Cassette-less systems are considered **direct digital radiography (DR)** because the detector and reader are a permanent part of a table or wall unit; therefore, a cassette is not needed. There are a number of detector configurations used in DR that employ either direct acquisition (without scintillator) or indirect acquisition (with scintillator) (Figure 25-1).

Indirect acquisition systems use a two-part process involving a scintillator (which converts incoming x-ray photons to light) and a photodetector (which converts light into an electronic signal). Indirect systems include those that use photostimulable storage phosphor imaging plates (IP), charged coupled devices (CCD), and silicon.

Direct acquisition systems directly convert incoming x-ray photons to an electronic signal. These systems use selenium and are sometimes referred to as direct radiography (DR) systems (Table 25-1).

The term **flat panel** (or **flat field**) **detectors** is also being used to describe both the indirect amorphous silicon and the direct amorphous selenium plates that are being used in some digital systems.

HISTORICAL DEVELOPMENT

Computed radiography (CR) first became available in the early 1980s when it was introduced by Fuji but, as happens with many new technologies, there were problems with high cost and poor image quality. As computer technology has advanced, so too has the ability of CR to produce images comparable to, and in many instances better than, film. Currently, a number of manufacturers produce CR

FIGURE 25-1 Image capture systems. *(Courtesy of Barry Burns, University of North Carolina, Division of Radiologic Science)*

TABLE 25-1. Most Common Computed Radiography/Digital Radiography Systems

Type		Detector	Scintillator	Charge Reader	Company
CR Indirect		Photostimulable phosphor		Laser	Fuji, Kodak, Agfa
DR Indirect	Flat panel	Amorphous silicon	CsI	TFT	Philips, Siemens, GE
DR Direct	Flat panel	Amorphous selenium		TFT	Kodak, Hologic
DR Indirect		Rare earth intensifying screen		CCD	Swiss ray
DR Indirect	Flat panel	Amorphous silicon	Rare earth screen	TFT	Canon

plates and processor systems. Many of them have Internet Web sites with a considerable amount of information on the advantages of their particular systems. (Commercial Web sites with information on computed radiography include *www.fujimed.com, www.kodak.com, www.agfaus.com, www.ge.com.*)

INDIRECT PHOTOSTIMULABLE PHOSPHOR IMAGING PLATE SYSTEMS

Photostimulable Imaging Plates

A photostimulable phosphor imaging plate is a rigid sheet with several layers that are designed to record and enhance transmission of the image from a beam of ionizing radiation. The layers include a protective layer, a phosphor layer, a support layer made of polyester, a conductor layer, and a light shield layer (Figure 25-2). The protective layer simply insulates the imaging plate from handling trauma. The phosphor layer holds the photostimulable phosphor, which is the active component in the plate. The support layer is simply a base on which to coat the other layers. The conductor layer grounds the plate to eliminate electrostatic problems and absorb light to increase sharpness. Finally, the light shielding layer prevents light from erasing data on the imaging plate or leaking through the backing, decreasing the spatial resolution. The imaging plate is loaded into a cassette that looks much like a radiographic film and intensifying screen cassette. Con-

sequently, computed radiography cassettes are sometimes referred to as "filmless cassettes."

In order for CR to function, the imaging plate material must have the ability to store and release the image information in a usable form. The most common phosphor with characteristics favorable for CR is barium fluorohalide bromides and iodides with europium activators (BaFBr:Eu and BaFI:Eu). The halides are approximately 85 percent bromide and 15 percent iodine. Due to the lower atomic number of barium, the K-edge attenuates best between 35 and 50 keV, somewhat lower than the typical K-edge for rare-earth intensifying screens, but well within the diagnostic range (35 keV is a typical average energy production from an exposure of 80 kVp). However, **the absorption efficiency above and below 35 to 50 keV is below that of rare-earth intensifying screens.** This means that more exposure may be needed in order to have similar quantum noise outside the optimal energy range. Also, the imaging plate phosphor will absorb more low-energy scatter than the rare-earth phosphor and film, which means appropriate kVp, and masking must be used to achieve optimal images. **This also makes the imaging plate more sensitive to scatter both before and after it is sensitized through exposure to the x-ray beam.**

Some other compounds that may be used in the PSP are BaSrFBr:Eu, RbBr:T1,RbCl, and CsBr:Eu.

Latent Image Production

The incident x-ray beam produces a latent image within the photostimulable fluorohalides that comprise the active layer of the imaging plate (IP) in the cassette. When the fluorohalides luminesce, they do not release all the energy absorbed from the incident x-ray beam. Although some light is emitted, the phosphors retain sufficient energy in the form of a latent image. It is this latent image that will be used to create a digital image for the computer to record and display.

This latent image is actually created by energy transfer during photoelectric interactions. The photoelectrons that are produced then excite a number of low-energy electrons to create "holes" in the crystal phosphor. Although about half of the electron holes will recompose and emit light photons, the fluorohalides will hold or trap the other half of the

FIGURE 25-2 Photostimulate phosphor imaging plate showing layers.

Protective layer
Phosphor layer
Conductor layer
Support layer
Light shield layer
Backing layer

electrons, thus creating the "holes" at the Europium sites. These Europium electron holes are the actual latent image. **The latent image will lose about 25 percent of its energy in 8 hours, so it is important to process the cassette shortly after exposure.** Cassettes stored for several days after exposure and before processing lose most of their latent image.

The latent image is processed by loading the cassette into an image reader device (IRD) where the imaging plate is scanned by a helium-neon laser beam. These laser beam scans cause the phosphors to emit the stored latent image in the form of light photons, which are detected by photosensitive receptors converted to an electrical signal, which is in turn converted to a unique digital value for that level of luminescence. Once the plate is read, it is erased to remove all vestiges of the latent image.

Image Acquisition

Image acquisition begins with x-ray exposure to the imaging plate. Since the imaging plate is placed in a cassette, it can be used tabletop or with a grid, similar to the use of film screen. The rules of positioning hold true for CR; areas that are clipped or poorly positioned cannot be corrected with this or any other system. **It is the responsibility of the radiographer to select proper technique; chronic overexposure should be avoided.** Radiation exposure causes fluorescence of the imaging plate but some of the energy of the beam is also stored in the plate. It is this stored energy that is used to create an image during reading and processing. Some of the electrons, which are excited by the absorbed energy, are trapped in the crystal structure of the phosphor at higher energy levels. Thus a latent image is stored in the imaging plate, similar to a latent image on film, but with wider latitude. The imaging plate then needs to be read to release the stored information, which can be manipulated by the computer and used in either soft or hardcopy form.

Reading Digital Radiography Data

Reading the imaging plate involves a finely focused laser beam that frees the trapped electrons, allowing them to return to a lower energy state, referred to as

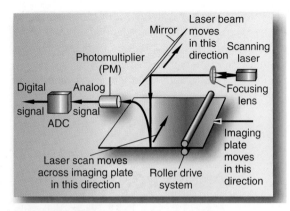

FIGURE 25-3 Photostimulable phosphor imaging plate reader. The plate is moved through the system while a focused laser scans the surface in a raster pattern. When the laser strikes the surface of the imaging plate, the emitted light is detected by the PM tube, which sends an analog signal to the ADC for conversion into a digital signal, which is then sent to the computer for processing and display.

photostimulated luminescence (PSL). Electrons moving to a lower energy state release blue-purple light photons in proportion to the absorbed radiation. The laser light beam is directed to the imaging plate through a series of components; this beam must be monitored since the intensity of the blue light from the imaging plate is dependent on the power of the laser beam. Scanning of the imaging plate by the laser occurs in a raster pattern as the plate is fed through the processor. The light liberated from the imaging plate is emitted in all directions and is collected by an optical system that directs it to one or more photomultiplier (PM) tubes, which are sensitive only to the blue light. The PM tube converts the visible light into an electronic signal whose output is in analog form. This analog signal must be converted into a digital signal before the computer can work with the image information. This is accomplished with an analog to digital converter (ADC). The entire reading process is illustrated in Figure 25-3. The PM tubes adjust the output signal range so it can be optimally handled during the digitization process. Any residual image left on the imaging plate is erased by exposure to an intense light to release any remaining trapped electrons.

Imaging
Plate (IP)

Stacker

Stacker

Erasure
unit

Laser

Laser
scanner

Image Reader

Laser Printer

FIGURE 25-4 Internal view of image reader and stacker with relationship to a chest unit and laser printer. Image can also be sent to PACS. *(Courtesy of FUJIFILM Medical Systems USA.)*

When the light is released from the plate along the line the laser has scanned, the PMT is performing a point-by-point readout along this line. There are two new techniques to speed up this process. One method would read the light from the PSP line by line to increase data acquisition speed. Another way to speed up the process and at the same time obtain more information is to use a dual-sided PSP, which has a screen on both sides that can be scanned and read simultaneously. The primary advantage of dual-sided reading is improved spacial resolution.

The reading and erasing of an imaging plate can occur in a single processor unit, as seen in Figure 25-4, or it can be accomplished with separate desktop processor and erasure units. The larger units typically allow stacking and loading of multiple cassettes, whereas a desktop processor requires the imaging plate to be removed from the cassette and fed into the processor. Plate throughput can average anywhere from 30 plates/hour to over 200 plates/hour depending on the type of processor used. Workload and cost will determine which unit will best serve department requirements. There are also tables and upright bucky units that contain multiple PSP plates and a reader in the

unit, so no cassette handling is required. The units move and process plates after each exposure, allowing the radiographer to view images in a monitor within the control booth. Fuji has these combined units, which can process over 200 images per hour.

The finely focused laser beam that scans each line of the imaging plate correlates to one line spacing or pixel dimension. The analog signal emitted by the PM tube has an infinite range of values that the ADC must convert into limited discrete values that can be stored as digital code. Pixel depth or the number of bits that represent an analog signal will determine the number of density values. Typically, there are 10 ($2^{10} = 1,024$), 12 ($2^{12} = 4,096$), and 16 ($2^{16} = 65,536$) bit ADCs, which will determine the density values for the analog signal and so the gray scale of the system. Therefore, the number of bits/pixels will determine how many density values can be present and so affect the density and contrast of an imaging system. Another important variable related to pixels is spatial resolution. **The smaller the pixel, the higher the spatial resolution.** Pixel size is dependent on the sampling frequency, which is expressed in pixels/mm.

The matrix size is dependent on the sampling frequency and the image receptor size. At 10 pixels/mm a 14" × 17" plate would have a matrix of ∼3,500 × 4,200, while at 5 pixels/mm the 14" × 17" would have a matrix of ∼1,750 × 2,100. Pixel size, matrix, and bit depth determine the size of the computer file for a given image.

To accomplish the task of changing the analog signal into the correct components for digital manipulation, the analog signal must be sampled in order to find the location and size of the signal. It must then be quantitized to determine the average value of the signal in the sample. During preprocessing, the CR system must also determine the orientation of the part on the plate as well as the number of projections present per plate. Locating the image data on the plate allows the system to sample and manipulate only the clinically useful information. This raw data from scanning will have a range of values related to how much radiation the plate received. Areas outside the lines of collimation will have the lowest exposure, therefore, the lowest values. The highest values will lie within the collimated field, allowing the system to locate the useful information or data and disregard the data outside these lines. This is why markers placed outside the collimated field may not appear in the processed image. The method used by Fuji to recognize the clinically useful area on the imaging plate is known as exposure data recognition (EDR), which has three modes: automatic (auto), semiautomatic (semi), and fixed. Automatic mode adjusts latitude and sensitivity for the image. It is also used when placing more than one image on a cassette.

There are certain expectations that need to be met when placing more than one image per plate. The plate can be programmed and then used for a number of different scanning detection patterns (Figure 25-5). **The beam and part should be centered within each pattern, and collimation should be parallel and equidistant from the edges of the imaging plate** (Figure 25-6). The semiautomatic mode automatically adjusts only sensitivity, while the reading latitude is fixed. It is used when the image is centered, but the collimation borders are not parallel or equidistant from the plate edges. **Fixed mode is similar to film screen processing in that latitude and sensitivity are fixed, requiring correct technique factors to be used to obtain a diagnostic image since this mode will not correct density problems.**

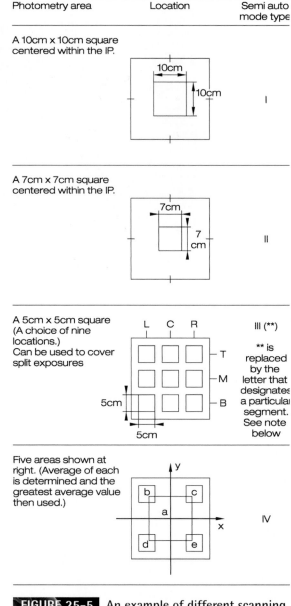

FIGURE 25-5 An example of different scanning detection patterns available on a Fuji system set for semiautomatic exposure data recognition (EDR) mode. *(Courtesy of FUJIFILM Medical Systems USA)*

FIGURE 25-7 Histogram of the gray scale generated from a computed radiography image by Laurie Cesar from the Mayo Clinic. The vertical axis represents the number of pixels. The horizontal axis represents the quantity of information (image density). Low density is to the left, high density to the right. *(Reprinted by permission of the American Society of Radiologic Technologists, 1997)*

FIGURE 25-6 Nonparallel collimation artifact. Histograms require that collimation edges be parallel to the sides of the imaging plate.

During initial processing a **histogram** is generated from the image data that allows the CR system to find the useful signal by locating the minimum and maximum signal within the anatomical regions of interest in the image. To generate a histogram, the scanned area is divided into pixels and the signal intensity for each pixel is determined. An example of a histogram is shown in Figure 25-7.

The shape of a histogram will correspond to the specific anatomy and technique used for an exam. This will be used to compare to the look-up table (LUT) data that has the standard contrast, speed, and latitude for that exam. Image processing will provide the proper gray scale, regardless of variations in kVp and mAs, resulting in consistent images. However, if the exposure values are extremely outside the normal range, the system cannot compensate and produce a diagnostic image.

The appropriate anatomical menu is selected by body part by the radiographer when the imaging plate is loaded into the reading unit. The histogram is also used to eliminate unnecessary information outside the collimated field, like scatter radiation, which degrades the final image. Once the true patient image data is identified, that information is rescaled to stabilize image density and contrast. This is when exposure errors are corrected. Algorithms, which are unique to each manufacturer, process the data once the exposed area is determined and the signal histogram is established. Fugi uses MFP (multi-objective frequency), tonescaling is used by Kodak, and Agfa is using a MUSICA (multi-scale image contrast algorithm) system.

The correct anatomical menu should be selected prior to processing the imaging plate; otherwise the image will not process the correct density and contrast. Most modern CR readers allow preprocessing of incorrectly run plates. Figure 25-8 is an example of a typical chest histogram with the various anatomical areas annotated on the histogram. Figure 25-9 illustrates how a computed radiography system can analyze a pediatric chest histogram and then display regions of interest outside the lung. Finally, it is critical to adhere to uniform positioning and collimation procedures when using a computed radiography system. The reading system must be given consistent data to analyze if it is to provide consistent diagnostic quality results.

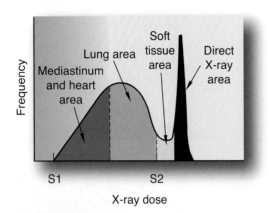

FIGURE 25-8 Example of a histogram that would be produced by a normal chest radiograph. *(Courtesy of FUJIFILM Medical Systems USA)*

FIGURE 25-9 Example of a histogram that would be produced by a pediatric chest with potential computerized enhancements possible by displaying density ranges typical of other regions of interest outside normal lung densities. *(Courtesy of FUJIFILM Medical Systems USA)*

The knee images in Figure 25-10 illustrate the ability of a CR system to adjust the histogram into the visible diagnostic density range. Look carefully at Figures 25-10A and B as compared to C and D and then to E and F. While it may appear that all three CR images (B, D, and F) have appropriate density ranges as compared to the conventional radiography images, a careful inspection will show that CR image 25–10B is extremely grainy and as a result is outside the acceptable range for detail. This is an example of the CR histogram adjusting for density but lacking adequate data to fill in an acceptable level of detail.

In the past, most CR systems relied completely on the technologist's accuracy of selecting the correct anatomical menu before the imaging plate was processed. This means that if an image of a knee was processed as a chest, the resulting image may not be of diagnostic quality (Figure 25-11). New generation CR readers store the "raw" data (pre-histogram analysis) in the workstation. This feature allows images that were processed with an incorrect anatomical menu to be re-processed using the correct anatomical menu with no loss of its original quality.

The raw data has to go through a number of manipulations to achieve the optimum gray scale range to give a useful diagnostic image. A gradation processing function maps the density values in a nonlinear curve as a basis for adjusting density and contrast. These gradation curves serve to match image contrast requirements to specific exam types or to emphasize specific densities, such as lung fields. The curves are manufacturer specific, but can function in much the same way as $D_{log}E$ curves of different film types. Programs within the computer can manipulate the contrast scale, or the slope of the $D_{log}E$ curve. For example, if the slope becomes steeper, contrast increases in the image. Most CR systems allow you to view the response ($D_{log}E$) curve on the workstation monitor as the image is manipulated.

Spatial frequency processing is also possible with CR systems. It should be used when it is necessary to increase image sharpness. Edge enhancement is obtained with an unsharp mask technique. In this technique the original image is blurred by a low-pass filter, which is subtracted from the original to leave only high spatial frequency signal. This signal is amplified and added back into the exam data to produce an image with higher frequencies

65 kVp	4 mAs
65 kVp	4 mAs
65 kVp	16 mAs
65 kVp	16 mAs

A   B   E   F

C   D

| 65 kVp | 8 mAs |
| 65 kVp | 8 mAs |

FIGURE 25-10 Comparison of conventional and computed radiography images of the knee. These images illustrate the ability of a CR system to adjust the histogram of the incoming data into the visible diagnostic density range. While it may appear that all three CR images (on the right side) have appropriate density ranges as compared to the conventional radiography images, a careful inspection will show that image B is extremely grainy and as a result is outside the acceptable range for detail. This is an example of the CR histogram adjusting for density but lacking adequate data to fill in an acceptable level of detail.

FIGURE 25-11 Histogram error artifact. Selection of an adult histogram used on a pediatric chest.

or edge enhancement. It is important to understand that edge enhancement techniques usually increase noise and as a result may produce lower quality images with higher base fog levels and lower contrast.

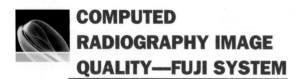

COMPUTED RADIOGRAPHY IMAGE QUALITY—FUJI SYSTEM

Although the image reader device analyzes the imaging plate exposure and adjusts the sensitivity of the receptors to ensure maximum data acquisition, it is still important for the radiographer to understand how to assess image quality. The computed radiography processing system indicates several values that are useful for this purpose. Although dif-

ferent manufacturers use different systems for this information, the basic concept is similar.

The Fuji computed radiography system uses an S number to assist in evaluating exposure. It is inversely proportional to the exposure reaching the imaging plate. For example, an S value of 200 indicates that the imaging plate received about 1 mR (approximately the same exposure necessary to produce a diagnostic density image with a typical 300 RS film-screen combination). A higher S value indicates that the imaging plate (IP) was underexposed, while a lower S value indicates overexposure of the IP. Properly exposed imaging plates should produce S values of 150–250. Figure 25-12 demonstrates a full range of over- and underexposed images.

Kilovoltage for computed radiography will control contrast similar to film radiography. However, some computed radiography manufacturers recommend avoiding the use of more than 80 kVp for non-grid imaging because higher kVp levels produce excessive fog that will decrease contrast significantly more than the same increase with a film-screen imaging receptor.

The Fuji system uses two types of CR plates with different speeds and resolution. The standard plate (ST-V) is used for exams that would typically use a 400 relative speed film-screen speed system and has resolution of around 5.0 lp/mm. The ST-V has a reflective layer between the phosphor layer and the conductive layer. For exams requiring lower speed and increased resolution, the high-resolution plate (HR) is used; it is comparable to a 100 film-screen speed system and has a resolution slightly greater than 5 lp/mm.

One advantage to CR is the wide dynamic range response of the imaging plate detector. Rather than the characteristic curve of film-screen systems, the response of an imaging plate to x-ray is linear. This linear response gives the imaging plate increased exposure latitude over film-screen (Figure 25-13). This means that areas that receive very little radiation can be enhanced by the computer instead of all the densities clumping around the toe of the $D_{log}E$ curve as they do when using a film receptor. Conversely, areas receiving greater exposure can be separated and brought down into the visible density range by the computer instead of all clumping around the shoulder of the $D_{log}E$ curve.

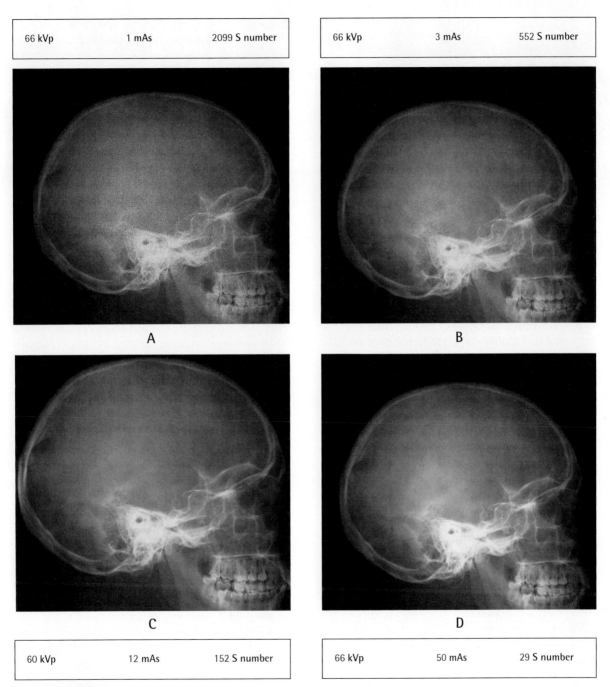

| 66 kVp | 1 mAs | 2099 S number |
| 66 kVp | 3 mAs | 552 S number |

A

B

C

D

| 60 kVp | 12 mAs | 152 S number |
| 66 kVp | 50 mAs | 29 S number |

FIGURE 25-12 A demonstration of over- and underexposure with a CR system. While it may appear that all four CR images have appropriate density ranges, a careful inspection will show that with the exception of image C, the Fuji S numbers are outside the optimal range of 150–250. Image A has an S number of 2099, which indicates that it was grossly underexposed, As a result, it exhibits excessive loss of detail and graininess. Image D has an S number of 29, which indicates that patient exposure was probably close to 10 times more than it should have been.

Density

—— Film-screen
—— Computed
radiograph

$D_{LOG}E$

FIGURE 25-13 Comparison of $D_{log}E$ curves of radiographic film and intensifying screens versus a digital computed radiography system. Note that the computed radiography system response is linear and does not have a toe or shoulder as the film–screen curve.

TOLERATION OF OVEREXPOSURE

An important extension of the density range occurs with CR with areas of much greater exposure because the imaging plate does not have a D_{max} curve. Instead it has a straight line that far surpasses the $D_{log}E$ curve of a film emulsion (see Figure 25-13). This creates a dangerous radiation safety problem because CR systems have an extremely high toleration for patient overexposure. When film is exposed beyond D_{max}, it actually reverses and begins to get lighter (as with duplicating film). The CR imaging plate continues to record the exposure and the computer can bring these densities down into the visible range. This is why a CR system can compensate for gross overexposure. This is also why the radiographer using CR must realize that **there is great danger in permitting personal professional standards to relax and routinely over-exposing all patients with the intention of the CR system adjusting the histogram to correct the** **exposure.** This practice is unethical, violates ALARA radiation protection guidelines, and is to be avoided at all times.

Digital processing requires the technologist to be knowledgeable in the details of CR image acquisition as well as post processing parameters and procedures. For example, many manufacturers state in their technical usage information that mAs has little effect on the visualization of image density. This can be a confusing statement for radiographers who are knowledgeable about the relationships between mAs and kVp and clearly understand how to control them when creating an optimal diagnostic image. What manufacturers are trying to convey is that the extended range of the straight line portion of the image receptor response curve allows a CR system to digitally process the image after exposure to bring the density into the visible range, even when the image receptor is grossly overexposed. This does not change the fact that changes in mAs will increase or decrease the quantity of photons received by the image receptor. These changes directly affect the quantity of information the image receptor passes on to the post processing system. Many images post processing systems may not require mAs settings as high as film-based image receptors did in the past, but this is why diagnostic quality images may now be produced with less mAs, not a reason to overexpose patients so the post processing system can adjust the display density downward.

Another important quality factor in digital processing is better known and tends to receive more attention because the results are immediately visible on the images: adequate mAs is required to activate any digital image receptor. Failure to use a high enough mAs setting produces quantum mottle, which produces a grainy, reticulated image for which digital post processing cannot compensate. This is why a minimum CR sensitivity number is required by many radiololgists to ensure they are diagnosing from an image that meets the minimum data requirements of the CR system.

There are multiple benefits inherent in this increased latitude, such as the ability to image structures of widely different attenuation values such as the chest, on the same image without loss of visibility of structures with widely different densities (such as lung vasculature and the mediastinum). (See

TABLE 25-2. Fuji Computed Radiography System Summary

System Limitations and Guidelines for Use

Corrects exposure errors >2X.

Images with low contrast or high mottle may be produced for exposure errors up to 50X.

To achieve optimal quality exposure must be set within a range of 2X.

Cannot compensate for low photon intensity (underexposure).

Cannot compensate for excessive scatter radiation.

The system cannot compensate for:

exposure >2X
insufficient mAs
insufficient kVp
excessive part size
excessive kVp
inadequate grid use

Photostimulable Phosphor Imaging Plates

Standard Plate (ST-V) ~ 300RS (~5.0 lp/mm)
High-Resolution Plate (HR) ~100RS (~5.0 lp/mm)

Exposure Data Recognition (EDR) Preprocessing Modes

AUTOmatic
entire image plate is scanned
requires beam and part centered to image plate
requires image margins parallel to image plate
requires image margins equidistant from edges

SEMIautomatic
center of image plate is scanned
requires image at center of image plate

FIXED
eliminates preprocessing
designed for use when anatomy cannot be centered to image plate
density and contrast depend on exposure set by radiographer

Image Labeling

L value
subject contrast (differential light intensities)
changes with kVp, scatter, part size
appropriate range 1.6–1.8
>2.2 = low inherent data contrast

S value
photomultiplier tube sensitivity used for final reading (exposure index)
Standard Plate (ST-V) appropriate range 150–250
<50 = gross patient overexposure
(may produce residual exposure on next use of image plate)
<100 = substantial patient overexposure
>400 = objectionable mottle
High-Resolution Plate (HR) appropriate range 50–100
<10 = gross patient overexposure (may produce residual exposure on next use of image plate)
<25 = substantial patient overexposure
>100 = objectionable mottle
inversely proportional to image plate exposure (reciprocal roentgen value)
2 = 100 mR
20 = 10 mR
200 = 1 mR (~400RS)
2,000 = 0.1 mR
20,000 = 0.01 mR

C values
baseline contrast and density shift values in image processing program

G setting
gradient

R setting
spatial frequency enhancement

Figures 25-8 and 25-9.) Another benefit is the increased margin for error in over- and underexposure to the receptor. CR can maintain a useful density over a wider latitude than allowable with film-screen. However, even though density can be maintained, the overall image quality may be poor if exposures range too far from optimal. **Images that are underexposed will show quantum mottle, even though the density is acceptable, while overexposed images will tend to suffer from low contrast.**

Table 25-2 provides a summary of the Fuji computed radiography system.

IMAGE ACQUISITION ELEMENTS

CR offers many advantages over traditional film-screen for obtaining diagnostic images; however, as with any system, there are pitfalls that must be recognized. To obtain high-quality images with minimal patient dose, a deeper understanding of CR is required. One of the big advantages of CR is the reduction of repeat exposures due to incorrect technique or to image various densities in the same anatomical region without repeat exposures. Two reasons CR has this advantage are the wide dynamic range of the imaging plate and the ability to use windowing and leveling in the image.

Computed radiography systems have a number of special elements as a result of their digitizing and processing of the image. Some of these special elements are functions of the digital acquisition of imaging data that occurs in the image receptor. Others are functions of the post processing software systems that handle the data output from the image receptor. Still others are functions of the digital display systems that create the final image that is visible to the technologist and physician. All of these special elements can directly affect the quality of the digital diagnostic image and must be understood by the radiographer in order to produce the highest possible quality image. Many manufacturers program their software with mathematical algorithms that will modify the data in a manner consistent with producing a desired result, such as images with high resolution, low contrast, rapid display, etc.

Sensitivity

The sensitivity of the various computed radiography image receptors is different for each manufacturer. Different manufacturers calibrate the response of their system with different beam qualities and report the results using parameters that have different dependencies on exposure. Therefore, it is extremely difficult to compare the sensitivity of one system with another. In addition, as manufacturers improve their systems they sometimes introduce entirely new image receptors and software enhancements that also cause sensitivity measures to change.

The exposure sensitivity of the imaging plate ranges from a minimum of 0.1 mR up to a maximum of 100 mR, a range of approximately 10,000:1. If soft tissue and bone densities are required, one exposure will give the information owing to the ability to change window levels. In order to evaluate the exposure for a CR image, most manufacturers have an exposure indicator that provides information on the average amount of radiation used for an image (Table 25-3).

Fuji uses a sensitivity number (S number) that is related to the amount of amplification required by the PM tube to adjust the digital image. The S number is inversely related to exposure in mR, so a large S number indicates a low exposure to the imaging plate, while a small S number reflects high mR. For example, an exposure of 1 mR has an S value of 200. Properly exposed images should have an S value around 150–250 for ST-V plates, reflecting appropriate patient dose.

Kodak's CR indicator system is called the exposure index, which is directly proportional to the radiation striking the imaging plate. An exposure of 0.1 mR has an exposure index of 1,000 while 1 mR in this system gives an exposure index of 2,000, and 10 mR results in an exposure index of 3,000. Properly exposed images should have an exposure index that ranges from 1,800 to 2,200.

The Agfa system uses log median exposure LgM; it compares the exposure level of an image to a baseline established for the department. Since it is based on a log system, an increase of 0.3 means the dose was doubled. Agfa also has a "speed class" that is similar to film-screen, like 200 and 400, that the radiographer selects before the plate is put in the reader. Techniques used by the radiographer will also need to reflect the speed class selected. Choosing the speed for the imaging plate will direct the

TABLE 25-3.	Exposure Index Numbers Relative to Imaging Plate Exposure				
Agfa LgM Speed Class			200		
Fuji S Value	2	20	200	2,000	20,000
Kodak Exposure Index		3,000	2,000	1,000	
mR	100	10	1	0.1	0.01

system to prepare for the relative amount of light to be read from the plate. This will allow the electronics in the system to be optimized to the appropriate range and result in a better image data set.

The increased latitude of the imaging plate allows for correction of exposure errors, but as the exposure error increases, image quality will decrease. If a substantial overexposure occurs, the resulting image will not offer optimum image quality. Basic principles regarding the production of poor low-contrast images when using film-screen do not change with the use of CR. Factors that produce low contrast include high kVp, no grid or inadequate grid efficiency, inadequate beam limitation, and increased part size or tissue thickness (Table 25-4). As with film-screen, kVp selection should be based on desired subject contrast and grid selection. It is recommended that kVp not exceed 80 for all non-grid radiography. Since CR plates have a wide dynamic range they are especially sensitive to fogging, from both scatter and background radiation. The lower K edge of the BaFBr phosphor contributes to the scatter sensitivity of CR when compared to the higher K edge of rare-earth intensifying screens. Because the imaging plate is so sensitive to background ionizing radiation, **it is recommended that plates be erased daily if not used to eliminate unwanted noise** from these sources.

Data Clipping

Most CR system do not send all the data acquired by the image receptor to the post-acquisition system because the quantity of data is far greater than the display system can provide for viewing. This element of CR is called data clipping because the software processing the data coming from the image receptor is programmed to recognize that some data represents exposure below the diagnostic imaging range, while other data represents exposure far above the diagnostic range. Essentially, the algorithm eliminates data that is clinically irrelevant to a particular examination. As you might expect, the algorithm must vary, depending on the body part or clinical diagnosis. This is one of many reasons why CR systems demand to know what examination is being performed before the image can be acquired, processed, and displayed.

Data clipping is an excellent example of why overexposure of patients is ethically wrong. Grossly overexposed images are often post-processed by algorithms that eliminate the overexposed portion of the image receptor output. It has long been established that the ALARA concept includes avoiding any exposure to human tissue that will not be viewed during the diagnostic process. Data clipping algorithms are a strong rationale for radiographers to use to justify decreasing mAs during CR exposures as long as settings remain well above the quantum mottle/reticulation range.

Spatial Frequency Processing— Edge Enhancement

Edge enhancement algorithms can create spectacularly enhanced contrast edges. It has been well established that edge enhancement overprints data at the edge line and this can compromise the accuracy of the image through obscuring details in these regions. For this reason edge-enhanced images should also be viewed without edge enhancement. Radiologists find it particularly useful for large structures in low-contrast regions, such as mediastinal airways or the inferior lateral cervical vertebra. Both the Fugi and Agfa CR systems use algorithms that emphasize high spatial frequencies for small objects (such as bony trabeculae) and low spatial frequencies for larger objects (such as the bowel and kidneys).

Spatial Frequency Processing— Image Blurring

Using a post-acquisition algorithm to blur objects can also be helpful. This feature is most commonly applied to high noise images, such as quantum mottle/reticulation images to make the sharp edges of the noise blur into the background.

TABLE 25-4.	Factors That Produce Low Contrast and Are Prone to Cause CR Imaging Plate Fogging
	high kVp
	no grid or inadequate grid efficiency
	inadequate beam limitation
	increased part size or tissue density

Look-up Table Adjustments

The CR system look-up table is a histogram of the luminance values (for image display) derived from the image receptor pixel values (from image acquisition). All CR systems allow the display to be adjusted from the look-up table. This permits changes in optical density or contrast that is often compared to adjusting the $D_{log}E$ curve of a film emulsion to enhance a particular portion of the image. Unfortunately, some manufacturers set their systems so that only authorized persons can access the look-up table adjustments. When used this way, the look-up table becomes a system calibration tool. However, accomplished CR users can use this feature to enhance pathologies such as fractures that are difficult to visualize, for example, periosteal tears in infants who have been abused.

Histogram Equalization

Some CR systems that are in dedicated environments, such as a chest unit, may have the histogram of the image receptor data modified to enhance a particular element. Chest CR systems can stack histogram-equalized images behind the normal image. This allows radiologists to view a normal display of a chest along with a bone-enhanced histogram image, a soft tissue enhanced image, etc. An image that is often cited for this process is a PA chest with a lung neoplasm hiding behind a rib. Although this lesion would be missed by most physicians, when a soft tissue enhanced image is viewed (which essentially removes all bony trabeculae from the ribs) the neoplasm is seen clearly. Because these are modified images, they should never be viewed for diagnosis without comparative images from the same data set in an unmodified state. This feature of CR creates a major imaging dilemma for radiologists because there is no end to the number of modified and enhanced images that can be created from a single image data set. Medical malpractice liability that assumes a radiologist is responsible for viewing all possible enhancements would require physicians to read from dozens of images for each standard projection and literally bring the practice of radiology to a halt. The American College of Radiology addresses this issue by issuing standard procedure guidelines that clearly indicate that digitally enhanced images

are not routine. This permits radiologists to view them as needed, much the same way that an angiogram might be recommended as a follow-up study to acquire more information after a CT of the brain.

Collimator Edge Identification

Most CR systems include algorithms designed to detect abrupt edges of exposure and nonexposure. These are assumed to represent collimator edges. It is possible to have an abrupt straight line of tissue density when there are prosthetic devices or other implants that may trigger these algorithms. Most CR systems have been developed to the point where it is rare for this to occur; nevertheless it is useful for the knowledgeable CR operator to remember that this algorithm functions during most post-acquisition processing.

Some algorithms produce an extremely light-gray background outside the collimation edges to reduce the glare from the unexposed areas during image display.

Image Stitching

It is possible to stitch together multiple images from some CR systems. This is especially useful for scoliosis studies of the spine, long bone studies, or angiographic imaging of peripheral vasculature. The algorithms that accomplish these images rely on overlapping exposures to verify registration marks and image contrast edges to align multiple exposures into a single image.

Grid Use

Grid use in CR occurs more often due to the sensitivity of the imaging plate to scatter. When performing chest radiography, a grid should be used when chest measurements exceed 24 to 26 cm for optimum images. Even when using a grid, if a substantial overexposure ($>2\times$) occurs, enough scatter may be generated to degrade the image. Selecting the proper grid will depend on part size, kVp desired, scatter cleanup desired, and grid frequency (lines per cm or inch). The imaging plate is scanned line by line; **if the scan frequency and the grid frequency are similar and oriented in**

A multihole grid pattern.

the same direction a Moire effect will be observed. Recommendations for grid frequency are 85 lines/in (33–34 lines/cm) for a 14×17 and 103 (40–44 lines/cm) for a 10×12. Multihole grids that avoid Moire pattern artifacts are available for CR systems (Figure 25-14). These grids filter the primary beam angle with circular holes instead of linear lead strips that CR image receptors and post-acquisition software may display in an overlapping Moire pattern that renders the information between the lines undiagnosable.

DIRECT EXPOSURE IMAGING SYSTEMS

Direct acquisition systems directly convert incoming x-ray photons to an electronic digital signal. These systems use amorphous selenium (a-Se) and are sometimes referred to as **direct radiography systems.** The term **flat panel** (or **flat field**) **detectors** is also being used to describe both the indirect amorphous silicon and the direct amorphous selenium plates that are being used in some digital radiography systems. Some of these systems employ a stationary high-frequency grid that is used on all exposures.

DIRECT SELENIUM FLAT PANEL IMAGING PLATE SYSTEMS

The active layer in the imaging plate is amorphous selenium, which is a semiconductor with excellent x-ray photon detection ability and spatial resolution of >20 lp/mm. Prior to the exposure, a high-voltage charge is applied from the top surface of the selenium layer. The ionization caused by the x-ray photons results in the selenium atoms freeing electrons for collection by the electrodes at the bottom of the selenium layer. The charge that is collected is then transmitted through thin film transistors (TFTs) to the computer for processing. This process is illustrated in Figure 25-15.

INDIRECT SILICON FLAT PANEL IMAGING PLATE SYSTEMS

Amorphous silicon (a-Si:H) cannot directly convert x-rays into an electric charge, but it does work as a light detector (photodiode) to capture fluorescent light. Because the atomic number of silicon is only 14, it is necessary to have a relatively thick silicon layer to provide adequate sensitivity to the incoming x-ray photons. Amorphous silicon requires a scintillator, such as cesium iodide (CsI)(which is currently used by Philips and General Electric) or a rare-earth intensifying screen composed of gadolinium and lanthanium with osysulfides (this system is currently used by Canon). Scintillators emit light isotropically, which can reduce spatial resolution. To minimize light spread, CsI is manufactured as structured crystals in the form of needles or columns 10 to 20 micrometers in diameter. This significantly reduces light spread and channels light toward the amorphous silicon photodiode. The Canon scintillator is designed as a thin screen to minimize light spread. Once the light reaches the amorphous silicon, it is converted into an electric signal. Figure 25-16 illustrates the design of an amorphous silicon system.

FIGURE 25-15 Direct conversion amorphous selenium flat panel imaging plate. The high-voltage charge at the top surface of the selenium layer results in the ionization caused by the x-ray photons to free electrons for collection by the electrodes at the bottom of the selenium layer. The charge that is collected is then transmitted through thin film detectors (TFTs) to the computer for processing.

Thin Film Transistors (TFTs)

Both the amorphous silicon and amorphous selenium flat plate detectors use thin film transistors (TFT) for electronic readout. The TFT collects the electric charges produced by either the selenium or silicon as an array or matrix of pixel-size detector elements. Each TFT element collects the charge and then, when a gate is activated by the computer, sends a signal. The TFTs are positioned in a matrix that allows the charge pattern to be read out on a pixel-by-pixel and column-by-column basis. Philips, General Electric, and Canon are all using TFTs.

FIGURE 25-16 Indirect amorphous silicon flat panel imaging plate system. When x-ray photons strike the CsI they are converted to light. The columns of CsI reduce the light spread interacting with the amorphous silicon.

Charge Coupled Device (CCD)

The CCD is a photodetector, a device that is capable of converting visible light into an electric charge and storing it in a sequential pattern. This stored charge can then be released line by line to the ADC. Typically, a screen is used as a scintillator and the light produced from x-ray interactions must be optically coupled to the CCD by lenses or fiber-optics. The electrical signal produced by the CCD is then sent to the computer for image processing.

DICOM STANDARD

The Digital Imaging and Communications in Medicine (DICOM) standard is a system of computer software standards that permit a wide range of digital imaging programs to understand one another. The DICOM-3 standard is currently in use and it is responsible for much of the acceptance of digital imaging modalities in recent years. Prior to the widespread use of DICOM-3, many medical imaging systems, especially those made by different manufacturers, were unable to communicate with each other. DICOM-3 permits the interfacing of diverse systems; for example, a diagnostic radiographic digital radiography system, a computed tomography unit, and a digital chest system can all share the same computer network and software filing system without conflict.

COMPUTED RADIOGRAPHY ARTIFACTS

As with all computerized imaging systems, computed radiography has unique artifact patterns as a result of errors in the systems. CR artifacts are classified according to where they occur in the image processing sequence.

Acquisition

- Phantom images may appear as a result of incomplete image plate erasure. This artifact requires troubleshooting of both the CR plate preparation system and the display systems (laser imagers and/or display monitors). Extreme overexposure may require two erasures cycles to completely remove the image.

- Scratches are permanent artifacts caused by damage to imaging plates. Replacement of CR plates is expensive, but it is the only solution because these artifacts cannot be repaired.

- Light spots are usually caused by dust or other foreign material on the imaging plate. CR plates can be cleaned but must be done carefully according to manufacturers' recommendations to avoid permanent damage.

- Dropout artifacts are reductions in resolution either overall or in specific areas of the image. They tend to be accompanied by contrast scale reductions, but this is difficult to assess because there are so many ways to modify image contrast and display monitors have inherent contrast deterioration over time. Dropout artifacts

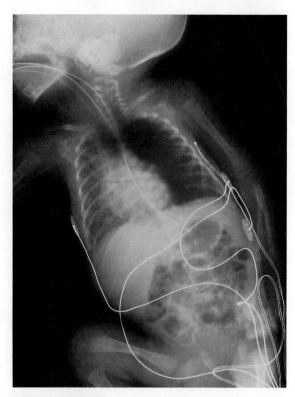

FIGURE 25-17   Heat blur artifact caused by the image receptor being exposed to intense heat.

are a result of dust accumulation in the CR or laser imaging unit components (polygonal mirror, light gate, or other reflective surfaces). Cleaning of these units on a regularly quality assurance schedule may avoid both image deterioration and early replacement of both CR and laser imaging equipment.

- Fogging due to imaging plates being much more sensitive than film

- Quantum mottle (or reticulation) caused by inadequate exposure (usually insufficient mAs)

- Heat blur (Figure 25-17) caused from image receptor being exposed to intense heat

Post Acquisition

- Algorithm artifacts cover a wide range of image problems that correspond to the post-acquisition processing functions that are available on a specific CR system. To control these artifacts, manufacturers restrict access or provide preset values in order to provide a reasonable level of consistency between images for diagnostic comparisons.

- Dropout artifacts are also possible at this stage but are limited to problems in laser imaging equipment.

- Laser film transport artifacts, including uneven scanning, distortion, and overlapping shading. These are all caused by uneven transport of film material through a laser imaging system.

- Histogram error (see Figure 25-11) due to incorrect preprocessing histogram selection - adult histogram used on pediatric chest.

- Nonparallel collimation (see Figure 25-6)—histograms require that collimation edges be parallel to the sides of imaging plate.

Display

- Density/brightness window level adjustments
- Contrast window width adjustments
- Electronic magnification/minification adjustments
- Image enhancement artifacts, usually a result of incorrectly set presets for edge enhancement, contrast range, spatial frequency filtration, etc.

SUMMARY

Digital radiography replaces traditional film with a reusable detector. Detectors currently used to acquire radiographic images include photostimulable storage phosphor imaging plates (IP), charge coupled devices (CCD), silicon, and selenium. These detectors are classified as either indirect conversion or direct conversion. Silicon and selenium receptors are also known as flat panel detectors.

Indirect conversion systems use a two-part process involving a scintillator (which converts incoming x-ray photons to light) and a photodetector (which converts light into an electronic digital signal). Indirect systems include those that use photostimulable storage phosphor imaging plates (IP), charged coupled devices (CCD), and silicon.

Direct conversion systems directly convert incoming x-ray photons to an electronic digital signal. These systems use selenium and are sometimes referred to as direct radiography (DR) systems.

In order for digital radiography to function, the imaging plate material must have the ability to store and release the image information in a usable form. The imaging plate is more sensitive to scatter both before and after it is sensitized. The latent image will lose about 25 percent of its

energy in 8 hours. Pixel size and quantity depend on the size of the phosphor plate being scanned. The smaller the pixels and the larger the matrix, the higher the spatial resolution.

When using the Fuji computed radiography systems, it is important to remember that the beam and part need to be centered within each pattern and collimation must be parallel and equidistant from the edges of the imaging plate, and the correct histogram algorithm must be selected prior to processing. The Fuji system uses an S number to assist in evaluating exposure. A higher S value indicates that the imaging plate was underexposed, while a lower S value indicates overexposure.

Kilovoltage for digital radiography will control contrast similar to film radiography, However, some digital radiography manufacturers recommend avoiding the use of more than 80 kVp because higher kVp levels produce excessive fog that will decrease contrast significantly more than the same increase with a film-screen imaging receptor. The primary advantage to digital radiography is the wide dynamic range response of the imaging plate detector. Rather than the characteristic curve of film-screen systems, the response to x-ray is linear, so the imaging plate does not have a D_{max}. When film is exposed beyond D_{max}, it actually reverses and begins to get lighter (as with duplicating film). The digital radiography imaging plate continues to record the exposure and the computer can bring these densities down into the visible range. This is why a digital radiography system can compensate for gross overexposure. This is also why the radiographer using digital radiography must realize that there is great danger in permitting personal professional standards to relax and routinely overexposing all patients with the intention of the digital radiography system adjusting the histogram to correct the exposure. This practice is unethical, violates ALARA radiation protection guidelines, and is to be avoided at all times.

Once the image has been converted into an electrical signal, it still needs to be converted into electronic pulses that are correlated to the image matrix for the computer. One method of accomplishing this signal is to place a charged coupled device (CCD) in contact with the scintillator. Both the amorphous silicon and amorphous selenium flat plate detectors use thin film transistors (TFT) for electronic readout. Each TFT element collects the charge and then, when a gate is activated by the computer, sends a signal.

Digital radiography has unique artifact patterns as a result of errors in the systems. Some of the more common digital radiography artifacts include fogging, quantum mottle, heat blur, histogram error, and nonparallel collimation.

REVIEW QUESTIONS

1. Give an example of the types of image receptors used for both a direct and indirect conversion digital radiography system.

2. Name the image receptors used in one of the flat panel detector systems.

3. Explain the function of two of the layers of a photostimulable phosphor imaging plate.

4. Why are imaging plates more sensitive to radiation than radiographic film?

5. Why do digital radiography cassettes stored for several days after exposure and before processing lose most of their latent image?

6. How is digital radiography spatial resolution controlled?

7. What data are collected during the creation of the histogram from a digital radiography exposure?

8. Why do digital radiography systems have significantly greater latitude than conventional film-screen radiography systems?

9. What elements of computed radiography systems make them prone to violations of ALARA radiation protection concepts?

10. Name as many digital radiography artifacts as you know.

REFERENCE AND RECOMMENDED READING

Bell, J. (1999). A direct image capture system: The future of digital x-ray. *Medical Imaging Technology, 17*(2), 105–109.

Burns, C. (1993). Using computed digital radiography effectively. *Seminars in Radiologic Technology, 1*(1), 24–35.

Bushberg, J., Seibert, J., Leidholdt, E., & Boone, J. (2003). *The essential physics of medical imaging.* Baltimore: Williams & Wilkins (2nd ed.).

Cesar, L. (1997). Computed radiography: Its impact on radiographers. *Radiologic Technology, 68*(3), 225–232.

Choatas, H., Dobbins, J., & Ravin, C. (1999). Principles of digital radiography with large-area electronically readable detectors: A review of the basics. *Radiology, 210*(3), 595–599.

Frey, G., & Sprawls, P. (1997). *The expanding role of medical physicists in diagnostic imaging: Proceedings of the 1997 AAPM summer school.* Madison, WI: Advanced Medical Publishing for American Association of Physicists in Medicine.

Fuji Photo Film Co., Ltd. (1996). *Fujifilm imaging and information: Chapter 2: Information capacity of FCR images.* (Ref. No. CR-008040C2 [CR-96-9]). Tokyo: Author.

Fuji Photo Film Co., Ltd. (1996). *Fujifilm imaging and information: Chapter 3: Auto density control (EDR)* (Ref. No. CR-008040C3 [CR-96-9]). Tokyo: Author.

Fuji Photo Film Co., Ltd. (1996). *Fujifilm imaging and information: Chapter 4: Image processing.* (Ref. No. CR-008040C4 [CR-96-9]). Tokyo: Author.

Fuji Photo Film Co., Ltd. (1996). *Fujifilm imaging and information: Chapter 5: Special image processing* (Ref. No. CR-008040C5 [CR-96-9]). Tokyo: Author.

Fuji Photo Film Co., Ltd. (1996). *Fujifilm imaging and information: Appendix 1: Clinical effects of FCR.* (Ref. No. CR-008040A1 [CR-96-9]). Tokyo: Author.

Fuji Photo Film Co., Ltd. (1996). *Fujifilm imaging and information: Appendix 2: Case studies.* (Ref. No. CR-008040A2 [CR-96-9]). Tokyo: Author.

Hamers, S., & Freyschmidt, J. (Eds.). (1998). Digital radiography with an electronic flat-panel detector: First clinical experience in skeletal diagnostics. *MedicaMunda, 42*(3), 2–6.

Hillman, B., & Fajardo, L. (1989). Clinical assessment of phosphor-plate computed radiography: Equipment, strategy, and methods. *Journal of Digital Imaging, 2*(4), 220–227.

Hindel, R. (1983). Digital imaging—the technology of the future. *The Canadian Journal of Medical Radiation Technology, 14*(4), 128.

Lim, A. (1996). *Image quality in film digitizers: Testing and quality assurance. Syllabus: A Course in Physics,* 183–193. Chicago: Radiological Society of North America.

Long, B. W. (1989). Computed radiography: Photostimulable phosphor image plate technology. *Radiologic Technology, 61*(2), 107–112.

Mixdorf, M., & Tortorici, M. (1993). Practical considerations in computed radiography. *Seminars in Radiologic Technology, 1*(1), 16–23.

Murphey, M., Quale, J., Martin, N., Bramble, J., Cook, L. & Dwyer, S. (1992). Computed radiography in musculoskeletal imaging: State of the art. *American Journal of Roentgenology, 158,* 19–27.

Neitzel, U. (1999, July). *Integrated digital radiography with a flat electronic detector.* Retrieved www.de.ms.philips.com/sections/rad/digbucky/news/html/neitzel.htm, 7-16-99.

Reiner, B. I., Siegel, E. L., & Carrino, J. A. (Eds.). (2002). *Quality assurance: Meeting the challenge in the digital medical enterprise.* Society for Computer Applications in Radiology (SCAR). Great Falls, VA.

Samei, E., & Flynn, M. J. (Eds.). (2003). *Advances in digital radiography: Categorical course in diagnostic radiology physics.* Radiological Society of North America, Oak Brook, IL.

Samei, E., Seibert, J., Willis, C., Flynn, M., Mah E., Junck, K. (2001). Performance evaluation of computed radiography systems. *Medical Physics, 28,* 3, p. 361–371.

Seibert, J., Bogucki, T., Ciona, T. (1998). *Acceptance testing and quality control of photostimulable storage phosphor imaging systems* (Report of Task Group #10.) College Park, MD. American Association of Physicists in Medicine.

Siegel, E., & Kolodner, R. (1999). *Filmless radiology.* New York: Springer-Verlag.

Solomon, S., Jost, R., Glazer, H., Sagel, S., Anderson, D., & Molina, P. (1991). Artifacts in computed radiography. *American Journal of Roentgenology, 157,* 181–185.

Sonoda, M. (1983). Computed radiography utilizing scanning laser stimulated luminescence. *Radiology, 148,* 833–838.

Wilson, P. (1984). Digital imaging: An introduction. *Radiography, 50*(590), 449.

Yamazaki, T., Satoh, M., Eguchi, Y., Yamada, K., Endo, Y., & Kaga, Y. (1998). *Image quality of the digital radiography system using the flat panel detector compared with the storage phosphor based computed radiography system.* (Scientific Exhibit 0499PH) Chicago: Radiological Society of North America.

CHAPTER 26

Digital Image Management

Barbara Smith

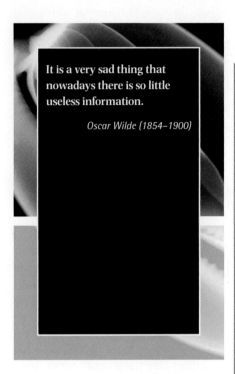

It is a very sad thing that nowadays there is so little useless information.

Oscar Wilde (1854–1900)

KEY TERMS

electronic medical record
hard copy
hospital information system (HIS)
picture archiving and communication system (PACS)
radiology information system (RIS)
soft copy

OBJECTIVES

Upon completion of this chapter, the student should be able to:

- Discuss advantages of using PACS in a medical imaging department.

- Explain why a PACS network may require a separate computer network from the one used throughout an institution.

- Describe the various types of laser printers that can be used for digital images.

- Explain soft-copy monitor display parameters.

- Identify types of storage available for digital images.

- Discuss the necessity for DICOM in medical imaging.

Introducing computers into diagnostic imaging brought about the possibility of a filmless environment. The ability of computer systems to handle large amounts of data makes it possible to acquire, distribute, display, and store images without film. Computed medical imaging first appeared in the 1980s when computers were unable to handle large amounts of data rapidly, image quality was poor, and it was expensive. Computers and networks now handle data much faster, display monitors have higher resolution, efficient storage exists, and communication format standardization has occurred. Although film remains an important part of medical imaging, it is no longer the primary recording and storage media.

There are many advantages to the digital environment over film. Digital images can be viewed in a variety of settings simultaneously, they can be manipulated without reexposing the patient, they can be retrieved rapidly, they require less physical storage space, and they can be sent to remote locations. These advantages are available due to the advent of a **picture archiving and communication system (PACS)**, which is a computer system that can manage images in an electronic form. PACS use begins with the integration of information from the **electronic medical record** (often from a **hospital information system [HIS]**) with the **radiology information system (RIS)**. This data is then correlated with the scanners and other equipment that creates the images in digital formats, such as digital radiography (which includes both computed radiography [CR] and direct radiography [DR]), computed tomography, magnetic resonance imaging, ultrasound, and others. The PACS then distributes images through a network infrastructure, which can be both within and outside a facility. The images can be displayed on monitors (**soft copy**) or printed onto film (**hard copy**). Finally, the images are stored in digital form, requiring much less space than film storage. The PACS is composed of the hardware and software components that are required to create this digital environment.

IMAGE ACQUISITION

Computers were used early on for computed tomography, magnetic resonance imaging, ultrasound, and nuclear medicine to capture, display, and move images between workstations and printers. These configurations are sometimes called mini PACS. This development was followed by digital fluoroscopy and angiography, where the video signal from the image intensifier was converted into a digital signal. Finally, radiographic images were converted to digital through the use of computed radiography and film digitizers.

Digital image capture in digital radiography (CR and DR) is discussed in Chapter 25, Digital Radiography. A film digitizer is used to convert an analog film image to a digital image that can then be used in a PACS. This allows patient film files to be converted to digital and combined with new digital images when hospitals transition to filmless operation. Film digitizers also allow images to be sent to outside institutions through teleradiology.

All film digitizers require a system that uses light transmitted through a film to a light sensor, where a signal can be acquired, digitally processed, and transmitted (archived) to a computer. The optical density of the film will affect the amount of light transmitted through the film and so the amount of signal that is generated. There are two systems available for digitizers; one uses a laser and the other a CCD linear array.

A laser film digitizer uses a laser beam that scans in a raster pattern across the film as it is transported through the digitizer. The laser light transmitted through the film is detected by a device that converts the light into a signal that is amplified and sent to an analog-to-digital converter (ADC). The CCD digitizer uses light focused in a line on the film, which then strikes a linear array CCD detector. When light strikes the CCD it causes electrons to leave in a signal that is proportional to the amount of light coming through the film. Once a film image is digitized it can be sent to remote locations and/or added to the patient's digital file.

IMAGE DISTRIBUTION

Network infrastructure and file management have a tremendous impact on how image data travels or is distributed. Once images are obtained they need to be transmitted over a network. Just as film images need to be sent to a radiologist to be read, stored, and often sent to clinicians, so do digital images. A PACS allows digital images to be sent from their acquisition point to a radiologist or other clinician to be diagnosed and then stored for retrieval. In order to move digital information, a network is required to allow computers in the system to communicate with one another.

Each digital acquisition system (CR, DR, CT, etc.) has a computer workstation that holds the images in files for the technologist to check for quality before sending them for diagnosis. The size of an image file will depend on matrix size and bit depth.

Gray scale bit depth ranges from 8 bits to 32 bits. A byte is equal to 8 bits, so the file size of a pixel is multiplied by the bit depth divided by 8. A gray scale bit depth of 8–32 equals a range of 1–4 bytes of storage that would be required per pixel in the image matrix. A gray scale bit depth of 12 produces 2^{12} gray levels. This represents 4,096 different shades of gray that are available, a spectacular diagnostic range that is far beyond the range of the human visual system.

Image file size is determined by the formula XY (B/8)

where: X = x-axis pixel matrix size
         Y = y-axis pixel matrix size
         B = gray scale bit depth

EXAMPLE: What is the anticipated image file size for a computed radiography digital image comprised of a 2,500 × 2,500 matrix with a 12–bit depth?

Answer:

XY (B/8)
2,500 × 2,500 (12/8) =
6,250,000 (12/8) =
6,250,000 (1.5) =
9,375,000 = 9.375 Mb

EXAMPLE: What is the anticipated file storage necessary for a computed tomography examination comprised of 2,500 images, each with a 512 × 512 matrix at 16–bit depth?

Answer:

XY (B/8)
512 × 512 (16/8) =
262,144 (16/8) =

262,144 (2) =
524,288 = 524.288 Kb
524.288 Kb × 2,500 images = 1,310,720 = 1.31072 Gb

Diagnostic radiography has a large matrix size for each image to increase resolution while a CT image has a lower matrix for each image, but many more images are obtained for each exam. A PACS transmits large amounts of data to a wide range of processing, storage, and display units.

To move image data from one place to another in a PACS requires a network with bandwidth capable of handling large data files. Bandwidth is measured in bits per second (bps) and describes how much data can be moved. Usually a PACS network is separate from other hospital information systems since the data files are large and need to move quickly. A local area network (LAN) connects all the computers in a system and often uses a special wiring system such as an Ethernet that can have a bandwidth of 10 Mbps. When information leaves the system to go to another location far away, such as teleradiology, it is over a wide area network (WAN), which often operates at much slower speeds. Many institutions are establishing wireless networks, which, although convenient, may operate even slower. Slower transmission systems require more time to display images with extremely large files, such as multiple detector CT or 3D echocardiography. Display times for these modalities may be too long to allow reasonable use via some of the networks. This factor, along with the special language and operating systems used by PACS, often causes problems in interfacing with patient HIS.

In a digital environment patient information needs to be computer accessible for use by the imaging department and PACS. Patient data is contained in an HIS database. The database specific to imaging departments is often called a radiology information system (RIS). The ideal goal is for patient information to be exchanged between an interconnected HIS and RIS so that data can be retrieved from both systems. The RIS can then send patient information to be communicated to PACS, allowing patient data and images to be connected within the systems. Using HIS and RIS to communicate with PACS allows for more uniform patient identification. In the filmless, paperless imaging department, the HIS can register patients and send orders to the RIS. The RIS produces a work list with examinations ordered for the day, which are then distributed to the imaging equipment where the examination is performed. Once the images are acquired, both image and patient data is sent through the PACS to the radiologist or other physician to be read and stored.

IMAGE DISPLAY

Image display devices are dependent on the purpose of the user. Traditionally, film was displayed on an illuminator viewbox. Digital images can still be produced on film (hard copy) with a laser printer. However, in a filmless environment the images are viewed on a monitor (soft copy). Digital images need to be displayed for the technologist to review and by the radiologist to read. They can also be displayed for clinicians throughout a hospital or clinic. Vendors are exploring methods of protecting patient confidentiality, necessary to offer access to authorized users via Internet and wireless gateways. There are numerous advantages to soft-copy display: multiple viewing of the same image, variation of image display parameters (such as density/brightness/sensitivity and contrast), and reduced numbers of lost films.

Hard-copy Display

Hard-copy display refers to images that are visualized on film. Hard-copy films are required for some applications, even in "filmless" departments, for physicians without soft-copy display, for orthopedic image measurements, and for operating rooms.

Laser Printers. Laser printers were introduced in 1983 as part of the Fuji CR system. Since that time many manufacturers and types of laser printers have been developed. There are three light sources for laser printers: infrared (780–820 nm), solid-state diode (~670–680 nm), and helium-neon (HeNe: 633 nm). The printers produce transilluminated hard-copy film images from computerized digital information. Printers work with either wet or

FIGURE 26-1 A laser printer calibration film demonstrates the full range of density and contrast for the unit. *(Courtesy of Jeff Lloyd, Spectrum Health)*

dry processors often have a bit depth or gray scale of 8 bits, while some detectors may have 10, 12, 15, or 16 bits. This requires a calibration from the larger bit size of the detector to the lower 8 bits for the printer. Calibration films can be printed to check the optical density range of the printer (Figure 26-1).

Generally, a laser printer, regardless of the manufacturer, has the following components: a laser source, collimator lens or beam-shaping optics, a beam modulator, deflecting mirror-shaping lenses, and a cylindrical reflection mirror (Figure 26-2). The printer also has an unexposed film storage with a mechanical transport to move the film through the printer as it is exposed line by line in a raster scan pattern by the laser. After passing through the laser area, the film is processed, either by wet or dry processing methods, and it is deposited into the exposed film receptor bin.

Conventional laser film is a wet-processing method that uses silver halide in the emulsion. The laser deposits energy on the film, creating latent image centers, just as the light from a screen on traditional radiographic film. However, wet laser film is designed to be sensitive to either red (HeNe) or infrared (diode) wavelengths rather than the green or blue of conventional film. This type of laser film

FIGURE 26-2   Schematic diagram of a film laser camera. A constant–intensity laser source is focused by a collimator lens, modulated according to the digital value of the image pixel, and directed at the film. The F-theta/toroidal lenses and the cylindrical mirror modify the shape of the beam to minimize distortion toward the periphery of the image. *(Permission of Bushberg, J.; Beth, J., Landholt, K.; and Boone, J. (2002).* The Essential Physics of Medical Imaging. *Philadelphia: Lippincott, Williams, Wilkins, 2nd edition, Fig. 17.12)*

cannot be exposed to a red safelight in the darkroom or it will be fogged. After the laser energy creates the latent image, the film is processed through developer, fixer, and, finally, the wash. The more laser energy striking the film, the higher the density.

Dry Processors.   Dry processors do not use developer, fixer, or wash to process an image on film, eliminating the need for chemicals and plumbing required by wet processing. This allows more flexibility in printer placement within an imaging department. Medical printers commonly use thermal processing for film-based images. Thermal processing involves the use of heat-sensitive film with silver-based emulsion, dye microcapsules, and carbon-based adherographic printing.

Silver-based dry film contains silver benhate that responds to light from a laser and heat from a thermal head. The laser beam produces latent image centers; only the activated silver halide grains develop when heated by the thermal head. Since the density results immediately after exposure to the laser and heat, it does not require wet processing, which leaves all the chemical compounds on the film. Potentially, the film could continue to develop density if exposed to high heat conditions, something referred to as "print-up." Manufacturers have developed films that minimize this condition, resulting in a stable film image in most circumstances. Unexposed dry-processing laser film has a shorter shelf life than conventional film since it is more sensitive to heat and humidity.

Heat-permeable microcapsules contain dye that is located in the film. The microcapsules become active when exposed to a laser light and become permeable to allow developing agents to enter them. The film passes over a thermal head to allow this processing to occur. Unexposed microcapsules are not permeable and so will not develop. As the film cools, the microcapsules become impermeable, stopping the chemical development process. High heat during storage of the processed image can increase film density over time. Adherographic processing uses selective adhesion of carbon particles onto a plastic base that is then sealed. The film is composed of multiple layers, which is exposed to a gallium arsenide laser. Wherever the laser exposes the film, carbon particles adhere. This becomes a distinct image when the layers are separated. This process was first developed by Polaroid Medical Imaging Systems in 1993. To protect the image and keep the carbon particles in place, a cover sheet is sealed or laminated onto the finished film.

Soft-copy Display

Soft-copy display refers to images visualized on monitors, either flat panel technology or older cathode ray tubes (CRTs).

A great advantage of digital imaging is the ability to manipulate the image without reexposing the patient. Images are best manipulated when they are displayed on a monitor. Additionally, images can be viewed in multiple locations simultaneously and can be quickly distributed to multiple locations when in digital format.

Monitor characteristics are determined by the requirements of the user. Technologists need to evaluate an image prior to sending it to PACS, while radiologists need to use images for diagnosis. Physicians will look at images either in the hospital or at remote locations. All of these uses will not need the same display quality. Diagnostic viewing by the radiologist requires a monitor with the highest spatial and contrast resolution (along with higher cost), while clinical viewing stations for physicians may be acceptable with lower resolution and less cost. Radiographers require monitors that will allow adequate visualization of contrast and resolution to determine if the image is of diagnostic quality for the physician.

There are two types of monitors on the market that are found in most imaging departments: the cathode ray tube (CRT) monitor and the liquid crystal display (LCD) monitor. The resolution of a monitor is based on how many pixels can be displayed in the horizontal and vertical dimensions. A 1 K CRT monitor would display $1,280 \times 1,024$ pixels, while a 2 K CRT monitor would display $2,048 \times 2,560$ pixels. The higher the number of pixels, the higher the resolution. LCD monitors may have resolutions as high as 3–5 megapixels. Typically, radiographers and physicians use lower resolution monitors, while the radiologist workstations provide higher resolution.

Traditional CRT monitors operate with an electron gun in the back of the unit that directs an electron beam toward the phosphor screen in the front (Figure 26-3). The gun operates in a raster pattern, scanning line by line (Figure 26-4). The phosphor emits light when struck by the electron beam and that is the picture displayed through the front of the monitor. The luminance of a CRT is less than that of a film on an illuminated viewbox, and over time the aging of the electron gun and display phosphor will also lower brightness. Because of the lower lumi-

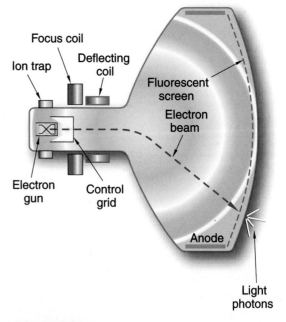

FIGURE 26-3 A video monitor (cathode ray tube [CRT]).

1st scan 2nd scan Entire frame

2621/2 lines
1/60 second

2621/2 lines
1/60 second

525 lines
1/30 second

FIGURE 26-4 A video monitor raster scanning pattern. The electron beam scans the diagonal lines as active traces, while the horizontal lines are inactive retraces to position for the next active trace. The electron beam scans 262 1/2 alternate lines every 1/60 second and the second set of lines the next 1/60 second. Consequently, the entire 525-line raster pattern is scanned every 1/30 second. This is 30 times per second, which is 15,720 scan lines per second.

nance ambient light has more impact on image display quality, affecting the perception of image contrast. CRT monitors are deeper than a film viewbox and require more space when replacing lightboxes on a desk or wall. Heat generated by the CRT monitor must also be considered when installing these devices. Black and white or monochrome CRT monitors are used for most imaging. However, color is required for some modalities, such as nuclear medicine and Doppler ultrasound images.

Image quality on a CRT monitor is affected by resolution, luminance, contrast, uniformity, and glare. Since these areas can affect the technologist and radiologist when viewing images, a QC program needs to be performed on a regular basis to ensure high quality is maintained. Acceptance testing of new equipment will establish a baseline for QC measurements that will be a reference for annual testing. There are phantoms available for QC testing, and a photometer for measuring luminance will be needed. Just as with a bank of film lightboxes, all monitors in a workstation should have the same level of luminance.

Resolution is related to the number of pixels in the horizontal and vertical dimensions. However, detail of a monitor with a large matrix may still be poor due to electron spot size changing or "blooming," causing pixel size to become larger than the nominal or state size. This blooming is affected by luminance and monitor age. A SMPTE test pattern can be used for a visual inspection of resolution, or more complex tests can be run.

Contrast should be set the same on all monitors so that the same gray scale is consistent throughout the department. Ambient light reflections on a monitor will have a negative impact on contrast. Monitors have design features to reduce this effect; however, it cannot be eliminated. Therefore, monitors should not be used in rooms with bright lighting. Acceptance testing will allow an acceptable test pattern image to be stored that can be retrieved for testing annually. Contrast is also a function of luminance, and the monitor must have adequate amounts of light from all areas. A luminance uniformity test uses a photometer to test the light from the center and outer corners of the monitor. This will pick up any deviation across the display.

Soft-copy veiling glare, often referred to as "glare," results from the internal process of a monitor, rather than the external light causing reflection off the monitor screen. Glare will also cause a decrease in contrast, producing lower image quality. There are a number of factors that cause glare, for example, light scattering on the faceplate, light leakage, and electron backscattering. All of these actions will cause light spread, which will decrease contrast. Veiling glare is discussed in detail in Chapter 14, Vision and Perception.

The use of CRT monitors requires a consistent power source since fluctuations in voltage will affect the electron gun and image display. Ambient room light must be reduced so as to maximize image contrast. Placing workstations with the corresponding monitors and control panels requires a different environment from using hard-copy film illuminator viewboxes.

Flat panel LCD monitors are an alternative to using CRT monitors. These monitors are much thinner than CRTs, which means they use less space on desks and counters. The LCD monitor regulates the image by using a light source behind the screen shining on individual pixels, which control the amount of light transmitted through. Liquid crystal and hydrogenated amorphous silicon (a-Si:H) thin film transistors (TFT) are contained between glass plates on the front of the monitor, which regulate pixel transparency. This allows rapid changes in voltage to alter a pixel from black (no light transmitted) to transparent (full light transmission). LCD monitors have a higher luminance than CRT monitors and do not have problems with veil glare. They also generate less heat than CRT monitors and are stable long term. Reflection tends to be less with LCD monitors, allowing higher ambient light levels to be used in areas where it may be impractical to lower room lights, such as in the emergency department. LCD monitors have restricted fields of view. This is the angle from which the display screen can be viewed. A special problem of LCD displays is that the field of view gradually deteriorates as the viewer moves away from the center of the screen. Similar to a CRT the LCD requires quality testing on a regular basis, starting with acceptance testing and continuing periodically throughout the life of the monitor. LCD monitors, though more expensive than CRTs, require less maintenance and are easier to install.

STORAGE

A major problem for all radiology departments is the storage of film as required by local legal precedents. Many institutions store all films for 5 to 7 years, with pediatric and litigation films retained indefinitely. Many hours of staff time and immense amounts of space are required to maintain these files. A PACS eliminates the need for most of the space for storage

and reduces the time requirements. Misfiling becomes much less likely and acquisition time can be reduced tremendously. In addition, PACS terminals permit access to images from remote locations (e.g., surgery, emergency units, etc.).

Image storage requires immense amounts of memory. Digital storage of images for a typical large radiology department that does 150,000 examinations per year (with about 100,000 of these diagnostic radiography and the 50,000 divided among CT, ultrasound, MRI, nuclear medicine, mammography, and vascular procedures) has been estimated at about 3.2 terabytes of computer memory per year. Considering a normal 3–5-year image storage requirement, a total memory of 10–16 terabytes (Tb)(10,000 Gb or 10,000,000-16,000,000 Mb) would be required for a complete digital PACS. With gigabytes and terabytes of memory now readily available, many radiology departments are beginning digital storage of many procedures.

Consideration must be given to short-term, long-term, and off-site storage for backup due to catastrophic data loss. Short-term storage is often on a local modality hard drive when an exam is completed. Upon completion of the exam, the image is sent to the PACS server and can be stored in a redundant array of independent discs (RAID) for a few weeks or months for quick retrieval. This is similar to keeping films in the radiology department prior to long-term storage. Once the necessity for quick access is not required, the image can be placed in long-term storage. This storage may be in a "jukebox," where either discs or tapes are retrieved by a robotic arm. Off-site storage is used to ensure data integrity if a catastrophic event were to occur that could destroy data at an institution. Transition to digital storage frees up space in the imaging department previously occupied by film storage.

DICOM

Most radiology departments do not have all equipment made by one manufacturer or vendor, which means that a method had to be developed to allow all systems to communicate in the digital environment. The American College of Radiology (ACR) and National Electrical Manufacturers Association (NEMA) began work on standards for PACS in 1982 and the first version was implemented in 1985. The name *DICOM* (Digital Imaging and COmmunication in Medicine) was developed in 1992. DICOM was designed so imaging equipment vendors could develop instruments that can communicate and participate in sharing medical information. The focus is on information exchange, interconnectivity, and communication. It is a standards-based protocol for exchanging and storing medical data, both as actual images and as text associated with images. Basically, DICOM provides a high level of structure for defining possible communications between systems. It is a protocol for exchanging and storing medical data as both images and the text associated with them. When purchasing any equipment for an imaging department, a conformance statement must provide documentation of the specific DICOM services and data types supported.

There are lots of files attached to each image, which contain data such as patient and image information. There is a large amount of raw data that needs to travel through the system, which needs to be converted, especially when traveling to equipment from different vendors. Just imagine, all the equipment speaks different languages and you need an interpreter. DICOM is an object-oriented standard that designates real-world objects that it models and the information objects used to achieve that modeling. There are two classes of information: object class, which contains information about study and patient, and service class, which describes what to do with objects. The service class includes image storage, image query, image retrieval, image print, storage resource, and examination. The object class includes normalized and composite information. The normalized object can contain information in areas such as patient, study, results, storage resource, and image annotation. The composite object will have the modality

TABLE 26-1.	DICOM Information Classes	
Service Class	**Object Class**
Image storage	Normalized
Image query	• Patient, study, results, storage resource, image annotation
Image retrieval	Composite
Image print	• CR
Storage resource	• CT
Examination	• MR
	• Digitized film
	• NM
	• US

used, such as CR, DR, CT, MR, digitized film, US, and NM. (See Table 26-1.)

The object class and service class combine to form units, or service object pairs (SOPs). The combination of a service, such as image storage, with an object, such as a CT exam, would constitute a SOP. Equipment can either "use" or "provide" a service, leading to the terms **service class user** (SCU) and **service class provider** (SCP). Whether equipment is a user or provider depends on how it is asked to function. For example, if the CT scanner wants to send an image to the workstation for storage, the CT scanner is the SCU (user) and the workstation is the SCP (provider). The CT scanner must know how to "send" the image data and the workstation must know how to "receive" it. Then the workstation can become a user when it wants to send the image for storage, while the storage is the provider. In this case the workstation can be either a provider or user depending on how it is asked to function. DICOM is an extremely complex software; this is only a simple explanation of how it can work.

SUMMARY

The introduction of PACS has changed everything about radiology. When fully implemented, PACS is designed to save time and space by eliminating all areas associated with the use of film. The digital environment allows faster image acquisition with fewer repeats and faster turnaround time with diagnosis. PACS provides wider and faster availability of images and may shorten hospital stays.

REVIEW QUESTIONS

1. What is the difference between digital acquisition of an image and digitizing a film?
2. Why are digital image data files so large?
3. What is the difference between RIS and HIS?
4. How does a laser film printer create an image?
5. What are some advantages of using soft-copy display?
6. Why do radiologist monitors have a higher resolution than the ones used by the technologist?
7. What affects image quality on a CRT monitor?
8. Why can higher ambient light be used with an LCD?
9. Why would an institution consider off-site storage for images?
10. What is the difference between object class and service class in DICOM?

REFERENCES AND RECOMMENDED READINGS

Alkhalifah K., Brindhaban A., Al' Ali H., & Alhuraibi A. (2005). The stability of dry and wet laser imaging systems. *Radiologic Technology.* 76(3), 192–196.

Chu R., Christian E., Eaton B. (1999). Stability of a dry laser imaging system. *Radiologic Technology,* 71(1), 29–34.

DeJarnette, W. T. (1999, September). PACS: The next generation. *Applied Radiology, 28,* 31–35.

Graf, B., Simon, U., Eickmeyer, F., & Fiedler, V. (2000). 1K versus 2K monitor: A clinical alternative free-response receiver operating characteristic study of observer performance using pulmonary nodules. *American Journal of Roentgenology, 174*(4), 1067–1074.

http://medical.nema.org/, DICOM, Digital Imaging and Communications in Medicine, NEMA. August 14, 2004.

Huang, H. PACS and Imaging Informatics. (2004). New York: John Wiley & Sons.

Huang, H. K. (1999). *PACS: Basic principles and applications.* New York: Wiley-Liss.

Huda, W., & Szeverenyi, (1999, February). The filmless radiology department: A primer. *Applied Radiology, 28,* 30–34.

Reiner, B. I., Siegel, E. L., & Carrino, J. A. (Eds.). (2002). *Quality assurance: Meeting the challenge in the digital medical enterprise.* Great Falls, VA: Society for Computer Applications in Radiology (SCAR).

Samei, E., & Flynn, M. J. (Eds.). (2003). *Advances in digital radiography: Categorical course in diagnostic radiology physics.* Radiological Society of North America, Oak Brook, IL.

Seibert, J. A., Filipow, L. J., & Andriole, K. P. (Eds.). (1999). *Practical digital imaging and PACS.* Madison, WI: Medical Physics.

Siegel, E. L., & Kolodner, R. M. (Eds.). (1999). *Filmless radiology.* New York: Springer.

Zahriger, M., Wassmer, G., Kurg, B. (2001). Image quality of digital chest x-ray wet versus dry laser printers. *Journal of Digital Imaging. 314,* 158–162.

UNIT IV
Analyzing the Image

The ability of the radiographer to analyze the image brings his or her professional skills to the highest levels possible. The process of analyzing demands a thorough knowledge of the scientific basis by which the image was produced as well as a significant amount of clinical experience. When these skills are applied via problem-solving techniques, the process of diagnosis results. **The radiographer diagnoses the image exactly as the physician diagnoses pathology.** This unit is designed to provide the analytical abilities in both diagnosis and treatment that make the radiographer an image expert.

The imaging process is remarkably similar for all radiologic and imaging sciences modalities. From conventional film and screen radiography through computed radiography to magnetic resonance imaging and ultrasound, the phases of acquiring, process-ing, archiving, and displaying the image have common parameters. This unit explores the process of analyzing the image from this common perspective.

Digital radiography acquires the image and then processes, archives, and displays it very differently from conventional radiography. Unit III is devoted to the specifics of these differences.

Before attempting to diagnose the quality of the image, it is important that the radiographer under-stands the imaging process, including a diagnostic problem-solving technique. Then it is important to ex-plore in depth each of the properties which affect ra-diographic quality to examine the controlling and influencing factors, their effect on the appearance of the image, how to assess them, and how to make ad-justments properly. Separate chapters on **density, contrast, recorded detail,** and **distortion** explore these elements. When a diagnostic process is applied to all of the properties together, an artistic skill in im-age evaluation results. A system that utilizes this process is presented as the **art of image critique.**

Finally, it is the responsibility of the radiographer to monitor and evaluate the performance of all radi-ographic equipment. This is accomplished through the process of **quality management.**

CHAPTER 27

The Imaging Process

[a] requirement of radiography when it is to be practiced as a personal art is the deliberate deviation from "average values." The practice of deviating from average values, settings, measurements, etc. is the mark of the successful professional man in almost any field, and is the principle reason for the esteem he enjoys in his community. His services are sought because he knows how and when to deviate from a standard solution of a problem.

Gerhart S. Schwarz, M.D.,
inventor of the XVS Unit-Step
Radiography System

KEY TERMS

acceptance limits
pyramid problem

OBJECTIVES

Upon completion of this chapter, the student should be able to:

- Describe the five phases of the imaging process.

- Describe the pyramid problem of geometrical progression as it relates to radiographic image quality.

- Apply the four steps of the diagnostic process to a clinical imaging problem.

- Explain how image acceptance limits may fluctuate due to various external factors.

THE IMAGING PROCESS

The imaging process is nearly the same for all radiologic and imaging sciences modalities. All modalities have phases such as where the image is acquired, processed, archived, and, finally, displayed for analysis.

The difference between conventional film/screen radiography and digital radiography, whether computed radiography (CR) or direct radiography (DR), is in the specifics of how these five phases are achieved. The parameters of image quality remain the same for the vast majority of factors. This includes image display, which is a major component of digital radiography but was neglected with conventional film/screen radiography because it was a simple process of viewing hard-copy images on an illuminated viewbox. Although considerable research had been done regarding controlling conditions for viewing hard-copy films, it was not until

digital radiography required a monitor display that the full technology of viewing the image was pursued with the same scientific rigor.

The five phases of the imaging process occur in a well-established sequence (Figure 27-1). The image begins with acquisition, proceeds through processing, then is archived, followed by display, and is then ready for analysis.

Image Acquisition

The image acquisition process is unique to each imaging modality. Figure 27-2 shows the image acquisition phase for both conventional film/screen imaging and digital imaging in this textbook.

The Imaging Process

FIGURE 27-1 The imaging process.

Image Acquisition Phase

FIGURE 27-2 Image acquisition phase.

The creation of the x-ray beam (see Chapters 2–7) and the creation of the x-ray image (see Chapters 15–18) are common to both conventional film/screen imaging and digital imaging. Conventional film/screen imaging is detailed in Chapters 19 to 23. Digital imaging is detailed in Chapters 24 to 26.

Image Processing

Image processing is divided into film/hard-copy and monitor/soft-copy. Figure 27-3 shows the image processing phase for both conventional radiographic imaging and digital radiography in this textbook. Chapters 19–21 detail film hard-copy processing. Chapters 24–25 detail digital image processing. Both film/screen and digital imaging can be processed either film/hard copy or monitor/soft copy. Conventional film/screen images can be recorded on film/hard copy or they can be digitized into DICOM format images that can be processed via monitor/soft-copy methods. Digital images can be processed for monitor/soft copy or they can be produced as film/hard copy by a laser or dry imaging system.

Image Archiving

Image archiving consists of storing images for reference. Film/hard copy can be physically stored (these issues are addressed in Chapter 19, Radiographic Film) or digitized and stored electronically. Monitor/soft-copy images can be stored through a variety of electronic storage options (which are detailed in Chapter 24, Digital Image Processing and Chapter 26–Digital Image Management). Figure 27-4 shows the image archiving phase for conventional and digital radiography.

Image Display

Image display is a critical element in both conventional film/screen and digital imaging. Although it was considered a minimal area for investigation and change when all images were viewed as film/hard copy on an illuminated viewbox, the advent of digital imaging required a monitor display and a focus of attention. Figure 27-5 illustrates the components of image display for both film/screen and digital imaging.

FIGURE 27-3 Image processing phase.

FIGURE 27-4 Image archiving phase.

Although considerable research had been done regarding controlling conditions for viewing hard-copy films, it was not until minor variations in spatial resolution, density/brightness, and contrast/dynamic range became obvious with the new technology that image display became a full phase for consideration.

Image Display Phase

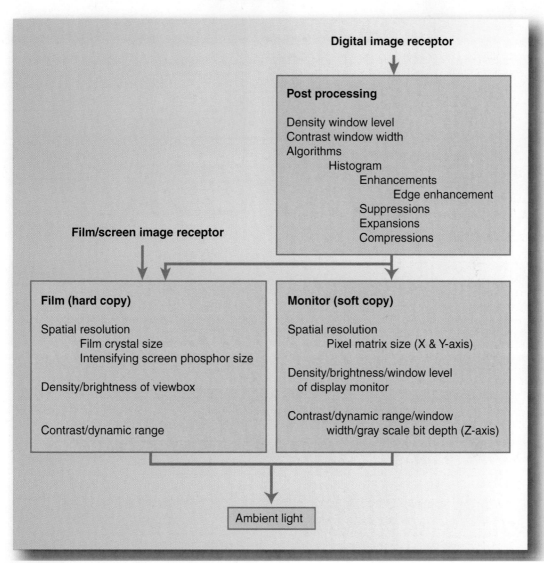

FIGURE 27-5   Image display phase.

Image Analysis

Analyzing the image (see Chapters 28–31) include the traditional image quality factors of density, contrast, recorded detail, and distortion. These factors are shown in Figure 27-6. These factors apply to how the x-ray beam is controlled by the radiographer prior to detection by the image receptor. Control of the beam remains the same for both conventional film/screen imaging and digital imaging. **Although there are differences in how conventional film/screen and digital imaging acquire the image, these are variations in how the image receptor responds to the incoming data, not fundamental changes in the quality factors of density, contrast, recorded detail,**

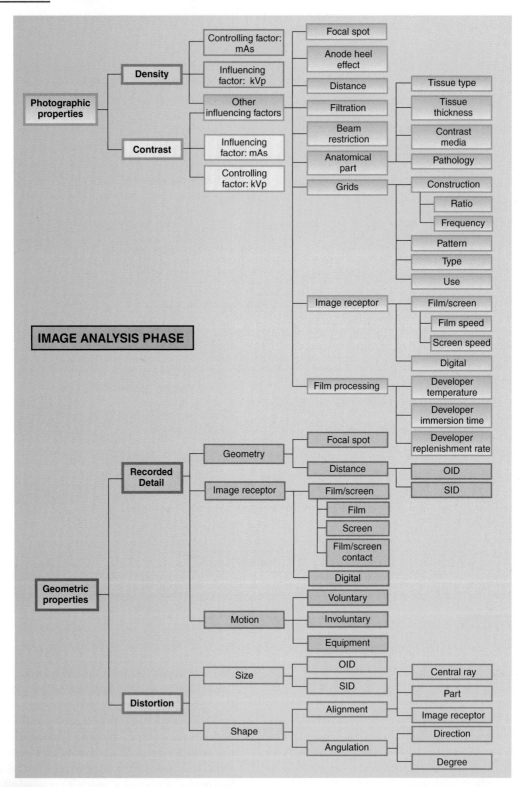

FIGURE 27-6 Image analysis phase.

and distortion. For example, just as a high-speed intensifying screen will respond differently from a wide latitude phosphor to the incoming x-ray photons, so will a direct digital image receptor.

PROFESSIONAL IMAGING STANDARDS

Just as all professionals are expected to adhere to the technical and ethical standards of their field, so radiographers are expected to establish personal imaging standards which satisfy the diagnostic needs of the radiologist and the quality needs of the supervisor. Additionally, they must not violate the personal ethical standards of radiation protection and patient care. Everyone makes mistakes, but professionals are able to correct their mistakes by using a careful analytical process to determine exactly what went wrong. In radiography, emphasis must be placed on learning how to look at images critically.

The Pyramid Problem

A major roadblock in overcoming complex problems such as establishing imaging standards is sometimes called the **pyramid problem.** An acceptable image is the result of a multitude of factors, including technical factor selection, subject density, contrast, pathology and film processing. Unfortunately, some factors can act upon each other, thus creating a pyramid of problems for the radiographer. When many factors are acting upon each other, the result is an astronomical number of possibilities.

THE ANALYTICAL PROCESS

Diagnosing and Treating the Image

Anyone working in a clinical setting quickly becomes acquainted with the process of medical diagnosis. Determining the cause of a problem is a fascinating process. Most medical professionals would welcome an opportunity to participate in this process but they are restricted by law. In fact, the *Scope of Practice of the American Registry of Radiologic Technologists* states "under no circumstances (shall a radiographer) give out oral or written diagnoses." However, the diagnosis of technical problems in the imaging process requires the same skills that a physician uses in medical diagnosis.

Physicians are experts in the science of anatomy and physiology. Radiologists are physicians who are expert in the art of diagnosing through anatomical images as well. But even radiologists are not trained in the finer points of creating and analyzing the image. In this area the radiographer is the true professional expert. The diagnosis and treatment of image quality is the domain of the radiography profession and radiographers are eminently qualified to practice this art and science.

The Diagnostic Process

A knowledge of the diagnostic process is necessary for the radiographer to diagnose and treat the image. The secret to solving any pyramid problem is a careful and meticulous breakdown of the whole into individual parts. The difference between being good and being great is often only a matter of attention to detail. Taking time to break down and analyze technical problems permits proper diagnosis to occur. When properly followed, the diagnostic process makes the treatment clear. Diagnosis involves the highest level of mental acuity. It requires the use of the skills of analysis, synthesis and evaluation to solve complex problems. A diagnostic problem-solving strategy includes four major steps.

Narrowing the Search Field. The first phase involves **narrowing the search.** Experts begin with a review of the entire image to avoid premature narrowing. During this review a search is made for anything that is different from a diagnostic quality image. When differences are noticed a pattern is sought, especially when there is more than one cue. These cues focus attention on a suspicious area, thus narrowing the search. An example would be an image that looks light, gray, and blurred. An inexperienced radiographer might jump to the conclusion that the image was too light and there was motion. However, an expert radiographer might notice additional cues, such as the loss of detail confined to a small region and proper image receptor exposure in other areas.

Hypothesis Activation. The second phase requires that the cues be used to **seek hypotheses.** An effort is made to formulate a hypothesis that will explain all the cues. Cues that do not fit the hypothesis should be held in reserve. In the example, the inexperienced radiographer might hypothesize that too little radiation was used and that the patient was breathing. The expert would realize that many hypotheses could account for the image, including several cases of "too little radiation," such as insufficient kVp, mA or time, excessive distance and improper film, screens or processing. They would also include several explanations for a blurred image, such as poor film/screen contact, increased object-to-image receptor distance and tube motion, as well as the patient motion hypothesis.

Information Seeking. The next phase demands that the hypotheses be tested by **seeking more information.** When stumped, radiographers should use general questioning to produce more cue information. It may be necessary to shift focus to other possible solutions when new cues are discovered. In the example, the novice radiographer might ask the patient if she held her breath. When the patient answers "yes," the novice radiographer might not believe her, rather than reject the hypothesis of patient motion. The expert, on the other hand, might notice during the questioning of the patient that her breast was superimposed over the area of interest. This additional cue could be used to return to the image. A new look at the image might show that the underexposed area was confined to the breast region.

Hypothesis Evaluation. The last phase of the diagnostic process is the **evaluation of the final hypothesis.** It is critical that the hypothesis used resolves the greatest amount of cue data. At this point the radiographer should be able to predict the solution to the problem. The inexperienced radiographer would apply the "too little radiation and patient motion" hypothesis and increase the mAs

while watching the patient closely. The expert radiographer would conclude that the most likely hypothesis was increased subject density, decreased subject contrast, and poor film/screen contact. The expert would then ask the patient to move the breast aside and use a different cassette with good film/screen contact. Of course, the expert would produce a diagnostic quality image. The novice would be left with an overexposed image of even poorer quality than the first one.

Remember, however, data shows that novices often do surprisingly well when using the diagnostic process. Diagnosing ability can be improved by:

1. Remembering that cues are not a diagnosis;
2. Being careful to separate observations from inferences;
3. Not jumping to conclusions at the first cue;
4. Looking for competing hypotheses;
5. Trying each cue with each hypothesis;
6. Validating the hypothesis with questioning, when possible;
7. Ruling out hypotheses one by one;
8. Being cautious of premature closure;
9. Being tentative in the diagnosis until experienced; and, most important,
10. **Being confident in your expert knowledge.**

 ## ACCEPTANCE LIMITS

Knowing how to diagnose an imaging problem is not helpful until the knowledge can be applied to radiographic quality analysis. This application involves establishing and adhering to quality imaging standards.

Graphing Acceptance Limits

The main goal must be to fix the limits of the radiographs that will be accepted against those that will not. This is much easier to understand by looking at the concept of **acceptance limits** graphically. The quality of all the radiographs produced by a technologist over a period has been graphed in Figure 24-7.

FIGURE 27-7 Radiographic image quality distribution curve. Note that the curve is skewed to the dark side. Standard practice dictates that a dark or low contrast image is always preferable to one that is too light or high contrast.

FIGURE 27-8 Typical acceptance limits of radiographic quality.

Although the radiographer's goal is to always produce a diagnostic quality image, suboptimal images are often accepted for diagnosis. There are many reasons for this practice, the most important being the knowledge that the prime cause of increased patient radiation dose is repeated exposure. Radiologists do not expect textbook results on every patient. They do, however, have the right to expect the radiographer to provide an image that permits them to see all the structures critical to their diagnosis. Figure 27-8 shows where a typical radiologist might draw the line on overexposed or underexposed images. The important thing to remember is that if the radiographer, supervisor, radiologist, or other physician determines that an image is not acceptable, **it is outside the acceptance limits of quality.** When this occurs, the radiographer is obligated to analyze the image and make a proper decision on what factor or factors caused the error. The technique and procedure must then be adjusted to bring the unacceptable image back to the **perfect center** of diagnostic quality.

Striving for Perfection

Too often there is a tendency to correct only enough to obtain a passable image (Figure 27-9). **All corrections should strive for perfection.** Attempt-

O = Original Image
R = Repeated Image

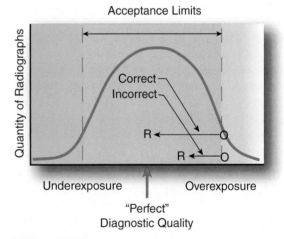

FIGURE 27-9 Correcting image quality.

ing to get by with minimal adjustments contributes to a negative image of the profession. The best radiographer can miscalculate and produce a poor image once, but competency is questioned when a radiographer is repeatedly unable to correct mistakes. The true professional completes the meticulous analysis by making a competent adjustment and achieves near perfection each time an exposure must be repeated.

Factors Affecting Acceptance Limit Curves

It is interesting to consider the factors that may affect the shape of the acceptance limit curve. Figure 27-7 is skewed to the overexposure side because these errors are more acceptable than underexposure mistakes. A bright light is capable of revealing information that is obscured in an overexposed image. However, when an image is underexposed there is no method to see information that is not present on the image receptor. There are many other factors that can modify the shape of the acceptance curve. When acceptance limits are very narrow, a high repeat rate occurs (Figure 27-10). However, if the radiographers are not producing many perfect images, the repeat rate will remain high (Figure 27-11) even when acceptance limits are very wide.

An interesting phenomenon has been observed over the years in many radiology departments. When a radiograph is hovering near the acceptance limits for the department, radiographers will often attempt to have it approved by a radiologist known to have wide acceptance limits. Departmental acceptance limits are simply a composite of the limits imposed by each radiologist, supervisor, and radiographer in the department. Narrow acceptance lim-

its may cause radiographers to produce more images near perfect center, thus changing the curve shape, as shown in Figure 27-12.

Conversely, wide limits may permit radiographers to become careless and produce fewer images near perfect center, thus changing the curve shape, as shown in Figure 27-11. Many factors can change

FIGURE 27-11 Wide acceptance limits may produce a high repeat rate by permitting radiographers to become careless and produce fewer images near perfect center.

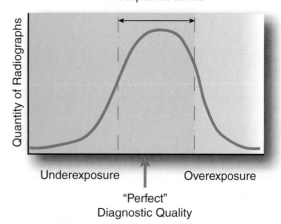

FIGURE 27-12 Narrow acceptance limits may cause radiographers to produce more images near perfect center.

FIGURE 27-10 Narrow acceptance limits may produce a high repeat rate.

the shape of the image quality curve. Among them are the positioning and technical abilities of the radiographer, the quality standards of everyone involved in the imaging chain, the condition of the equipment, the stress level of the department, and on and on. Awareness of these factors, combined with high professional standards, can help one's personal curve appear as in Figure 27-13.

Practical Considerations

In actual clinical practice the achievement of a diagnostic quality image the first time is not as hard as it might at first appear. Each factor must be varied within set limits to see a noticeable change in the image. It is important not only to learn the rules pertaining to image quality but to be sure they are used in clinical practice. The real problem is in learning **to make large enough changes to cause visible differences** on the image. Radiographers who are unsure of their ability often make timid changes that cannot be seen in the repeat image. When a decision is made to repeat a procedure (and doubly expose the patient), a change large enough to bring

FIGURE 27-13 Ideal acceptance limits.

the image to the center of diagnostic quality must be made. Shifting the image from just outside the acceptance limits to just inside them is inexcusable. As professionals, radiographers must always strive toward perfection.

SUMMARY

Professional imaging standards can be established by overcoming the pyramid problem. Evaluating imaging problems is the true professional expertise of the radiographer. The analytical process of diagnosis is appropriate for use in solving these problems. The diagnostic process involves narrowing the search field, hypothesis activation, information seeking, and hypothesis evaluation.

The concept of acceptance limits is helpful in understanding how repeated radiographs must be corrected. All repeated radiographs should strive for perfection by attempting to reach the "diagnostic quality" center of the acceptance limit curve. When a decision is made to repeat a procedure, a change large enough to bring the image to the center of diagnostic quality must be made.

REVIEW QUESTIONS

1. What is the pyramid problem?
2. What are the four steps in the diagnostic problem-solving strategy?
3. What is the purpose of a cue in narrowing the search?
4. When is an image determined to be outside acceptance limits?
5. Why are acceptance limit curves skewed to the dark side?

REFERENCES AND RECOMMENDED READING

American Registry of Radiologic Technologists. (1987). *Article I, Section D. Rules and regulations as revised August 1987*. Minneapolis, MN: Author.

Berman, L., De Lacey, G., Twomey, E., Twomey, B., Welch, T., & Eban, R. (1985). Reducing the errors in the accident department: A simple method of using radiographers. *British Journal of Radiology, 290*, 421–422.

Bowman, S. (1991). Introducing an abnormal detection system by radiographers into an accident and emergency department: An investigation into radiographers' concerns about the introduction of such a system. *Research in Radiography, I*(I), 2–20.

Carlton, R. R. (1992). Another dimension of quality assurance in radiology. In L. T. Gurley & W. J. Callaway, (Eds.), *Introduction to radiologic technology* (3rd ed, pp. 149–166). St. Louis, MO: C. V. Mosby.

Carlton, R. R., & McKenna, A. (1989). Repeating radiographs: Setting imaging standards. In *Postgraduate advances in radiologic technology*. (Editor—Eugene Frank) Berryville, VA: Forum Medicum.

Carnevali, D. L., Mitchell, P. H., Woods, N. F., & Tanner, C. A. (1984). *Diagnostic reasoning in nursing*. Philadelphia: J. B. Lippincott.

Cheyne, N., Field-Boden, W., Wilson, I., & Hall, R. (1987). The radiographer and the front line diagnosis. *Radiography, 53*(609), 114.

Cullinan, A., & Cullinan, J. (1994). *Producing quality radiographs* (2nd ed.). Philadelphia: J. B. Lippincott.

Cullinan, J. E. (1981). A 'perfect' chest radiograph—or a compromise? *Radiologic Technology, 53*(2), 121.

Dowd, S. B. (1995). *Encyclopedia of radiographic positioning*. Philadelphia: W. B. Saunders.

Edwards, J., & Bowman, S. (1994). The expanding role of the radiographer. *Radiologic Science and Education, 1*(1), 14–20.

Goldman, L. W. (1977). Effects of film processing variability on patient dose and image quality. *Second Image Receptor Conference: Radiographic Film Processing: Proceedings of a Conference held in Washington, DC, March 31–April 2, 1977*. (HEW Publication [FDA] 77-8036, 55-63). Rockville, MD: U.S. Department of Health, Education, and Welfare, Public Health Service, Food and Drug Administration, Bureau of Radiological Health.

Hendee, W. R., & Ritenour, R. (2002). *Medical imaging physics* (3rd ed.). New York, New York: Wiley.

Mumford, L. C. (1980). Radiographic quality 'a seminar'. *The Canadian Journal of Medical Radiation Technology, 11*(1), 10.

Prior, J. A., Silberstein, J. S., & Stang, J. M. (1981). *Physical diagnosis: The history and examination of the patient*. St. Louis, MO: C. V. Mosby.

Singer, B. H. (1971). The aesthetic method in radiographic exposure. *Radiologic Technology, 42*(6), 411.

Swinburn, K. (1971, March 20). Pattern recognition for radiographers. *The Lancet*, Vol. 7699, pp 589–90.

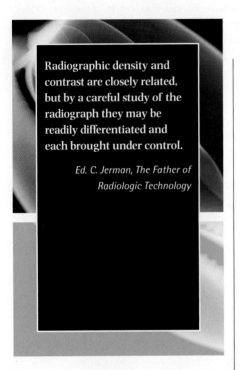

CHAPTER 28

Density

> Radiographic density and contrast are closely related, but by a careful study of the radiograph they may be readily differentiated and each brought under control.
>
> *Ed. C. Jerman, The Father of Radiologic Technology*

KEY TERMS

brightness
density
exposure
  maintenance
  formula
window level

OBJECTIVES

Upon completion of this chapter, the student should be able to:

- Identify density as a prime component of the photographic properties controlling visibility of detail of radiographic image quality.

- Define density/brightness.

- Describe the effects of density changes on image appearance.

- Describe the process of evaluating image density.

- Explain why mA and time are the controlling factors of film density.

- Explain how each influencing factor affects image density.

- Assess density on various images.

- Recommend appropriate adjustments to compensate for variation in the controlling and influencing factors that affect image density.

ASSESSING DENSITY

Density is one of the two photographic properties that comprise visibility of detail. Visibility of detail refers to the fact that the image is visible to the human eye only because sufficient density (and contrast) exists to permit the structural details to be perceived. **The traditional definition of density was the degree of overall blackening from the black metallic silver deposited in the emulsion** of film. This will now be described as film **density. Brightness** describes the concept of density as it is displayed on a soft-copy monitor for digital images. It is the proper term for the level of the display monitor light emission. **Window level** describes the digital processing that produces changes in density/brightness, so it also is appropriate to use when controlling image density. Unless otherwise specified, the term *density* refers to image density/brightness.

The physical concept of density is discussed in detail in previous chapters (particularly in Chapter 21, Sensitometry). In this chapter the concept of density is approached in an artistically professional manner aimed at diagnosing the image. The art of radiography is a clinical one and must be practiced as such. It is extremely important that this information be used in a clinical setting concurrently with its study.

The major consideration in assessing density is verification that proper densities are visible throughout the anatomical area of interest on the image. Of course, these densities must be well within the range of human visibility (usually OD 0.25–2.50). Much of this ability to verify proper densities is a result of clinical experience (Figure 28-1). It is obvious that the proper density for lung tissue is not as great as the proper density for the thoracic spine, even though they are both thoracic structures. Common sense and a trained professional eye are the primary tools of the radiographer when evaluating density. The ability to assess density is a result of continued conscientious evaluation of images during clinical experiences. The radiographer who becomes professionally interested in the process of diagnosing the image quickly gains and refines this ability.

A

B

FIGURE 28-1 Clinical experience in assessing film density: (A) Although this image is not acceptable for the clavicle, it is a diagnostic quality image of the acromioclavicular joints; (B) Although this image is not acceptable for the thoracic spine, it is a diagnostic quality image of the chest.

Information is recorded on an image that is overexposed but may not exist at all on a radiograph that is underexposed. The overexposed image has received too many photons and, as a result, has recorded too much information. A bright light or scanner can eliminate the excess information and reveal details within the range of human visual ability. With a digital imaging system, this is very easily accomplished by adjusting the window level. This is not the case with a film that is underexposed. The underexposed image has not received the information in the first place and is not capable of being manipulated to reveal details that were never recorded. Consequently, **whenever a choice must be made between excess and insufficient density, the wise decision is always the choice that will produce the overexposed image.**

EFFECTS ON IMAGE APPEARANCE

The effects of mAs and the other influencing factors on density are not exact because of the multiple variables that are part of the imaging system. Many of the variables affect the density of the image in a nonlinear fashion under some conditions. For example, the typical D log E curve is only somewhat linear in the straight line portion. If exposure conditions push into the toe or shoulder regions of the curve, dramatic film density changes can be seen. Similarly, density changes can sometimes be seen from only a slight nonlinearity in the intensifying screen phosphor response curve, the film silver halide response, the thermionic emission of the x-ray tube filament, etc. A digital response curve can be preset or adjusted to compensate for these problems.

Fortunately, these variables have a statistical tendency to balance one another. But in cases where conditions cause a majority of the variables to increase or decrease exposure a total of more than 30 percent, an unexpected change in film density may become visible. Even when unexpected density changes exceed the 30 percent necessary to become visible, they seldom place the image outside the acceptance limits.

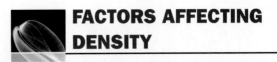

FACTORS AFFECTING DENSITY

A wide variety of factors affect density (Figure 28-2). These factors are classified as either controlling or influencing factors. The controlling factor should be used as the principle method for adjusting for insufficient or excessive density.

Milliampere-Seconds as the Controlling Factor

While the relationship between mAs and exposure is a direct proportional one, the relationship of these two factors to density is much more complex. Density is determined by the characteristics of the image receptor. A D log E sensitometric curve or a digital response curve expresses the relationship between exposure and density. For film, the log-relative exposure is plotted on the x axis and density (D) plotted on the y axis. The relationship between exposure and density determines the shape and position of the D log E curve for a given film under specific processing conditions. This relationship is described in detail in Chapter 21. Recall that film density is the $\log_{10}$ of opacity and opacity is the relationship of incident light to transmitted light. For example, if a region of a radiograph has an OD of 1.0, only 10 percent or 1/10 of the incident light is transmitted through the radiograph in this region. The opacity of the region would be 10. If the OD number is increased to 1.3, the opacity is doubled (to 20) and the percentage of light transmitted through the film is halved (to 5 percent or 1/20). Increments of 0.3 changes in OD numbers represent a doubling or halving of opacity.

The important part of the D log E curve is that portion between the toe and the shoulder (the diagnostic range of the film). In this central straight line portion, the film density is approximately proportional to the log relative exposure. This is because a straight line will always have a constant ratio. If the slope of the straight line portion is at a 45° angle, the average gradient will measure 1.0. In this example, a doubling of exposure will result in a doubling of the opacity. (Note that the term *doubling of*

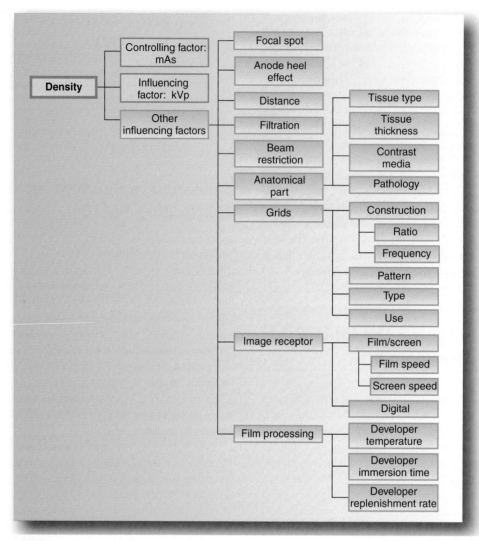

FIGURE 28-2 Image analysis: factors affecting density.

film density is not used because density is a log number. A change of 0.3 in density reflects a doubling or halving of opacity.) **A common misnomer in radiography is that doubling the exposure will double the film density.** This is not true for a typical radiographic film/screen system.

For digital image receptor systems, changes in mAs no longer control density. Image density/brightness on the display monitor is controlled by window leveling. **Setting the correct mAs is still critical in determining proper digital image receptor**

exposure. Despite the ability to control image density through post-processing parameters, it is still the responsibility of the radiographer to provide the digital image receptor with an appropriate exposure for a given procedure.

Digital image histograms are graphic representations of the exposure to the image receptor. They are explained and illustrated in Figures 25-7 through 25-10. The manipulation of the histograms during input and output (post processing) provides opportunities to enhance the image to fa-

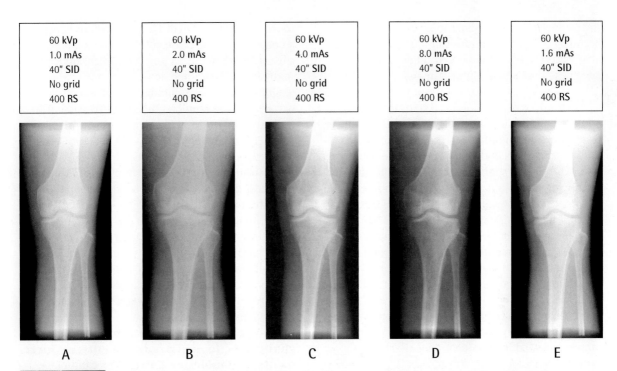

60 kVp	60 kVp	60 kVp	60 kVp	60 kVp
1.0 mAs	2.0 mAs	4.0 mAs	8.0 mAs	1.6 mAs
40" SID	40" SID	40" SID	40" SID	40" SID
No grid	No grid	No grid	No grid	No grid
400 RS	400 RS	400 RS	400 RS	400 RS
A	B	C	D	E

FIGURE 28-3 The effects of mAs change on film density images A–D demonstrate the effect of increasing mAs. Each image is double the mAs of the previous one. Image E represents a 20 percent decrease in mAs from image B.

cilitate diagnosis. These same features also allow information to be obscured and can impede diagnosis. Because the use of the histogram is a dangerous two-edged sword, most manufacturers have elected to restrict most users from manipulating this portion of the digital system. As radiographers become more knowledgeable about digital acquisition and post processing, some manufacturers are opening portions of this feature to users. There are some digital units that offer preset histograms that either must or may be changed by the radiographer. Advanced users are also provided access to create custom histograms for specific clinical situations, which can then be displayed as presets to all users. There is an increasing tendency for radiographers to assert their professional knowledge base in this area that is well worth the effort for both patient and professional.

If the exposure to an image receptor is increased, the density to that receptor will increase to a point.

Since density is primarily determined by the amount of exposure a receptor receives, and since exposure is directly proportional to mAs, **mAs is used as the primary controller of image receptor exposure and film density.** As mAs increases, x-ray exposure increases proportionally and film density also increases (Figure 28–3). The direct proportional relationship between mAs and exposure is used to calculate mAs changes necessary to maintain consistent image density when one or more technical factors are altered. By maintaining a specific exposure relative to the speed of the image receptor, consistent density can be achieved.

When applied to x-rays, the reciprocity law can be restated to say film density should remain unchanged as long as the intensity and duration of the x-ray exposure (controlled by mAs) remains unchanged. Remember that the reciprocity law fails for extremely short (less than 0.01 second) or long (more than a few seconds) exposure times. Within the range of normal radiographic exposures, it can become a factor in special situations (such as pediatric extremities or high-speed angiography). This law does not apply to digital systems.

Film density should remain unchanged as long as the total exposure to the image receptor and all other conditions remain unchanged. If the mAs used to create one image is the same as the mAs used to create a second image of the same structure, then both images should have the same film density. As long as mAs is constant, any combination of mA and exposure time values will create the same film density and image receptor exposure. This was demonstrated previously by the radiographs in Figure 11-1. Of course, accurate results depend on using equipment that is properly calibrated and maintained through an effective quality control program.

The control of density in most instances rests with the radiographer. An appropriate mAs setting may be selected from a technique chart developed for the particular x-ray unit in use. An automatic exposure system will control the time but the mA and the exact density setting will be decided by the radiographer. Computerized exposure systems will provide a suggested technique setting, which can then be modified. Other variables, such as generator phase or falling loads, may also affect the final decision. The experienced radiographer will adapt the suggested mAs setting for the individual patient. Experience and study of various body habitus, pathologies, positioning, and equipment quickly provide the radiographer with clinical knowledge that can be used for these adjustments.

The minimum change necessary to cause a visible shift in film density is 30 percent of mAs, or any other influencing factors that would equal this change. This rule is essentially true for most digital system response curves. However, it is important to realize that the digital histogram can be manipulated to make a very slight change in exposure, cause a huge change in density/brightness. Although it is not normal for a histogram to produce results outside normal usage, it is certainly possible. Various authors over the years have set the minimum for a visible density change at values between 25 and 35 percent of mAs. Although studies of vision have demonstrated that

some people can detect changes in film density as small as 1 percent, this level of perception is not possible when viewing a complex clinical image with many widely separated densities. Some trained professionals, such as radiologists and radiographers, can perceive as small a change as 10 percent on a radiograph but this is extraordinary. In clinical practice a change as small as 30 percent is seldom justified. A comparison between Figures 28-3B and E illustrate a 20 percent change in mAs. This change is difficult to see and would not compensate for improper film density.

An image must be outside the acceptance limits to require repeating the exposure. All acceptance limits permit some degree of variation—at least 30 percent over or underexposed. In these instances the image would have to be significantly more than 30 percent over or underexposed than a diagnostic quality image.

The general rule of thumb for mAs changes is to make adjustments in increments of doubles or halves. For example, a repeated image that is too light at 10 mAs should be repeated at 20, 40, or 80 mAs, depending on the circumstances. Of course, determining which circumstances require 20 mAs, which require 40 mAs, and which require 80 mAs is something that is acquired only through experience and further study. Figures 28-3(A–E) illustrate the doubling and halving rule.

Regardless of variations in equipment output, anatomy, physiology, or pathology, the idea is to adjust the intensity to permit the same amount of radiation to reach the image receptor, thus creating the same density. From this perspective, the art of radiography does not look especially difficult. However, many other factors are yet to be added to the simple task of determining appropriate density.

One clinical practice that should be avoided is attempting to adjust density by increasing or decreasing "a step in time." Due to wide variation in x-ray unit controls, "a step in time" may be a 10 percent change on one unit but a 20 percent or even 30 percent change on another. In fact, time stations are often not linear on the same unit. This makes the "step in time" rule dangerous because of its inconsistency. In addition, in many instances "a step in time" will not even accomplish a visible density change.

Essentially, if the image does not require doubling or halving of the exposure, it seldom requires repeating. Exceptions to this rule are special studies where a fine adjustment of barely 30 percent is crucial to demonstrating a small vessel or pathological condition. The radiographer will often adjust his or her technique chart by a 30 percent margin, but will seldom subject the patient to a second exposure for such a minor change. Making exposure adjustments should be a case of taking bold action (at least doubling or halving) or taking no action at all.

Kilovoltage as an Influencing Factor

Kilovoltage alters the intensity of the beam reaching the image receptor in two ways. Kilovoltage controls the energy and, therefore, the strength of the electrons striking the target of the x-ray tube for any given mAs. More important, kilovoltage controls the average energy of the x-ray photons produced at the anode target. Therefore, a change in kilovoltage alters the intensity of the beam when the mAs and other factors remain the same. Kilovoltage also affects the production of scatter radiation. Because of this, a change in kilovoltage alters the intensity of the beam after it enters the subject (or object) but before it forms the image.

Both the quantity and quality of the x-ray beam will vary significantly with changes in kilovoltage. As a result, kVp has a tremendous impact on density. Research has been done to determine a practical formula which takes both the quantity and quality factors into account. The primary finding is that there are too many variables to be quantified into a reliable formula. A visible change in film density can usually be detected with a 4–5 percent change in kVp in the lower ranges (30–50 kVp), but an 8–9 percent change is required in the middle ranges (50–90 kVp), and a 10–12 percent change in the higher ranges (90–130 kVp).

Because the radiographer must have a method of using kilovoltage to adjust and compensate for film density changes, the rough guide known as the **15 percent rule** has been developed. The 15 percent rule is used as a guide to maintain the same image receptor exposure/film density when kilovoltage changes, as follows:

A 15 percent increase in kilovoltage causes a doubling of exposure to the image receptor. A 15 percent decrease in kilovoltage causes a halving of exposure to the image receptor.

EXAMPLE: A radiograph of the elbow is produced using 4 mAs at 60 kVp. What kVp would be required to halve the exposure to the image receptor?

Answer:

60 kVp − (60 kVp × 15%)
60 kVp − (60 kVp × 0.15)
60 kVp − (9 kVp) = 51 kVp

The 15 percent rule is somewhat accurate within the range of 60 to 100 kVp. Of course, this does not include the entire diagnostic radiography range, which may run from 30 to 150 kVp. The percentage of kVp required to halve the exposure to the image receptor is always greater as the kVp increases. This is primarily due to the increased scatter radiation produced at higher kilovoltages. However, the greatest variable in the production of scatter is the thickness of the part. Therefore, image receptor exposure is increased when radiographing a thick subject (Figure 28-4). Consequently, a 20 percent rule may be more accurate when radiographing a 5 cm wrist, while a 15 percent rule may be more accurate when radiographing a 20 cm abdomen. Another factor which has a mathematical effect on the 15 percent rule is the starting kVp. The percentage change for doubling or halving decreases slightly as the starting kVp increases. In actual fact, **the 15 percent rule may vary from a 15 percent rule to a 25 percent rule** within the diagnostic radiography range of kVps and the diagnostic range of image densities. The 15 percent rule is commonly applied by radiographers because it can be used without producing images outside the acceptance limits. However, understanding the variability of the rule will do much to increase awareness of potential problems when radiographing extremely large or small objects, or with unusually low or high kVp settings. Changing kilovoltage is the primary method of changing image contrast. **Consequently, the 15 percent rule will always change the contrast of the image.** When a contrast change is desirable, the 15 percent

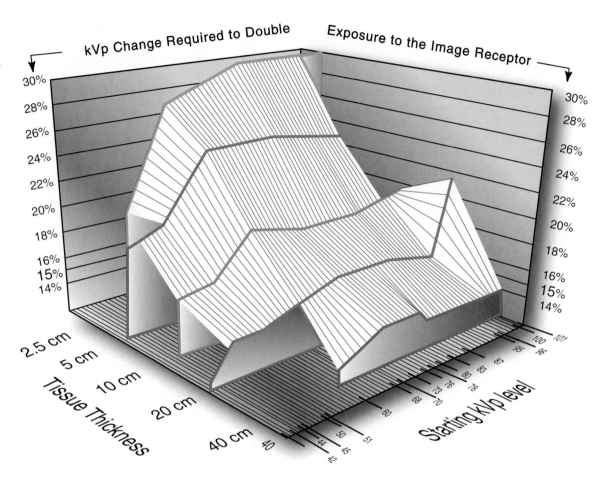

FIGURE 28-4 The relationship of kVp and tissue thickness to image receptor exposure. Note that the line representing a 15 percent increase in kVp is not within the range of some part thicknesses and kVps used in routine diagnostic radiography. It is apparent that the 15 percent rule is not a constant and must be applied with careful consideration of other factors, especially tissue thickness and starting kVp. *(Data extracted from "Kilovoltage Conversion in Radiography" The X-Ray Technician, 31: 373–379, 436, 1960 by Gerhart S. Schwartz, courtesy of the American Society of Radiologic Technologists. Graphics courtesy of Chris Innskeep, Rhodes State College)*

rule is a useful method of maintaining film density. However, when only a film density change is desired, the 15 percent rule should not be used because it causes a contrast change as well. When film density changes are desired, the method of choice is to vary the mAs because it is the controlling factor for film density.

The configuration of the generator is another important consideration in how kVp affects image receptor exposure/film density. The total number of higher energy photons in the

x-ray tube emission spectrum is controlled by the amount of ripple in the waveform. For example, a single-phase, 2-pulse (1φ2p) waveform has a significantly lower average photon energy than a 3-phase, 12-pulse (3φ12p) waveform, resulting in less density (see Chapter 7).

Compensation for the configuration of the generator is most commonly accomplished by considering only the phasing and number of pulses. Conversion factors have been developed for these compensations (Table 28-1).

TABLE 28–1. Conversion Factors Effect of Generator φ on Image Receptor Exposure

When Converting Generator Phase From:	To:	To Maintain Exposure Multiply mAs by a Conversion Factor of:
1φ2p	3φ6p	0.6
1φ2p	3φ12p/ high frequency	0.5
3φ12p/ high frequency	1φ2p	2.0
3φ12p/ high frequency	3φ6p	1.2

Derived from DuPont Bit System, 12th edition, E.I. DuPont Nemours, Inc., Wilminton, DE.

EXAMPLE: If 80 kVp and 20 mAs produce a satisfactory exposure on a 1φ2p unit, what mAs should be used with the same patient and examination on a 3φ12p unit?

Answer:

mAs × conversion factor
20 mAs × 0.5 = 10 mAs

Other Influencing Factors

Focal Spot Size. Larger focal spots utilize a greater incident electron stream than small focal spots. Most manufacturers carefully compensate for this effect by adjusting the actual mA at the filament for dual-focus tubes. The actual mA received by the filament when set at 100 mA for a large focal spot is less than the actual mA received when set at 100 mA for a small focal spot. There should be no difference between large and small focal spots when the unit has been calibrated properly. However, this effect may differ by the 30 percent necessary to alter image density in an improperly calibrated unit.

Large focal spots tend to bloom more at higher milliamperages and may occasionally reach a point where they alter the image receptor exposure. Blooming occurs with large milliamperages because the incident electron beam is not as easily fo-

cused by the focusing cup. It is rare for blooming to cause a visible film density difference.

Because properly calibrated units will not exhibit film density changes when focal spots are changed, differences of this type should be reported as a quality control procedure. If film density differences are perceived due to focal spot blooming, replacement of the tube may be indicated.

Anode Heel Effect. The anode heel effect alters the intensity of radiation, and therefore the density, between the anode and cathode ends of the x-ray tube. Depending on the angle of the anode, this effect can cause an image receptor exposure variation of up to 45 percent between the anode and cathode ends of the image. Image receptor exposure is always greater at the cathode end. The anode heel effect is more pronounced when the collimator is open wide than when it is closed because a greater portion of the peripheral beam, and therefore a greater portion of the intensity difference, reaches the image receptor when the collimator is wide open. The anode heel effect is also more significant when using extremely small angle anodes (12° or less).

When the anode heel effect becomes apparent, it can be minimized or converted to an advantage. It is minimized by collimating the beam and eliminating as much of the intensity difference at the periphery as possible. If a given film size is required (i.e., 14″ × 17″) collimation may be achieved by using a greater SID.

The anode heel effect may be converted to an advantage in examinations of objects with greater subject density at one end than at another. The advantage is utilized by placing the portion of the object with the greatest subject density toward the cathode end of the tube. This utilizes the greater intensity for the greater subject density and leaves the lesser intensity of the anode end of the tube for the lesser subject density. The anode heel effect can often be used to advantage in a number of examinations (Table 28-2).

Distance (SID and OID). Source-to-image receptor distance (SID) alters the intensity of the beam reaching the image receptor, according to the inverse square law. The inverse

TABLE 28-2.	Projections That May Use the Anode Heel Effect to Advantage	
Projection	**Body Part to Be Placed Toward**	
	Cathode End of Tube	Anode End of Tube
Femur (AP/lateral)	hip	knee
Lower leg (AP/lateral)	knee	ankle
Humerus (AP/lateral)	shoulder	elbow
Forearm (AP/lateral)	elbow	wrist
Thoracic spine (AP)	abdomen	neck
Thoracic spine (lateral)	neck	abdomen
Lumbar spine (AP/lateral)	pelvis	abdomen

square law affects exposure in inverse proportion to the square of the distance. This is represented by the formula:

$$\frac{I_1}{I_2} = \frac{D_2^2}{D_1^2}$$

where: I_1 = old intensity
I_2 = new intensity
D_1^2 = old distance squared
D_2^2 = new distance squared

The law states that the intensity (exposure) varies inversely with the square of the distance.

The inverse square law formula expresses the change in intensity when the distance changes. For example, as distance increases, radiation intensity and film density decrease. However, the most common situation in radiography is a need to maintain an acceptable image receptor exposure/film density while changing the distance. To maintain image receptor exposure, mAs (or an influencer) must be changed to compensate for the exposure change. The **exposure maintenance formula** is used for

this purpose. This formula is based on the inverse square law but is reversed to a direct square law because mAs must increase when distance increases, and vice versa, in order to maintain image receptor exposure.

$$\frac{mAs_1}{mAs_2} = \frac{D_1^2}{D_2^2}$$

where: mAs_1 = original mAs
mAs_2 = new mAs
D_1^2 = old distance squared
D_2^2 = new distance squared

EXAMPLE: If a satisfactory exposure is obtained with 20 mAs at 72″, what mAs will be required to maintain the same exposure at 40″?

Answer:

$$\frac{mAs_1}{mAs_2} = \frac{D_1^2}{D_2^2}$$

$$\frac{20 \text{ mAs}}{mAs_2} = \frac{72^2}{40^2}$$

$$\frac{20 \text{ mAs}}{mAs_2} = \frac{5,184}{1,600}$$

$$mAs_2 = \frac{20 \text{ mAs} \times 1,600}{5,184}$$

$$mAs_2 = \frac{32,000}{5,184}$$

$$mAs_2 = 6.2 \text{ mAs}$$

It is more useful when algebraically changed to solve for the new mAs, which is the most common factor that must be calculated in clinical practice:

$$mAs_2 = \frac{mAs_1 \times D_2^2}{D_1^2}$$

EXAMPLE: If a satisfactory PA chest radiograph is made at 72″ with 4 mAs, what mAs will be required at 56″?

Answer:

$$mAs_2 = \frac{mAs_1 \times D_2^2}{D_1^2}$$

$$mAs_2 = \frac{4 \text{ mAs} \times 56^2}{72^2}$$

TABLE 28-3. mAs Change Factors for Approximate Exposure Maintenance When Distance Changes

To calculate the new mAs, multiple the old mAs by the factor in the corresponding box to the distance change.

Old Distance	New Distance 36" 90 cm	40" 100 cm	48" 120 cm	56" 140 cm	72" 180 cm
36" (90 cm)	–	1.23	1.77	2.42	4.00
40" (100 cm)	0.81	–	1.44	1.96	3.24
48" (120 cm)	0.59	0.69	–	1.36	2.25
56" (140 cm)	0.41	0.51	0.73	–	1.65
72" (180 cm)	0.25	0.31	0.44	0.60	–

$$mAs_2 = \frac{4\ mAs \times 3{,}136}{5{,}184}$$

$$mAs_2 = \frac{12{,}544}{5{,}184}$$

$$mAs_2 = 2.5\ mAs$$

The exposure maintenance formula is only accurate within a moderate acceptance range. **The nonlinearity of some components in the imaging system makes it impossible to exactly quantify the relationship between radiation beam intensity and film density.**

Table 28-3 illustrates the mAs change factors for the most common distances employed in radiography. The vast majority of diagnostic radiography today is done at 40" to 72". In addition 56", which is halfway between 40" and 72", is useful in mobile radiography when circumstances do not permit either of the two preferred distances. A useful rule of thumb for doubling and halving distances can be derived from this table by considering the 30 percent range necessary to produce a visible film density difference in the image:

Use only the distances 40", 56", and 72". When increasing distance, double the mAs for each change. When decreasing distance, halve the mAs for each change. For example, halve the mAs when changing from 72" to 56" and halve it again when changing from 56" to 40".

Distance doubling and halving will bring image receptor exposure within roughly 50 percent of the original exposure and usually within image acceptance limits. This is only a rough rule of thumb for clinical practice. The exact conversion factors will produce much better mAs estimates.

Object-to-image receptor distance (OID) has an effect on image receptor exposure/film density. The air-gap technique uses an increased OID to prevent scatter radiation from reaching the image receptor. This scatter radiation would normally cause a visible decrease in film density when radiographing large patients. In most instances, OID variations are insufficient to cause visible film density changes.

Filtration. Filtration and its ability to alter beam intensity affect image receptor exposure and film density. All types of filtration—inherent, added, and total—alter film density. Film density decreases when filtration is increased.

X-ray units are calibrated with inherent, added, and total filtration in place. When added filtration is changed, which is rare, a half-value layer calculation should be made to permit adjustment of mAs or other factors to maintain exposure. When compensating filtration is used, film density must be established for both filtered and unfiltered regions. As with any other exposure problem, this is a matter of measurement of part size and clinical experience.

Beam Restriction. Restricting the beam, collimating, or reducing the primary beam field size reduces the total number of photons available. This reduces the amount of scatter radiation and therefore reduces the overall image receptor exposure and film density.

Scatter production is dramatically increased with large anatomical part size and high starting kVp levels (see Figure 28-4). Therefore, these two factors also determine when compensation must occur for beam restriction. However, the effect of beam restriction on film density depends on how much scatter reaches the image receptor, not how much scatter is produced. Some of the scatter that is produced, especially in very large patients or when using high ratio grids, may not reach the image receptor and therefore will not affect the film density. For example, a high-efficiency grid may be capable of removing as much as 95 percent of the scatter, leaving very little to affect film density.

Technical factor compensation for changes in film density is required only under the following circumstances:

- **large anatomical part**
- **high kilovoltage**
- **low grid efficiency**
- **nongrid examinations**

Figure 28-5 demonstrates that only extremely small beam restrictions (4″ × 4″ or smaller) when used with no grid or a low efficiency grid require mAs compensation to maintain image receptor exposure and film density. **The compensation necessary in mAs for the effect of beam restriction on image density is less than 30 percent (a visible difference) for nearly all images produced with grids at 8″ × 10″ or larger beam sizes** (Figure 28-6).

FIGURE 28-5 The effect of beam restriction on mAs compensation required to maintain film density. *(Courtesy of Barry Burns, University of North Carolina, Chapel Hill, NC)*

Anatomical Part. Because the patient is the prime attenuator of the beam, the anatomical part being examined has a great deal of influence on image receptor exposure and film density. The amount of attenuation is dependent on the thickness and type of the tissue being imaged. The tissue type is affected by the average atomic number and the density (quantity of matter per unit volume) of the tissue. The use of contrast media will alter the average atomic number of the tissue and can affect film density. Pathology can alter tissue thickness and/or type.

There is an inverse relationship between tissue thickness/type and image receptor exposure/film density. In other words, as tissue thickness, average atomic number of the tissue, and/or tissue density increases, film density decreases. **This is not a linear relationship** because of the multitude of variations in tissue composition. Depending on the type of contrast media or the type of pathology, an inverse or a direct relationship may exist.

Adjustments for changes in the anatomical part depend on the radiographer's ability to assess the tissue thickness and tissue type while also considering the pathology and the use of contrast media. This ability is achieved only through clinical experience. Technique charts are designed to compensate for most changes in tissue thickness and type. Radiolucent contrast media (such as air) will increase film density, while radiopaque contrast media (such as barium and iodine) will decrease film density. Pathology can have either an additive or a destructive effect. Additive conditions decrease film density, while destructive conditions increase film density.

A special problem related to part thickness occurs whenever severe tube angles (more than 15″) are used. The geometry of a severe tube angle causes a significant difference in tissue thickness between the edges of the image (Figure 28-7). Measurement of body parts for angles must occur at the central ray to average these differences. However, in some instances more than a 30 percent exposure difference may occur between the central ray and both ends of the image (more than a 60 percent difference between the ends of the image). Careful consideration of technical factors and use of the anode heel effect, when possible, may prevent some of these problems.

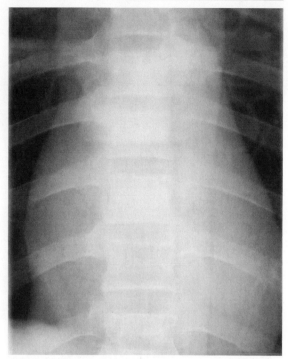

85 kVp	1.0 mAs	40" SID
12:1 No grid	400 RS	29.8 mR

85 kVp	1.0 mAs	40" SID
12:1 No grid	400 RS	31.6 mR

FIGURE 28-6 The effect of beam restriction on film density. Although both radiographs were produced at the same technical factors, A was collimated to 14″ × 17″ while B was collimated to 4″ × 8″.

Casting materials present during orthopedic radiography affect the thickness of the anatomical part. Casting materials differ somewhat in composition but they attenuate the beam in a manner very similar to normal tissue attenuation. **Adjustments for cast materials should be made for the increased thickness of the body part exactly as if an uncasted part of the same size were being radiographed.** No adjustment should be made for the casting material itself.

Grids. Grids absorb scatter, which would otherwise add exposure to the image receptor and density to the film. The more efficient the grid, the less the image receptor exposure/film density. Grids with high ratios, low frequency and dense interspace material; moving grids and improperly used grids (incorrect focal distance, etc.) all reduce image receptor exposure/film density.

Compensation for varying grid ratios is generally accomplished by increasing mAs. The amount of mAs needed can be calculated using the grid conversion factors (see Table 18-2). Changes between grids, which is the most common clinical problem, are accomplished by using the following formula:

$$\frac{mAs_1}{mAs_2} = \frac{GCF_1}{GCF_2}$$

where: mAs_1 = original mAs
mAs_2 = new mAs
GCF_1 = original grid conversion factor
GCF_2 = new grid conversion factor

Because the primary purpose of a grid is the improvement of contrast, compensating for film density changes by varying the kVp is not recommended because it may change the contrast in the opposite direction, thus negating the reason for using the grid in the first place.

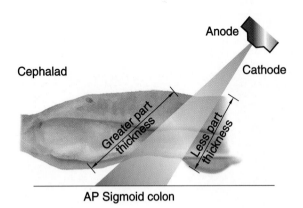

Anode

Cephalad

Cathode

Greater part thickness

Less part thickness

AP Sigmoid colon

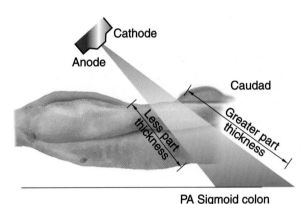

Cathode

Anode

Caudad

Less part thickness

Greater part thickness

PA Sigmoid colon

FIGURE 28-7 The effect of severe tube angle on film density. Note the changes in part thickness from the superior to inferior edges of the primary beam field.

Image Receptor. Both film and intensifying screens alter film density. When the intensifying screen phosphors convert x-ray photons to the light photons that will expose the silver halides in the film, they attenuate the intensity of the light that has become the imaging beam. When the silver halide crystals in the film emulsion form latent image centers, they establish the physical foundation for the black metallic silver that is the definition of density. Relative speed (RS) numbers are the most useful parameters for intensifying screen combinations.

Relative speed (RS) numbers have been developed by manufacturers to permit easy adjustment of technical factors when changing film/screen combinations (see Chapter 23). As relative speed increases, the amount of exposure required to maintain the same film density decreases. Compensations for changes in relative speed can be made by adjusting mAs because exposure is directly proportional to mAs. Film density can be maintained by using the following formula:

$$\frac{mAs_1}{mAs_2} = \frac{RS_2}{RS_1}$$

where: mAs_1 = old mAs
mAs_2 = new mAs
RS_1 = old relative speed
RS_2 = new relative speed

Of course, the relative speed conversion formula may also be algebraically expressed as:

$$mAs_2 = \frac{RS_1 \times mAs_1}{RS_2}$$

EXAMPLE: What is the proper mAs for use with an 80 RS system when technical factors of 55 kVp and 5 mAs produce an acceptable image with a 200 RS system?

Answer:

$$\frac{mAs_1}{mAs_2} = \frac{RS_2}{RS_1}$$

$$\frac{5}{mAs_2} = \frac{80}{200}$$

$$mAs_2 \times 80 = 5\ mAs \times 200$$
$$mAs_2 \times 80 = 1,000\ mAs$$

$$mAs_2 = \frac{1,000\ mAs}{80}$$

$$mAs_2 = 12.5\ mAs$$

Digital radiographic systems can be varied in their sensitivity to the income x-ray photons. Because radiographers need a reference point in order to produce quality images, most digital radiography system manufacturers calibrate the sensitivity processing algorithms to both the histogram control features as well as provide a sensitivity index or exposure value for each image. The digital radiography chapter discusses both of these factors at length with the obvious implications for controlling the density of the image in addition to the traditional controlling factor of mAs and the influencing factors of kVp and the other elements of the practice of radiography.

Film Processing. The condition of the film processing solutions can dramatically alter film density. Establishment of density, contrast and base plus fog parameters for the film processing system is part of the quality control program. Ascertaining that film processing density, contrast and base plus fog values are within parameters can remove film processing as a density factor.

Film density will increase when the developer solution temperature increases, immersion time increases or replenishment rates increase. Film density will decrease when the above factors decrease, as well as when contamination decreases solution strength.

SUMMARY

Density is one of the two photographic properties that comprise visibility of detail. Visibility of detail refers to the fact that the radiographic image is visible to the human eye only because sufficient density (and contrast) exists to permit the structural details to be perceived. Film density is the degree of overall blackening from the black metallic silver deposited in the emulsion. **Brightness** describes the concept of density as it is displayed on a softcopy monitor for digital images. It is the proper term for the level of the display monitor light emission. Window level accurately describes the digital processing that produces changes in density/brightness.

When mAs is decreased, the resulting film density will be decreased and vice versa. The effects of mAs and the other influencing factors on density are not exact because of the multiple variables that are part of the imaging system.

A wide variety of factors affect density. These factors are classified as either controlling or influencing factors. The controlling factor is mAs and it should be used as the principle method for adjusting for insufficient or excessive image receptor exposure/film density. The influencing factors include kilovoltage, focal spot size, anode heel effect, distance, filtration, beam restriction, anatomical part, grids, image receptors and film processing.

When the controlling or any of the influencing factors are altered, some change in image receptor exposure/film density will occur. However, with some of the factors, the effect is often negligible. Table 28-4 illustrates the effect on image receptor exposure/film density when the various factors are changed.

REVIEW QUESTIONS

1. Define film density.

2. What is the controlling factor of density and how does it affect it?

3. How are density adjustments made for changes in kilovoltage?

4. How do the inverse square law and the exposure maintenance formulas differ from one another?

5. How do variations in the anatomical part affect density?

6. What are the relationships to density of grid ratio, frequency, interspace material and grid use?

7. What is the relationship to density of relative speed for film/screen combinations?

8. How does film processing affect density?

TABLE 28-4.	Effect on Image Receptor Exposure/ Film Density When Factors Are Changed

+ = increases density
− = decreases density
∅ = negligible effect

Controlling Factor

+ Increasing milliamperage–seconds
− Decreasing milliamperage–seconds

Influencing Factors

+ Increasing kilovoltage
− Decreasing kilovoltage
+ Increasing number of pulses in the generator waveform
− Decreasing number of pulses in the generator waveform
∅ Focal spot size
∅ Anode heel effect
− Increasing distance
+ Decreasing distance
− Increasing filtration
+ Decreasing filtration
− Increasing beam restriction/collimation
+ Decreasing beam restriction/collimation
− Increasing anatomical part thickness or tissue type
+ Decreasing anatomical part thickness or tissue type
+ Using radiolucent contract media
− Using radiopaque contrast media
− Additive pathological conditions
+ Destructive pathological conditions
− Increasing grid ratio
+ Decreasing grid ratio
+ Increasing film/screen combination relative speed
− Decreasing film/screen combination relative speed
+ Increasing film processing developer time, temperature and/or replenishment rate
− Decreasing film processing developer time, temperature and/or replenishment rate

REFERENCES AND RECOMMENDED READING

Bauer, R. G. (1970). High kilovoltage chest radiography with an air gap. *Radiologic Technology, 42,* 10–14.

Bierman, A. & Boldingh, W. H. (1951). The relation between tension and exposure times in radiography. *Acta Radiologica, 35,* 22–26.

Bloom, W. L., Hollenbach, J. L., & Morgan, J. A. (1965). *Medical radiographic technic* (3rd ed.). Springfield, IL: Charles C Thomas Publishers.

Bryan, G. J. (1970). *Diagnostic radiography: A manual for radiologic technologists.* Baltimore: Williams & Wilkins.

Cahoon, J. B. (1961). Radiographic technique: Its origin, concept, practical application and evaluation of radiation dosage. *The X-Ray Technician, 32,* 354–364.

Carlton, R. R. & McKenna, A. (1989). *Repeating radiographs: Setting imaging standards, Postgraduate Advances in Radiologic Technology.* Edited by Eugene Frank. Berryville, VA: Forum Medicum.

Carroll, Q. B. (1993). *Evaluating radiographs.* Springfield, IL: Charles C Thomas Publishers.

Carroll, Q. B. (2003). *Fuchs's radiographic exposure, processing, and quality control* (7th ed.). Springfield, IL: Charles C Thomas Publishers.

Chow, M. F. (1988). The effect of a film's sensitivity to its speed, contrast, and latitude. *The Canadian Journal of Medical Radiation Technology, 19*(4), 147.

Clark, K. C. (1953). An introduction to high-voltage technique. *Radiography, 19,* 2–33.

Cullinan, A. & Cullinan, J. (1994). *Producing quality radiographs* (2nd ed.). Philadelphia: J. B. Lippincott.

Distance—technique relationship of angulated projections. (1980). *Radiologic Technology, 52*(3), 301.

Eastman Kodak Company. (1980). Health sciences markets division. *The Fundamentals of Radiography* (12th ed.). Rochester, NY: Kodak Publication M1–18.

Eastman, T. R. (1975). Technique charts: The key to radiographic quality. *Radiologic Technology, 46,* 365–368.

Eastman, T. R. (1973). Measurement: The key to exposure with manual techniques. *Radiologic Technology, 45,* 75–78.

Eastman, T. R. (1969). Chest technique through body habitus. *Radiologic Technology, 41,* 80–84.

Epp, E. R., Weiss, H., & Laughlin, J. S. (1961). Measurement of bone marrow and gonadal dose from the chest x-ray examination as a function of field size, field alignment, tube kilovoltage and added filtration. *British Journal of Radiology, 34,* 85–100.

Files, G. W. (1952). *Medical radiographic technique.* Springfield, IL: Charles C Thomas Publishers.

Files, G. W. (1935). Maximum tissue differentiation. *The X-Ray Technician, 7,* 17–24.

Fuchs, A. W. (1958). *Principles of radiographic exposure and processing.* Springfield, Illinois: Charles C Thomas Publishers.

Fuchs, A. W. (1950). The rationale of radiographic exposure. *The X-Ray Technician, 22,* 62–68, 76.

Fuchs, A. W. (1949). Control of radiographic density. *The X-Ray Technician, 20,* 271–273, 291.

Fuchs, A. W. (1948). Relationship of tissue thickness to kilovoltage. *The X-Ray Technician, 19,* 287–293.

Fuchs, A. W. (1947). The anode 'heel' effect in radiography. *Radiologic Technology, 18*(4), 158.

Fuchs, A. W. (1940). Balance in the radiographic image. *The X-Ray Technician, 12*(3), 81–84, 118.

Funke, T. (1966). Pegged kilovoltage technic. *Radiologic Technology, 37,* 202–213.

Geiger, J. (1960). The heel effect. *Radiologic Technology, 32*(1), 55.

Gratale, P., Turner, G. W., & Burns, C. B. (1986). Using the same exposure factors for wet and dry casts. *Radiologic Technology, 57*(4), 325–328.

Gratale, P., Wright, D. L., & Daughtry, L. (1990). Using the anode heel effect for extremity radiography. *Radiologic Technology, 61*(3), 195–198.

Hiss, S. S. (2003). *Understanding radiography* (4th ed.). Springfield, IL: Charles C Thomas.

Jenkins, D. (1980). *Radiographic photography and imaging processes.* Lancaster, England: MTP Press Limited.

Jerman, E. C. (1928). *Modern x-ray technic.* St. Paul, MN: Bruce.

Kebart, R. C., & James, C. D. (1991). Benefits of increasing focal film distance. *Radiologic Technology, 62*(6), 434–441.

Lauer, O. G., Mayes, J. B., & Thurston, R. P. (1990). *Evaluating radiographic quality: The variables and their effects.* Mankato, MN: The Burnell Company.

Mattsson, O. (1955). Practical photographic problems in radiography. *Acta Radiologica Supplementum, 120,* 1–206.

Morgan, J. A. (1977). *The art and science of medical radiography* (5th ed.). St. Louis, MO: Catholic Hospital Association.

Schwarz, G. S. (1959). Kilovoltage and radiographic effect. *Radiology, 73,* 749–760.

Schwarz, G. S. (1960). Kilovoltage conversion in radiography. *The X-Ray Technician, 31,* 373–379, 436.

Schwarz, G. S. (1961). *Unit-step radiography.* Springfield, IL: Charles C Thomas.

Seeman, H. E. (1968). *Physical and photographic principles of medical radiography.* New York: Wiley & Sons.

Shephard, C. (2003). Radiographic image production and manipulation. New York: McGraw Hill.

Tortorici, M. (1992). *Concepts in medical radiographic imaging.* Philadelphia: W. B. Saunders.

United States War Department. (1941, July 3). *Technical manual: Roentgenographic technicians* Washington, DC (TM 8–240).

Williams, W. A. (1956). Radiographic effect formula: Its practical application. *The X-Ray Technician, 28,* 1–6, 67.

Wilsey, R. B. (1921). The intensity of scattered x-rays in radiography. *American Journal of Roentgenology, 8,* 328–338.

(Courtesy of Dr. Marion Frank)

The Case of the Animal with the Large Calcified Tumor-Like Mass

What is the huge mass in the lower abdomen of this animal?

Answers to the case studies can be found in Appendix E.

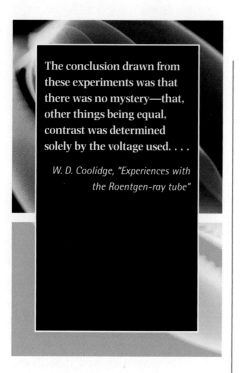

CHAPTER 29   Contrast

The conclusion drawn from these experiments was that there was no mystery—that, other things being equal, contrast was determined solely by the voltage used. . . .

W. D. Coolidge, "Experiences with the Roentgen-ray tube"

KEY TERMS

contrast
contrast mask
dynamic range
image recepter (film)
scale of contrast
window width

OBJECTIVES

Upon completion of this chapter, the student should be able to:

- Identify contrast as a prime component of the photographic properties controlling visibility of detail of image quality.

- Explain the various terms used to describe contrast/dynamic range.

- Define *contrast* and the factors that affect it.

- Describe the factors that affect image receptor (film) contrast.

- Describe the factors that affect subject contrast.

- Describe the effect of fog on contrast.

- Describe the effects of contrast changes on image appearance.

- Determine the technical factor changes necessary to achieve optimal contrast.

- Assess contrast on various radiographic images.

- Recommend appropriate adjustments to improve contrast under various conditions.

417

- Explain why kilovoltage peak is the controlling factor of contrast.

- Explain how each influencing factor affects contrast.

ASSESSING CONTRAST

Contrast is one of the two properties that comprise visibility of detail. Visibility of detail refers to the fact that the image is visible to the human eye only because sufficient contrast (and density) exists to permit the structural details to be perceived. **Image contrast is the difference between adjacent densities.** It can be mathematically evaluated as the percentage or ratio of the differences between densities. These differences can range from clear white through various shades of gray to black.

The term **dynamic range** describes the concept of contrast as it is displayed on a soft-copy monitor for digital images. It is the proper term for the range of density/brightness of the display monitor light emission. For radiographic images the term contrast/dynamic range can be applied. The term **window width** accurately describes the digital processing that produces changes in the range of density/brightness, so it also is appropriate to use when controlling image contrast. Finally, the term contrast/dynamic range/window width is applied to gray scale bit depth (also known as the z axis). Sufficient difference in exposure to the receptor are necessary for the individual pixels to exhibit different exposure values. These exposure differences are displayed through various bit depth values along the z-axis of the image.

Because contrast consists of various densities, a thorough knowledge of the factors that control density is a prerequisite to understanding it. Although contrast must be considered an independent factor, the fact that it is composed of densities makes it very difficult to separate it from the evaluation of overall density. Any change in overall density will affect contrast. This makes contrast the most difficult of the prime technical factors to evaluate and adjust.

Describing Contrast

When the differences between adjacent densities that comprise contrast are great, the image is described as high contrast. The result is fewer discernible shades of gray. Conversely, when the differences are minimal, the image is described as low contrast. This produces more discernible shades of gray. Figure 29-1F has the fewest shades of gray and therefore has the highest contrast.

In Figure 29-1A–F, there are progressively less discernible shades of gray. Figure 29-1A has the lowest contrast image. This is analogous to a gray scarf on a gray coat, which has low contrast, versus a black scarf on a white coat, which has high contrast. Table 29-1 summarizes the relationships between the various terms used to describe contrast.

As the differences between adjacent densities increase, there are fewer shades of discernible gray and the contrast is increased. Increasing contrast produces a high contrast image. As the differences between adjacent densities decrease, there are more shades of discernible gray and the contrast is decreased. Decreasing contrast produces a low contrast image.

The term *good contrast* is often applied to high contrast, but this is a misnomer and should be avoided because high contrast is not necessarily the most desirable. In fact, in most instances low contrast provides more information. Low contrast provides more differences in density even though the difference between densities is less. As long as the differences remain within the visible range of densities, low contrast provides more diagnostic information. Figures 29-2A and B are good examples of how high contrast fails to provide all the information that is obtained from a low contrast image.

TABLE 29-1. Relationship between Terms Used to Describe Contrast

High Contrast	Low Contrast
Few shades of gray	Many shades of gray
Increased contrast	Decreased contrast
Low kVp	High kVp
Short scale contrast	Long scale contrast
Short (narrow) dynamic range/window width	Large (wide) dynamic range/window width

FIGURE 29-1   Pure contrast changes in a digital abdomen image produced with a fixed density point. These computerized images vary only in contrast as shown in the accompanying D log E curves. From A to F the contrast curve becomes steeper and shorter, but the density point does not move up or down. C is considered optimal contrast for a diagnostic image. *(Computed radiography images courtesy of Bruce Long, Indiana University Medical Center, Indianapolis)*

A

B

FIGURE 29–2 High and low contrast (A) Chest radiograph produced using 80 kVp. (B) Chest radiograph of same patient using 110 kVp.

Contrast is a psychovisual perception. In other words, the psychological effects of the relationships between the densities produce a visual perception that we call contrast. The perception problem is greater because not only do individuals have different physiological visual abilities, but individual background experiences also affect the final perception. Perhaps it would be better to think of contrast in terms of an individual's "contrast sensitivity."

Although high contrast images may be perceived as more pleasing to the untrained eye, radiographers and radiologists realize that, although the lower contrast image is not as dramatic in its presentation, it often demonstrates more information. Without contrast there would be no image because all densities would appear identical. More information is visible simply because more densities are present, thus forming more possibilities for contrast differences.

Scale of contrast is the number of useful visible densities or shades of gray. Short scale contrast refers to an image that demonstrates considerable or maximal differences between densities and has a minimal total number of densities. Conversely, long scale contrast refers to an image that demonstrates slight or minimal differences between densities but has a maximal total number of densities (Figure 29-3). **Short**

scale contrast is also called high contrast, or increased contrast, while long scale contrast is called low contrast, or decreased contrast.

The advent of computerized digital processing has made it useful to sometimes describe contrast as **physical** and **visible.** Physical contrast is the total range of density values recorded by the image receptor. It is the maximum contrast possible and is the most accurate representation of the varying intensities present in the x-ray beam after it has passed through the subject. Visible contrast is the total range of density values that can be perceived by the human eye in a single image. It is a portion of the physical contrast and comprises the information from which diagnosis is made. Digital imaging allows radiographers access to the entire range of densities available. Radiographers manipulate the physical contrast available into the visible range to produce the diagnostic image.

Manipulating Contrast

The image receptor records many densities that cannot be seen by the human eye. Depending on the desired contrast, the recorded densities are compressed or expanded to form a range of visible den-

| 40 KVP | 50 KVP | 60 KVP | 70 KVP | 80 KVP | 90 KVP | 100 KVP | 110 KVP | 120 KVP |

FIGURE 29-3 Variations in scale of contrast. The number of shades of gray, the scale or range of contrast, increases as kVp increases.

sities. This can be accomplished by changes in the film's $D_{log} E$ curve, adjustments in kVp, or by the use of digital window width adjustments. Compression or expansion of the range of densities separates the physical contrast that is actually recorded by the image receptor from the visible contrast that can be perceived by the viewer on a single image.

It is important to realize that the digital response curve can be manipulated to make a very slight change in exposure, cause a huge change in contrast/dynamic range/window width/gray scale bit depth. Although it is not normal for a response curve to produce results outside normal usage, it is certainly possible.

IMAGE CONTRAST

Image contrast is the total amount of contrast acquired from both the anatomical part and the image receptor. These are described as **subject** and **image receptor (film)** contrast, respectively.

Image Receptor Contrast

Film contrast is the range of densities that the film is capable of recording. Mathematically, this is expressed as the slope of the D log E curve. Film con-

trast depends on four factors: the use of **intensifying screens, film density, the D log E curve,** and **processing.**

Intensifying Screens. Intensifying screens create an inherently higher contrast image. Although the exact reason is unknown, contrast is always lower for a film exposed to x-rays only than it is for the same film exposed to light from intensifying screens. It is most likely related to the way in which the film responds to the x-ray photons. The D log E curve changes dramatically when a film designed for exposure by light is exposed directly to x-rays. Changing screen speed has a negligible effect on contrast.

Film Density. Film contrast also changes with changes in film density. The exact effect is shown in Figure 29-4. There is an optimal range of densities that permits contrast to be visualized at a maximum. Excessive or inadequate film density decreases contrast. This is especially true in the toe and shoulder regions of the curve. If the kVp remains constant, mAs and distance will determine the actual value of exposure, thereby determining the location of the exposure on the log relative exposure axis of the curve. If a film is exposed correctly, the film densities will fall within the visible

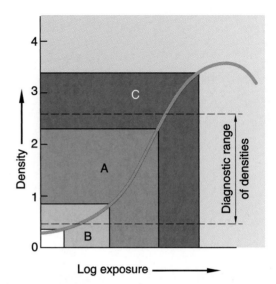

FIGURE 29-4 Contrast index for film density ranges (1–6). Note that the maximum contrast (range 4) is essentially the straight line portion of the curve. Contrast is decreased for toe and shoulder measurements but is maximized for the straight line portion of the D log E curve (OD) 1.2–1.5. (Also note that this range corresponds to the speed point [OD 1.2].) *(Courtesy of Barry Burns, University of North Carolina, Division of Radiologic Science)*

FIGURE 29-5 The effect of film density on contrast. (A) When the film is correctly exposed, the densities fall within the visible range. (B) An underexposed film occurs when the exposure places the developed densities into the toe. (C) An overexposed film occurs when the exposure places the developed densities into the shoulder. The decrease in contrast of underexposed and overexposed films occurs because the slope is not as steep in the toe and shoulder.

range of the D log E curve. If the exposure places the developed densities on the toe (an underexposed film) or shoulder (an overexposed film), the slope is not as steep, resulting in a decrease in contrast (Figure 29-5).

D log E Curve. The primary determinant of the shape of the D log E curve is the physical composition of the film emulsion. As the slope of the curve becomes steeper, contrast is increased. For example, in Figure 29-6, film A possesses higher contrast than film B. Because of the steeper slope of the curve, the visible density range is compressed into a narrower exposure range. Film A is a high contrast, narrow latitude film. Film B is a low contrast, wide latitude film because the visible density range is expanded across a wider exposure range.

Film Processing. Increasing film developer time, temperature, or replenishment rate will increase the chemical fog on the film. These changes produce a decrease in the slope of the curve especially in the

toe region (Figure 29-7). When any processing factor causes a change in base fog, contrast is affected. Developer temperature and immersion time, replenishment, and developer contamination are the primary processing factors that cause objectionable fog levels. Increased developer temperature, time, and replenishment rates cause increased fog and decreased contrast. As shown in Figure 21-10, film processing has an optimal range and any factor that causes processing to deviate from optimal values will decrease contrast. Developer contamination by fixer causes increased fog and decreased contrast because the chemical ability of the developer reducing agents is seriously impaired by the pH change in the solution.

Digital Image Receptors. The primary method for adjusting contrast with digital imaging systems, is through window width manipulations. Digital response curves can be varied in their sensitivity to

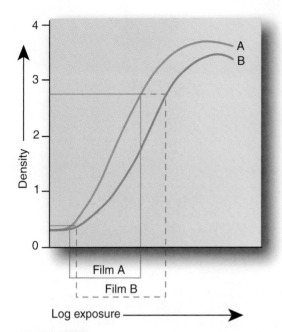

FIGURE 29-6 The effect of the D log E curve on contrast. As the slope of the curve becomes steeper, contrast is increased. Film A possesses higher contrast than Film B, because Film A compresses the visible density range into a narrower exposure range.

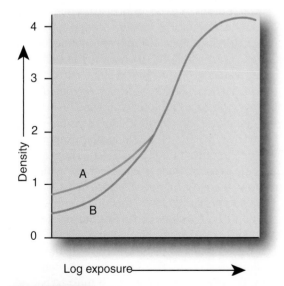

FIGURE 29-7 The effect of processing fog on contrast. In curve A, increased fog raises the toe of curve and decreases its slope, thus decreasing contrast.

the incoming x-ray photons and therefore to the range of densities available for acquisition processing and/or display. Because radiographers need a reference point in order to produce quality images, most digital radiography system manufacturers calibrate the sensitivity processing algorithms to provide a reasonable linear range of density/brightness for each image. Chapter 25, Digital Radiography, discusses both of these factors at length with the obvious implications for controlling the density and contrast of the image.

Subject Contrast

Subject contrast is the range of differences in the intensity of the x-ray beam after it has been attenuated by the subject. It is dependent on kilovoltage and the amount and type of irradiated material.

Kilovoltage. Kilovoltage peak (kVp) is the primary controller of subject contrast. As kVp increases, a wider range of photon energies is produced (Figure 7-6). The wider the range of photon energies, the greater the ability of the photons to penetrate the body tissues. This leads to a wider range of exposures on the image receptor, which results in an overall lower contrast.

As long as the kVp is adequate to penetrate the part being examined, low kVp will produce high subject contrast. When the kVp is too low, most of the photons do not reach the image receptor because they are absorbed in the patient. Low kVp produces higher subject contrast because most of these low energy photons are absorbed by thicker parts while more penetrate the thin part. With high kVp, subject contrast is decreased because more uniform penetration occurs between thick and thin parts.

The effect of kVp on subject contrast can be detailed by examining the D log E curve. Figure 29-8 shows the range of transmitted photon intensities forming the exposure to the film for both high and low kVp techniques for the same film type. High kVp produces a compressed range of relative exposures, which the slope of the D log E curve reflects within the visible density range. Low kVp produces an expanded range of relative exposures, which the slope of the D log E curve is unable to reflect within the visible density range. This causes some of the lowest

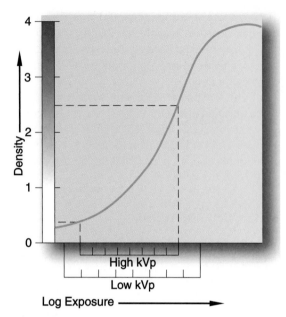

FIGURE 29-8   The effect of kVp on subject contrast. The range of transmitted photon intensities for high kVp produces a compressed range of relative exposures, which are reflected within the visible density range by the slope of the curve. The expanded range of exposures produced by low kVp is too wide for the curve to reflect within the visible density range. This causes some of the lowest and highest photon intensities not to be visible when low kVp is used.

FIGURE 29-9   The effect of scatter radiation on contrast. Scatter radiation producing image density (and incorrect information) in a region of high subject density (under the vertebral column). The scatter interferes with the ability of the bone to cast a light shadow on the image.

and highest exposures to fall outside the visible density range. Increasing kVp causes density differences that were previously undetectable to become visible, resulting in an increase in the diagnostic information provided by the image.

This concept is demonstrated nicely by comparing chest radiographs to radiographs of the ribs. In chest radiography high kVps result in a wide range of image densities that fall within the visible range. Both the air-filled lungs and the bony structures are demonstrated within the visible range. No structures appear under or overexposed. In rib radiography low kVps are used to enhance the differences between the air-filled lungs and the overlying bony structures. The air-filled lungs demonstrate increased film density, while the bony structures demonstrate decreased film density compared to the chest image.

In addition to kVp, radiation fog has a significant effect on contrast. It is the result of x-ray interactions with matter, primarily Compton scatter. As kVp increases the percentage of Compton interactions increases. As a result of this increase in the amount of scatter reaching the image receptor, contrast is decreased. Scatter raises the base plus fog (the toe) and decreases the slope of the curve (Figure 29-7). These changes cause the lightest film densities to be "fogged over" so they can no longer be distinguished from one another (see Figure 29-9). The resulting image no longer includes a clear or pure "white" region, and therefore has less contrast.

Fog can be caused by factors other than scatter radiation. These include subjecting film to heat, low level ionizing radiation, or chemical fumes. Developer temperature, replenishment, and developer contamination may also cause objectionable fog levels. The effect of fog on contrast must be considered during clinical radiography because it sets the acceptance limits for contrast regulation. The radiographer should remember that any factor that results in an increase in fog will decrease contrast.

Amount of Irradiated Material. The amount of irradiated material depends on the thickness of the body part and the field size. Both these factors influence the number of x-rays transmitted to the image receptor. As body part thickness increases, x-ray absorption increases. Conversely, as body part thickness decreases so does absorption. This difference in absorption between various thicknesses influences subject contrast. When the difference between adjacent thicknesses of various body parts is great, subject contrast is increased. When little difference exists in the thickness of adjacent body parts, subject contrast is decreased.

When the overall thickness of a body part increases, or when field size increases, the amount of scatter created will increase. This results in a decrease in subject contrast. A decrease in overall body part thickness or field size results in increased subject contrast.

Type of Irradiated Material. The type of irradiated material is influenced by the atomic number of the material and its tissue density. Both these factors influence subject contrast.

Materials with a higher atomic number, such as lead and iodine, absorb a greater percentage of the x-ray beam than low atomic number materials, such as hydrogen, carbon, and calcium. This results from the presence of a greater number of electrons, which enables more interactions to occur. When the difference between the average atomic number of adjacent tissues is great, subject contrast is increased. When little difference exists between them, subject contrast is decreased. For example, bone has a higher average atomic number than soft tissue. Therefore, subject contrast between bone and soft tissue is greater than the contrast between adjacent soft tissue structures. Contrast media increase subject contrast by introducing greater differences in atomic number variations than those that exist naturally.

Tissue density describes how tightly the atoms of a given substance are packed together. When the difference between the densities of adjacent tissues is great, subject contrast is increased. When little difference exists between them, subject contrast is decreased. For example, bone tissue is a denser substance than lung tissue. Therefore subject contrast between bone and lung tissue is greater.

EVALUATING CONTRAST

The major consideration in evaluating visible contrast is **verification that a proper range of densities is visible throughout the anatomical area of interest** on the image. Proper density alone is not enough. The anatomical structures of interest are visible only when sufficient contrast between the densities exists. Of course, these densities must be well within the range of human visibility (OD 0.25–2.50).

Unlike the evaluation of density, contrast assessment requires more than just sufficient density within the visibility range. Adequate contrast must demonstrate enough distinctly different densities within the range to satisfy diagnostic quality requirements for the particular examination. Much of this ability is the result of clinical experience. It is obvious that proper contrast is not the same for all tissues. Knowledge of anatomy and physiology, both normal and abnormal, as well as pathology and technical factors, is critical for proper contrast evaluation. Only when these skills are combined with an experienced and trained professional eye, can proper contrast evaluation occur.

Because there is more information recorded on an image than is seen, the diagnostic importance of contrast is a matter of how many densities are included in the visible contrast range. To some extent, it can be said that low contrast images have more information. However, the critical point is that the various densities must be discernible.

The human eye is limited in its ability to discern light and dark. This essentially establishes a value for the lightest and darkest visible shades of gray. When additional shades of gray are added to the visible range of contrast, they must fit between these two densities. Each additional shade of gray reduces the magnitude of the density difference, or the contrast, between the lightest and darkest grays. Eventually, a point is reached where additional shades of gray do not have enough density difference to be visible (see Figure 29-1A). Of course, this occurs at different points, depending on individual visual abilities. A 30 percent exposure difference has been used as the minimum change to cause a visible difference because this magnitude is discernible by nearly everyone. However, some professionals may be able to discern as little contrast as a 15 percent difference, which means they are capable of seeing twice as many shades of gray as someone who can discern only a 30 percent change.

Discerning contrast can be extremely difficult for even the experienced radiographer when the image exhibits poor density. **Contrast evaluation can be made only when sufficient density exists to permit the range of contrast to be seen.** The eye tends to consider nearby densities and contrast when evaluating image quality. It is so difficult for the eye to ignore nearby factors that a **contrast mask** is often helpful (Figure 29-10). A contrast mask is a simple tool to help focus on the contrast in a selected area. When a contrast mask is used with an image, adjacent information is eliminated. This makes the evaluation much easier as the contrast problem becomes evident as well as easier to evaluate (Figure 29-11). Because of the difficulty in ignoring nearby density problems (ei-

ther too light or dark) even the experienced radiographer will find a contrast mask useful in making some evaluations.

Selecting the Appropriate kVp

There are no established rules concerning how much contrast is desirable in all situations. Experience and knowledge enable the radiographer to determine when a change in contrast will increase the diagnostic quality of an image. Many radiologists

FIGURE 29-10 A contrast mask.

A

B

FIGURE 29-11 Using a contrast mask. (A) A radiograph of a chest that appears too light, making contrast evaluation difficult. (B) The same radiograph with the contrast mask applied to the right upper lobe of the lung, making contrast evaluation easier.

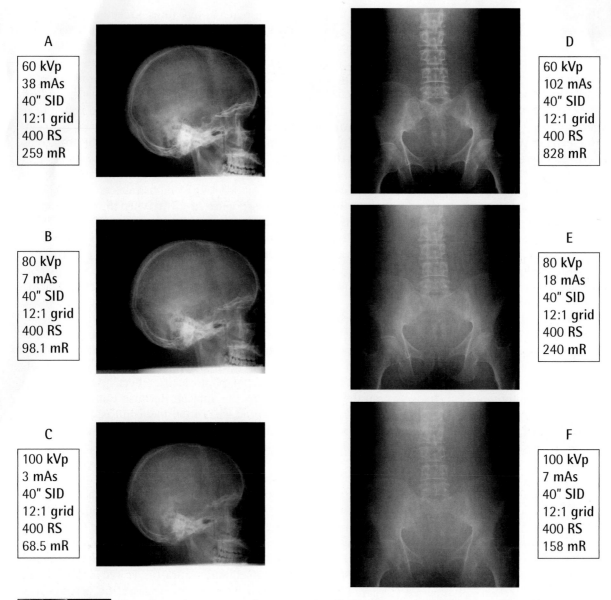

A

60 kVp
38 mAs
40" SID
12:1 grid
400 RS
259 mR

B

80 kVp
7 mAs
40" SID
12:1 grid
400 RS
98.1 mR

C

100 kVp
3 mAs
40" SID
12:1 grid
400 RS
68.5 mR

D

60 kVp
102 mAs
40" SID
12:1 grid
400 RS
828 mR

E

80 kVp
18 mAs
40" SID
12:1 grid
400 RS
240 mR

F

100 kVp
7 mAs
40" SID
12:1 grid
400 RS
158 mR

FIGURE 29-12   The effect of contrast on image quality. Skull radiographs produced at (A) 60 kVp; (b) 80 kVp; (C) 100 kVp. Abdomen radiographs produced at (D) 60 kVp; (E) 80 kVp; (F) 100 kVp. Compare these images, noting contrast changes due to anatomical part differences.

find it desirable to have uniform contrast throughout a single examination to permit comparisons between projections. Low contrast can be achieved to some degree by utilizing a fixed kilovoltage technique system. Other radiologists prefer a higher contrast. This can be achieved to some degree by utilizing a variable kilovoltage technique system.

The radiographs in Figures 29-1 and 29-12 illustrate the effect of contrast on image quality. Notice in Figure 29-12 that the contrast varies as the kVp varies. Also notice that the contrast varies for the same kVp with different body part thickness (different subject densities). The exposure factors for these images used different mAs values to compensate for the differences in scatter radiation as the kVp was changed.

The images in Figure 11-2 illustrate the effect of kVp on image density. To perceive a contrast change, density should be maintained at a uniform level. The 15 percent rule is an acceptable method of achieving uniform image receptor exposure/film density when changing contrast. **A visible change in contrast will not be perceived until kVp is changed by 4–12 percent, depending on the kVp range** (Table 29-2). There is no reason to repeat an exposure for contrast reasons unless at least a 4–5 percent change is made, although higher kVps require even greater changes. The effects of mAs and the influencing factors on image contrast are not exact because of the wide variety of variables that are part of the imaging system. Many of the variables affect the contrast of the image as a side effect of other changes.

Both the quantity and quality of the x-ray beam will vary with changes in kilovoltage. There are too many variables to be quantified into a reliable formula. Because the 15 percent rule is used so much when maintaining exposure, it is convenient to use it as the minimum practical change within the diagnostic range. Remember that the 15 percent rule is a misnomer as the actual changes necessary to maintain exposure vary from 15–25 percent (Figure 28-4).

When a radiograph is outside acceptance limits, it needs to be repeated. All acceptance limits permit some degree of variation, at least 8–15 percent change in contrast. **The rule for contrast changes is to make adjustments in increments of 15 or 8 percent.** If the radiograph does not require an 8 percent change in kVp and contrast, it seldom requires repeating. Exceptions to this rule are fine adjustments of 8 percent that are crucial to demonstrate small structures. Radiographers may adjust technique charts by an 8 percent margin, but will seldom subject the patient to a second exposure for such a minor change. As with density adjustments, contrast changes require bold action or no action at all.

In some instances it may be desirable to decrease kVp to increase contrast when mAs must be increased. A radiograph of a 20 cm abdomen produced at 90 kVp demonstrates a relatively low contrast (Figure 29-13B). When the same abdomen is radiographed at 70 kVp, a significantly higher contrast results (Figure 29-13A). The reduced kVp produced less scatter radiation, thus producing higher contrast. The natural tendency to increase kVp for thicker parts will not produce satisfactory radiographs if the effect of increased Compton scatter on contrast is not considered first.

Radiographic image contrast occurs due to the photoelectric effect's total absorption of photons in the subject. High contrast is directly related to the number of photoelectric effect interactions that occur in the subject. Because Compton interactions produce scatter, low contrast is directly related to the amount of Compton scatter that occurs in the subject. Image contrast can be controlled by adjusting kVp. The kVp controls the relationship between the number of photoelectric versus Compton interactions.

Contrast can be determined by matching the average incident photon energy with the average inner-shell binding energy of the predominant subject material, as shown in Figure 12-8. For example, when maximum contrast is desired for bone tissue, technical factors that increase the percentage of photoelectric interactions should be used. Photoelectric effect interactions increase as kVp decreases.

FACTORS AFFECTING CONTRAST

The controlling and influencing factors that affect contrast are shown in Figure 29-14. **The controlling factor that affects contrast has the most di-**

TABLE 29-2.	Changes Necessary to Produce Visible Contrast Differences	
Level	Change Necessary to Produce Visible Change	Change Equal to Percent Change
30–50 kVp	4–5 percent	1–3 kVp
50–90 kVp	8–9 percent	4–8 kVp
90–130 kVp	10–12 percent	9–16 kVp

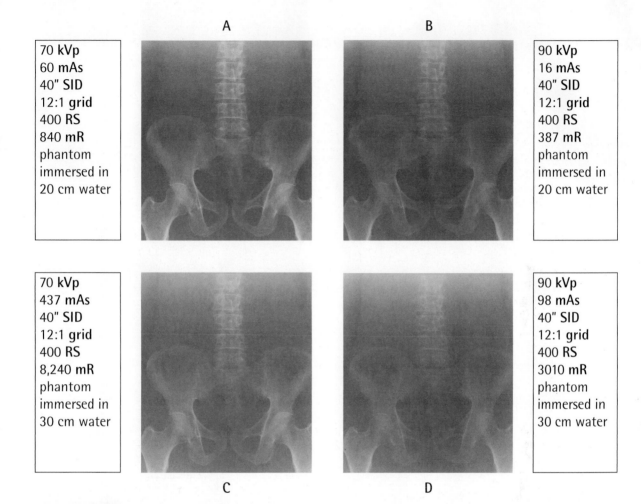

70 kVp
60 mAs
40" SID
12:1 grid
400 RS
840 mR
phantom
immersed in
20 cm water

90 kVp
16 mAs
40" SID
12:1 grid
400 RS
387 mR
phantom
immersed in
20 cm water

70 kVp
437 mAs
40" SID
12:1 grid
400 RS
8,240 mR
phantom
immersed in
30 cm water

90 kVp
98 mAs
40" SID
12:1 grid
400 RS
3010 mR
phantom
immersed in
30 cm water

FIGURE 29-13   Increased contrast on 20 and 30 cm abdomens. (A) 20 cm abdomen at 70 kVp; (B) 20 cm abdomen at 90 kVp; (C) 30 cm abdomen at 70 kVp; (D) 30 cm abdomen at 90 kVp. All images were exposed with the same AEC and have the same overall density values. (Note the differences in mAs and mR dose.)

rect effect on the image. When it is changed, the image will change as a primary result. The influencing factors that control contrast have a **less direct effect** on the image or change other factors as well as contrast. When the influencing factors are changed the contrast is affected, but not as directly as with the controlling factor. With some of the factors this change is so small that it is essentially negligible.

Kilovoltage as the Controlling Factor

Kilovoltage peak (kVp) is the controller of contrast. As kVp increases contrast decreases. As kVp decreases contrast increases. In most instances the control of contrast rests with the radiographer by selecting an appropriate kVp setting

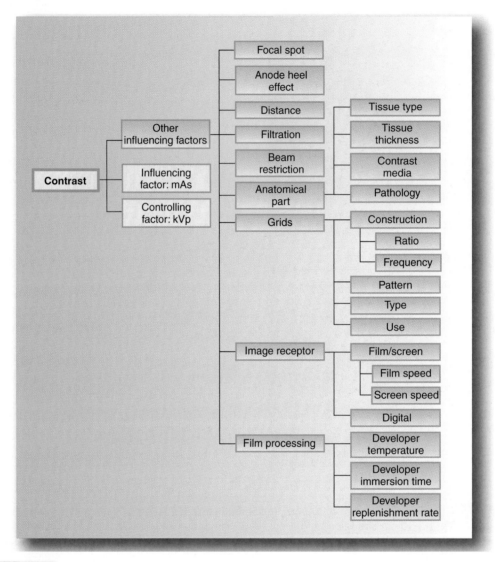

FIGURE 29-14 Image analysis: factors affecting contrast.

from a technique chart developed for the particular x-ray unit in use. Other variables such as generator configuration (phase, falling load, or frequency) may also affect the final decision. A generator configuration that increases the effective kVp will result in a decrease in contrast. For example, for a given kVp a three-phase generator will produce a lower contrast than a single-phase unit.

Kilovoltage also controls the amount of scatter radiation produced. Increasing kVp increases the amount of radiation fog, thereby decreasing contrast.

The radiographer must adapt the suggested kVp setting for the individual procedure. Experience and study of various body habitus, pathologies, positioning, and equipment quickly provides the radiographer with clinical knowledge that can be used for these adjustments.

Influencing Factors

Influencing factors include milliampere-seconds (mAs), focal spot size, anode heel effect, distance, filtration, beam restriction, anatomical part, grids, film/screen combinations, and processing.

Milliampere-Seconds (mAs). Milliampere-seconds alters image receptor exposure and film density of the image and therefore affects contrast. When the change is sufficient to move film density differences out of the range of human vision, either over or underexposed, the contrast is decreased (see Figure 29-5).

Focal Spot Size. The possibility of the focal spot size altering contrast enough to be visible is extremely unlikely. Focal spot sizes have such a small effect on exposure that it is unlikely that their effect on contrast could be detected.

Anode Heel Effect. The anode heel effect alters the intensity of radiation and therefore affects image receptor exposure and film density, which can affect contrast. The intensity of radiation is greater at the cathode end of the tube. This difference would become visible only with open collimation and a small anode target angle (less than 12°). The anode heel has very little effect on contrast.

Distance. Source-to-image receptor distance (SID) alters the intensity of the beam reaching the image receptor according to the inverse square law. This affects film density and therefore contrast. Greater distance decreases density while less distance increases it. As distance alters exposure, it can change the contrast exactly as does mAs.

Object-to-image receptor distance (OID) also has an effect on image receptor exposure/film density and contrast. An air-gap technique increases object-to-image receptor distance and this permits scatter radiation to avoid the image receptor. This scatter radiation would normally contribute radiation fog to the exposure. Removing scatter from the image will increase contrast.

Filtration. Filtration increases the effect of kVp by changing the average photon energy of the beam. All types of filtration—inherent, added, and total—alter image receptor exposure/film density and contrast. Filtration affects contrast by changing the average photon energy and decreasing beam intensity. The increase in the average photon energy causes more Compton scatter production and this decreases contrast. The decreased intensity decreases image receptor exposures and film density, which decreases contrast. This change is negligible, however, because most of these low energy photons do not exit the patient to contribute to the image receptor exposure. The predominant effect of filtration is caused by changes in average photon energy, therefore increased filtration decreases contrast.

Beam Restriction. Restricting the beam, collimating, or reducing the primary beam field size reduces the total number of photons available. This reduces the amount of scatter radiation and therefore increases contrast.

Anatomical Part. Because the patient is the prime attenuator of the beam, both the amount and type of tissue being examined greatly influence density and contrast. As the anatomical part size increases, the amount of scatter created by the part also increases, resulting in a decrease in contrast. As tissue density increases, the amount of scatter increases, which also results in a decrease in contrast. As average atomic number increases (i.e., using contrast media), there is more photoelectric absorption, resulting in higher or increased contrast.

As with density adjustments, compensation for anatomical part changes depends on an ability to assess tissue type, thickness, pathology, etc. This ability is achieved only through clinical experience.

Grids. The primary function of a grid is contrast improvement (Figure 29-15). Grids improve contrast by removing scatter before it reaches the image receptor. The contrast improvement factor (K) is the best measure of how well a grid accomplishes this function. The contrast improvement factor is

80 kVp	3.2 mAs	40" SID
No grid	400 RS	45.2 mR

80 kVp	17 mAs	40" SID
12:1 grid	400 RS	226 mR

A

B

FIGURE 29-15 The effect of a grid on contrast. (A) 80 kVp without a grid; (B) 80 kVp with a grid. Both images were exposed with the same AEC and have the same overall density values. (Note the differences in mAs and mR dose.)

dependent on the amount of scatter produced, which is controlled by the kVp and the amount and type of irradiated tissue. As the amount of scatter radiation increases, the lower the contrast and the lower the contrast improvement factor. The contrast improvement factor K is measured by using the average gradient (or gamma) of the straight line portion of the D log E curve:

$$K = \frac{\text{average gradient with the grid}}{\text{average gradient without the grid}}$$

If K = 1, then no improvement in contrast has occurred. Most grids have contrast improvement factors between 1.5 and 3.5 so their contrast is 1.5–3.5 times better than an identical non-grid image. The higher the K factor, the greater the contrast improvement.

Higher ratio grids remove more scatter and therefore have a greater contrast improvement factor. This results in a higher contrast image.

Image Receptor. With film/screen image receptor systems, the primary determinant of the shape of the D log E curve is the physical composition of the film emulsion. As the slope of the curve becomes steeper, contrast is increased. Intensifying screens create an inherently higher contrast image. Contrast is always lower for a film exposed to x-rays only than it is for the same film exposed to light from intensifying screens.

With digital image receptor systems, sufficient differences in exposure to the receptor are necessary for the individual pixels to exhibit different exposure values. **These exposure differences are dis-**

played through various bit depth values along the z-axis of the image. These can then be adjusted on the monitor through the manipulation of the window width.

Processing. Increasing film developer time, temperature, or replenishment rate from the optimal range will increase the chemical fog on the film. These changes produce a decrease in the slope of the curve, which results in a decrease in contrast. Decreasing film development time, temperature, or replenishment rate from the optimal range will decrease the film's density, which in turn will decrease contrast.

SUMMARY

Contrast is one of the two photographic properties that comprise visibility of detail. Visibility of detail refers to the fact that the radiographic image is visible to the human eye only because sufficient contrast (and density) exists to permit structural details to be perceived. Image contrast is the difference between adjacent densities. It can be mathematically evaluated as the percentage or ratio of the differences between densities. These differences can range from clear white through various shades of gray to black.

Dynamic range describes the range of contrast as it is displayed on a digital image. Window width describes the process that produces changes in the range of density/brightness. Sufficient differences in exposure to the receptor are necessary for the individual pixels to exhibit different exposure values. These exposure differences are displayed through various bit depth values along the z-axis of the image.

When the differences between adjacent densities that comprise contrast are great, the image is described as high contrast. The result is fewer discernible shades of gray. Conversely, when the differences are minimal the image is described as low contrast.

Short scale contrast is also called high contrast, or increased contrast, while long scale contrast is called low contrast, or decreased contrast. Physical contrast is the total range of density values recorded by the image receptor whereas visible contrast is the total range of density values that can be perceived by the human eye in a single image.

Image contrast is the total amount of contrast acquired from both the anatomical part and the image receptor. These are described as image receptor contrast and subject contrast respectively. Image receptor (film) contrast is the range of densities that the film is capable of recording. Film contrast depends on four factors: the use of intensifying screens, film density, the D log E curve, and film processing. Digital image receptor contrast is adjusted through window width manipulations. Subject contrast is the range of differences in the intensity of the x-ray beam after it has been attenuated by the subject. It is dependent on kilovoltage and the amount and type of irradiated material.

The major consideration in evaluating visible contrast is verification that a proper range of densities are visible throughout the anatomical area of interest on the image. Proper density alone is not enough. The anatomical structures of interest can be visualized only when sufficient contrast between the densities exists. To perceive a contrast change, exposure should be maintained at a uniform level. The 15 percent rule is an acceptable method of achieving this.

A wide variety of factors affect contrast. These factors are classified as either controlling or influencing factors. The controlling factor is kVp and it should be used as the principle method for altering the contrast. The influencing factors include milliamperage-seconds, focal spot size, anode heel effect, distance, filtration, beam restriction, anatomical part, grids, image receptors, and film processing.

TABLE 29-3.	Effects of Changing Factors on Contrast

+ = increases contrast

− = decreases contrast

∅ = negligible effect

Controlling Factor

− Increasing kilovoltage

+ Decreasing kilovoltage

− Increasing number of pulses in the generator waveform

+ Decreasing number of pulses in the generator waveform

Influencing Factors

∅ Increasing milliamperage-seconds*

∅ Decreasing milliamperage-seconds*

∅ Focal-spot size changes

∅ Anode heel effect

∅ Increasing SID

∅ Decreasing SID

+ Increasing OID

− Decreasing OID

− Increasing filtration

+ Decreasing filtration

+ Increasing beam restriction/collimation

− Decreasing beam restriction/collimation

− Increasing amount of irradiated tissue

+ Decreasing amount of irradiated tissue

− Increasing atomic number or density of tissue

+ Decreasing atomic number or density of tissue

+ Using contrast media (increasing or decreasing atomic number)

− Additive pathological conditions

+ Destructive pathological conditions

+ Increasing grid ratio

− Decreasing grid ratio

∅ Increasing film/screen combination relative speed

∅ Decreasing film/screen combination relative speed

+ Use of intensifying screens

− Increasing or decreasing film processing developer time and temperature beyond optimal

*For example, changing mAs while maintaining density by SID changes.

When the controlling factor or any of the influencing factors is altered, some change in contrast will occur; however, with some of the factors the effect is often negligible. Table 29-3 illustrates the effect on contrast when the various factors are changed. For the purpose of this review, assume that compensation has been made for the changes in the density. Remember that if no compensation is made for the changes in density, and the resulting image is over or underexposed contrast will always decrease.

REVIEW QUESTIONS

1. Define contrast.
2. How do high contrast images differ from low contrast images?
3. What is the difference between physical and visible contrast?
4. What factors affect image receptor (film) contrast and subject contrast?
5. How does film density affect image receptor contrast?
6. What is the controlling factor of subject contrast and how does it affect it?
7. How do variations in the anatomical part affect contrast?
8. What is the effect of a grid on contrast?
9. How does film processing affect contrast?

REFERENCES AND RECOMMENDED READING

Abildgaard, A., & Notthellen, J. A. (1992). Increasing contrast when viewing radiographic images. *Radiology, 185*(2), 475–478.

Bauer, R. G. (1970). High kilovoltage chest radiography with an air gap. *Radiologic Technology, 42,* 10–14.

Bierman, A., & Boldingh, W. H. (1951). The relation between tension and exposure times in radiography. *Acta Radiologica, 35,* 22–26.

Bloom, W. L., Hollenbach, J. L., & Morgan, J. A. (1965). *Medical radiographic technic* (3rd ed.). Springfield, IL: Charles C Thomas.

Bryan, G. J. (1970). *Diagnostic radiography: A manual for radiologic technologists.* Baltimore: Williams & Wilkins.

Cahoon, J. B. (1961). Radiographic technique: Its origin, concept, practical application and evaluation of radiation dosage. *The X-Ray Technician, 32,* 354–364.

Carlton, R. R., & McKenna, A. (1989). Repeating radiographs: Setting imaging standards. In *Postgraduate advances in radiologic technology.* (Eugene Frank, ed.) Berryville, VA: Forum Medicum.

Carroll, Q. B. (1993). *Evaluating radiographs.* Springfield, IL: Charles C Thomas.

Carroll, Q. B. (2003). *Fuchs's radiographic exposure, processing, and quality control* (7th ed.). Springfield, IL: Charles C Thomas.

Chow, M. F. (1988). The effect of a film's sensitivity to its speed, contrast, and latitude. *The Canadian Journal of Medical Radiation Technology, 19*(4), 147.

Clark, K. C. (1953). An introduction to high-voltage technique. *Radiography, 19,* 21–33.

Cullinan, A., & Cullinan, J. (1994). *Producing quality radiographs* (2nd ed.). Philadelphia: J. B. Lippincott.

Distance—technique relationship of angulated projections. (1980). *Radiologic Technology, 52*(3), 301.

Eastman Kodak Company. (1980). Health Sciences Markets Division. *The fundamentals of radiography* (12th ed.) (Kodak Publication M1–18) Rochester, NY: Author.

Eastman, T. R. (1969). Chest technique through body habitus. *Radiologic Technology, 41,* 80–84.

Files, G. W. (1935). Maximum tissue differentiation. *The X-Ray Technician, 7,* 17–24+.

Files, G. W. (1952). *Medical radiographic technique.* Springfield, IL: Charles C Thomas.

Fuchs, A. W. (1940). Balance in the radiographic image. *The X-Ray Technician, 12*(3), 81–84, 118.

Fuchs, A. W. (1948). Relationship of tissue thickness to kilovoltage. *The X-Ray Technician, 19,* 287–293.

Fuchs, A. W. (1950). The rationale of radiographic exposure. *The X-Ray Technician, 22,* 62–68, 76.

Fuchs, A. W. (1958). *Principles of radiographic exposure and processing.* Springfield, IL: Charles C Thomas.

Funke, T. (1966). Pegged kilovoltage technic. *Radiologic Technology, 37,* 202–213.

Gratale, P., Turner, G. W., & Burns, C. B. (1986). Using the same exposure factors for wet and dry casts. *Radiologic Technology, 57*(4), 325–328.

Hiss, S. S. (1993). *Understanding radiography* (3rd ed.). Springfield, IL: Charles C Thomas.

Jenkins, D. (1980). *Radiographic photography and imaging processes.* Lancaster, England: MTP Press Limited.

Jerman, E. C. (1928). *Modern x-ray technic.* St. Paul, MN: Bruce.

Kelsey, C. A. (1982, June). Comparison of nodule detection with 70 kVp and 120 kVp chest radiographs. *Radiology,* 609.

Kodera, Y., Schmidt, R. A., Chan, H., & Doi, K. (1984, January). Backscatter from metal surfaces in diagnostic radiology. *Radiology,* 231.

Koenig, G. F. (1957). Kilovoltage as a qualitative factor. *The X-Ray Technician, 29,* 1–4, 13.

Lauer, O. G., Mayes, J. B., & Thurston, R. P. (1990). *Evaluating radiographic quality: The variables and their effects.* Mankato, MN: The Burnell Company.

Mattsson, O. (1955). Practical photographic problems in radiography. *Acta Radiologica Supplementum,* 1201–1206.

McEnerney, P. (1960). Evaluation of radiographic contrast after uncompensated factor changes. *Radiologic Technology, 32*(1), 23.

Mitchell, F. (1991). Scattered radiation and the lateral lumbar spine part 1: Initial research. *Radiography Today, 57*(644), 18–20.

Mitchell, F., Leung, C., Ahuja, A., & Metreweli, C. (1991). Scattered radiation and the lateral lumbar spine part 2: Clinical research. *Radiography Today, 57*(645), 12–14.

Morgan, J. A. (1977). *The art and science of medical radiography* (5th ed.). St. Louis, MO: Catholic Hospital Association.

Morgan, R. H. (1946a). An analysis of the physical factors controlling the diagnostic quality of roentgen images: Part III. Contrast and the intensity distribution function of a Roentgen image. *American Journal of Roentgenology and Radiation Therapy, 55*(1), 67–89.

Morgan, R. H. (1946b). An analysis of the physical factors controlling the diagnostic quality of roentgen images: Part IV. Contrast and the film contrast factor. *American Journal of Roentgenology and Radiation Therapy, 55*(5), 627–633.

Newman, H. (1933). Relation of kilovolts to thickness of part—x-ray technic. *The X-Ray Technician, 5,* 21–26.

Roderick, J. F. (1950). Photographic contrast in roentgenology. *The X-Ray Technician, 22,* 141–150, 163.

Schwarz, G. S. (1959). Kilovoltage and radiographic effect. *Radiology, 73,* 749–760.

Schwarz, G. S. (1960). Kilovoltage conversion in radiography. *The X-Ray Technician, 31,* 373–379, 436.

Schwarz, G. S. (1961). *Unit-step radiography.* Springfield, IL: Charles C Thomas.

Seeman, H. E. (1968). *Physical and photographic principles of medical radiography.* New York: Wiley & Sons.

Spiegler, G. (1950). The story of contrast and definition. *Radiography, 41*(189), 177–182.

Thompson, M. A., Hattaway, M. P., Hall, J. D., & Dowd, S. B. (1994). *Principles of imaging science and protection.* Philadelphia: W. B. Saunders.

Tortorici, M. (1992). *Concepts in medical radiographic imaging.* Philadelphia: W. B. Saunders.

Trout, E. D., Graves, D. E., & Slauson, D. B. (1949). High kilovoltage radiography. *Radiology, 52,* 669–683.

United States War Department. (1941, July 3). *Technical manual: Roentgenographic technicians,* Washington, DC: (TM 8–240).

Wegelius, C. (1954). The diagnostic use of high voltage rays in relationship to the physical background of mass absorption. *Acta Radiologica Supplementum. 116,* 589–597.

Wilks, R. J. (1981). *Principles of radiological physics.* Edinburgh: Churchill Livingstone.

Wilsey, R. B. (1921). The intensity of scattered x-rays in radiography. *American Journal of Roentgenology, 8,* 328–338.

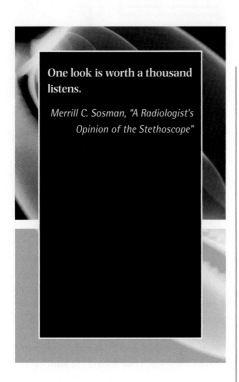

Recorded Detail

CHAPTER 30

One look is worth a thousand listens.

Merrill C. Sosman, "A Radiologist's Opinion of the Stethoscope"

KEY TERMS

aliasing
definition
detail
edge spread function (ESF)
imaging noise
line spread function (LSF)

modulation transfer function (MTF)
nyquist criterion
point spread function (PSF)
quantum mottle
quantum noise
recorded detail

sharpness
spatial resolution

OBJECTIVES

Upon completion of this chapter, the student should be able to:

- Define recorded detail, including synonymous terms and derived units.

- Explain the effect of various distances on recorded detail.

- Describe the factors that affect penumbra/point spread function size.

- Describe the effect of film/screen combinations on the resolution of recorded detail.

- Discuss the relationship of the three intensifying screen factors to recorded detail.

- Explain digital image receptor factors that control recorded detail.

- Describe appropriate techniques to prevent patient motion.

- Synthesize various geometrical factors into a clinical protocol for improving resolution.

- Recommend techniques for reducing motion, including immobilization devices.

ASSESSING RECORDED DETAIL

Recorded detail is one of the two geometric properties of image quality. Unlike the photographic properties of density and contrast, which control the visibility of detail, the geometric properties control detail itself. **Recorded detail is the degree of geometric sharpness or accuracy of the structural lines actually recorded in the image.** Good detail exists even when it cannot be seen due to poor visibility of detail or, in other words, when the density and/or contrast are poor. Recorded detail is one of the easiest of the prime technical factors to evaluate and adjust.

Recorded detail is also referred to as **definition, sharpness, spatial resolution, or simply as detail.** When the term *detail* is used by itself, it usually refers to the recorded detail of the radiographic image. Detail is easily quantified and even has a derived unit. The term *spatial* resolution is applied to quantified discussions of recorded detail.

The primary film/screen **unit of resolution** is line pairs per millimeter (lp/mm) or cycles per mm. A radiographic resolution tool is composed of pairs of lines a set distance from one another (Figure 30-1). The point at which the viewer can discern the closest pair of lines from each other represents the lp/mm reading. Most human visual acuity is limited to the range of 5 lp/mm. At this level each line is 0.1 mm wide, so a structure of this size could be discerned. Unfortunately, most radiographic imaging systems do not provide this level of resolution.

Digital imaging recorded detail (or spatial resolution as it is more commonly called) is determined primarily by matrix size, pixel size, and gray scale bit depth. These correspond to the x, y, and z-axis of the digital image. Digital imaging recorded detail is most commonly described in terms of spatial frequency. Spatial frequency is usually discussed as high or low. A shorter wavelength signal (with higher frequency) represents pairs of lines that can be visualized very close together. This is high resolution. The opposite is true for low frequency spatial resolution as this signal has longer wavelength (and lower frequency) representing

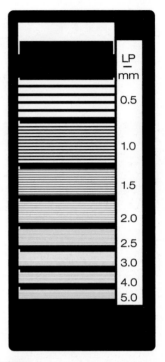

FIGURE 30-1 A resolution tool. The tool is read by discerning the point at which the finest lines are still visible as separated from one another. This point is then compared to the scale to determine the lp/mm reading. High spatial resolution represents a high-frequency signal that is capable of imaging smaller objects. Low spatial resolution represents a lower frequency signal that can only image larger objects. *(Courtesy of Fluke Biomedical)*

pairs of lines that are further apart. This is low resolution. Spatial resolution is measured by several different units, including point spread function (PSF) line spread function (LSF), modulation transfer function (MTF), and system noise.

All radiographic images have less recorded detail than the object itself. In other words, the radiographic image exhibits some, but never all, of the detail of the anatomical part. The art of radiography involves controlling the degree of **unsharpness** so that it does not interfere with image diagnosis.

The effect of poor resolution on the image is seen as a lack of sharp definition of fine detail. This is

A

B

FIGURE 30-2 Assessing resolution. (A) A pediatric wrist exhibiting good resolution. (B) An adult knee exhibiting fair resolution in the tibia and poor resolution in the femur.

caused by unacceptable levels of penumbra as compared to the umbral shadows that are expected from the part. Point spread function (PSF) measures penumbra and is used to quantify digital system spatial resolution. Evaluation of resolution is best accomplished when an image has high contrast and a diagnostic quality density.

Recorded detail is usually evaluated during quality control testing by imaging a resolution test tool. In a clinical situation, small structures are the easiest to examine to evaluate recorded detail. The trabeculae of bone is an excellent guidepost to image resolution. Much of the ability to assess when the resolution is too poor to be of diagnostic quality is a matter of clinical experience (Figure 30-2).

Spatial Resolution

Digital imaging requires a more specific term for resolution. Spatial resolution describes the ability of an imaging system to accurately display objects in two dimensions. Spatial resolution is higher when two objects can be demonstrated to be smaller or closer together.

Spatial resolution for digital images can be expressed in terms of three dimensions of the image. These are known as the x axis, y axis, and z axis. Understanding how each of these dimensions is displayed can become extremely complex when different sources of data (such as CT and MRI) must be considered. However, there are common imaging parameters or measures that form the basis of all modalities, and these are fairly easy to understand. Although each measure must be considered separately, together they express the quality of the spatial resolution of the image. The spatial resolution quality measures are summed in Table 30-1.

To understand each measure, it is important to remember that most medical images use a two-dimensional format to illustrate a three-dimensional region of interest in the human body. However, these two-dimensional images contain three dimensions of information in that not only can structures be located according to height and width in an x-y grid matrix, but individual pixels are also represented by various shades of gray (the gray scale) (Figure 30-3).

The x-y grid matrix dimensions make up the spatial resolution because this information is

TABLE 30-1. Spatial Resolution Quality Measures

Spatial Resolution	Object Size	Object Distance	Unit(s) of Measurement	Modulation Transfer Function) (MTF)	Point Spread Function (PSF)
High	Small	Close	High lp/cm or lp/mm	High (near 1.0)	Low
Low	Large	Distant	Low lp/cm or lp/mm	Low (0.0 to <1.0)	High

Gray scale bit depth (z-axis)

x-axis →

y-axis

FIGURE 30-3 Spatial resolution and gray scale bit depth. Horizontal x axis, vertical y axis, and the z axis that are represented by the value of the information collected in a single pixel (according to the gray scale shade displayed).

TABLE 30-2. Gray Scale Bit Depth (Z-Axis)

Bits	Exponential Representation	# Shades of Gray
1	2^1	2
6	2^6	64
8	2^8	256
10	2^{10}	1,024
12	2^{12}	4,096
16	2^{16}	65,536
24	2^{24}	16,777,216
32	2^{32}	4,294,967,296

A 1-bit pixel is capable of displaying 2 shades of gray (2^1)

represented through various points in space. The gray scale (sometimes called the z axis) represents a depth to the information in the image. The gray scale is a summation of the information in the voxel that is represented by each pixel. Digital image quality is very much concerned with the gray scale bit depth, which is a measure of how many shades of gray can be displayed by each z-axis pixel in the x-y matrix. Gray scale bit depth (z-axis) values are shown in Table 30-2.

There are a number of different measures of spatial resolution. Those used most often to describe and compare imaging systems are point spread function, line spread function, spatial frequency,

modulation transfer function, and noise. Although these sound intimidating, it is possible to understand why each is important as it relates to digital imaging without using a graduate degree in medical physics to calculate their values.

Point Spread Function (PSF). Point spread function (PSF), line spread function (LSF), and edge spread function (ESF) all express the boundaries of an image. In conventional radiography this aspect was called penumbra or blur. PSF is determined by complex mathematical measurement of the image produced from a single point. Figure 30-4 illustrates how a single point from a line extending through the imaging plane is isotropically imaged by an imaging system. The raw data for PSF measurements in imaging is usually in μm, but the PSF itself is valid only after application of an appropriate PSF, LSF, or ESF formula. For x-ray imaging (such as computed radi-

FIGURE 30-4   Point spread function. (A) A vertical line creates a point when it intersects the horizontal imaging plane. (B) 3D graphic representation of the imaging receptor response to the point is the point spread function (PSF). Note that the imaging receptor responds isotropically. (Note. From The Essential Physics of Medical Imaging (2nd ed., p. 264), by J. Bushberg, J. Seibert, E. Leidholdt and J. Boone, 2002, Philadelphia: Lippincott. Reprinted with permission)

FIGURE 30-5   Spatial resolution can be measured by how close together pairs of lines can be displayed (top), by the units measuring the distance between the line pairs (lp/mm or cm), by a sine wave representing this distance (which is actually the spatial frequency), or by the spatial frequency in cycles per unit of length (c/mm or cm).

ography) a point is made by drilling a tiny hole in a sheet of lead and then producing an x-ray image of the hole. Nuclear medicine uses a point source of radioactivity; computed tomography, a thin metal wire; sonography, a monofilament; and MRI, a small water-filled hole in a tissue equivalent phantom.

Spatial Frequency.   High spatial resolution represents a high-frequency signal that is capable of imaging smaller objects. Low spatial resolution represents a lower frequency signal that can only image larger objects. This parameter is determined by measuring the distance between pairs of lines that can be imaged as distinct from one another. The test tools are simply pairs of lines that are different distances from one another. The tool is imaged by the system, and the viewer determines the smallest pair of lines that can be visualized. The pairs of lines are then measured as line pairs per unit of length (usually mm or cm). Figure 30-5 illustrates how pairs of lines are transferred to the spatial frequency unit of cycles per unit of length. This is similar to the more common frequency measurements in cycles per unit of time, as with electrical power at 60 cycles per second. The higher the spatial frequency, the closer together the sine waves, and the closer together the line pairs.

Modulation Transfer Function (MTF).   **Modulation transfer function (MTF)** measures the accuracy of an image compared to the original object on a scale of 0 to 1. This is sometimes called the fidelity (or trueness) of the image. Mathematically, MTF measures the percentage of object contrast that is recorded. Because this measurement varies according to the size of the object (a greater percentage of object contrast is recorded for larger objects), MTF is more useful when represented as a graph of MTF versus the size of the object (the spatial frequency), as shown in Figure 30-6.

An MTF of 0 represents no signal and therefore no image. An MTF of 1 represents a signal of such extremely high fidelity that it records the image perfectly. MTF values for imaging modalities can reach 1.0 for large objects such as those with a spatial frequency of 1.0 lp/cm for computed tomography or 1.0 lp/mm for computed radiography. As the spatial frequency of objects rises, the MTF decreases. For example, a CT system may demonstrate an MTF of 1.0 for a spatial frequency of 1.0 lp/cm but drop to an MTF of 0.4 for a spatial frequency of 2.0 lp/cm (see Figure 30-6).

FIGURE 30-7 Noise. Imaging noise is represented as increasing from A through B to C. When the noise level rises, more complex computer processing algorithms may be necessary. When their limits are reached, degradation of the image occurs. *(Note. From* The Essential Physics of Medical Imaging *(2nd ed., p. 273), by J. Bushberg, J. Seibert, E. Leidholdt, and J. Boone, 2002, Philadelphia: Lippincott. Reprinted with permission)*

FIGURE 30-6 A typical modulation transfer function (MTF) curve measures the accuracy of an image compared to the original object on a scale of 0.0 to 1.0. Because this measurement varies according to the size of the object, MTF curves are plotted according to the size of the object (the spatial frequency). This graph demonstrates that when the spatial frequency is 1.0 lp/cm, the MTF is close to a perfect 1.0. However, when the spatial frequency rises to 3.0 lp/cm, MTF drops to around 0.10. The CT system represented by this graph produces relatively low imaging resolution for objects with a spatial frequency greater than 2.0 lp/cm.

Noise. **Imaging noise** is simply background information that the image receptor receives. As long as the background noise is significantly less than the amount of information that is coming from the image receptor, computer processing algorithms can easily filter out the noise. When the noise level rises, as shown in Figure 30-7, more complex algorithms may be necessary. When their limits are reached, degradation of the image occurs.

Quantum noise refers to a lack of sufficient incoming data for processing. The word "quantum" means "counted or measured," and the term has been used in radiography to indicate an insufficient number of incoming x-ray photons reaching the image receptor. This results in a blotchy or mottled image. For this reason, the phenomena is also called **quantum mottle.** The solution to the problem remains the same—increase the number (or quanta) of incoming signals, whether it requires increasing the mAs of an x-ray beam (the most common solution), or a stronger signal from an ultrasound transducer, radioactive isotope, or RF coil in an MRI unit.

Digital Sampling (Nyquist Criterion) and Aliasing (Moiré Pattern)

Digital systems are susceptible to a few imaging problems that are unique to the way they collect information. Because all digital systems sample the incoming signal at discrete points, they do not collect as much information as an analog system. Digital imaging requires that the spatial resolution frequency signal be sampled twice from each cycle. This is known as the **Nyquist criterion** or limit because it is the processing algorithm that averages the incoming analog data by using the distance between the imaging detector elements (to ensure that data is not missed or double-sampled. This is some-

A

Analog input signal →

Sampling 2x/cycle produces accurate (same level) digital signal

B

Analog input signal →

Sampling < 2x/cycle produces aliased (inaccurate) digital signal

FIGURE 30-8   Aliasing. Improper sampling not in accordance with the Nyquist criterion produces aliasing (often visualized as a moiré pattern). (A) Nyquist criterion sampling 2x/cycle produces an accurate level high-frequency digital signal. (B) Violation of the Nyquist criterion sampling <2x/cycle produces an inaccurate fluctuating low-frequency digital signal.

FIGURE 30-9   Motion unsharpness. The diaphragm, heart, and bowel are all unsharp due to motion of this pediatric patient.

times stated as signal averaging over the detector aperture width.

Aliasing occurs when the Nyquist criterion is violated. This occurs when the spatial frequency exceeds the Nyquist frequency and the incoming data is sampled less than twice per cycle. Data collected under these conditions is said to be aliased (Figure 30-8). These images look like a moiré pattern. When a computed radiography image demonstrates this pattern, the first reaction of experienced radiographers is to troubleshoot the grid, especially a reciprocating grid mechanism, for malfunction. The image is more often the result of inadequate sampling of the incoming data. Essentially what occurs in the computer is that a low-frequency aliased image wraps around over the high-frequency image. This creates a visual impression of two slightly out of alignment images in a moiré pattern.

 EFFECTS ON IMAGE APPEARANCE

Resolution affects the image appearance by demonstrating fine detail structures, often very close to the size limits of the naked eye. When fine detail is lacking, the image will often appear blurred.

Motion unsharpness is often not perceived by the beginning student, partially because students must learn to critically examine each image in a methodical manner. Another reason is that a thorough knowledge of how various anatomical structures should appear radiographically is necessary in order to recognize when motion causes them to appear unacceptable (Figure 30-9). The assessment of motion is a matter of obtaining sufficient clinical experience. Progress in professional competence has been achieved when the beginning radiographer easily discerns motion unsharpness.

FACTORS AFFECTING RECORDED DETAIL

The factors that control recorded detail are shown in Figure 30-10. Close consideration of these factors will reveal that recorded detail is improved only through factors that increase the patient dose. This makes consideration of how much resolution is necessary for a particular study a patient radiation protection issue. Resolution problems should be approached in this order:

1. Eliminate **motion**;
2. Reduce **OID** (OFD);
3. Reduce **focal spot size**;
4. Reduce **intensifying screen phosphor size and concentration**; and
5. Increase **SID** (FFD).

Geometry

The geometry of the beam is the most important factor in establishing the level of resolution desired for recorded detail. Because the x-ray beam em-

anates from a small point (the focal spot), the further the photons move from their source, the further they diverge. In Figure 30-11 note how much more tissue is imaged and exposed at the level of the spine than at the level of the collimator light beam. This is the basis of the inverse square law and it applies to the geometry of the beam as well.

Distance. The distances between the source or focal spot (S), object or part (O), and image receptor (I) are critical in establishing sufficient recorded detail. These distances are referred to, as shown in Figure 30-12, so that SOD + OID = SID. **Resolution is improved when OID decreases** and degraded whenever it increases. This is why the affected side or part of interest is always positioned as close to the receptor as possible.

Resolution is improved when SID increases and degraded when it decreases. Increasing SID improves the recorded detail of the image enough that numerous leaders in radiography are currently advocating a routine 48″ (120 cm) distance in place of the current 40″ (100 cm) distance.

When it is necessary to make adjustments in order to improve detail, OID should be evaluated first. **The minimum OID should be used to improve detail.** The details of the positioning and the equip-

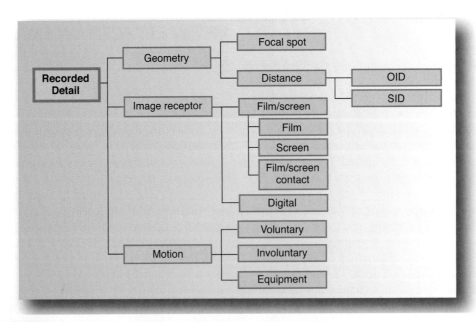

FIGURE 30-10 Image analysis: factors affecting recorded detail.

ment in use should be carefully considered. In many instances a change in positioning will accomplish a remarkable improvement in detail. In fact, most positioning routines were established with OID as a critical factor. For example, the PA chest projection is preferred because it places the heart closer to the

FIGURE 30-11   Divergence of the x-ray beam. More tissue is imaged and exposed at the level of the spine (point B) than at the level of the collimator light beam (point A).

image receptor than does the AP projection. The left lateral stomach, AP kidney and AP lumbar projections were all developed for the same reason.

The OID can also be minimized by considering the distance between the surface supporting the part and the image receptor. Differences between the **table-top-to-Bucky tray distance can have a considerable influence on OID.** Of course, the minimal OID is obtained with non-Bucky procedures that place the part directly on the cassette, as is routine in extremity radiography. However, once the need for a grid supersedes the resolution that is lost by using a Bucky tray, careful consideration can still result in significant differences in detail. For example, whereas a head unit will often permit an OID of 1–2 cm, a floating top table may permit an OID of only 10 cm. The differences in image quality are significant (Figure 30-13).

Once the OID has been minimized, **resolution is improved when SID increases** and degraded when it decreases. Again, positioning routines were established to take advantage of this relationship. For example, the lateral cervical is usually performed at 72″ (180 cm) instead of 40″ (100 cm) because the OID cannot be reduced due to the distance between the neck and shoulder. Increased SID is the only method that can produce a lateral image comparable to the AP and oblique projections, which have a much smaller OID.

Source to object distance (SOD)

Source to image receptor distance (SID)

Object to image receptor distance (OID)

FIGURE 30-12   Critical distances in radiography.

80 kVp	10 mAs	40" SID
8:1 grid	400 RS	57.3 mR

80 kVp	10 mAs	40" SID
8:1 grid	400 RS	57.3 mR

A   B

FIGURE 30-13 (A) 7 cm OID (OFD); (B) 14 cm OID (OFD).

Focal Spot Size. Focal spot size is controlled by the line focus principle (see Figure 6-13). A multitude of tube designs have been used over the years to minimize the effective focal spot while maximizing the actual focal spot to absorb the heat.

The umbra is the distinctly sharp area of a shadow or the region of complete shadow. **The penumbra is the imperfect, unsharp shadow surrounding the umbra.** With light, it is the region of partial illumination that surrounds the complete shadow. It is also referred to as the edge gradient. Digital systems are evaluated for this factor as part of spatial resolution by measuring their point spread function (PSF) and line spread function (LSF).

The focal spot size is a major controller of image resolution because it controls penumbra. The fact that the source of the x-ray photons is not a point source, although it is sometimes convenient to think of it as such, is what causes penumbra. Figures 30-14A and B illustrate the umbra and penumbra caused by the focal spot size and configuration. As the focal spot decreases in size, penumbra also decreases, thus increasing resolution. Focal spots are usually not capable of imaging structures smaller than the focal spots themselves.

The width of the penumbra (unsharpness) can be mathematically calculated using the following formula:

$$P = \frac{\text{Focal Spot Size} \times \text{OID}}{\text{SOD}}$$

EXAMPLE: Calculate the penumbra for an image taken with a 1.0 mm focal spot, at a 40" distance and an OID of 3".

Answer:

$$P = \frac{\text{Focal Spot Size} \times \text{OID}}{\text{SOD}}$$

If the SID is 40" and the OID is 3", then the SOD = 40" − 3" = 37".

$$P = \frac{1.0 \times 3"}{37} = \frac{3}{37} = 0.08 \text{ mm}$$

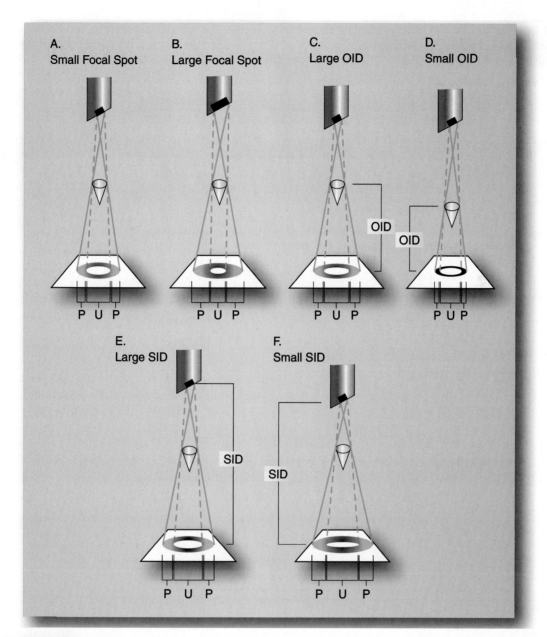

FIGURE 30-14 Umbra and penumbra. The umbral area receives essentially no photons. The penumbral area receives more photons at the outer edges with progressively fewer photons toward the umbral area, thus creating an imperfect, unsharp shadow around the umbra. (A and B) The effect of focal-spot size on resolution. The geometry of the beam reduces penumbra and increases resolution as focal-spot size decreases. (C and D) The effect of object-to-image receptor distance (OID) on resolution. As the OID decreases, penumbra is reduced and resolution increases. (E and F) The effect of source-to-image distance (SID) on resolution. As SID increases, penumbra is reduced and resolution increases.

EXAMPLE: Calculate the penumbra for an image taken with a 2.0 mm focal spot, at a 40" distance and an OID of 3".

Answer:

$$P = \frac{\text{Focal Spot Size} \times \text{OID}}{\text{SOD}}$$

If the SID is 40" and the OID is 3", then the SOD = 40" − 3" = 37".

$$P = \frac{2.0 \times 3"}{37} = \frac{6}{37} = 0.16 \text{ mm}$$

EXAMPLE: Calculate the penumbra for an image taken with a 1.0 mm focal spot, at a 40" distance and an OID of 8".

Answer:

$$P = \frac{\text{Focal Spot Size} \times \text{OID}}{\text{SOD}}$$

If the SID is 40" and the OID is 8", then the SOD = 40" − 8" = 32".

$$P = \frac{1.0 \times 8"}{32} = \frac{8}{32} = 0.25 \text{ mm}$$

EXAMPLE: Calculate the penumbra for an image taken with a 1.0 mm focal spot, at a 72" distance and an OID of 3".

Answer:

$$P = \frac{\text{Focal Spot Size} \times \text{OID}}{\text{SOD}}$$

If the SID is 72" and the OID is 3", then the SOD = 72" − 3" = 69".

$$P = \frac{1.0 \times 3"}{69} = \frac{3}{69} = 0.04 \text{ mm}$$

From these examples, it is evident that penumbra decreases when the focal spot decreases, when the OID decreases and when the SID increases.

Figures 30-14C and D illustrate that as OID decreases, penumbra also decreases. Figures 30-14E and F illustrate that as SID increases, penumbra decreases. When penumbra decreases, resolution is increased.

Penumbra is increased by another phenomenon known as attenuation or absorption unsharpness. Because of the divergence of the incident x-ray beam, only an object that is trapezoidal would have a perfectly sharp edge (Figure 30-15A). A trape-

FIGURE 30-15 Attenuation unsharpness. The D line represents the amount of density that would occur in the image receptor under each object. (A) A trapezoidal object shaped congruent to the divergence of the beam. (B) A square object produces density shadings that form the penumbra. (C) A round object produces a penumbra that is incorporated into the continuously varying density of the shape itself.

zoidal object would have a relatively equal object thickness that would attenuate the beam, causing an equal proportion of the beam to reach the image. A square object would project an edge with a gradually increasing attenuation (Figure 30-15B). Circular objects, which predominate in the human body, have an attenuation that varies throughout the entire object, reaching a maximum at a single point (Figure 30-15C). Consequently, the attenuation of the object itself causes a continuously varying projected density, which, when added to the penumbra, causes structures in the human body to have gradual instead of sharp abrupt edges.

Image Receptor

Film/Screen Image Receptor Systems. Film/screen combinations are most commonly classified by speed. Within a single phosphor type, there is an inverse relationship between film/screen combination speed and resolution. In other words, a slow film/screen combination will demonstrate better resolution than a fast one. This is such a definite relationship that many slow film/screen combinations are labeled as detail combinations.

Once the geometrical considerations of recorded detail have been maximized, the most common source of better resolution is the film/screen combination. Most institutions utilize at least two differ-

ent film/screen combinations in recognition of the better detail required by extremity examinations. This policy permits higher speed film/screens to be used to reduce patient dose for other examinations that do not require such high resolution.

Although various types of film have a wide variety of resolving capabilities, in radiography the intensifying screen always has poorer resolution than the film. Radiographic film usually has resolving capabilities in the range of 100 lp/mm, far beyond the ability of any screen or human eye. As long as the film is sensitive to the light emitted by the screens, film speed and resolution are not important issues in radiographic imaging.

Although obsolete due to excessive patient dose, nonscreen or direct exposure film possesses the highest resolution possible. Direct exposure film often required 20–100 times the mAs of a film-screen exposure.

Adjustment of film speed is seldom considered for resolution purposes. However, when a decision is made to use a higher resolution intensifying screen, its slower speed may be somewhat compensated for by using a higher speed film to help reduce patient dose.

The resolving power of an intensifying screen depends on three factors: **phosphor size, phosphor layer thickness,** and **phosphor concentration.** The relationship of these factors to recorded detail, patient dose, and density is shown in Table 30-3. As

TABLE 30-3.   Effects of Intensifying Screen Factors on Resolution

Phosphor Change	Effect on Image Resolution	Effect on Patient Dose	Effect on Film Density
Phosphor size			
increases	decreases	decreases	increases
decreases	increases	increases	decreases
Layer thickness			
increases	decreases	decreases	increases
decreases	increases	increases	decreases
Phosphor concentration (Packing density)			
increases	increases	decreases	increases
decreases	decreases	increases	decreases

phosphor size and layer thickness decrease, resolution increases along with patient dose; however, increasing phosphor concentrations will result in an intensifying screen that is better able to record details while reducing patient dose. Overall, as intensifying screen speed is decreased, there is a gain in resolution but patient dose must be increased. This creates a classical confrontation in radiography that pits recorded detail against patient dose. The decision is often left to the radiographer, who must consider all elements of both sides of the issue. Detail-speed screens can resolve about 15 lp/mm, regular-speed screens about 10 lp/mm, and high-speed screens about 7 lp/mm. These differences in recorded detail are easily visualized (Figure 23-3).

Recall that because of their higher conversion efficiency, rare-earth phosphors have significantly better resolving abilities than similar speed calcium tungstate screens.

Quantum mottle is a phenomenon that may dramatically affect recorded detail when high-speed intensifying screens are used with extremely low mAs. Modern intensifying screen technology is so advanced that it is now possible to obtain screens that are so sensitive that sufficient radiographic density can be achieved at extremely low mAs. If the total number of incident photons reaching the intensifying screen are insufficient to activate enough phosphors to emit light to cover the entire surface of the film, quantum mottle results (Figure 22-6). When using diagnostic radiographic intensifying screens, quantum mottle is corrected **only** by increasing mAs.

When resolution is unsatisfactory and the geometric solutions have been exhausted, a higher resolution film/screen combination should be used. It is important to remember that this decision includes a significant increase in patient dose. Conversely, if resolution is more than satisfactory for the examination, a lower resolution film/screen combination should be considered to reduce patient dose.

The radiographic film and intensifying screens are sandwiched together in the cassette by pressure pads that keep them in immediate direct contact with one another. When the film/screen contact is broken, even over a small area of the cassette, the image detail is not as sharp because of increased penumbra (Figure 22-5).

The only adjustment for poor film/screen contact is repairing or discarding the cassette. The procedures for testing cassettes for film/screen contact are part of a quality control program.

Digital Image Receptor Systems. The primary factors affecting the recorded detail of digital imaging systems are the detector geometric properties and the image processing system. Table 25-2 provides a comparison of the differences in the detector systems for each of the most common CR/DR systems.

Photostimulable phosphor systems, which are often called Computed Radiography (CR), have recorded detail limitations very similar to film/screen intensifying screen phosphor systems. This is because they depend on a phosphor to acquire incoming x-ray photon data. The factors are phosphor size, layer thickness, and concentration. Additional limits on recorded detail may occur in CR systems during the scanning of the phosphor screen and during the processing phase. **The major factors that limit photostimulable phosphor systems are the intensifying screen and scanning system.**

Indirect digital radiography (flat panel) systems are of two types. One uses an intensifying screen with a CCD detector while the other uses a silicon detector with a CsI scintillator. The screen/CCD system has the same limitations that effect recorded detail in film/screen intensifying systems (phosphor size, layer thickness, and concentration). The silicon/scintillator/TFT system also has limitations due to the fill factor. The fill factor is the area of the detector that is light sensitive. A high fill factor produces higher resolution. Each interface between system elements reduces recorded detail, for example, silicon detector to CsI scintillator to TFT charge reader. The processing phase is also a factor. **The major factor that limits indirect digital systems is the size of the detector element.**

Direct digital radiography (flat panel) selenium detectors can be made much thicker because photons traveling through them maintain a much more vertical path than in silicon detectors. There is virtually no blurring during direct detection of photons. However, they cannot be made as small as silicon detectors. **The major factor that limits direct digital systems is the size of the detector element.**

The image processing system also sets a limit on recorded detail (spatial resolution) depending on the acquisition and display matrix size, pixel size, and gray scale bit depth. These correspond to the x, y, and z-axis of the digital image (Figure 30-3).

Motion

Motion affects recorded detail because it fails to permit enough time for a well-defined image to form. Instead, the image is spread over a linear distance and appears as a blurred series of densities in which no fine detail can be perceived.

Voluntary Motion. Voluntary motion is that which is under the direct control of the patient. For the most part, this comprises the voluntary nervous system in cognizant adults (children and incognizant adults may be excepted in some cases). For **all** patients, including children and incognizant adults, **communication,** especially in a manner that establishes a professional and competent atmosphere, is the best method of controlling voluntary motion. There are a few examinations, such as most headwork, where immobilization greatly decreases the potential need for a repeated exposure.

For most examinations, when the radiographer effectively communicates positioning instructions, the patient is able to cooperate in reducing motion. Instructions must be given in a kindly and concerned manner. They must be in an understandable language, which includes avoiding medical terminology when appropriate, using proper pronunciation of foreign language instructions, at a proper volume and properly enunciated. Even infants and incognizant adults will respond to a kindly tone of voice and gentle handling. Never assume that your patient is unable to understand your instructions. Many young children can be amazingly cooperative when they wish to be and incognizant adults will often remember fragments of conversations when they regain full cognizance.

Involuntary Motion. Involuntary motion is not under the conscious control of the patient. For the most part, involuntary motion is controlled by the involuntary nervous system and is physiological in nature. Heartbeat and peristalsis are the most common examples. Involuntary motion can be best reduced by decreasing exposure time.

Equipment Motion. Although often overlooked, motion of equipment can also be an occasional problem. If the movement of the reciprocating grid mechanism is not dampened, it can cause vibration of the cassette in the Bucky tray. If the x-ray tube suspension system is not balanced and isolated from other moving devices, especially overhead suspended units, it can vibrate or drift. This type of motion is extremely difficult to detect. It is usually suspected only when a variety of patients examined with the same x-ray unit appear to have motion problems.

Communication. The best method of reducing motion is patient communication. It is assumed that appropriate aids to positioning, such as foam pads, angle sponges, and sandbags, are already in use. The radiographer should consider the instructions that are given to be sure that they are clear, concise, and understandable.

Exposure Time Reduction. When the patient is unable to cooperate, the best method is a reduction in exposure time with a corresponding increase in mA to maintain sufficient mAs and film density. Involuntary motion can be best reduced by a reduction in exposure time. Other methods of decreasing exposure time while maintaining exposure include using higher speed film and screens, decreasing SID and increasing kVp. Increasing kVp is not a preferred method because of the accompanying contrast change. Table 30-4 summarizes the pros and cons of each method.

Immobilization. When communication and exposure time reduction are not sufficient to reduce motion, partial immobilization must be considered. Immobilization devices, such as foam pads, angle sponges, and sandbags, should be considered routine positioning aids. Patient motion can be expected when these aids are not provided. If students find it uncomfortable or difficult to hold radiographic positions during laboratory positioning practice, imagine how an ill patient who is in pain (most likely lying

TABLE 30-4. Effects of Various Methods for Reducing Exposure Time to Avoid Motion

Method	Density	Contrast	Resolution	Distortion
mA increase	maintains	maintains	maintains	maintains
kVp increase	maintains	decreases	maintains	maintains
Film/screen speed increase	maintains	maintains	decreases	maintains
SID decrease	maintains	maintains	decreases	increases

on the most acute area) must feel. The use of positioning aids is part of professionalism. Even when they are in short supply, the radiographer should try to locate the proper aids for the patient.

For some examinations, especially headwork, immobilization greatly reduces the potential need for repeated exposures and should be used routinely. A wide range of immobilization devices and techniques have been developed over the years; some are available commercially while others are homemade.

Experienced radiographers often say that tape is the radiographer's best friend. Tape should certainly be carried at all times by radiographers and used freely when warranted. A strip of tape across the forehead (folded sticky side out across skin surfaces) has avoided many repeated cranial exposures.

Some devices, especially in pediatrics, are designed to immobilize the entire body. Pediatric boards, mummy wrapping techniques, Pig-O-Stats™, and compression bands are common examples. Individual parts can usually be immobilized with combinations of tape, sandbags, long-handled paddles, compression bands, and sheet wrapping. As a **last** resort, human immobilizers may be used to hold the patient in position. Male relatives are the first choice, female relatives second, then nonradiology hospital personnel and nonprofessional radiology personnel. Radiographers are the last choice. Under no circumstances should anyone be expected to routinely hold patients.

SUMMARY

Recorded detail is one of the two geometric properties of radiographic image quality. Unlike the photographic properties of density and contrast, which control the visibility of detail, the geometric properties control detail itself. Recorded detail is the degree of geometric sharpness or accuracy of the structural lines actually recorded in the radiographic image. Good detail exists even when it cannot be seen due to poor visibility of detail or, in other words, when the density and/or contrast are poor.

Recorded detail is also referred to as definition, sharpness, resolution, or simply as detail. When the term detail is used by itself, it usually refers to the recorded detail of the radiographic image. Detail is easily quantified and even has a derived unit. The term resolution is applied to quantified discussions of recorded detail. The unit of resolution is line pairs per millimeter (lp/mm) or cycles per mm.

The factors that affect recorded detail are geometry, including SID, OID, and focal spot size; image receptor and motion.

When the factors that affect recorded detail are altered, some change in the recorded detail will occur. No effect will occur unless one of these factors is altered. Table 30-5 illustrates the effect on recorded detail when the various factors are changed.

TABLE 30-5. Effect of Changing Factors on Recorded Detail

| + = increases recorded detail (resolution) |
| - = decreases recorded detail (resolution) |

Geometry

+	Increasing SID
-	Decreasing SID
-	Increasing OID
+	Decreasing OID
-	Increasing patient thickness
+	Decreasing patient thickness
-	Increasing focal–spot size
+	Decreasing focal–spot size

Film/Screen Combination

-	Increasing film/screen speed
+	Decreasing film/screen speed
+	Good film/screen contact
-	Poor film/screen contact

Motion

| - | Increasing motion |
| + | Decreasing motion |

REVIEW QUESTIONS

1. What is recorded detail?

2. How is resolution measured?

3. How do the SID and the OID affect recorded detail?

4. What is the relationship between focal spot size and recorded detail?

5. What is the difference between umbra and penumbra?

6. What three factors affect the resolving power of intensifying screens?

7. What is the difference between voluntary and involuntary motion?

8. What are the methods which can be used to reduce the possibility of motion?

REFERENCES AND RECOMMENDED READING

American Registry of Radiologic Technologists. (1987). Use of 'penumbra' studied. *Radiologic Technology, 58*(1), 74.

Ball, J., & Price, T. (1989). *Chesneys' radiographic imaging.* Oxford: Blackwell Scientific.

Bushong, S. C. (2004). *Radiologic science for technologists: Physics, biology, and protection* (8th ed.). St. Louis, MO: C.V. Mosby.

Cahoon, J. B. (1961). Radiographic technique: Its origin, concept, practical application and evaluation of radiation dosage. *The X-Ray Technician, 32,* 354–364.

Carroll, Q. B. (1993). *Fuchs's radiographic exposure, processing, and quality control* (5th ed.). Springfield, IL: Charles C Thomas.

Crooks, H. E. (1973). Some aspects of radiographic quality with special reference to image sharpness. *Radiography, 39*(468), 317–327.

Cullinan, A., & Cullinan, J. (1994). *Producing quality radiographs* (2nd ed.). Philadelphia: J. B. Lippincott.

Eastman Kodak Company. (1977a). *Image insight 1: The quality image* (Publication M3-182). Rochester, NY: Author.

Eastman Kodak Company. (1977b). *Image insight 2: Geometry of image formation: Detail* (Publication M3-184). Rochester, NY: Author.

Eastman Kodak Company. (1980). Health Sciences Markets Division. *The Fundamentals of Radiography* (12th ed.) (Kodak Publication M1-18). Rochester, NY: Author.

Engel, T. L. (1979). Effect of kilovoltage and milliamperage on focal spot size. *Radiologic Technology, 50*(5), 559–561.

Files, G. W. (1935). Maximum tissue differentiation. *The X-Ray Technician, 7,* 17–24+.

Files, G. W. (1952). *Medical radiographic technique.* Springfield, IL: Charles C Thomas.

Fodor, J., & Malott, J. C. (1993). *The art and science of medical radiography* (7th ed.). St. Louis, MO: C. V. Mosby.

Fuchs, A. W. (1940). Balance in the radiographic image. *The X-Ray Technician, 12*(3), 81–84, 118.

Fuchs, A. W. (1950). The rationale of radiographic exposure. *The X-Ray Technician, 22,* 62–68, 76.

Fuchs, A. W. (1958). *Principles of radiographic exposure and processing.* Springfield, IL: Charles C Thomas.

Geometrical fallacies. (1983). *Radiologic Technology, 54*(4), 297.

Godderidge, C. (1995). *Pediatric imaging.* Philadelphia: W. B. Saunders.

Haus, A. G. (1980, October). Effects of geometric and screen-film unsharpness in conventional and 350 kVp chest radiography. *Radiology, 197.*

Haus, A. G. (1985). Evaluation of image blur (unsharpness) in medical imaging. *Medical Radiography and Photography, 61*(1–2), 42–53.

Hiss, S. S. (2003). *Understanding radiography* (4th ed.). Springfield, IL: Charles C Thomas.

Jenkins, D. (1980). *Radiographic photography and imaging processes.* Lancaster, England: MTP Press Limited.

Jerman, E. C. (1928). *Modern x-ray technic.* St. Paul, MN: Bruce.

Lauer, O. G., Mayes, J. B., & Thurston, R. P. (1990). *Evaluating radiographic quality: The variables and their effects.* Mankato, MN: The Burnell Company.

Morgan, J. A. (1977). *The art and science of medical radiography* (5th ed.). St. Louis, MO: Catholic Hospital Association.

Morgan, R. H. (1945a). An analysis of the physical factors controlling the diagnostic quality of roentgen images: Part I. Introduction. *American Journal of Roentgenology and Radiation Therapy, 54*(2), 128–135.

Morgan, R. H. (1945b). An analysis of the physical factors controlling the diagnostic quality of roentgen images: Part II. Maximum resolving power and resolution coefficient. *American Journal of Roentgenology and Radiation Therapy, 54*(4), 395–402.

Morgan, R. H. (1949). An analysis of the physical factors controlling the diagnostic quality of roentgen images: Part V. Unsharpness. *American Journal of Roentgenology and Radiation Therapy, 62*(6), 870–880.

Seeman, H. E. (1968). *Physical and photographic principles of medical radiography.* New York: Wiley & Sons.

Sparks, O. J. (1960). Possibilities and limitations of definition. *Radiologic Technology, 32*(2), 148.

Spiegler, G. (1950). The story of contrast and definition. *Radiography, 41*(189), 177–182.

Stears, J. G., Gray, J. E., & Frank, E. D. (1989). Radiologic exchange (resolution by focal spot size). *Radiologic Technology, 60*(5), 429–430.

Stockley, S. M. (1986). *A manual of radiographic equipment.* Edinburgh: Churchill Livingstone.

Sweeney, R. J. (1975). Some factors affecting image clarity and detail perception in the radiograph. *Radiologic Technology, 46*(6), 443.

Thompson, M. A., Hattaway, M. P., Hall, J. D., & Dowd, S. B. (1994). *Principles of imaging science and protection.* Philadelphia: W. B. Saunders.

Tortorici, M. (1992). *Concepts in medical radiographic imaging.* Philadelphia: W. B. Saunders.

United States War Department. (1941, July 3). *Technical manual: Roentgenographic technicians* (Washington DC: TM 8-240).

Wilks, R. J. (1981). *Principles of radiological physics.* Edinburgh: Churchill Livingstone.

CHAPTER 31 | # Distortion

> Hans Castorp peered through the lighted window, peered into Joachim Ziemssen's empty skeleton. The breastbone and spine fell together in a single dark column. The frontal structure of the ribs was cut across by the paler structure of the back. Above, the collar-bones branched off on both sides, and the framework of the shoulder, with the joint and beginning of Joachim's arm, showed sharp and bare through the soft envelope of flesh. The thoracic cavity was light, but blood-vessels were to be seen, some dark spots, a blackish shadow.
>
> *Thomas Mann, Der Zauberberg*
> *(The Magic Mountain)*

KEY TERMS

caudad
cephalad
distortion
elongation
foreshortening

OBJECTIVES

Upon completion of this chapter, the student should be able to:

- Define size and shape distortion.
- Explain the effects of SID and OID on image distortion.
- Discuss various methods of minimizing distortion through variation of SID and OID.
- Explain why elongation and foreshortening are relational definitions.
- Describe the routine relationships between central ray, anatomical part, and image receptor.
- Explain the proper terms used to describe angulation direction and degree.

- Differentiate distorted images from routine projections.
- Calculate the magnification factor when given SID and SOD.
- Calculate the actual size of an object when given the projected size, SID, and OID.
- Describe adjustments of SID, and OID that will minimize magnification.
- Describe adjustments of central ray, anatomical part, and image receptor that will minimize shape distortion.

455

ASSESSING DISTORTION

Distortion is the second of the two geometric properties affecting radiographic image quality. Unlike the photographic properties of density and contrast, which control the visibility of detail, the geometric properties control detail itself. **Distortion is a misrepresentation of the size or shape of the structures being examined.** It creates a misrepresentation of the size and/or shape of the anatomical part being imaged. This misrepresentation can be classified as either size or shape distortion. Distortion, like detail, exists even when it cannot be seen due to poor visibility or, in other words, when the density and/or contrast are poor. The evaluation and adjustment of distortion require a thorough familiarity with normal radiographic anatomy. Unless the normal size and shape of a structure are known, comparison of the size and shape cannot be accomplished. Distortion can be difficult to determine even when normal sizes and shapes are known. Because the objective of radiography is to provide accurate images of structures, methods of minimizing distortion are important to diagnosis.

The factors that control distortion are shown in Figure 31-1. Careful examination of these factors will reveal that distortion is directly related to positioning. Only careful attention to the distances, direction, and angulation between the anatomical part, central ray, and image receptor can minimize distortion.

FACTORS AFFECTING SIZE DISTORTION

Size distortion can be only magnification with film/screen radiography. With traditional film/screen systems, minification is impossible, due to the divergent property of x-ray photons. Since it is not possible to reflect or refract x-ray photons by ordinary methods, they can only diverge from their point source. Thus, only magnification is possible and all size distortion is controlled by the radiographic distances, SID and OID. In digital image receptor systems, both minification and magnification are possible. This is all done through post-processing parameters.

In all instances, **reduced magnification size distortion increases the resolution of recorded detail.** Therefore, the objective in most radiography is to minimize magnification as much as possible. Magnification radiography is an exception to this rule. In this instance, the principles of magnification geometry are used to increase the size of structures that are too small to be easily visualized. Special conditions must be created to achieve diagnostically acceptable magnification images.

Magnification size distortion is controlled by positioning the body part and tube to maximize SID while minimizing OID. This can be accomplished by various procedures and by positioning. For example, an upright oblique cervical vertebra projection can be performed at 72″ (180 cm), while a supine projection is performed at 40″ (100 cm). An AP

FIGURE 31-1 Image analysis: factors affecting distortion.

chest may place the heart 6″ (15 cm) from the image receptor, while a PA projection would place it 2″ (5 cm) away.

Source-to-Image Receptor Distance

The SID has a major effect on magnification (Figure 31-2). **The greater the SID, the smaller the magnification,** because as SID increases the percentage of the total distance that makes up OID decreases. The OID is the critical distance for magnification and resolution.

Although 40″ (100 cm) has developed as the current routine SID, this was not always so. The popular SID has been increasing since the advent of radiography and will probably continue to do so. The first x-ray techniques book in the United States is generally recognized to be the 1918 *Extract from the United States Army X-Ray Manual,* in which 20″ (50 cm) is discussed as a reasonable SID. When Ed Jerman developed the first positioning and technique book, *Modern X-Ray Technic,* in 1928, he recommended distances varying from 25″ (63 cm) to 36″ (90 cm). Of course, in those days shorter distances were necessary because the x-ray tubes were not capable of handling the load required to provide sufficient density with the film and screens of the time. As generator technology advanced, the SID increased.

Glenn Files' 1945 book, *Medical Radiographic Technic,* established the 40″ (100 cm) SID. For over 50 years this has remained the standard distance, but now there are institutions that use 48″ (120 cm) as a routine distance and the movement appears to be growing. Although a change demands new grids as well as careful consideration of x-ray unit design so that tube-to-tabletop distances can be achieved, and low table design so that radiographers can reach the tube, the increased resolution is worth the expense and trouble.

For many, many years chest radiography has routinely been performed at 72″ (180 cm) because the erect positioning arrangement permits a horizontal beam to be used and the increased SID effectively minimizes the magnification of the heart shadow. Any examination that permits a horizontal beam to be used can easily be established at an SID greater than 40″ (100 cm), and in many places the lateral cervical vertebral examination is performed at 72″ (180 cm) as well.

The source-to-object distance (SOD) is seldom discussed because it is included in descriptions of SID and OID, which are more critical. The SID is the distance that must be established by the radiographer when positioning.

The SID must be maximized to decrease magnification. Examinations of body parts with large inherent OID, such as the lateral cervical vertebra and the chest, use large SID whenever possible. In addition, the historical trend to increase the routine SID should be continued.

Large size   Small size

FIGURE 31-2 The effect of SID on image size magnification. Magnification size distortion is minimized by increasing SID.

Object-to-Image Receptor Distance

The OID is also a critical distance in both magnification and resolution. Figure 31-3 illustrates two major facets of OID. First, when objects within a structure are at different levels (Figure 31-3, objects A and B) they will be projected onto the image as different sizes. This is similar to the manner in which the eye processes information for depth perception; smaller objects are perceived as more distant and larger objects as closer.

The radiographer should develop a stereoscopic perception of the radiographic image, which is difficult because radiographic perceptions are in reverse of the normal information the eye is accustomed to processing. This is because objects that are further from the image receptor will be magnified. For example, in a chest radiograph the ribs are seen as wider as they become more posterior. This effect should make them appear closer, which is the opposite of the truth for the PA projection. Nevertheless, the perception of three-dimensionality can be developed and then used to determine object-to-image receptor distance visually. When describing objects, it is important to remember that the size and distance relationship in a radiographically projected image is the opposite of that perceived visually.

A more important size relationship that is controlled by OID is shown in Figure 31-3 between objects B and C, where object C appears identical in size to object B. This is an illusion because object C is much smaller but is magnified more because of its location in the part. This illustrates that a thorough knowledge of normal radiographic anatomy is a prerequisite to making judgements about size relationships. This is also one of the reasons radiographic examinations must include two projections, as close to 90° from one another as possible. When AP and lateral projections cannot be performed because of superimposing structures, as in an examination of the kidneys, it is important to include two oblique projections at 90° to one another. The two 90° opposing images can be used to verify the positional relationship of structures. This is also a shape distortion issue.

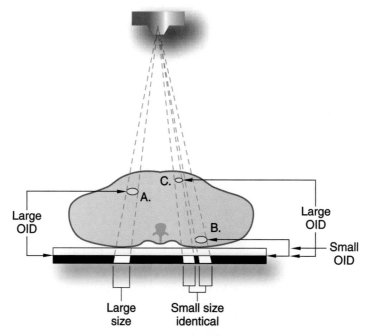

FIGURE 31-3 The effect of OID on image size magnification. Objects A and B are identical in size but their images as projected on the receptor are of significantly different sizes. Object C is significantly smaller than B, yet the image sizes are identical because of C's greater OID.

The OID is also important in dosimetry because it establishes the source-to-entrance skin distance that is the benchmark maximum exposure to the patient. Because OID varies with the part size and position of the patient, it accounts for the increased exposure that is part of many examinations. For example, there is a significant difference in the OID between an AP and a lateral projection (Figure 31-4). Note that the SOD changes dramatically in the figure as well. Obviously the entrance skin exposure would be greater with the lateral, even if the same exposure factors were used. Consequently, larger patients receive a greater exposure simply because their entrance skin surface is closer to the source, making their SOD much less. The increased mAs that is often used to provide sufficient image receptor exposure then increases the patient entrance skin exposure even more.

The OID must be minimized to decrease magnification. Examinations of body parts with large inherent OID, such as the kidneys and chest, use positioning techniques to achieve as small an OID as possible.

Calculating Size Distortion

Size distortion is present in any radiographic image and can be measured very accurately by using simple geometry. **Magnification, or size distortion, can be assessed by calculation of the magnification factor.** The magnification factor is the degree of magnification and is calculated by:

$$M = \frac{SID}{SOD}$$

where: M = magnification factor

The mnemonic device shown can be used (see discussion of Ohm's law in Chapter 3).

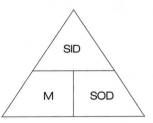

EXAMPLE: If the SID is 40" (100 cm) and the SOD is 30" (75 cm), what is the magnification factor?

Answer:

$$M = \frac{SID}{SOD}$$

$$M = \frac{40"}{30"} \text{ or } M = \frac{100 \text{ cm}}{75 \text{ cm}}$$

$$M = 1.33$$

The magnification will be 33 percent or the image will be 133 percent of the object size.

A.   B.

FIGURE 31-4   Variation in OID with size and projection. (A) Short OID, large SOD, low entrance skin exposure. (B) Large OID, short SOD, high entrance skin exposure.

EXAMPLE: If the SID is 40″ and the OID is 2″, what is the magnification factor?

Answer: Since the SOD is not supplied, it must be found by using the formula:

$$SID = SOD + OID$$
$$40″ = SOD + 2″$$
$$SOD = 40″ - 2″$$
$$SOD = 38″$$

then

$$M = \frac{SID}{SOD}$$
$$M = \frac{40″}{38″}$$
$$M = 1.05$$

The magnification factor permits calculation of the actual size of an object that is projected as an image by using the formula:

$$0 = \frac{I}{M}$$

where: 0 = object size
$\quad\quad\;\; I$ = image size
$\quad\quad M$ = magnification factor

The following mnemonic device can be used.

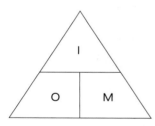

EXAMPLE: If a projected image measures 5″ and the magnification factor is 1.02, what is the size of the actual object?

Answer:

$$0 = \frac{I}{M}$$
$$0 = \frac{5″}{1.02}$$
$$0 = 4.9″$$

EXAMPLE: If object B in Figure 31–3 is 2″ in diameter on the image and is measured to be 3″ from the image receptor (by using a lateral projection), what is its actual size if the SID is 40″?

Answer: Since the SOD is not supplied, it must be found by using the formula:

$$SID = SOD + OID$$
$$40″ = SOD + 3″$$
$$SOD = 40″ - 3″$$
$$SOD = 37″$$

then

$$M = \frac{SID}{SOD}$$
$$M = \frac{40″}{37″}$$
$$M = 1.08$$

then

$$0 = \frac{I}{M}$$
$$0 = \frac{2}{1.08}$$
$$0 = 1.85″$$

If the image size and the object size are known, the percent of magnification can be determined using the following formula:

$$\frac{I - 0}{0} \times 100 = \text{percent of magnification of the object}$$

EXAMPLE: If an object measures 5 cm and the image measures 6 cm, what would be the percent magnification of the object?

Answer:

$$\frac{I - 0}{0} \times 100 = \text{percent magnification of the object}$$

$$\frac{6 - 5}{5} \times 100 = \text{percent magnification of the object}$$

$$\frac{1}{5} \times 100 = \text{percent magnification of the object}$$

$$0.2 \times 100 = 20 \text{ percent of magnification of the object}$$

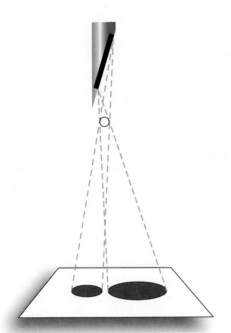

Objects smaller than the focal spot itself cannot be imaged due to penumbral overlap. The entire image is composed of overlapping penumbra with no umbra to define the edges.

Shape distortion due to unequal magnification. Note how the alignment of the part appears different depending on the degree of distortion. *(Note. Adapted with permission from Producing Quality Radiographs, by A. M. Cullinan, copyright 1987, Philadelphia: J. B. Lippincott)*

The magnification formula assumes that the focal spot is a point source. Because it is not, when the object size approaches the effective focal spot size or smaller, special problems develop from penumbral overlap (Figure 31-5). Therefore, **objects smaller than the effective focal spot cannot be demonstrated** and the magnification formula must be modified to consider the width of the focal spot.

 FACTORS AFFECTING SHAPE DISTORTION

Shape distortion is the misrepresentation by unequal magnification of the actual shape of the structure being examined (Figure 31-6). Shape distortion displaces the projected image of an object from its actual position and can be described as either elongation or foreshortening. **Elongation** projects the object so it appears to be longer than it really is, while **foreshortening** projects it so it appears shorter than it really is. Elongation occurs when the tube or the image receptor is improperly aligned. Foreshortening occurs only when the part is improperly aligned. Changes in the tube angle cause elongation, never foreshortening.

Shape distortion often results because structures lie normally at different levels within the body. Shape distortion also occurs because of the divergence of the x-ray beam. The projected length varies, depending on the angle between the object and the diverging beam (Figure 31-7).

Adjustment of shape distortion requires careful consideration of the beam-part image receptor geometry involved in the projection. This information must be combined with a knowledge of the normal projection of the structures to determine exactly how improvements can be achieved.

Alignment

Shape distortion can be caused or avoided by careful alignment of the central ray with the anatomical part and the image receptor. Proper positioning is achieved when the central ray is at right angles to the anatomical part and to the image receptor. This means the part and the image receptor must be parallel. When the position of the body part or object within the body does not permit this alignment, cre-

ative positioning must be utilized. The half-axial 30° angulation of the cranium to demonstrate the occipital bone, the 25° cephalad angulation of the pelvis to demonstrate the sigmoid colon, and the 10° caudad angulation of the coccyx, are all examples of routine procedures that were developed to minimize distortion.

Alignment adjustments involve bringing the tube central ray, the part and the image receptor back into their correct relationship—part and image receptor parallel to one another with the central ray perpendicular to both. Incorrect centering may occur from off-centering the tube (misalignment of the central ray), incorrectly positioning the part or off-centering the image receptor (Figure 31-8).

Central Ray. The central ray is the theoretical photon that exits from the exact center of the focal spot. Ideally the central ray is intended to be projected **perpendicular to both the anatomical part and the image receptor.** Whenever the central ray is not perpendicular, some degree of shape distortion will result. This occurs in every image because only the central ray is truly perpendicular. Any structure that is not positioned at the central ray will be distorted because of the divergence of the beam—**the farther from the central ray, the greater the distortion.** This applies as distance from the central ray increases transversely as well as longitudinally. For example, an AP pelvis will have

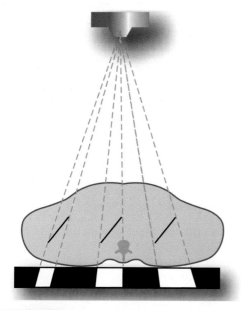

FIGURE 31-7 Shape distortion due to the angle between the object and the diverging beam. Although all three objects are at the same angle to the image receptor, the project length varies according to the angle between the object and the diverging beam.

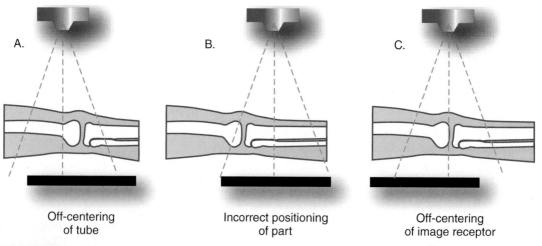

A. Off-centering of tube

B. Incorrect positioning of part

C. Off-centering of image receptor

FIGURE 31-8 Incorrect centering.

more distortion of an object near the right greater trochanter than an object near the symphysis pubis. This is why it is so important to position according to standardized central ray locations.

Long bone length studies are an example of a procedure developed to ensure accurate central ray centering. The procedure shown in Figure 31-9 uses a radiopaque ruler, positioned from above the hip joint to below the ankle joint, as a measurement control. Spot exposures of the critical joints—hip, knee and ankle—are then made with the central ray perpendicular to the joint space to ensure accurate measurement.

Centering away from the specified central ray entrance point is equivalent to angling the tube away from perpendicular because the entire perspective of the anatomical part is distorted. Some projections take advantage of this type of distortion. For example, a PA lumbar projection uses the divergence of the beam to open the lordotically curved intervertebral joints (Figure 31-10).

The central ray is normally positioned perpendicular to the anatomical part and to the image receptor. When the part is superimposed over other structures, central ray angulation can be a useful

A. PA projection

B. AP projection

FIGURE 31-10   Divergence of the beam used to advantage. The lordotic curvature of the lumbar spine and the divergence of the beam can be used to open the intervertebral joints in a PA projection.

FIGURE 31-9   A long bone leg length study. Exact central ray location is critical to ensuring an accurate measurement of the bone lengths. (A) Inaccurate leg lengths due to beam divergence at the joints from a single exposure. (B) Accurate leg lengths with three spot exposures, each perpendicular to a joint.

FIGURE 31-11 Foreshortening and magnification due to anatomical part and image receptor alignment. (A) Normal relationship between part and image receptor. (B and C) Foreshortening and magnification due to changes in anatomical part alignment. (D and E) Elongation and magnification due to changes in part/image receptor and central ray/image receptor alignment.

tool to provide a projection that would otherwise be impossible to differentiate from overlying structures. The use of the semiaxial AP projection of the skull to project the occipital region free of facial bone superimposition is an example. Failure to maintain the correct relationship between the part and the image receptor will produce a projected image that may not be comparable to norms and is therefore useless in the diagnostic process.

Anatomical Part. The long axis of the anatomical part, or object, is intended to be positioned perpendicular to the central ray and parallel to the image receptor. When these positions are incorrect, distortion may occur. Elongation occurs when there is poor alignment of the tube and/or image receptor. Foreshortening occurs only when there is poor alignment of the part (Figure 31-11). Figure 31-11A shows the intended relationships of central ray, part, and image receptor. In Figure 31-11B the entire object is fore-shortened because of the improper part-to-image receptor relationship. In addition to the entire object being foreshortened, one end is more magnified due to increased OID, which indicates that size distortion is also occurring.

In Figure 31-11C the entire object is again fore-shortened with one end being more magnified due to increased OID. However, because of the differences in the actual size of the two ends, the increased size distortion of the smaller end makes both ends appear the same size.

Note especially the vast differences in the projected images of these anatomical part relationships. Figure 31-11A projects an accurate image. Figure 31-11B projects distortion of both size and shape so the entire object is foreshortened and the large end appears larger than it really is. Figure 31-11C also projects distortion of both size and shape but has distorted the relationship so both ends appear the same size.

The anatomical part is normally positioned with its long axis perpendicular to the central ray and parallel to the image receptor. As with the central ray, some routine projections are designed to vary from this standard to avoid superimposition. Failure to maintain the specified relationships between the central ray and the image receptor can result in an image that is not comparable to norms and therefore of limited value in the diagnostic process.

Image Receptor. The image receptor is intended to be positioned perpendicular to the central ray and parallel to the anatomical part. As long as the image receptor plane is parallel to the object, the only result of off-centering of the image receptor is the clipping of a portion of the area of interest. Although this will usually result in a repeated exposure, there is no distortion of image size or shape.

However, when the image receptor plane is not parallel to the object, or if the central ray is not centered to the part, serious shape distortion results exactly as if the object were not parallel. Figures 31-11D and E illustrate for the image receptor the same examples shown for the object in Figures 31-11B and C above.

The image receptor plane is normally positioned perpendicular to the central ray and parallel to the anatomical part. Even in routine projections designed to vary from this standard, the specified relationships must be maintained to obtain a useful diagnostic image.

Angulation

Angulation refers to the direction and degree the tube is moved from its normal position perpendicular to the image receptor. Numerous radiographic projections utilize angulation to avoid superimposition of parts. The semiaxial AP projection of the cranium, tangential os calcis, and axial clavicle are all examples.

The angulation of the tube is designed to cause a controlled or expected amount of shape distortion to avoid superimposition. As long as the specified angulation is applied, the image is comparable to norms and is of diagnostic quality. Angulation of the tube also changes the SID, which, unless compensated for by a new SID, will produce a decrease in image receptor exposure.

Direction

The most common direction of tube angle is longitudinal. Longitudinal angulations are usually termed **cephalad** when the tube is angled toward the head of the patient, and **caudad** when it is angled toward the patient's feet. Some radiographic tubes can also be angled transversely (sometimes referred to as "roll"). Transverse angulations are usually identified as right and left (in reference to the patient).

The direction of the tube angle is specified according to patient position and must be maintained as specified. When the patient position is reversed, the direction of tube angle must also be reversed to maintain the relationship. For example, 25° cephalad for an AP projection is identical to 25° caudad for a PA projection.

Degree. Degree is simply a method of describing the exact amount of angulation **and is usually stated as the angle between the central ray and the image receptor plane from the standard reference point of perpendicularity.** Because the standard reference point is 90° from the patient's head, radiographic angles must be added or subtracted from that point. For example, 5° cephalad is 5° from perpendicular as is 5° caudad. It is important to maintain the correct degree of angle specified for a given procedure. Tube angulations also change SID, which will produce changes in magnification. Table 31-1 provides conversions for common tube angulations.

TABLE 31-1.	SID Compensations for Common Tube Angulations	
Tube Angulation	Overhead Scale	True SID
5°	39.8″	40″
10°	39.4″	40″
15°	38.6″	40″
20°	37.6″	40″
25°	36.2″	40″
30°	34.6″	40″
35°	32.8″	40″

Note. From *Radiologic Technology, 52* pp. 3, 304, by Robert J. English 1980, by permission of the American Society of Radiologic Technologists.

Evaluating Shape Distortion

Shape distortion is a more subjective evaluation than size. It is much more difficult to assess because there is no effect that can be calculated, as in the magnification factor for size distortion. Instead, the entire assessment relies on the radiographer's knowledge of normal anatomy and the normal projected images for each position.

EFFECT ON IMAGE APPEARANCE

Size

Size distortion is generally a matter of magnification (Figure 31-12). All magnification involves a degree of loss of resolution, even when special systems are designed to minimize the loss.

A

B

FIGURE 31-12 Magnification size distortion. (A) Minimal heart size magnification in a PA chest. (B) An AP projection of the same patient demonstrating greater heart size magnification. *(Courtesy of Tracy Thegze, RT(R), Community Hospital, Munster, IN)*

Shape

Shape distortion involves both elongation and foreshortening and is a serious alteration in the projected image (Figure 31-13). There are situations where shape distortion can be used to advantage, as in a tangential os calcis.

60 kVp	15 mAs	72" SID
No grid	100 RS	11.9 mR

A

60 kVp	15 mAs	72" SID
No grid	100 RS	11.9 mR

B

60 kVp	15 mAs	72" SID
No grid	100 RS	11.9 mR

C

FIGURE 31-13   Shape distortion. (A) This radiograph was taken with the central ray perpendicular and centered to the center of the image receptor. (B) This radiograph was taken with the central ray perpendicular but off center to the left (away from the pelvis). The effect on distortion is not significant; however, changes in the image appearance are evident, particularly when studying the pelvis, which was furthest from the central ray. (C) This radiograph was taken with a central ray angle of 25° and centered to the center of the image receptor. Notice the significant distortion created by angling the central ray.

SUMMARY

Distortion is the second of the two geometric properties affecting image quality. Unlike the photographic properties of density and contrast, which control the visibility of detail, the geometric properties control detail itself. Distortion is the difference between the structures being examined and the recorded image. It creates a misrepresentation of the size and/or shape of the anatomical part being imaged. This misrepresentation can be classified as either size or shape distortion. Distortion, like detail, exists even when it cannot be seen due to poor visibility or, in other words, when the density and/or contrast are poor. The evaluation and adjustment of distortion require a thorough familiarity with normal radiographic anatomy. Unless the normal size and shape of a structure are known, comparisons of size and shape cannot be accomplished.

When the factors that affect size and shape distortion are altered, some change in distortion will occur. No change will occur unless one of these factors is altered. Table 31–2 illustrates the effect on distortion when the various factors are changed.

TABLE 31–2. Effect of Changing Factors on Distortion

+ = increases distortion	
− = decreases distortion	
Size Distortion	
−	Increasing SID
+	Decreasing SID
+	Increasing OID
−	Decreasing OID
+	Increasing patient thickness
−	Decreasing patient thickness
Shape Distortion	
+	Improper central ray alignment
+	Improper anatomical part alignment
+	Improper image receptor alignment
+	Improper direction of central ray angle
+	Improper degree of central ray angle

REVIEW QUESTIONS

1. What is distortion?
2. What is the difference between size and shape distortion?
3. How do the SID and the OID affect size distortion?
4. What is the magnification factor formula?
5. What is the difference between elongation and foreshortening?
6. How does the alignment of the anatomical part affect shape distortion?
7. How do the direction and degree of angulation affect shape distortion?
8. How can shape distortion be used to advantage?

REFERENCES AND RECOMMENDED READING

Ball, J., & Price, T. (1989). *Chesneys' radiographic imaging.* Oxford: Blackwell Scientific.

Bushong, S. C. (2004). *Radiologic science for technologists: Physics, biology, and protection* (8th ed.). St. Louis, MO: Elsevier.

Cahoon, J. B. (1961). Radiographic technique: Its origin, concept, practical application and evaluation of radiation dosage. *The X-Ray Technician, 32,* 354–364.

Carroll, Q. B. (2003). *Fuchs's radiographic exposure, processing, and quality control* (7th ed.). Springfield, IL: Charles C Thomas.

Cullinan, A., & Cullinan, J. (1994). *Producing quality radiographs* (2nd ed.). Philadelphia: J. B. Lippincott.

Distance—technique relationship of angulated projections. (1980). *Radiologic Technology, 52*(3), 301.

Distortion in imaging. (1989). *Radiography Today,* 55(628), 31.

Eastman Kodak Company. (1977). *Image insight 2: Geometry of image formation: Detail* (Publication M3-184). Rochester, NY: Author.

English, R. J. (1980). Distance-technique relationship of angulated projections. *Radiologic Technology, 52*(3), 301–304.

Files, G. W. (1952). *Medical radiographic technique.* Springfield, IL: Charles C Thomas.

Haus, A. G. (1980, October). Effects of geometric and screen-film unsharpness in conventional and 350 kVp chest radiography. *Radiology,* 197.

Haus, A. G. (1985). Evaluation of image blur (unsharpness) in medical imaging. *Medical Radiography and Photography, 61*(1–2), 42–53.

Hiss, S. S. (2003). *Understanding radiography* (4th ed.). Springfield, IL: Charles C Thomas.

Jenkins, D. (1980). *Radiographic photography and imaging processes.* Lancaster, England: MTP Press Limited.

Jerman, E. C. (1928). *Modern x-ray technic.* St. Paul, MN: Bruce.

Lauer, O. G., Mayes, J. B., & Thurston, R. P. (1990). *Evaluating radiographic quality: The variables and their effects.* Mankato, MN: The Burnell Company.

Morgan, J. A. (1977). *The art and science of medical radiography* (5th ed.). St. Louis, MO: Catholic Hospital Association.

Morgan, R. H. (1945a). An analysis of the physical factors controlling the diagnostic quality of roentgen images: Part I. Introduction. *American Journal of Roentgenology and Radiation Therapy, 54*(2), 128–135.

Morgan, R. H. (1945b). An analysis of the physical factors controlling the diagnostic quality of roentgen images: Part II. Maximum resolving power and resolution coefficient. *American Journal of Roentgenology and Radiation Therapy, 54*(4), 395–402.

Morgan, R. H. (1949). An analysis of the physical factors controlling the diagnostic quality of roentgen images: Part V. Unsharpness. *American Journal of Roentgenology and Radiation Therapy, 62*(6), 870–880.

Pearson, G. R. (1951). Radiographic projection studies. *Radiologic Technology, 23*(1), 1.

Petersen, T. D., & Rohr, W. (1987). Improved assessment of lower extremity alignment using new roentgenographic techniques. *Clinical Orthopaedics, 219,* 112–119.

Riles, G. W. (1943). *Medical roentgenographic technique.* Springfield, IL: Charles C Thomas.

Seeman, H. E. (1968). *Physical and photographic principles of medical radiography.* New York: Wiley & Sons.

Stockley, S. M. (1986). *A manual of radiographic equipment.* Edinburgh: Churchill Livingstone.

Tarrant, R. M. (1952). Maintaining desired anode-film distance and alignment after angling the x-ray tube. *Radiologic Technology, 23*(5), 349.

Thompson, M. A., Hattaway, M. P., Hall, J. D., & Dowd, S. B. (1994). *Principles of imaging science and protection.* Philadelphia: W. B. Saunders.

Tortorici, M. (1992). *Concepts in medical radiographic imaging.* Philadelphia: W. B. Saunders.

United States War Department. (1941, July 3). *Technical manual: Roentgenographic technicians,* Washington DC: (TM 8–240).

Wilks, R. J. (1981). *Principles of radiological physics.* Edinburgh: Churchill Livingstone.

CHAPTER 32 The Art of Image Critique

> If all the factors involved in the making of a . . . radiograph are known, it then becomes a simple matter, by means of . . . (a) method of analysis, to decide what may be done to improve the quality of that radiograph.
>
> *Ed. C. Jerman, The Father of Radiologic Technology*

OBJECTIVES

Upon completion of this chapter, the student should be able to:

- Discuss the elements of a diagnostic image as they relate to the art of image critique.

- Identify the steps of the decision-making process.

- Describe an effective image critique method, incorporating critical problem-solving skills.

- Use an effective image critique method.

- Explain the differences among technical factor problems, procedural factor problems, and equipment malfunctions.

- Apply an effective image critique method to a wide range of problems specific to clinical situations beyond those presented in this chapter.

IMPLEMENTING IMAGING STANDARDS

Radiographers are required to make critical decisions every day about the quality of their radiographic images. Critiquing an image is a very complex process which requires a thorough knowledge of all aspects of radiography. Deciding if an image is acceptable or unacceptable should be approached in a logical, organized manner. Image critique is an analytical process that involves many of the steps of diagnostic decision making, including critical problem solving.

The Diagnostic Image

The art of image critique revolves around the concept of deciding exactly where in the diagnostic quality spectrum a particular radiographic image lies. A practical technical definition of a diagnostic quality image has never been established because the artistic elements involved to produce the required medical information vary so much from one situation to another. The exponential number of variables involved make radiography as much an art as a science.

The production of a diagnostic image involves an overwhelming number of variables, including such elements as patient anatomy, pathological conditions, radiographic positioning, patient preparation, radiation protection, x-ray equipment, prime technical factor selections, collimation, image receptors, processing, density and contrast perceptions, detail and distortion. In other words, nearly all of the elements of anatomy, positioning, physics, and principles of exposure are involved. **The art of image critique is the application of scientific knowledge to an analysis of the image.**

The Analytical Process

It is important to remember that not even radiologists are trained in the finer points of creating and analyzing the quality of a radiographic image. The radiographer is the expert and has the responsibility of proceeding with image analysis. Only with an acceptable image can a radiologist make an accurate diagnosis. It is the radiographer's professional responsibility to create the best possible image given each individual circumstance.

To determine whether an image is of diagnostic quality, the steps of an analytical decision making process must be followed.

The process begins with a review of the entire image. This is essential to avoid premature narrowing. During the review the radiographer watches for anything that is different from a diagnostic quality image. When differences are noticed, a pattern is sought, especially when there is more than one cue. Cues and patterns focus attention on a suspicious area, thus narrowing the search. Cues and patterns are then used to seek hypotheses. An effort is made to formulate a hypothesis that will explain all the cues. Cues that do not fit the hypothesis are held in reserve. The hypothesis is then tested by guided information seeking, with general questioning to produce more cue information. The last step is an evaluation of the final hypothesis. The hypothesis attempts to resolve the greatest number of cues and patterns.

There are myriad factors that can affect the quality of a radiographic image and these factors can act upon each other to create an astronomical number of possible imaging problems. An image critique system uses the diagnostic problem solving process to critically think through the problem and help resolve the situation.

IDENTIFYING AN IMAGING PROBLEM

The identification of an imaging problem requires the use of a full range of radiographic expertise. The radiographer must first recall that the purpose of the radiographic image is to provide information about the medical condition of the patient. The information needed may vary greatly, depending on the suspected medical problem and the anatomical region to be examined. For example, alignment of a nail during a hip-pinning operation requires a type of information different from that needed for detection of a small blood vessel constriction during cerebral angiography.

The meaning of the expression "diagnostic quality image" is quite different in these two cases. The hip pinning requires two images at right angles to one another as fast as possible with a major consideration being patient dose. The cerebral angiograph requires maximum visibility of detail and resolution from a high-speed exposure with less consideration of patient dose. Any definition of a diagnostic quality image must consider the clinical situation while providing a good balance between visibility of detail (density and contrast) and the geometry of the image (recorded detail or distortion).

The primary problem encountered by radiographers in successfully critiquing images is the tendency to glance at images instead of critically evaluating them for image quality. The professional approaches each image as a window in the diagnostic process.

In her introductory text for radiologists, *Fundamentals of Radiology*, Dr. Lucy Frank Squire emphasizes to aspiring radiologists that, "While the single-glance approach has its value, it is full of danger to the patient, because the presence of a very obvious abnormality tends to suppress psychologically your search for more subtle changes." She suggests that students utilize a systematic approach to evaluating images, primarily by looking at various structures in a deliberate order, concentrating on each structure while excluding the superimposed shadows of other structures. Radiographers should adopt an identical process by looking at each technical and procedural factor in a systematic fashion before jumping to any "glancing" conclusions.

AN EFFECTIVE IMAGE CRITIQUE METHOD

An effective image critique method is a three-step process involving:

1. **the classification of the image,**
2. **the determination of the cause of the problem and**
3. **the recommendation of corrective action** (Figure 32-1).

This approach is designed to provide the radiographer with an organized and systematic protocol for critiquing an image. When consistently used, the system will be found to be a thorough and dependable method for establishing and maintaining professional skills at the very highest level of competence. The form in Figure 32-2 illustrates the application of this image critique method.

Classification of the Image

The first step in classifying the image is to evaluate it to determine if it is within the diagnostic acceptance limits. If the image is within the acceptance limits it should be critically examined to determine if it is of **optimal** diagnostic quality. If it is satisfactory in every respect, the pride of professional competence is the radiographer's reward. If the image is within acceptance limits but not of optimal diagnostic quality, the radiographer should continue the critique to refine his or her technical skills. Although the image may be submitted for diagnosis, a continued critique provides an opportunity to improve the quality of care for future patients.

If the image is outside the acceptance limits, a continued critique is mandatory prior to attempting to repeat the exposure. Failure to continue the critique is ethically unacceptable for a radiographer because it subjects the patient to additional radiation exposure without ascertaining how to produce an acceptable image.

Determination of the Cause of the Problem

The actual diagnostic problem solving begins with determination of the cause of the unacceptable or suboptimal image. In most instances there is more than one cause and this can complicate the problem-solving process immensely. Searching for cues or patterns is primarily a matter of clinical experience. It is best to slowly narrow the search process by first trying to classify the problem into one of three major categories:

1. **a technical factor problem,**
2. **a procedural factor problem or**
3. **an equipment malfunction problem.**

All of these categories are then further subdivided in an effort to determine the exact cause of the problem.

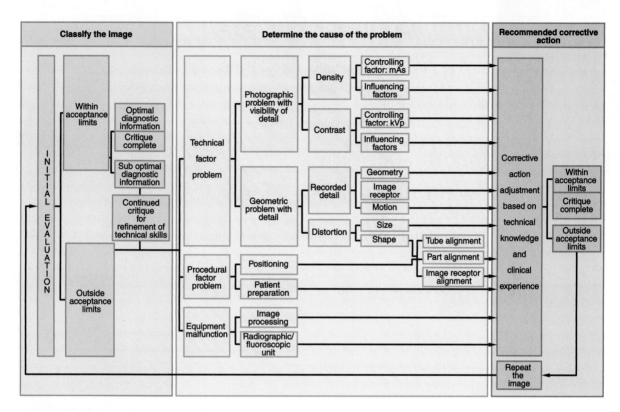

FIGURE 32-1   An effective image critique method.

Technical Factor Problems. Technical factor problems can be arranged into two categories: **a photographic problem with visibility of detail or a geometric problem with detail.** (Of course, some images will have problems with both visibility of detail and detail.) The photographic problems concern maintaining sufficient density and contrast to make the detail of the image visible. Even with good detail present, anatomical structures cannot be visualized unless appropriate density and contrast are also present. An image that appears totally black may still possess good detail; it is simply beyond the ability of the human eye to discern it. Geometric problems directly concern the production of detail (also called definition, sharpness, and resolution). (See Figure 27-6 Image Analysis Phase)

Photographic problems with visibility of detail are further classified as **density** or **contrast** problems. Density problems may be the result of the mAs selection and/or a variety of other influencing fac-

tors, including the image receptor, the selected kVp level, distance, grid selection, beam restriction, a pathology problem, etc. Contrast problems are the result of the kVp selection and/or a variety of influencing factors, including field size, patient thickness, grid selection, etc.

Geometric problems with detail are further classified as **recorded detail** or **distortion** problems. Recorded detail problems are the result of the geometry of the beam (focal spot size, SID, or OID), the image receptor, and/or patient motion. Distortion is further classified as size distortion (magnification) or shape distortion. Size distortion problems are the result of SID or OID. Shape distortion problems are the result of improper tube, part and/or image receptor alignment.

Procedural Factor Problems. A procedural factor problem can be classified as one that involves **patient positioning** or **patient preparation** for

IMAGE CRITIQUE FORM

I. **CLASSIFY THE RADIOGRAPHIC IMAGE AS:**
☐ **WITHIN ACCEPTANCE LIMITS**
  ☐ Optimal diagnostic information (critique is complete)
  (all checkmarks below this line require completion of section II and III)
  ☐ Suboptimal diagnostic information
☐ **OUTSIDE ACCEPTANCE LIMITS**

II. **DETERMINE THE CAUSE OF THE PROBLEM AS:**
☐ A: **Technical Factors**
  ☐ Photographic problem with visibility of detail
    ☐ Density
      ☐ mAs_____
      ☐ Influencing factor (specify) _____
    ☐ Contrast
      ☐ kVp _____
      ☐ Influencing factor (specify) _____
  ☐ Geometric problem with detail
    ☐ Recorded detail
      ☐ Geometry (specify) _____
      ☐ Image Receptor _____
      ☐ Motion _____
    ☐ Distortion
      ☐ Size (Magnification) (specify)_____
      ☐ Shape (Part/Image Receptor/Tube Alignment) (specify) _____
☐ B: **Procedural Factors**
  ☐ Patient Positioning
    ☐ Tube Alignment _____
    ☐ Part Alignment _____
    ☐ Image Receptor Alignment _____
  ☐ Patient Preparation (specify) _____
☐ C: **Equipment Malfunction**
  ☐ Processing Equipment (specify) _____
  ☐ Radiographic/Fluoroscopic Equipment (specify) _____

III. **RECOMMENDED CORRECTIVE ACTION** For each cause specified above:
_____
_____
_____

FIGURE 32-2 Form used for image critique.

the x-ray examination. Proper patient positioning results when the part, the image receptor, and the tube (central ray) are correctly aligned with one another. The result is an image which demonstrates the anatomical structures of interest from the proper perspective. Of course, a thorough knowledge of the anatomy being visualized for a given radiographic procedure is essential to determine if the positioning is accurate. When studying an image for accuracy in positioning, three alignment factors should be reviewed separately:

1. the tube alignment,
2. the part alignment and
3. the image receptor alignment.

The second procedural factor problem involves preparation of the patient for the examination. Proper patient preparation includes removing radiopaque objects from the area of interest (e.g., jewelry, safety pins, etc.), proper bowel cleansing for a gastrointestinal study, recording a thorough history, communicating clear instructions to the patient, etc.

Equipment Malfunction. The last major category in the classification of the causes of an imaging problem is equipment malfunction. While the technical and procedural factors may have been correctly determined, a problem can still result when the equipment being used for the examination does not function properly. Problems normally occur with the processing equipment or with the radiographic/fluoroscopic equipment. These problems can be kept to a minimum through an effective quality control program.

Recommendation of Corrective Action

Each identified cause requires an appropriate corrective action that will resolve the problem. Corrective action adjustments are based on knowledge and clinical experience. Clinical experience is gained through careful attention to problems and successes. Remember that clinical knowledge is gained by critiquing acceptable but suboptimal images, analyzing repeated images, and recording successful results.

It is recommended that radiographers purchase or make a personal technique system booklet that can be easily carried while performing clinical examinations. This booklet should record appropriate technical factors, including the specific tube used (by room number or location), kVp, mAs, distance, grid, the relative speed of the film/screen combination (if applicable), anatomical projection, part thickness, and any other variable factors (adjustable filtration, focal spot size, etc.). By using a personal technique system booklet, the radiographer has a quick reference for establishing the technical and procedural factors for a specific examination. Additionally, this guide can be useful for determining accurate adjustments in order to correct a problem.

APPLYING THE IMAGE CRITIQUE METHOD

Figure 32-3 illustrates how to use the image critique method that has been outlined. The radiograph in Figure 32-3A is classified as an image which is outside the acceptance limits of image quality. To determine the cause of this problem, the entire image should be studied for technical and procedural accuracy as well as for potential equipment malfunction problems.

From this review, it is determined that the image exhibits a technical factor problem and a procedural problem but no apparent equipment problem. Further searching narrows the technical factor problem to a photographic problem of visibility of detail and the procedural problem to patient positioning. This narrowing is based on observations that the image is overexposed and that not all of the anatomical structures of interest are demonstrated on the image. These two cues narrow the search by eliminating geometric problems of detail, patient preparation, and equipment malfunction as probable causes. Once suspected problem areas are defined, the cues and patterns should be used to form a hypothesis about the probable cause of the problem.

A

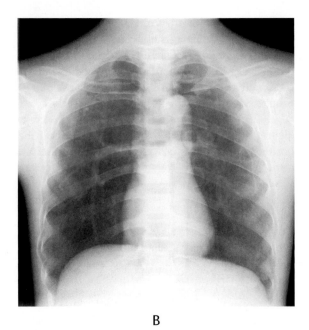

B

FIGURE 32-3 (A) Original radiograph. (B) Repeated radiograph.

The photographic problem of visibility of detail can be further narrowed to an exposure problem. The possible causes of excessive exposure are then reviewed to determine the most likely cause. Although too much mAs is the most common cause, a number of secondary factors, such as the film/screen combination, the grid selection and the kVp level, need to be considered and checked to test the hypothesis. This is a necessary part of evaluating the hypothesis.

Next, the procedural problem should be reviewed to determine the most likely cause. The problem is first narrowed to a patient positioning problem and then to an alignment problem.

The possible causes of alignment problems should then be reviewed to determine the most likely cause. Careful review of the image reveals that the central ray was not correctly aligned to the center of the image receptor. Because of this improper central ray alignment, some of the anatomical structures of interest (the lower lungs and costophrenic angles) are not visualized.

The final step is recommending corrective action. In the example, the corrective action involves changes in technical factor selection and patient positioning. The mAs is reduced by one-half the original amount to correct the density problem and the central ray is properly aligned to the midline of the image receptor. Figure 32-3B illustrates the result after these adjustments were made.

A thorough understanding of the concepts involved in producing an acceptable diagnostic quality image is important. Because of the large number of variables in the imaging process, acceptable images will not always result from the initial exposure. Even the best of radiographers will be required to repeat images because of the vast number of variables. By applying a systematic image critique method, radiographers are practicing one of the most complex skills of the profession. This analytical and effective image critique method will help to ensure the best possible patient care by minimizing the need to repeat an exposure.

SUMMARY

Critiquing an image is a very complex process which requires a thorough knowledge of all aspects of radiography. Deciding if an image is acceptable or unacceptable should be approached in a logical, organized manner. Image critiquing is an analytical process that involves many of the steps involved in diagnostic decision making, including critical problem solving.

To determine whether an image is of diagnostic quality, the steps of an analytical decision-making process must be followed.

The process begins with a review of the entire image to avoid premature narrowing. When differences are noticed, a pattern is sought, especially when there is more than one cue. Cues and patterns focus attention on a suspicious area, thus narrowing the search. Cues and patterns are then used to seek hypotheses. An effort is made to formulate a hypothesis that will explain all the cues. The hypothesis is then tested by guided information seeking, with general questioning to produce more cue information. The last step is an evaluation of the final hypothesis. The hypothesis attempts to resolve the greatest number of cues and patterns.

An effective image critique method is a three-step process involving: (1) the classification of the image; (2) the determination of the cause of the problem; and (3) the recommendation of corrective action.

In the first step, the image is classified to determine if it is within the diagnostic acceptance limits. If the image is within acceptance limits but not of optimal diagnostic quality, the radiographer should continue the critique to refine his or her technical skills. If the image is outside the acceptance limits, a continued critique is mandatory prior to attempting to repeat the exposure.

The actual diagnostic problem solving begins with determination of the cause of the unacceptable or suboptimal image. Searching for cues or patterns is primarily a matter of clinical experience. It is best to slowly narrow the search process by first trying to classify the problem into one of three major categories: (1) a technical factor problem; (2) a procedural factor problem; or (3) an equipment malfunction problem.

Each identified cause requires an appropriate corrective action that will resolve the problem. Corrective action adjustments are based on knowledge and clinical experience. Clinical experience is gained through careful attention to problems and successes.

Even the best of radiographers will be required to repeat images. Using an effective image critique method will help to ensure the best possible patient care by minimizing the need to repeat an exposure.

REVIEW QUESTIONS

1. What is the purpose of image critique?

2. During the analytical process of critiquing a radiograph, how are cues and patterns used?

3. What are the three steps in an effective image critique method?

4. What are the three classifications of imaging problems?

5. What are the two categories of technical factor problems?

6. A necklace is seen on a chest radiograph. What type of imaging problem would this be?

7. A film is jammed in the processor and destroyed. What type of imaging problem would this be?

8. How does a radiographer determine the appropriate corrective action for an imaging problem?

REFERENCES AND RECOMMENDED READING

Adler, A. M., & Carlton, R. R. (1989). Repeating radiographs: Critiquing the image. *Postgraduate Advances in Radiologic Technology.* Berryville, VA: Forum Medicum.

Adler, A. M., & Carlton, R. R. (1990). Perceiving the radiographic image. *Postgraduate Advances in Radiologic Technology.* (Eugene Frank, ed.) Berryville, VA: Forum Medicum.

Carlton, R. R., (1992). Another dimension of quality assurance in radiology. In L. T. Gurley, & W. J. Callaway (Eds.), *Introduction to Radiologic Technology* (3rd ed., pp. 149–166). St. Louis, MO: C. V. Mosby.

Carlton, R. R., & McKenna, A. (1989). Repeating radiographs: Setting imaging standards. *Postgraduate Advances in Radiologic Technology.* Berryville, VA: Forum Medicum.

Carnevali, D. L., Mitchell, P. H., Woods, N. F., & Tanner, C. A. (1984). *Diagnostic reasoning in nursing.* Philadelphia: J. B. Lippincott.

Cullinan, A., & Cullinan, J. (1994). *Producing quality radiographs* (2nd ed.). Philadelphia: J. B. Lippincott.

Cullinan, J. E. (1981). A 'perfect' chest radiograph—or a compromise? *Radiologic Technology, 53*(2), 121.

Dowd, S. B. (1995). *Encyclopedia of radiographic positioning.* Philadelphia: W. B. Saunders.

Goldman, L. W. (1977). Effects of film processing variability on patient dose and image quality. *Second Image Receptor Conference: Radiographic Film Processing: Proceedings of a Conference held in Washington, DC, March 31–April 2, 1977* (HEW Publication [FDA] 77-8036, 55–63). Rockville, MD: U.S. Department of Health, Education, and Welfare, Public Health Service, Food and Drug Administration, Bureau of Radiological Health.

Hiss, S. S. (2003). *Understanding radiography* (4th ed.). Springfield, IL: Charles C Thomas.

Jerman, E. C. (1926). An analysis of the end-result: The radiograph. *Radiology, 6,* 59–62.

Lauer, O. G., Mayes, J. B., & Thurston, R. P. (1990). *Evaluating radiographic quality: The variables and their effects.* Mankato, MN: The Burnell Company.

Novelline, R. A. (1997). *Squire's Fundamentals of radiology* (6th ed.). Cambridge: Harvard University Press.

Singer, B. H. (1971). The aesthetic method in radiographic exposure. *Radiologic Technology, 42*(6), 411.

CHAPTER 33

Quality Management

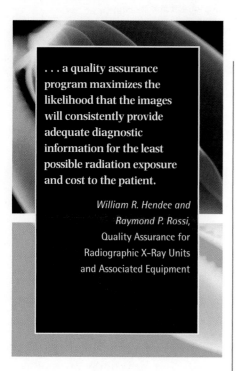

> . . . a quality assurance program maximizes the likelihood that the images will consistently provide adequate diagnostic information for the least possible radiation exposure and cost to the patient.
>
> *William R. Hendee and*
> *Raymond P. Rossi,*
> Quality Assurance for
> Radiographic X-Ray Units
> and Associated Equipment

KEY TERMS

external beam
   evaluation
film processing
   system
quality assurance
quality control
total repeat rate

OBJECTIVES

Upon completion of this chapter, the student should be able to:

- Define quality assurance and quality control and discuss their relationship to excellence in radiography.
- Describe the process of identifying imaging requirements, developing equipment specifications, selecting equipment, installing and testing equipment, and training the technical staff.
- Describe the objectives and responsibilities of monitoring equipment performance.
- Discuss primary automatic film processor quality control monitoring and maintenance procedures.

- Discuss primary quality control tests for external radiation beam monitoring of diagnostic radiographic systems, fluoroscopic systems, tomographic systems, and automatic exposure controls.
- List primary quality control tests for miscellaneous ancillary equipment, including cassettes and view boxes.
- Explain the rationale behind the data collection process and the basic analysis of a radiographic repeat-rate study.
- Describe a basic troubleshooting procedure.

QUALITY ASSURANCE AND QUALITY CONTROL

Regulation and Accreditation

In the United States, the federal government initiated radiologic and imaging sciences quality management regulations after the Radiation Control and Safety Act of 1968. The 1981 Consumer-Patient Radiation Health and Safety Act added considerably to the scope of this effort as did the 1990 Safe Medical Devices Act (SMDA) and the 1992 Mammography Quality Standards Act (MQSA). Today these acts and others relating to radiologic and imaging sciences are developed and enforced by the Center for Devices and Radiological Health (CDRH), which is part of the Food and Drug Administration (FDA) under the Department of Health and Human Services (HHS).

Of the acts currently in place, the SMDA and MQSA have had the greatest impact on the practice of the radiologic and imaging sciences. SMDA mandates that any serious injury or death due to a medical device be reported. MQSA requires mammography facilities to be approved by the FDA.

There are also voluntary accreditation procedures available and they are used by the vast majority of hospitals in the United States. The largest hospital accreditation agency is the Joint Commission on the Accreditation of Healthcare Organizations (JCAHO). Their approval is linked to many medical activities, most importantly to reimbursement by the federal and state governments and many insurance companies. Accreditation agencies establish quality standards, assess them, and provide certification that individual institutions have met the agency's standards.

Although there are numerous quality measurement consultants, books, and process methods, one is worthy of remembering in all medical settings. The Hospital Corporation of America's FOCUS-PDCA method has gained great acceptance. It functions as shown in Table 33-1.

Quality management consists of a coherent system designed to monitor equipment performance

TABLE 33-1. FOCUS-PDCA Method
Find and define a problem.
Organize a team to work on improvement.
Clarify the problem with current knowledge.
Understand the problem and its causes.
Select a method to improve the process.
Plan implementation.
Do the implementation and measure change.
Check the results.
Act to continue improvements.

through a variety of quality assurance and quality control standards or benchmarks.

Quality Assurance

Quality assurance consists of activities that provide adequate confidence that a radiology service will render consistently high-quality images and services. It is an evolutionary process that assesses everything that affects patient care. It may be medically, technically or managerially oriented. Quality assurance includes evaluating activities such as interpretation of examinations, maintenance of equipment, performance of procedures, filing systems, staff development, scheduling of examinations, and supply lines.

The quality assurance process operates by identifying problems or potential problem areas, monitoring the problem, and then resolving it. Monitoring problems involves several steps, including establishing criteria, performing monitoring, and collecting, analyzing, and evaluating data. It is these steps of the monitoring process that are of greatest concern to the quality assurance radiographer.

Quality Control

Quality control is the aspect of quality assurance that monitors technical equipment to maintain quality standards. The concept of quality control is rooted in the need to stabilize the various equipment components of the radiographic imaging chain. From incoming line current through x-ray production to the processing of the radiograph, erratic equipment performance causes repeat radiographs and unnecessary patient exposure to radiation. The term *quality control* is sometimes used to describe the evaluation of individual radiographs according to acceptance limits standards. It is probably better to think of this image evaluation process as image critiquing or quality checking rather than quality control, although the quality control process is certainly a critical part of the critique evaluation.

Technical expertise will not ensure success in radiography unless the equipment is reliable. Because radiographic equipment changes as it ages, there are often great differences between the results obtained on one unit and those obtained on another. The same unit cannot be counted on to produce exactly the same beam for the radiographer to control and analyze unless it is properly checked on a regular basis. The system of checks to accomplish a measure of consistency in beam output is the quality control.

Ensuring the quality of the radiographic image is a prime responsibility of the radiologic technologist. Every patient expects to receive the highest possible quality, or excellence, of service, from a medical facility. No one wants to be exposed to ionizing radiation by a radiographer incapable of producing excellent images.

It is important that quality control be seen as a method of controlling the radiographic image from start to finish. To do this requires a series of procedures (Figure 33-1). Unfortunately, some quality control begins with the last step instead of the first. An effective program cannot be achieved simply by monitoring equipment performance, although this is unquestionably the most involved step. The thought process preceding equipment purchase is critical.

PURCHASING EQUIPMENT

Identification of Imaging Requirements

It is not always apparent exactly what type of equipment is needed when new purchases are being considered. Historically, this decision was made by the chief radiologist or administrative technologist.

FIGURE 33-1   A total quality control system. *(Adapted from W. R. Hendee and R. P. Rossi, Quality Assurance for Radiographic X-Ray Units and Associated Equipment. (HEW Publication FDA 79-8094, 1979), Rockville, MD: U.S. DHEW, PHS, FDA, Bureau of Radiological Health)*

Rarely are the actual operators of the equipment, the radiographers, consulted. The result has been that nearly every x-ray department owns a radiological monstrosity that is avoided by radiographers and radiologists alike. These units are often inconvenient, overly sophisticated, or unable to produce quality images. Careful identification of imaging requirements can prevent these problems.

It is not necessary to be an expert in imaging physics and technology in order to be capable of contributing to the process of identifying the imaging requirements. Each member of the radiological team can contribute his or her expertise. The person who will make the final decision should interview the radiologists, administrators, supervisors, and staff technologists who will use the equipment. In many instances the needs of the radiologist will determine the basic parameters for the purchase. Administrators must often impose financial and space restraints, although they can also create new funds and space when necessary. Supervisors are often able to provide important information on patient flow and staffing needs. After the radiologists, the radiographers are the most important persons to have input because their experiences with equipment provide a wealth of information.

Development of Equipment Specifications

Generic equipment specifications should be developed from the interview information. It is important that the person formulating the specifications have the technical background to state exactly what is needed to meet the imaging requirements. An imaging physicist should be involved at this point. The best specifications include detailed statements of what the equipment should be capable of doing. For example, "Maintain mA linearity within ± 10 percent to produce a consistent exposure when mAs is maintained but mA is varied." This must include a change from highest to lowest setting. When the specifications are complete they are sent to vendors for bidding.

Selection of Equipment

The actual selection of equipment becomes simple if the investigation into the first two steps has been thorough. When the bids arrive they can be compared for meeting specifications, cost, and service. The actual decision is then academic. A pitfall in the process can occur when radiologists in the institution show a preference to a particular vendor, thus weakening the bargaining position of the department administrator. In many institutions this pitfall should be expanded to include interference by administrative officers unfamiliar with imaging equipment.

Installation and Acceptance Testing of Equipment

Installation and acceptance testing of equipment is the responsibility of the vendor and/or manufacturer. The quality control technologist must verify

that the equipment specifications have been met. Normally this includes supervising the testing procedures and results. It is suggested that the exact methods for acceptance testing be included in the original specifications. The data from these tests will form the standard for all future quality control monitoring.

Continuing Education

It is normally the responsibility of the vendor to familiarize the users of the equipment with its proper operation. With simple equipment, such as ancillary devices, the equipment manual may be sufficient for use in in-service training. More complex equipment should be demonstrated and explained by the vendor **to at least two persons** as part of the purchase contract. Continuing education **must** be an ongoing procedure. It is advisable to include both the quality control and in-service education coordinators in the initial training demonstrations. A good in-service program will include an orientation procedure as well as periodic updates on all complex equipment.

MONITORING EQUIPMENT PERFORMANCE

The final procedure of a total program is commonly considered to be the whole of quality control. Monitoring equipment performance includes routine checks of all radiographic equipment. Although they are interdependent, monitoring can be divided into two parts: (1) **film processing systems** and (2) **external beam evaluation.** Objectives for a performance monitoring system are to:

1. monitor the quality of the image processing systems,

2. measure the quality of the external radiation beams and

3. specify faults within these systems to allow corrective measures to be taken.

Evidence shows that a properly working quality control system will reduce equipment downtime and the number of repeated exposures. This will also reduce patient dose, patient waiting time, and supply costs, as well as increase confidence in diagnostic consultation and boost departmental morale.

Responsibility

Professional service personnel or medical physicists are not required to perform routine quality control procedures. Many procedures must be done daily, and to use these experts would be too costly. Radiographers, who are more available and knowledgeable about potential problems, should do the equipment monitoring. An initial cost outlay for testing equipment is required. To maintain a program, staff technologists must be given time to perform the procedures and to evaluate them.

Processor Monitoring

Processor monitoring is designed to permit an automatic film processor to fluctuate within set limits. These tests may be performed by anyone who has been oriented to the use of the equipment involved. Only a radiographer or processor maintenance person should perform the corrective actions.

Action must be taken to correct problems whenever the limits are exceeded. A quality control program that is not backed up by a commitment to shut down processors that are outside limits is of little value. Manufacturers' suggestions should be followed for the start-up and for the regular maintenance of the processor.

There are also several monitoring tests that should be done on a daily basis. These include a darkroom fog test, also known as a safelight test, and processor sensitometry to monitor speed, contrast, and base fog of film. See Chapters 19, 20, and 21 for details.

External Beam Evaluation

The second part of performance monitoring involves the evaluation of the external primary radiation beam. These tests must be performed by a radiographer who has a knowledge of the physical operation of the equipment and all related accessories. Corrective action should be taken only by an authorized service person.

FIGURE 33-2 Radiographic quality control equipment. Clockwise from upper left: wire mesh film/screen contact tool, collimator accuracy tool, pinhole focal spot camera, digital dosimeter with computer, synchronous spinning top and penetrometer tool, and kVp test cassette with star pattern focal spot tool. In center: noninvasive beam evaluator (NERO™ computerized unit with ionization chamber) and resolution pattern focal spot test tool.

Some monitoring equipment can be made very inexpensively; other equipment must be purchased. A dosimeter is an essential piece of equipment, and reasonable quality control cannot be performed without one. Computerized dosimeters are available that permit readouts and printouts of many quality control parameters from a single exposure. Figure 33-2 illustrates common quality control equipment. A room log should be kept to record test results, maintenance, and repairs performed on each x-ray tube and other system in each room.

Diagnostic Radiographic Systems. The tests that should be performed on diagnostic radiographic systems should be done on a **semiannual** schedule. The tests for x-ray tubes should include:

Focal spot size estimation. An estimate of focal spot size is important so that it is kept within acceptable limits to ensure proper image detail. There are three types of focal spot test tools: line pair resolution tools, star test patterns, and pinhole cameras. Both line pair resolution tools and star test patterns

2.0 mm   1.0 mm   1.0 mm

FIGURE 33-3 Focal spot images produced on dental x-ray film with a pinhole camera. *(Courtesy of J. E. Gray and M. Trefler, Pinhole cameras: Artifacts, modifications, and recording of pinhole images on screen film systems.* Radiologic Technology *52:3, 277-282, 1980 by permission of the American Society of Radiologic Technologists from* Quality Control in Diagnostic Imaging, *Aspen Publishers, Inc., Rockville, MD, 1983 by permission of the Mayo Foundation for Medical Education and Research)*

function by imaging a resolution pattern on a film. The image can then be analyzed to estimate the focal spot size. A pinhole camera permits measurement of the focal spot by creating an image of the effective focal spot on a film (Figure 33-3).

The National Electrical Manufacturers Association (NEMA) specifies that focal spots of 0.3 mm and smaller may be measured with a star test pattern. Focal spots larger than 0.3 mm should be measured with a pinhole camera. In clinical quality control assurance testing a pinhole camera is avoided because it is difficult to use accurately and requires massive tube loading. A star test pattern will satisfactorily monitor focal spot size growth in most instances. When the focal spot grows to an unacceptable size, the x-ray tube must be replaced. NEMA specifies that focal spots smaller than 0.8 mm may be 50 percent larger than the stated nominal size. Focal spots between 0.8 mm and 1.5 mm may be 40 percent larger than nominal, and focal spots larger than 1.5 mm may be 30 percent larger than nominal. For example, a 0.5 mm focal spot may actually be 0.75 mm and still be considered acceptable.

Half-value layer. The amount of total filtration in the primary beam is important for both radiation protection and image quality. Radiation protection is ensured by eliminating low-energy photons that are incapable of reaching the image receptor. Image quality is ensured by making appropriate contrast adjustments. Half-value layers are measured by us-

ing dosimetry equipment to detect the quality of aluminum filtration that will reduce the beam intensity to half the original value. Computerized quality control dosimeters provide a digital readout of the half-value layer. Half-value layer recommendations or requirements vary depending on the kVp. If insufficient filtration is present, the tube housing must be modified to supply additional aluminum filtration.

Collimator, central ray, and Bucky tray accuracy. The congruence of the projected centering light field and the central ray with the actual collimated primary x-ray beam and Bucky tray is of critical importance for radiation protection. Radiation protection is ensured by avoiding repeated images due to over-collimation errors and by avoiding irradiation of tissue unless it will be imaged. A collimator test tool is simply a lead marker for each corner of the light beam plus crosshairs or a lead marker, placed several centimeters above the cassette surface, for the central ray. A 2 percent SID error is allowed between the primary-beam image and the light field size (this is a U.S. federal standard). The centering mark should be within 1 percent of the light field central ray. The positive beam limitation (PBL) mechanism should not permit the primary beam to be larger than the cassette in the Bucky tray unless the override lock is activated. When these margins of error are exceeded, the collimator light or PBL mechanism must be adjusted.

Distance and centering indicators' accuracy. Many older x-ray units have inaccurate distance indicators located on tube support stands or overhead readouts. In addition, both distance and centering locks, stops, and detents may not be accurate. Assurance that distance and centering are accurate avoids the need for repeated exposures due to the inverse square law, misalignment of the central ray, and primary beam collimation. Distance indicators should be checked with a tape measure (point zero should be measured from the focal spot, which is approximately 1 cm from the bottom of the tube housing end cap). Centering indicators can be checked by visual inspection of the collimator light beam (assuming a collimator and central ray accuracy test has been done). Distance indicators should be ±10 percent, and centering indicators should be ±2 percent. If the indicators are not within these limits they should be adjusted.

Angulator or protractor accuracy. X-ray tables, Bucky units, and tubes with angulators or protractors must provide accurate readings for positioning baselines. They can be evaluated by using a large protractor for angle measurements and a level to verify that locks, stops, and detents are set to establish horizontal and perpendicular surfaces. Angles should be ± 1 percent, with adjustments made when necessary.

The tests for x-ray generators should include:

Kilovoltage accuracy. Kilovoltage settings tend to drift over time, primarily as a result of tube aging. Their accuracy is essential in maintaining image quality. The scale of contrast and density cannot be predicted unless the kVp is accurate. Verification and calibration of the kVp ensure that technique exposure charts will produce diagnostic quality images. Computerized dosimeters provide digital readouts or printouts of average and single-pulse kVp. If the settings drift beyond the ± 5 kVp of the labeled setting, the generator must be recalibrated.

Timer accuracy. Exposure time settings also tend to drift over time. Their accuracy is essential in maintaining image quality because exposure cannot be predicted unless the time is accurate. Verification and calibration of the timer ensure that technique exposure charts will produce diagnostic quality images. Computerized dosimeters provide digital readouts or printouts of the exposure time, or a spinning top may be used to measure 1ϕ generators and a motorized synchronous top may be used for 3ϕ units. The tops are less accurate, more time-consuming, and difficult to use. Exposure time settings should be maintained within ± 5 percent of the label. If the settings drift beyond this limit, the timing circuit or mechanism must be recalibrated.

mR/mAs and milliamperage linearity. Milliamperage settings also tend to drift over time, primarily as a result of tube aging. Their accuracy is essential to maintaining image quality because exposure cannot be predicted unless the mA is accurate. Assurance is needed that technique exposure charts will accurately produce diagnostic quality images. Milliamperage cannot be measured by noninvasive quality control methods. Consequently, mA station accuracy must be inferred by comparing mR/mAs measurements after both time and kVp accuracy have been verified. Comparative measurements are made for the same mAs at different mA and time settings to evaluate the linearity of the mA stations. Computerized dosimeters provide digital readouts or printouts of mR/mAs. Milliamperage stations should be maintained within ± 10 percent of each other, but some sources recommend maintaining the entire generator within ± 10 percent. If the settings drift beyond the established limit, the generator must be recalibrated.

Exposure reproducibility. Generators must be capable of repeating exposures accurately. This is ensured by measuring the mR/mAs of several different exposures with the same technical factors. Computerized dosimeters provide digital readouts or printouts of mR/mAs. Reproducibility should be maintained within ± 5 percent. If the readings are beyond this limit, the entire series of tube and generator tests should be analyzed to attempt to isolate the problem.

Specialized radiographic systems, such as fluoroscopy, tomography, and automatic exposure controls, require additional tests.

Fluoroscopic Systems. The tests for fluoroscopic systems should include:

Exposure reproducibility. Fluoroscopic spot film devices use automatic exposure controls (AECs) and they should be evaluated according to the AEC tests below.

Exposure rate. Fluoroscopic exposure rates are measured by a dosimeter exactly as diagnostic mR/mAs. The exposure rate should not exceed 5 R/min. If the rate exceeds this limit, the automatic brightness control or other systems may require calibration or repair.

Field size accuracy and beam alignment. As with collimation accuracy in diagnostic radiography, fluoroscopic units should not be capable of irradiating tissue outside the image receptor area. In addition to the evaluation performed for a diagnostic unit, fluoroscopic units should display everything within 1 cm of the edges of the image intensifier tube, and the primary beam should be aligned to the center of the image intensifier. Correction of the tube collimation, image intensification system, or video display system may be required (further testing by a service engineer is necessary).

Source-to-skin distance limits. Fluoroscopic units should not be capable of placing the tube target closer than 15″ (38 cm) (or 12″ [30 cm] for a mobile fluoroscopy unit) to the patient's skin surface (this is a U.S. federal requirement). Without making any exposure, the source-to-image receptor distance should be verified. If it is not within limits, the unit should not be used until a mechanical device is fitted to set a minimum source-to-skin distance.

Intensifier viewing system resolution. Because fluoroscopic resolution is much poorer than radiographic resolution, periodic assurance that it has not deteriorated is critical in maintaining confidence in diagnosis. A fluoroscopic mesh test tool or a resolution pattern test tool can be imaged to permit visualization of the maximum resolving ability of the system. If the resolution appears to be deteriorating, a service engineer should be consulted.

Intensifier viewing system contrast. Because fluoroscopic contrast is much higher than radiographic contrast, it is important to periodically determine approximately how low contrast a structure may be imaged. Special low contrast fluoroscopic test tools are available that consist of two plates of aluminum with holes of 1–7 mm drilled in one of the plates. When the plates are sandwiched together and imaged on a fluoroscopy system, low contrast evaluation can be made based on the smallest visible hole.

TV monitors and recorders. The vast majority of modern fluoroscopic systems use video systems for image display because of the reduction in patient dose. Although a video signal generator is the test tool of choice, its expense and limited application in radiography usually prohibit its use for routine testing. A fluoroscopic mesh test tool or a resolution test tool and a piece of wire mesh are more commonly used. The resolution test tool can be imaged on the fluoroscopy unit to permit visual measurement of the system resolution. The wire mesh can be imaged to permit visualization of distortion (Figure 33-4). When degradation in resolution or distortion is observed, a service engineer should be consulted.

Automatic brightness control. Although there are a number of types of automatic brightness controls, the term is used here in a generic sense. These controls are designed to function like an AEC

in that variations in subject density are automatically compensated for, resulting in a relatively uniform image density. A computerized dosimeter can be used to measure exposure after the beam passes through a phantom. When the phantom thickness is decreased by half, the exposure should be similarly reduced. If there is a great discrepancy between phantom thickness and exposure reduction, a service engineer should be consulted.

Tomographic Systems. The tests for tomographic systems should include:

Uniformity and completeness of motion. Tomography relies on the motion of the tube during exposure to produce a sectional image of the subject. Assurance of the uniformity and completeness of tube motion are basic tests. The test tool is simply a lead mask with a pinhole that is positioned several centimeters above the tomographic fulcrum. If the pinhole is centered to the image receptor and then imaged with a full tomographic motion, images similar to Figure 33-5 may be obtained. Erratic tube motion is demonstrated by the uneven densities. If the motion were incomplete, there would not be a full length of the tracing. If the motion is erratic or incomplete, the mechanisms involved in the tomographic motion should be cleaned (rails, guide-

FIGURE 33-5 Tomographic uniformity and completeness of motion test with a pinhole trace image. Both exposures were erratic, as demonstrated by the uneven densities along the entire pinhole exposure. *(By permission of Mayo Foundation for Medical Education and Research. All rights reserved)*

wheels, etc.) and the test repeated. If the problem continues, a service engineer should be consulted.

Section depth indicator accuracy. Tomographic units are designed to provide an image that is sharp (possessing good detail) only at the fulcrum level. Assurance that the fulcrum indicator is accurate is essential in diagnosing the location of structures within the subject. Commercial test tools are available or a penetrometer with lead numbered steps can be used. When a tomographic image is made of the test tool, the number that was at the level of the fulcrum should appear sharp. If it does not, the fulcrum indicator should be adjusted to the appropriate level. Additional testing may be required to ascertain the proper adjustment.

Section thickness accuracy. The sharp section of a tomograph should be of a known thickness, depending on the total arc of the tomographic motion (exact section thickness per arc is usually stated in the equipment manual). Commercial test tools are available or an angled wire mesh can be used. When the angled resolution mesh is imaged, the section thickness can be determined by measuring the region of sharpness on the image. If the section thickness is inaccurate, the pinhole trace

should be consulted. If it appears unacceptable, a service engineer should be consulted.

Resolution. Tomographic resolution is determined by imaging a resolution test pattern at the fulcrum level. The resulting image can be visually inspected to determine the resolving capability of the system. When resolution deteriorates, standard diagnostic quality control measures should be consulted first, then a service engineer.

Automatic Exposure Controls. The tests for automatic exposure controls (AECs) should include:

Exposure reproducibility. The same reproducibility standards for diagnostic radiography systems are applied to AECs. Using the same procedure, with the addition of a subject phantom, densitometer readings of images produced with the AEC should be within OD ±0.1 in the same areas. Reproducibility cannot be achieved on an AEC with dosimeter mR/mAs readings. Radiographs must be produced and measured with a densitometer. If the readings are not within limits, the generator AEC circuits must be calibrated.

Ion chamber sensitivity. Most AECs utilize three ion chambers and permit activation of various combinations during exposures. It is important to ensure that each ion chamber is equally sensitive by comparing the reproducibility of each chamber individually. Exact chamber locations should be verified by producing an image of the ion chambers by using the AEC without a subject at extremely low kVp. After this step is completed, the test is done by using a lead brick to block all chambers but the one to be tested. The AEC reproducibility test is then performed for the unblocked chamber. If all chambers do not respond within ±10 percent, a service engineer should be consulted to recalibrate the generator AEC circuitry.

Density variation control accuracy. Nearly all AEC units provide controls to decrease and increase density by changing the sensitivity of the ion chamber. These controls vary tremendously from one unit to another. Consultation of equipment manuals will provide the percentage of change each control is designed to produce. A computerized dosimeter can then be employed to obtain mR/mAs measurements to verify the intensity differences for each control. If the controls are not accurate, the generator AEC circuits must be calibrated.

Response capability. Each AEC has a minimum response capability (which varies with manufacturer and model). If the AEC cannot respond at the minimum time, there is no assurance that diagnostic quality images can be produced. Response capability is best evaluated by using a computerized dosimeter readout or printout to determine exposure time for AEC exposures made with a small lucite phantom. As the phantom thickness is reduced, the AEC should produce exposures within ±10 percent mR/mAs of one another until a time below the minimum exposure time is used. If the minimum response time is greater than specified, the AEC should not be used until the problem is corrected.

Backup timer verification. Occasionally, even the best radiographers will forget to activate the proper tube or AEC. When this occurs, patient radiation protection requires that AEC backup timers be functioning to terminate exposures and protect both patient and tube. When a lead plate is placed over the AEC ionization chamber and an exposure is made, the backup timer should terminate the exposure and a visual and an audible warning should occur. If the backup timer or signals fail, the AEC should not be used until the problem is corrected.

ANCILLARY EQUIPMENT

Ancillary equipment must also be monitored on a regular basis. This includes cassette cleaning, film/screen contact tests and view boxes and display monitors.

Cassette Cleaning and Inspection

During normal use, radiographic intensifying screens are exposed to dust and other foreign particles as cassettes are opened during loading and unloading of film. Periodic cleaning of the screens with a specially formulated antistatic solution removes these artifacts and eliminates the potential for misdiagnosis. At the time they are cleaned, cassettes should also be inspected for wear at corners, edges, and especially at hinges. When excessive wear is observed, the cassette should be tested to see

if it is lightproof. All cassettes should have a leaded identification number to assist in locating the source of artifacts during use.

Film/Screen Contact

Cassette backs and fronts may warp due to improper storage or traumatic handling. This can lead to loss of contact between the film and the intensifying screen. When poor film-to-screen contact exists, the diverging light photons from the screen cause loss of detail and contrast. A wire mesh test tool should be imaged and the radiograph examined for areas of poor detail. Although rescreening cassettes will replace the pressure pads and sometimes resolve the problem, many institutions prefer to replace the entire cassette.

View Box Uniformity

View boxes, or illuminators, should emit a uniform intensity of light. One of the greatest sources of misunderstanding between radiographers and radiologists is the difference in light intensity of different view boxes because it directly affects the perceived radiographic density. When radiographs consistently exhibit different densities on different view boxes, they become difficult to evaluate. View boxes should be monitored with a light meter periodically to alleviate this problem. View boxes are measured in NITs, the unit of luminance (1 NIT = 1 candela/m^2). Normal view boxes emit around 1,700 NIT, while mammography view boxes should be in the 3,500 NIT range. When inconsistencies are discovered, they should be brought to the attention of all professional staff.

Correction of the problem, when many view boxes are involved, can be expensive because most institutions have collected view boxes of different models and manufacturers over many years. The thickness and translucency of the plastic surface must be identical for all view boxes. Differences in the plastic are the most common cause of illumination problems. Old view boxes may require painting of their reflectors so the exact tone and reflecting ability of the paint matches newer models. Finally, the bulbs of all view boxes must not only be of the same manufacture and model but should be from the same production run. Attempts to solve view box problems should be carried out in the above order.

Display Monitors

Digital imaging display monitors require regular quality assurance to ascertain image quality and to monitor phosphor decay. These factors are sometimes referred to as monitor degradation. Both spatial resolution and optical density/brightness must be evaluated on a regular basis.

Spatial resolution is evaluated through the display of a standardized image the SMPTE test pattern (as shown in Figure 26-1) and a gray scale tool. All three display axis must be evaluated (x, y, and z). The x and y axes are evaluated by imaging spatial resolution test tools to evaluate point spread function (PSF), line spread function (LSF), and modulation transfer function (MTF). This measures the matrix and pixel size accuracy. These factors are discussed in detail in Chapter 30. The z-axis is evaluated through imaging a gray scale performance tool that is often generated form the storage memory of the monitor itself. This measures the gray scale bit depth. As with all quality assurance, the change in results over time is the critical test. Consequently it is important to maintain a log of the test results for each monitor and to use it to predict when calibration and replacement should be scheduled.

Optical density/brightness is evaluated through measurements of dynamic range with a luminance meter in unit of foot-Lamberts (fL) or candela per square meter (cd/M^2). Dynamic range is measured by setting the greatest visible black and white level by using the monitor contrast and brightness controls. Readings from both levels are obtained with a luminance meter. The dynamic range is calculated from the formula:

$$OD = \log (L_{max}/L_{min})$$

The SMPTE test pattern includes a 10 step gray scale that can be used to construct a DlogE curve. This curve can be used to monitor gray scale performance over time. Brightness uniformity is the difference between luminance measurements at the center of the display compared to the corner edges. The brightness uniformity specification is 15%. When a workstation has more than one monitor, the recommendation is that the luminance measurements match within 5%.

PACS SYSTEMS

Because each imaging modality has developed quality assurance measures, the primary quality issue for a PACS system is the accuracy of the interface between the specific modality system and the electronic medical record (EMR) in the Hospital Information System (HIS) and Radiology Information System (RIS). Some experts in PACS Management recommend that data from any system be held in a storage area (sometimes called the fix-queue or penalty box) until it can be matched with the modality, HIS, and RIS data or until human intervention resolves the mismatched data. This avoids problems with incomplete patient information being dumped into the PACS where it adds to unfinished work lists, skews data, and contributes to misfiled patient information. It is also important that a quality check is done on the interface between each element of the PACS system. This should include an item list that is developed with the manufacturer to assure the expectations of the clinical site are being met. One example that is often used is the proper setting for modality autosend switches. These features are designed to permit real-time transmission of images from a modality to the PACS system as the technologist or sonographer completes them. However, service technicians and modality operators may turn them off to increase the speed of the modality functions and may forget to reactivate them so physicians and radiologist assistants have immediate access to the images.

REPEAT IMAGE STUDIES

The careful analysis of repeated images has proven a valuable aid in diagnosing the radiographic process. Repeated radiographs are also referred to as reject, retake, or double-dose studies. Even excellent repeat image studies need take little time or effort to pinpoint conditions that may be easily corrected. Significant reductions in patient dose, radiographer time and effort and supply costs can be achieved with properly executed repeat image studies.

TABLE 33-2. Causes of Repeated Image

Total exposure	55 percent
Underexposure	34 percent
Overexposure	21 percent
Positioning	30 percent
Motion	3 percent

Obtaining Data

A repeat image study involves retaining all repeated radiographs, regardless of cause, for analysis. Any image outside the acceptance limits and scrap film should be included. Boxes labeled as to cause of repeat should be provided near each processor and the room and tube used should be noted on each image before it is discarded. Typical causes of repeats are shown in Table 33-2.

The most important rule when analyzing repeated images is to not discipline radiographers based on the information obtained. The analysis must be used in a constructive manner to improve working conditions and to point out areas where further technical training may be helpful. Radiographers must be informed of the intent of the study and asked to cooperate in a positive manner to improve both patient care and working conditions. Most radiographers are aware of numerous items they believe contribute to repeat radiographs and welcome an opportunity to find justification for their change. Incompetent radiographers should be disciplined through normal administrative procedures based on actual performance, not as a finding of a repeat image study. Failure by management to follow this suggestion may result in inaccurate repeat-study data when images are not submitted for analysis.

Analysis of Data

The analysis of collected data begins with the classification and counting of images by cause of repeat, room, tube, and radiographer. Data should also be separated according to time (weekly is most common). The compiled data should be examined for obvious problems. For example, a large number of

TABLE 33-3. Retake Percentage By Room

	Room #				
Reason	1	2	3	4	5
Overexposure	29	37	36	33	33
Underexposure	(45)	31	32	32	37
Positioning	20	18	18	19	17
Centering	10	11	(20)	9	9
Motion	6	7	6	5	5
Other	8	6	7	7	6
Total:	118	110	119	105	107

Technique exposure chart error?	Collimator misaligned?

Retake percentage by room.

TABLE 33-4. Retake Percentage by Technologist

	Technologist #				
Reason	1	2	3	4	5
Overexposure	35	31	32	30	43
Underexposure	32	31	31	34	30
Positioning	20	18	18	(30)	17
Centering	13	12	11	12	11
Motion	5	(11)	4	4	4
Error	(10)	4	5	3	3
Other	5	7	6	6	7
Total:	120	112	107	119	115

Need to be more careful?	Using long exposure times?	Has difficulty with some exams?

Retake percentage by radiographer. (Tables 33-3 and 33-4 adapted from *Analysis of Retakes: Understanding, Managing and Using an Analysis of Retakes Program for Quality Assurance.* (HEW Publication FDA 79-8097, 1979), Rockville, MD: U.S. DHEW, PHS, FDA, Bureau of Radiological Health.

images from a single room with an artifact in the same location might indicate a barium or iodine stain on a grid or table. Once obvious problems are addressed, the data should be examined for unequal distribution of repeats. Tables 33-3 and 33-4 illustrate how distributions can be diagnosed.

The **total repeat rate** is a valuable figure to monitor over long periods of time. It is calculated as a percentage of the total number of images produced during the period of the study. The total image figure can be extracted from institutional data in some cases or can be estimated by multiplying the number of examinations by the average number of images produced per examination. For example, a chest unit that produced 600 examinations in a week could be calculated to have produced 1,200 images (PA + lateral × 600). Repeat rates may suffer from a start-up effect where data may not be reliable for the first three weeks due to unfamiliarity with the requirements of the study or various psychological phenomena from stress to hypermotivation. Data indicates that radiographer repeat rates should be between 3 and 10 percent, with the average at 8 percent. One study demonstrated the student reject rates average to be slightly above 9 percent. Data also appear to indicate that when the rate drops below 3 percent there is a problem in data collection or an extremely wide acceptance limit in effect. It is important to realize that repeat rates are not only affected by processing equipment, x-ray equipment, patient condition, and radiographer competence, but also by the acceptance limits of the radiologists. In some instances a high repeat rate may indicate extremely high-quality standards in the institution while the same rate may also indicate poor-quality radiographers. Caution in interpretation is essential, and all aspects of the analysis should be carefully studied before conclusions are drawn.

TROUBLESHOOTING

Troubleshooting (locating problems when equipment malfunctions) is a diagnostic process. The same reasoning process that a physician uses to diagnose a disease can be applied to radiographic equipment. Beginning with the symptoms, the radiographer can work step-by-step through a problem-solving procedure to eliminate possible problems until the source of trouble is isolated.

Although radiographers are not qualified to perform invasive procedures on electronic equipment, they can often pinpoint the general source of the problem. For example, an increase in exposure could be caused by nearly all equipment in the radiographic imaging chain. However, a problem-solving approach may discover that all radiographs have increased exposure, not just the radiographs from a single unit. This might focus attention on the film processor. If the developer temperature is checked and found to be within normal limits, the radiographer might then check the replenishment tank only to discover that it is empty. To solve the problem, the radiographer might fill the tank, remove air locks from the replenishment lines, and restock the developer tank solution. A complete troubleshooting guide is provided in Appendix B.

SUMMARY

Quality assurance consists of activities that provide adequate confidence that a radiology service will render consistently high-quality images and services. Quality assurance includes evaluating activities such as interpretation of examinations, maintenance of equipment, performance of procedures, filing systems, staff development, scheduling of examinations, and supply lines. The quality assurance process operates by identifying problems or potential problem areas, monitoring the problem, and then resolving it.

Quality control is the aspect of quality assurance that monitors technical equipment to maintain quality standards. The concept of quality control is rooted in the need to stabilize the various equipment components of the radiographic imaging chain. From incoming line current through x-ray production to the processing of the radiograph, erratic equipment performance causes repeat radiographs and unnecessary patient exposure to radiation.

Equipment purchasing decisions should involve each member of the radiological team. Specific imaging requirements should be identified and equipment specifications should be developed. Once the equipment is selected, it is then installed and tested.

Monitoring equipment performance is an integral part of quality assurance. It involves the processing systems as well as the external radiation beams. Ancillary equipment should also be checked.

Monitoring the quality of the processing systems includes routine processor sensitometry and darkroom safelight testing. External beam evaluations involve monitoring the diagnostic radiographic systems, fluoroscopic systems, tomographic systems, and automated exposure controls. A wide variety of tests on each of the systems are performed to ensure equipment accuracy. Ancillary equipment, such as cassettes view boxes, and display monitors are also evaluated. PAC system interface accuracy is also important.

A careful analysis of repeat radiographs is also a valuable aid in diagnosing the radiographic process. Significant reductions in patient dose, radiographer time and effort, and supply costs can be achieved with properly executed repeat-image studies.

REVIEW QUESTIONS

1. Why are quality assurance and quality control so important?

2. What factors should be considered when making equipment purchasing decisions?

3. How should film processing systems be monitored?

4. How often should tests be performed on diagnostic radiographic systems?

5. What tests should be performed routinely on the x-ray generator?

6. What tests should be performed routinely on automatic exposure controls?

7. Why are repeat image studies a valuable part of quality assurance?

REFERENCES AND RECOMMENDED READING

Adams, M. J., Barsotti, J. B., Kohler, T. D., & Reel, L. A. (1994). Film processor quality assurance: Increasing reliability while decreasing costs. *American Journal of Roentgenology, 163*, 709–710.

Adler, A. M., & Carlton, R. R. (1989). Repeating radiographs: Critiquing the image. *Postgraduate Advances in Radiologic Technology.* Eugene Frank, ed. Berryville, VA: Forum Medicum.

Adler, A. M., Carlton, R. R., & Wold, B. (1992a). An analysis of radiographic repeat rate data. *Radiologic Technology, 63*(5), 308–314.

Adler, A. M., Carlton, R. R., & Wold, B. (1992b). A comparison of student radiographic reject rates. *Radiologic Technology, 64*(1), 26–32.

American Association of Physicists in Medicine. (1978). *Diagnostic radiology committee task force on quality assurance protocol: Basic quality control in diagnostic radiology* (AAPM Report No. 4). Chicago: Author.

American College of Radiology. (1981). *Quality assurance in diagnostic radiology and nuclear medicine—the obvious decision.* (HEW Publication [FDA] 81–8141) Rockville, MD: U.S. Department of Health, Education, and Welfare, Public Health Service, Food and Drug Administration, Bureau of Radiological Health.

Ardran, G. M., & Crooks, H. E. (1968). Checking diagnostic x-ray beam quality. *British Journal of Radiology, 41*, 193.

Ardran, G. M., Crooks, H. E., & James, V. (1969). Testing x-ray cassettes for film-intensifying screen contact. *Radiography, 35*(414), 143.

Barber, T. C., & Thomas, M. (1983). *Radiologic quality control manual.* Reston, VA: Reston.

Basart, J. A. (1974). Developer pH: Its significance in quality control. *Radiographic Technology, 45*(6), 413.

Berry, G. C., Starchman, D. E., & Howland, W. J. (1980). Objective equipment selection and performance evaluation. *Radiology Management, 2*(5), 14.

Bowers, J., Lin, P., & Rogers, L. (1978, May 12–13). Impact of equipment specifications on purchases.

Workshop in Purchase Specifications and Performance Evaluation of Radiologic Imaging Equipment Proceedings. Chicago: Midwest Chapter American Association of Physicists in Medicine, Northwestern University Medical School and Northwestern Memorial Hospital.

Brookstein, J. J., & Steck, W. (1971). Effective focal spot size. *Radiology, 98,* 31–33.

Burkhart, R. L. (1983). *A basic quality assurance program for small diagnostic radiology facilities.* (HHS Publication FDA 83–8218) Rockville, MD: U.S. Department of Health and Human Services, Public Health Service, Food and Drug Administration, National Center for Devices and Radiological Health.

Carlton, R. (1980). Establishing a total quality assurance program in diagnostic radiology. *Radiologic Technology, 52,* 23–38.

Carlton, R. R. (1992). Another dimension of quality assurance in radiology. In L. T. Gurley, & W. J. Callaway (Eds.), *Introduction to radiologic technology* (3rd ed., pp. 149–166). St. Louis, MO: C. V. Mosby.

Carlton, R. R., & McKenna, A. (1989). Repeating radiographs: Setting imaging standards. *Postgraduate Advances in Radiologic Technology.* Eugene Frank, ed. Berryville, VA: Forum Medicum.

Carroll, Q. B. (1993). *Fuchs's radiographic exposure, processing, and quality control* (5th ed.). Springfield, IL: Charles C Thomas.

Chu, W. K., Ferguson, S., Wunder, B., Smith, R., & Vanhoutte, J. J. (1979). A two-year reject/retake profile analysis in pediatric radiology. *Health Physics, 42*(1), 53–59.

Corr, B. (1978). A basic quality control system—Part 1. *The Canadian Journal of Medical Radiation Technology, 9*(3), 129.

Corr, B. (1985). Quality control in radiology: An administrative overview. *The Canadian Journal of Medical Radiation Technology, 16*(1), 4.

Crooks, H. E. (1975). Control of image quality, voltage, and filtration. *Radiography, 41*(481), 3.

Crooks, H. E. (1980). A device for checking the speeds and quality of x-ray films and efficiency of film processors. *Radiography, 46*(545), 128.

Cullinan, A., & Cullinan, J. (1994). *Producing quality radiographs* (2nd ed.). Philadelphia: J. B. Lippincott.

Cullinan, J. E. (1981). A 'perfect' chest radiograph—or a compromise? *Radiologic Technology, 53*(2), 121.

Dodd, B. C. (1983). Repeat analysis in radiology: A method of quality control. *The Canadian Journal of Medical Radiation Technology, 14*(2), 37.

Dreyer, K., Mehta, A., & Thrall, J. (2002) PACS: A Guide To The Digital Revolution. New York: Springer Verlag.

Eastman, T. R. (1993). Technique charts are vital to quality. *Radiologic Technology, 65*(1), 19.

Eisenberg, R. L., Akin, J. R., & Hedgcock, M. W. (1980, March). Optimal use of portable and stat examination. *American Journal of Roentgenology,* 523–524.

Engel, T. L. (1979). Effect of kilovoltage and milliamperage on focal spot size. *Radiologic Technology, 50*(5), 559.

Everson, J. D., & Gray, J. E. (1987). Focal-spot measurement: Comparison of slit, pinhole, and star resolution pattern techniques. *Radiology, 165*(1), 261–264.

Fairbanks, R., & Doust, C. (1979). Methods for studying the focal spot size and resolution of diagnostic x-ray tubes. *Radiography, 45*(533), 89.

Finney, W. (1999). Introduction to radiographic quality assurance. In P. W. Ballinger, *Merrill's atlas of radiographic positions and radiologic procedures* (7th ed., pp. 305–320). St. Louis, MO: C. V. Mosby.

Gilbert, M., & Carlton, W. (1978). Performance evaluations for diagnostic x-ray equipment. *Radiologic Technology, 50,* 243–248.

Gildenhorn, H. L., Rehman, I., Pape, L., & Baker, S. (1960). Standardization of physical factors in radiographic exposures. *Radiology, 75,* 262–267.

Goldman, L. W., & Beech, S. (1979). *Analysis of retakes: Understanding, managing, and using an analysis of retakes program for quality assurance* (HEW Publication [FDA] 79–8097). Rockville, MD: U.S. Department of Health, Education, and Welfare, Public Health Service, Food and Drug Administration, Bureau of Radiological Health.

Gray, J. E., & Trefler, M. (1980). Pinhole cameras: artifacts, modifications, and recording of pinhole images on screen film systems. *Radiologic Technology, 52*(3), 277.

Gray, J. E., Winkler, N. T., Stears, J. G., & Frank, E. D. (1983). *Quality control in diagnostic imaging: A quality control cookbook.* Rockville, MD: Aspen.

Guglielmo, J. (1980). Processor quality control science. *Radiology Management, 2*(4), 2.

Hall, C. L. (1977). Economic analysis from a quality control program. *Proceedings of the Society of Photo-optical Instrumentation Engineers, 127,* 271–275.

Hangiandreou, N. J., Fetterly, K. A., & Felmlee, J. P. (1999). Optimization of a contrast-detail-based method for electronic image display quality evaluation. *Journal of Digital Imaging, 12*(2): 60–7.

Haus, A. G. (1993). *Film processing in medical imaging.* Madison, WI: Medical Physics.

Hendee, W. R., & Ritenour, R. (1993). *Medical imaging physics* (3rd ed.). St. Louis, MO: C. V. Mosby.

Hendee, W. R., & Rossi, R. P. (1979). *Quality assurance for radiographic x-ray units and associated equipment* (HEW Publication [FDA] 79–8094). Rockville, MD: U.S. Department of Health, Education, and Welfare, Public Health Service, Food and Drug Administration, Bureau of Radiological Health.

Hendee, W. R., & Rossi, R. P. (1980). *Quality assurance for conventional tomographic x-ray units* (HEW Publication [FDA] 80–8096). Rockville, MD: U.S. Department of Health, Education, and Welfare, Public Health Service, Food and Drug Administration, Bureau of Radiological Health.

High and Normal Speed Rotors: Effect on Focal Spot Size, Resolution and Density. (1981). *Radiologic Technology, 53*(1).

Irfan, A. Y., Pugh, V. I., & Jeffery, C. D. (1985). Some practical aspects of peak kilovoltage measurements. *Radiography, 51*(599), 251–254.

Joint Commission on Accreditation of Healthcare Organizations Diagnostic Radiology Services. (1994). *Accreditation manual for hospitals.* Chicago: Author.

Kalivoda, F. J. (1979, Fall). Ancillary audits in the radiology services: Improving patient care. *Radiology Management,* 2–10.

Kebart, R. C., & James, C. D. (1991). Benefits of increasing focal film distance. *Radiologic Technology, 62*(6), 434–441.

Lam, R. W., & Price, S. C. (1989). The influence of film-screen color sensitivity and type of measurement device on kVp measurements. *Radiologic Technology, 60*(4), 319–321.

Langston, P., Crawley, M. T., & Whiting, G. (2001). Management of an equipment quality control programme in diagnostic radiology. *Radiography, 7*(3): 171–9.

Lowthian, J., & McFadden, B. (1989). Quality control for chest radiography. *Canadian Journal of Medical Radiation Technology, 18*(2), 93–97.

MacLean, B. (1984). Quality Control Report 1981–82: 9 months of operations. *The Canadian Journal of Medical Radiation Technology, 15*(1), 4.

Martell, B., & Gale, J. (2002). Quality assurance on imaging monitors: design and implementation. *Canadian Journal of Medical Radiation Technology, 33*(4): 3–12.

McEntee, M. F., Brennan, P. C., & Connor, G. O. (2004). The effect of X-ray tube potential on the image quality of PA chest radiographs when using digital image acquisition devices. *Radiography, 10*(4): 287–92.

McFadden, B. (1989). Half value layer calibration. *Canadian Journal of Medical Radiation Technology, 20*(2), 67–74.

McKinney, W. (1988). *Radiographic processing and quality control.* Philadelphia: J. B. Lippincott.

McKinney, W. E. J. (1993). Another look at film processor quality. *Radiologic Technology, 64*(4), 211–212.

McLemore, J. M. (1981). *Quality assurance in diagnostic radiology.* Chicago: Yearbook Medical.

Moores, B. M., Henshaw, E. T., Watkinson, S. A. A., & Pearcy, B. J. (1987). *Practical guide to quality assurance in medical imaging.* New York: Wiley.

National Electrical Manufacturers Association. (1985). Measurements of dimensions and properties of focal spots of diagnostic x-ray tubes. (NEMA Standards Publication No. XR-5-1984). Rosslyn, VA: Author.

Nelson, M. T. (1994). Continuous quality improvement (CQI) in radiology: An overview. *Applied Radiology, 23*(7), 11–16.

Nelson, R. E., Barnes, G. T., & Witten, D. M. (1977). Economic analysis of a comprehensive quality assurance program. *Radiologic Technology, 49,* 129–134.

Paleen, R., Skundberg, P. A., & Schwartz, H. (1989). How much is quality assurance costing your department? *Radiology Management, 11*(1), 24.

Pirtle, O. L. (1994). X-ray machine calibration: A study of failure rates. *Radiologic Technology, 65*(5), 291–298.

Potsaid, M. S., Rhea, J. T., Llewellyn, H. J. (1978, June). Quality assessment and assurance in diagnostic imaging. *Radiology,* 583–588.

Price, R. (1981). The continuous assessment of x-ray tubes and generators. *Radiography, 47*(553), 2.

Pugin, M. (1986). Teaching quality control in radiological imaging. *The Canadian Journal of Medical Radiation Technology, 17*(4), 14.

Rhatigan, L., & Montague, E. (1987). Computerized quality assurance. *Radiologic Technology, 58*(6), 523.

Roehrig, H. (1999). Image quality assurance for CRT display systems. *Journal of Digital Imaging, 12*(1): 1–2.

Roehrig, H. (1999). Image quality assurance for CRT display systems—Part II. *Journal of Digital Imaging, 12*(2): 49.

Rogers, K. D., Matthews, I. P., & Roberts, C. J. (1987). Variation in repeat rates between 18 radiology departments. *The British Journal of Radiology, 60,* 463–468.

Rouse, S., & Cowen, A. R. (1983). Quality assurance of fluorographic camera systems. *Radiography, 49*(587), 251.

Rozenfeld, M., & Jette, D. (1984, January). Quality assurance of radiation dosage: Usefulness of redundancy. *Radiology,* 241.

Siegel, E., & Kolodner, R. (2001). Filmless Radiology. New York: Springer.

Stears, J. G., Gray, J. E., Webbles, W. E., & Frank, E. D. (1985). X-ray waveform monitoring for radiographic quality control. *Radiologic Technology, 57*(1), 9–15.

Stears, J. G., Gray, J. E., Webbles, W. E., & Frank, E. D. (1989). Radiologic exchange (kVp measurements). *Radiologic Technology, 60*(3), 233–236.

Stein, K. M. (2000). Quality assurance in CT. *Radiologic Technology, 72*(1): 67.

Sweeney, R. J. (1983). *Radiographic artifacts: Their cause and control.* Philadelphia: J. B. Lippincott.

Thompson, M. A., Hattaway, M. P., Hall, J. D., & Dowd, S. B. (1994). *Principles of imaging science and protection.* Philadelphia: W. B. Saunders.

Thornhill, P. J. (1987). Quality assurance in diagnostic radiography: Are we using it correctly and what is its future? *Radiography, 53*(610), 161–163.

Watkinson, S., & Moores, B. M. (1984). Reject analysis: Its role in quality assurance. *Radiography, 50*(593), 189–194.

Watkinson, S., Shaw, M., Moores, B. M., & Eddleston, E. (1983). Quality assurance: A practical programme. *Radiography, 49*(578), 27.

Watkinson, S. A. (1985). Economic aspects of quality assurance. *Radiography, 51*(597), 133.

Wheeler, W. N. (1980). Equipment specifications and performance standards for equipment pertaining to the nuclear medicine department. *Radiology Management, 2*(5), 43.

World Health Organization. (1982). *Quality assurance in diagnostic radiology.* Geneva: Author.

Zimmer, E. A. (1960). *Artifacts and handling and processing faults on x-ray films.* New York: Grune & Stratton.

UNIT V Comparing Exposure Systems

Once a thorough background knowledge has been acquired, the radiographer must then analyze the clinical conditions and synthesize the information into a workable exposure system. The objective is to provide a method of producing consistent image quality. Consistency facilitates the diagnostic process by permitting more valid comparisons between examinations and confidence in the amount of information presented in the image. A balance must exist between image quality, patient situation, and dose.

This unit presents various exposure systems that have been developed and assists in evaluating which system is most appropriate for particular clinical situations. All radiographers must have a thorough understanding of how an exposure system functions if it is to be used successfully. The practice of radiography involves so many nonroutine situations, unusual conditions, and unique patients that simply following guidelines established by someone else does not permit the radiographer with the necessary skills to provide the patient with the best quality of care.

It is even more important to establish appropriate exposure factors when using computed or digital radiography systems and automatic exposure control (AEC) devices (phototimers). These automated systems cannot function unless the incoming photons are at the correct intensity and proper attenuation ranges to permit the computer or mechanical system to provide an appropriate range of input data for the processing of the image.

Because of the tremendous number of variables in the radiographic imaging chain, the most successful exposure systems maintain them all except a single variable for a given range of conditions. For example, a variable kVp system maintains all factors except kVp, which is varied to obtain appropriate exposures for different subject densities and contrasts. This unit begins with a technical discussion on **developing exposure charts** as a guide to establishing functional systems for clinical practice. This is followed by specific details in the development of **fixed kVp systems** and **variable kVp systems,** the most popular exposure systems. **Automatic exposure controls** follows and is used for more exposures than any other system. A full chapter of **exposure conversion problems** provides methods for solving complex problems similar to the nonroutine situations that arise in practice.

CHAPTER 34

Developing Exposure Charts

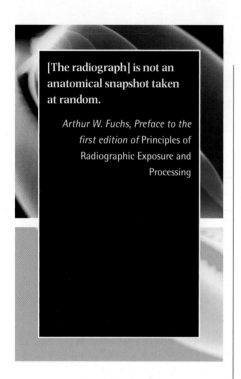

[The radiograph] is not an anatomical snapshot taken at random.

Arthur W. Fuchs, Preface to the first edition of Principles of Radiographic Exposure and Processing

KEY TERMS

anatomically
   programmed
   radiography
caliper

OBJECTIVES

Upon completion of this chapter, the student should be able to:

- Compare various exposure systems.
- Describe the advantages and disadvantages of fixed and variable kVp systems.
- Discuss other exposure systems that have influenced radiographic technique.
- Explain why measurement of part thickness is critical to the accurate use of technique charts.
- Describe the function of the radiographer when using automatic exposure control systems.

- Describe how programmed exposure control systems function.
- State the steps necessary to establish a technique chart.
- Explain a basic phantom testing procedure.
- Describe the process of selecting an optimal image range.
- Extrapolate a technique chart from a limited number of phantom test images.
- Describe the clinical trial and fine-tuning processes.

SYSTEM SELECTION

The foundations of the principles of radiographic exposure technique were laid in the 1920s by Ed. C. Jerman, known as the father of radiologic technology in the United States, and were developed into a scientific system in the 1940s by Arthur W. Fuchs.

Because radiographic exposure is such a complex process, technique systems function best when the large number of variables can be held constant while a single factor is permitted to vary. The goal of any radiographic exposure system is to provide a method of consistency in the quality of image production. Each type of exposure system functions in a different way to accomplish this goal, but all require the routine use of technique charts. Radiographers should consult a technique chart prior to making each exposure. Failure to follow this practice results in a higher personal repeat rate and excessive, unwarranted patient dose.

A radiography department can expect to produce consistent results only when accurate technique charts are provided for each x-ray unit. Monitoring and revising these charts are part of the quality control function. Institutions that develop and enforce policies requiring radiographers to utilize posted technique charts experience lower repeat rates. Radiographers are advised to follow posted technique charts and to bring inaccuracies to the attention of quality control personnel immediately to avoid continued poor-quality images and excessive patient dose. Utilizing technique charts is even more important with digital imaging systems.

Comparing Exposure Systems

Each exposure system has its advantages and disadvantages, and professionals quickly develop a rationale for their favorite system. The student must study each system in detail to learn its advantages and disadvantages before forming a personal professional judgment. It is important to recognize that any exposure system is designed to provide consistency in image quality and requires that all users of equipment in a single institution adhere to the same technique charts. Although personal philosophy may differ from institutional procedures and poli-

cies, the professional must let personal preference become secondary to the primary goal of widespread consistency in image quality. The following information outlines the various exposure systems that are explained in detail in this unit.

Fixed Kilovoltage Systems

Fixed kVp systems were developed by Fuchs in 1943 during World War II. They have strong theoretical support in the literature and among many radiographers because they tend to decrease patient dose, provide more information on the image, increase the consistency of image receptor exposure, lengthen exposure latitude, reduce x-ray tube wear, decrease time settings and therefore patient motion, and are easier to remember. However, these systems produce more scatter radiation, which tends to provide a lower contrast than a variable kilovoltage system. Low contrast is usually perceived as less pleasing to the eye and for this reason many institutions have not adopted the fixed kVp system.

Variable Kilovoltage Systems

Variable kVp systems were the first methodical approach to radiographic technique. They were proposed by Jerman in 1925 and predominated until x-ray generators became powerful enough to support fixed kVp techniques in the 1940s. They permit small incremental changes in exposure to compensate for variation in body part thickness. Most x-ray generators permit finer adjustment of kVp stations than of time or mA settings. Variable kVp systems produce higher contrast images, which enhance the visibility of fine detail and increase the perception of resolution. Institutions that have not adopted a variable kVp system cite the overwhelming advantages of fixed kVp to patient dose, image information, tube wear, etc.

Other Exposure Systems

Over the years since the work of Jerman and Fuchs, there have been many attempts to refine exposure systems. During the 1950s and 1960s attempts were made to use mathematical formulas to quantify the relationship between the primary factors, especially kVp and mAs. A number of these formulas have been proven invalid. Only the systems based on $\log_{10}$ survived, although there has been support for body habitus and proportional anatomy systems. However, several exposure systems have been developed that have either had a major effect on thinking about radiographic technique or have proven to be accurate in clinical situations.

Bit System. The Bit System was called the Du Pont Bit System because it was developed, by computer analysis, by Robert Trinkle of E. I. Du Pont de Nemours and Company, Inc. (now part of AGFA Corporation). Du Pont published the system in the 1970s and has supported it through numerous editions. The Bit System is a log-based system that utilizes points to quantify a vast number of radiographic variables, such as density and contrast, distance, anatomical thickness, kVp, mAs, pathology, grids, development time, etc. The concept was simply that each projection required an established number of bits. Any balanced combination of variables that equaled the required bits would produce a diagnostic-quality image. The Bit System even permits calculation of approximate entrance skin exposure.

XVS System. The X-Ray Value Scale (XVS) system was designed by Gerhart Schwarz in 1960. It was patterned after the photographic Exposure Value Scale (EVS) system but with the addition of research into the effect of part thickness on kVp's effect on image density. The system was the first used to quantify the primary radiographic variables. It permitted variance of exposure factors, much as with the Bit System. The basis of the system was a caliper that measured part thickness in XVS numbers. Any total of XVS numbers that equaled the caliper measurement could be obtained from special markings on the x-ray machine's distance, mA, time, and kVp indicators. The lack of standardization of all but a single factor resulted in too many variables for consistent diagnostic confidence. In addition, when manufacturers began to build units with XVS numbers, replacing technical controls, radiographers experienced difficulty in adapting to specific clinical situations.

Siemens Point System. The Siemens Point System was designed as a parallel system to the XVS system. It predated the Bit System, and although it was not as sophisticated, it permitted the radiographer to control the exposure variables much better than with the XVS system.

Supertech™ Calculator. In 1973 a log-based, slide rule technique calculator was developed by Brice Kratzer, patented, trademarked, and marketed as the Supertech™ Calculator by Supertech, Inc. Circular and slide rule calculators had been presented in the radiographic literature by C. W. Reed in 1939 and 1949, and William A. Williams had developed a circular calculator technique system in 1960. Several of these calculators were distributed by commercial companies, but only the Supertech™ Calculator has survived to the present and is updated continually. An acrylic penetrometer with a calibration master film for elementary quality control testing of machine output is utilized. After a short testing procedure, each machine can be assigned a correction factor that takes into account such variations as kVp, mA, time, part thickness, patient age, projection, distance, grid, pathology, etc. A computer disk provides a technique data reference to accompany the system. The Supertech™ Calculator remains a viable technique system, especially in low-volume clinics, physician's offices, and in ancillary radiographic service situations, such as chiropractics and podiatry.

Proportional Anatomy Systems. A body habitus system for chest radiography was proposed by Terry Eastman in 1969. Proportional anatomy systems were presented by Quinn Carroll in 1985 and by Eugene Frank and Norlin T. Winkler in 1987. These systems classify body parts and habitus into groups of similar subject density and contrast. The body habitus system determined technical factors for the chest from patient height and weight. The proportional anatomy systems use ratios or conversion factors to extrapolate a technique chart for the entire body from a control exposure.

Measurement of Part Thickness

Nearly all variables in exposure systems are changed according to the thickness of the anatomical part being radiographed, and no exposure system can be expected to function accurately unless the radiographer measures part thickness. Part thicknesses for various regions in the average adult were detailed by Arthur Fuchs (Table 34-1).

Failure to measure consistently will cause unnecessary repeated exposures, resulting in excessive patient dose. The device used to measure a part thickness is a **caliper.** Improper use of a caliper will result in improper technical factors and a repeated exposure. Caliper measurements are made either by central ray entrance and exit or by thickest part. It is critical that all radiographers using a particular technique chart measure by the same method and in exactly the same manner.

Central ray measurements should be made from the point of central ray entrance to exit. For example, in Figure 34-1, the chest should be measured at point B, not point A or C. Thickest part measurements should be made at the thickest part of the area of interest. If another special measurement point or method has been established, it must be followed by all users of the chart.

Automatic Exposure Control (AEC) Systems

When automatic exposure control (AEC) systems are used, the selection of exposure time factors, and thereby mAs selection, are eliminated. The

FIGURE 34-1   Proper caliper measurement of part thickness by using the central ray entrance-to-exit method as shown in B.

TABLE 34-1.   Average Adult Part Thickness By Region

Region	Average Thickness Adult—CMS AP	PA	Lat	Percent Frequency
Thumb, Fingers		1.5–4		99
Hand	3–5			99
			7–10	93
Wrist	3–6			99
			5–8	98
Forearm	6–8			94
			7–9	92
Elbow	6–8			96
			7–9	87
Arm	7–10			95
			7–10	94
Shoulder	12–16			79
Clavicle		13–17		82
Foot	6–8			92
			7–9	91
Ankle	8–10			86
			6–9	96
Leg	10–12			85
			9–11	89
Knee	10–13			92
			9–12	92
Thigh	14–17			77
			13–16	76
Hip	17–21			76
Cervical Vertebrae C1–3	12–14			77
Cervical Vertebrae C4–7	11–14			98
Cervical Vertebrae C1–7			10–13	90
Thoracic Vertebrae	20–24			76
			28–32	81
Lumbar Vertebrae	18–22			69
			27–32	77
Pelvis	19–23			78
Skull		18–21		96
			14–17	88
Sinuses Frontal		18–21		97
Sinuses Max.		18–22		88
			13–17	96
Mandible			10–12	82
Chest	20–25			82
			27–32	84

Reprinted with permission of the American Society of Radiologic Technologists from Arthur W. Fuchs's Relationship of tissue thickness to kilovoltage. *The X-ray Technician* [now *Radiologic Technology*] 19:6, 287–293, 1948.

radiographer must still exercise professional judgment to determine all other factors, including mA (which can be used to influence the time), kVp, distance, etc. Part of the art of phototiming is learning when to use AECs and when to avoid them.

ANATOMICALLY PROGRAMMED RADIOGRAPHY

Anatomically programmed radiography is a commonly utilized computerized exposure control systems. These systems are simply computerized technique charts utilizing existing exposure systems but storing the data in a memory bank that is an inherent part of the x-ray control console. Many of these units have anatomically based programming (Figure 34-2). For example, when the radiographer pushes a button to indicate a lumbar spine, a screen may provide a choice of projections. When the lateral projection is indicated, a suggested series of technical factors may be set on the x-ray console. If the exposure is begun, the computerized factors will be used. However, if the radiographer determines that nonroutine conditions exist, the technical factors can be modified prior to exposure. The computerized control can be programmed to display any desired exposure system and then be fine-tuned to meet existing needs. If the programmed console or consoles are monitored and maintained to display accurate techniques, they can be consulted for techniques for an entire department. Only an mAs correction factor would be needed for each room to make the chart accurate.

ESTABLISHING A TECHNIQUE CHART

The process of establishing a technique chart begins with collecting exposure data. The first step is to make a single exposure that produces an optimal diagnostic quality image. This original image must be at the optimal center of the acceptance limits curve. Although any projection can be used as a starting point in collecting data, it is preferred that the first

FIGURE 34-2 A programmed, computerized exposure control console. *(Courtesy of GE Healthcare)*

data be from a subject part size and kVp in the middle of the diagnostic range. Ideal part sizes are 10–25 cm and ideal kilovoltage is in the 60–80 range.

Figure 34-3 illustrates the steps in setting up a radiographic technique chart for any exposure system.

Initial Phantom Images

Initially, a series of test exposures is made to determine the optimal quality image. This is accomplished by using an appropriate phantom to produce images at a variety of technical factor combinations both above and below the average level. It is essential that the exposure remain the same at a control point to avoid misperception of the contrast range. It is preferred that the images be produced using an AEC to control the exposure. If an AEC is not available, or cannot be used due to other cir-

FIGURE 34-3 A systematic approach to establishing a technique chart.

[Flowchart contents:]
Produce phantom images

Select optimal phantom image

Extrapolate technique chart according to selected exposure system guidelines
- fixed kVp system
- variable kVp system
- other exposure systems

Perform phantom testing using extrapolated technique chart

Perform clinical trials

Perform clinical fine tuning

Continue ongoing fine tuning

image quality control checking. These professionals should not be asked to select the best image but to select those images they believe to be outside acceptance limits, because when any group of professionals is asked to select the best image there will be differences of opinion, leaving no consensus as to which is the best image. Conversely, elimination of those images that are not acceptable will often result in a series of images that are acceptable to all, although "perfect" to only a few.

Extrapolate Technique Chart

Next, a series of preliminary clinical trials should be performed by preparing a technique chart that adjusts current technical factors to those that are newly established as optimal. This is normally done by using the 15 percent rule and other guides for part thickness adjustments for particular exposure systems. Particular attention should be given to projections that have a narrow range of part thicknesses or few choices of technical factors. For example, the variations in a wrist or PA chest chart both require careful calculation, the wrist because the normal thickness range encompasses only about 3 cm and the PA chest because the extremely high kVp with a normal thickness range of only about 5 cm amplifies minute changes in mAs.

Phantom Testing

The new chart is then tested with a phantom to verify its effectiveness. Minimum phantom testing should include a median, small, and large part thickness. At this point the chart is completed for all part thicknesses for each projection.

Clinical Trials

Finally, a limited series of clinical trial examinations should be performed using the new chart. Each examination should be recorded and all repeated images should be saved for analysis. The series of clinical examinations should then be shown to each person who participated in the determination of the original standards. If the new image quality is accepted, a new exposure technique chart should be designed and implemented. If the new image quality experiences limited acceptance, adjustments

cumstances, an exposure or density reference control point must be established and measured with a densitometer. For example, the exact center of the body of L4 could be measured on each image. It would be necessary to adjust milliampere-second values until all images exhibited control point densities within OD 0.3 of one another.

Select Optimal Phantom Image

Once the series of phantom test images has been produced, it must be shown to all radiologists, who will be asked to diagnose the images, and to the supervisory radiographers, who will be responsible for should be made to satisfy deficiencies and all of the phantom testing and clinical trial steps should be repeated. Under no circumstance should clinical trials be performed until phantom testing and the other preliminary steps have been properly completed. Whenever new equipment is added to the imaging chain, especially a new x-ray tube or a new image receptor system, the phantom testing and/or clinical trial steps should be repeated until confidence in the chart is reestablished.

Clinical Fine-Tuning

Clinical fine-tuning requires that the technical factors for each exposure be recorded, regardless of whether the image is within acceptance limits. Each image is then used to fine-tune the chart. Excellent quality images permit technical factors for the part

thicknesses to be verified, while all other images permit adjustments of the technical factors for their respective part sizes.

Ongoing Fine-Tuning

It is important that a system of ongoing fine-tuning be established as a quality control monitoring method. The quality control radiographer should be consulted whenever a technique chart produces an unacceptable exposure and the cause is not evident. A series of unexplained rejected images may signify a change in one of the system's components that can be determined by quality control testing. The problem can often be fixed by a service engineer, although aging processes (such as filament wear, focal spot deterioration, and tube gas) may require adjustments of the technique chart.

SUMMARY

The goal of any radiographic exposure system is to provide a method of consistency in the quality of image production. Each type of exposure system functions in a different way to accomplish this goal, but all require the routine use of technique charts. Radiographers should consult a technique chart prior to making each exposure. Failure to follow this practice results in a higher personal repeat rate and excessive, unwarranted patient dose.

A radiography department can expect to produce consistent results only when accurate technique charts are provided for each x-ray unit. Monitoring and revising these charts are part of the quality control program. Institutions that develop and enforce policies requiring radiographers to utilize posted technique charts experience lower repeat rates.

Each exposure system has its advantages and disadvantages, and professionals quickly develop

a rationale for their favorite system. It is important to recognize that any exposure system is designed to provide consistency in image quality and this requires that all users of equipment in a single institution adhere to the same technique charts. The two most popular exposure systems are the fixed kVp system and the variable kVp system. Other exposure systems include the Du Pont Bit System, the XVS System, the Siemens Point System, the Supertech™ Calculator, and various proportional anatomy systems.

A systematic process for establishing a technique chart involves producing initial phantom images, selecting the optimal phantom image, extrapolating a technique chart for a given exposure system, performing phantom testing using the extrapolated technique chart data, performing clinical trials, clinical fine-tuning and, finally, establishing a system of ongoing fine-tuning.

REVIEW QUESTIONS

1. What is the principal goal of a radiographic exposure system?

2. Why is it important for radiographers to utilize technique charts?

3. What are some of the advantages of the fixed kVp system?

4. What are some of the advantages of the variable kVp system?

5. What are the two methods used for taking caliper measurements?

6. What are the steps involved in establishing a technique chart?

7. What should be done when a technique chart produces an unacceptable image and the cause is not evident?

REFERENCES AND RECOMMENDED READING

Cahoon, J. B. (1961). Radiographic technique: Its origin, concept, practical application and evaluation of radiation dosage. *The X-Ray Technician, 32*, 354–364.

Carroll, Q. B. (1993). *Fuchs's radiographic exposure, processing, and quality control* (5th ed.). Springfield, IL: Charles C Thomas.

Compton, S. (1987). Bit conversion of technical factors in vascular procedures. *Radiologic Technology, 58*(5), 413.

Cullinan, A. & Cullinan, J. (1994). *Producing quality radiographs* (2nd ed.). Philadelphia: J. B. Lippincott.

Dyke, W. P. (1975). Depth resolution: A mechanism by which high kilovoltage improves visibility in chest films. *Radiology, 117*, 159–164.

Eastman Kodak Company Health Sciences Markets Division. (1980). *The fundamentals of radiography* (12th ed.) (Kodak Publication M1-18). Rochester, NY: Author.

Eastman, T. R. (1969). Chest technique through body habitus. *Radiologic Technology, 41*, 80–84.

Eastman, T. R. (1971). Automated exposures in contemporary radiography. *Radiologic Technology, 43*(2), 80–83.

Eastman, T. R. (1973). Measurement: The key to exposure with manual techniques. *Radiologic Technology, 45*, 75–78.

Eastman, T. R. (1975). Technique charts: The key to radiographic quality. *Radiologic Technology, 46*, 365–368.

Eastman, T. R. (1978, July/August). A history of radiographic technique. *Applied Radiology*, 97–100.

Eastman, T. R. (1979). *Radiographic fundamentals and technique guide*. St. Louis, MO: C. V. Mosby.

Eastman, T. R. (1994). Technique charts improve x-ray quality. *Radiologic Technology, 65*(3), 183–186.

Files, G. W. (1952). *Medical radiographic technique*. Springfield, IL: Charles C Thomas.

Fodor, J., & Malott, J. C. (1993). *The art and science of medical radiography* (7th ed.). St. Louis, MO: C. V. Mosby.

Fuchs, A. W. (1934). Radiography of entire body employing one film and a single exposure. *Radiography and Clinical Photography, 10*, 9–14.

Fuchs, A. W. (1948). Relationship of tissue thickness to kilovoltage. *The X-Ray Technician, 19*, 287–293.

Fuchs, A. W. (1949). Control of radiographic density. *The X-Ray Technician, 20*, 271–273, 291.

Fuchs, A. W. (1950). The rationale of radiographic exposure. *The X-Ray Technician, 22*, 62–68, 76.

Funke, T. (1966). Pegged kilovoltage technic. *Radiologic Technology, 37*, 202–213.

Gyss, E. E. (1957). A medical radiographic technique chart based on constants. *Radiologic Technology, 29*(2), 76.

Hiss, S. S. (1975). Technique management. *Radiologic Technology, 46*(5), 369.

Hiss, S. S. (2003). *Understanding radiography* (4th ed.). Springfield, IL: Charles C Thomas.

Hochschild, T. J., & Cremin, B. J. (1975). Technique in infant chest radiography. *Radiography, 41*(481), 21.

Jenkins, D. (1980). *Radiographic photography and imaging processes*. Lancaster, England: MTP Press Limited.

Jerman, E. C. (1926a). Extremity technic. *Radiology, 6*, 252–254.

Jerman, E. C. (1926b). Potter-Bucky diaphragm technic. *Radiology, 6*, 336–338.

Jerman, E. C. (1928). *Modern x-ray technic*. St. Paul, MN: Bruce.

Lauer, O. G., Mayes, J. B., & Thurston, R. P. (1990). *Evaluating radiographic quality: The variables and their effects*. Mankato, MN: The Burnell Company.

Lex, J. K. (1957). The x-ray exposure chart. *The X-Ray Technician, 28*(4), 250.

Mattsson, O. (1955). Practical photographic problems in radiography. *Acta Radiologica Supplementum, 120*, 1–206.

McFadden, B. (1985). Principles of radiographic exposure: A new approach. *The Canadian Journal of Radiography, Radiotherapy, and Nuclear Medicine, 16*(2), 45–54.

Morgan, J. A. (1977). *The art and science of medical radiography* (5th ed.). St. Louis: Catholic Hospital Association.

Nemet, A., Cox, W. F., & Hills, T. H. (1953). The contrast problem in high kilovoltage radiography. *British Journal of Radiology, 26,* 185–192.

Revesz, G., Shea, F. J., & Kundel, H. L. (1982). The effects of kilovoltage on diagnostic accuracy in chest radiography. *Radiology, 142,* 615–618.

Schwarz G. S. (1958). A simple universal unit system of radiographic exposures suited to departmental, national, and international standardization. *Radiology, 71,* 573–574.

Schwarz, G. S. (1959a). Extended range radiography. *Radiology, 69,* 419–423, 1957.

Schwarz, G. S. (1959b). Kilovoltage and radiographic effect. *Radiology, 73,* 749–760.

Schwarz, G. S. (1960). Kilovoltage conversion in radiography. *The X-Ray Technician, 31,* 373–379, 436.

Schwarz, G. S. (1961). *Unit-step radiography.* Springfield, IL: Charles C Thomas.

Seeman, H. E. (1968). *Physical and photographic principles of medical radiography.* New York: Wiley & Sons.

Thomas, J. B. (1959). High kilovoltage equipment and technique. *The X-Ray Technician, 30*(6), 500.

Thompson, M. A., Hattaway, M. P., Hall, J. D., & Dowd, S. B. (1994). *Principles of imaging science and protection.* Philadelphia: W. B. Saunders.

United States Army. (1955, March). *Principles of radiographic exposure* (TM 8-282) (Washington, D. C.: United States Army).

United States War Department. (1941, July 3). *Technical manual: Roentgenographic technicians* (TM 8-240) (Washington, D. C.: United States War Department).

Williams, W. A. (1960). Standardization of x-ray technique. *The X-Ray Technician, 32*(2), 137.

CHAPTER 35

Fixed Kilovoltage Systems

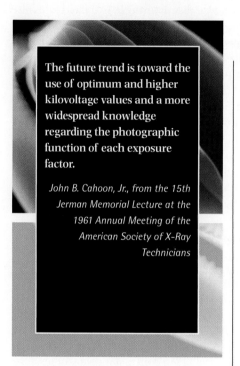

The future trend is toward the use of optimum and higher kilovoltage values and a more widespread knowledge regarding the photographic function of each exposure factor.

John B. Cahoon, Jr., from the 15th Jerman Memorial Lecture at the 1961 Annual Meeting of the American Society of X-Ray Technicians

KEY TERM

optimal kVp

OBJECTIVES

Upon completion of this chapter, the student should be able to:

- Describe the principles of fixed kVp technique theory.

- Discuss the primary advantages and disadvantages of fixed kVp technique systems.

- Define optimal kilovoltage.

- Explain how to establish fixed kVp for various subject parts.

- Describe the steps in establishing a fixed kVp technique chart.

- Synthesize a fixed kVp technique chart from control radiographs.

PRINCIPLES OF FIXED KILOVOLTAGE EXPOSURE SYSTEMS

Because radiographic exposure is such a complex process, technique systems function best when the large number of variables can be held constant while a single factor is permitted to vary. **In a fixed kilovoltage system, the kVp is held constant for a given range of subject densities and contrasts while the mAs is varied to achieve an appropriate image receptor exposure.** The kVp has a profound effect on many radiographic factors, such as contrast, type of interaction, production of scatter radiation, and average photon energy. In addition, it varies depending on generator phase, filtration, machine calibration, intensifying screen phosphor conversion efficiency, subject inner shell binding energy range, etc. Consequently, a technique chart that makes kVp a constant eliminates the effects of these variables on the exposure system. The basis of a fixed kilovoltage exposure system therefore becomes the concept of the optimal kilovoltage peak.

In keeping with the goal of any radiographic exposure system to provide consistency in the quality of image production, a fixed kilovoltage system provides a relatively uniform contrast and an easily remembered series of kilovoltages to which mAs values can be added to produce images within established acceptance limits. The uniform contrast contributes to radiologists' confidence in the information in the image as they do not have to contend with a variable gray scale.

Advantages and Disadvantages

There are a number of advantages to the fixed kilovoltage technique systems. These systems tend to decrease patient dose, because the kilovoltage is always at the maximum possible level, and this permits decreased mAs in compensation. The decreased mAs contributes to decreased patient dose. In addition, the consistency in kVp levels results in uniform contrast, permitting the radiologist to compare images of a given projection or patient, and provides more confidence in the diagnostic process. The higher average kVps that the optimal kVp concept produces lengthen exposure latitude. It also decreases mAs, thereby decreasing the average mA, which lowers x-ray tube heating and extends tube life, and/or decreasing time, which reduces the possibility of patient motion.

There are also disadvantages to a fixed kilovoltage technique system. These systems tend to provide a lower overall contrast than do variable kilovoltage systems and this is usually perceived by radiologists as less pleasing to the eye. Without question, the lower contrast produces much more scattered radiation and images that are less artistically beautiful. Additionally, small incremental changes in exposure for variations in body part thickness may not be possible with systems that fix kVp and vary mAs, due to less variety in mA stations and exposure times as compared to the kVp settings.

Optimal Kilovoltage Peak

The optimal kVp is the maximum kVp level that will produce images with appropriate contrast that are consistently within acceptance limits. This kVp level must ensure sufficient penetration of the subject as well as provide acceptable image contrast. Insufficient penetration of the area of interest, especially in contrast media studies, limits the diagnostic region to the edges of the contrast media. Sufficient penetration permits visualization through the contrast media and increases the diagnostic information available.

The use of the maximum kVp as optimal causes a corresponding decrease in the mAs required to produce acceptable image receptor exposure/film density. The mAs reduction contributes to both reduced mA and time. Reduced mA decreases x-ray tube heating and prolongs filament and anode life. Reduced time minimizes the possibility of patient motion. **The optimal kVp produces lower contrast and the minimum patient dose.** The fixed kVp system takes advantage of the only situation in radiography where image quality can be increased (low contrast and therefore more diagnostic shades of gray) and patient dose decreased (less mAs and therefore less mR/mAs).

Establishing Optimal Kilovoltage Peak

A number of optimal kVps are established for a fixed kVp system; each is specific for a range of subject densities and contrasts. In other words, the so-called fixed kVp is fixed only for a specific range of part thicknesses for a particular procedure. For example, where 80 kVp may be selected as the optimal kVp for noncontrast media abdominal examinations, 50 kVp may be determined to be the maximum for contrast that is acceptable for imaging the trabeculae of the smaller extremities. The optimal kVp should not be changed unless the conditions under which it was set have changed, or the acceptance limits are changed.

TABLE 35-1.	Common Optimal kVp Ranges for the Major Body Regions
Region	**Optimal kVp Range**
Small extremities	50–60
Iodine-based contrast media studies	68
Large extremities	70
Skull	80
Abdomen and ribs	80
AP vertebral column	80
Lateral vertebral column	90
Chest	120
Barium-based contrast media studies	120

ESTABLISHING A FIXED KILOVOLTAGE PEAK TECHNIQUE CHART

The specific steps to setting up a fixed kVp technique chart follow the basic outline provided in Chapter 34.

Initial Phantom Images

Setting up a fixed kVp system requires that a series of test exposures be obtained to determine the optimal kVp. This is accomplished by using an abdomen or pelvis phantom to produce images at a variety of kVps above and below the average level. It is essential that the exposure remain the same at a control point to avoid misperception of the contrast range (Figure 35-1). It is preferred that the images be exposed using an AEC, although an exposure or density reference control point can be used.

Select Optimal Phantom Image

Once the series of phantom test images has been produced, the optimal phantom image must be selected. The objective of optimal kVp is to determine the **highest** kVp and **lowest** contrast that is within acceptance limits, not the best image. The optimal kVp is the highest of the acceptable images. Remember that this process is one of elimination, not

of selection. In other words, radiologists and quality control radiographers should be asked to eliminate unacceptable images, not to choose the single best quality image.

Careful consideration must be given to the variety of subject densities and contrasts in the human body before establishing the optimal kVps for other procedures. Table 35-1 illustrates common optimal kVp ranges for the major body regions, but individual requirements often vary.

Extrapolate Technique Chart

Once the optimal kVp has been determined, an extrapolated technique chart should be obtained by adjusting current technical factors to the newly established optimal kVp. This is normally done by using the 15 percent rule to modify existing technical factors until the desired kVp has been achieved.

Milliampere-seconds is designed to be the primary variable for a fixed kVp exposure system. The mAs values for the technique chart must be set at minimum increments of 30 percent because values less than 30 percent are not significant.

Because there is no linearity with some of the exposure variables, no accurate formula can be given for extrapolating mAs values. However, most systems have been found to operate in the range of doubling or halving the mAs for every 5 cm of subject

60 kVp

80 kVp

A

B

100 kVp

120 kVp

C

D

FIGURE 35-1 A series of chest images produced at 60, 80, 100, and 120 kVp to determine the optimal kVp. While 60 kVp may be selected as optimal for ribs, 120 kVp may be determined to be optimal for the chest.

thickness. For example, if 80 mAs produces a diagnostic quality image of a 20 cm part, a 15 cm part will require about 40 mAs, while a 25 cm part will require about 160 mAs. This is often applied to variable kVp technique charts as a "2 kVp/cm rule," which is fairly consistent with the 15 percent rule and ensures sufficient penetration.

Phantom Testing

Phantom testing is recommended prior to performing patient examinations. As a minimum, phantom testing should be done for a medium, small, and large part size. Because of the nonlinearity of the exposure

systems and the inadequacy of the 15 percent rule, phantom testing should always be employed when the part size is less than 10 cm or the kVp is outside the median diagnostic range of 60–80.

Phantom testing also serves as a fine-tuning mechanism for the extrapolated chart prior to clinical use. Once several mAs values have been set, extrapolation of the mAs for subject thickness can be done accurately. For example, if 68 kVp is set as the optimal fixed kVp for iodine-based contrast media abdominal work, a technique chart might be established from a base diagnostic quality 20 cm phantom image at 50 mAs (Table 35-2). Step 1 illustrates a blank chart with the phantom technique. Using

TABLE 35-2.   Fixed kVp Technique Chart

Blank Chart with Phantom Technique		Extrapolation of Additional mAs Values	Fine-Tuning of Extrapolated mAs Values	Extrapolation of Final mAs Values
cm	kVp	Step 1 mAs	Step 2	Step 3	Step 4
16	68				30
17	68				35
18	68				40
19	68				45
20	68	50	50	50	50
21	68				60
22	68				70
23	68				80
24	68				90
25	68		100	100	100
26	68				115
27	68				130
28	68				145
29	68				160
30	68		200	180	180
31	68				215
32	68				250
33	68				285
34	68				320
35	68		400	360	360

the 15 percent rule, several additional mAs values can be extrapolated for phantom testing, as shown in Step 2. Upon phantom testing, the extrapolated mAs values may require fine-tuning, as shown in Step 3. Once phantom fine-tuning is accomplished, the extrapolation of the final mAs values can be completed, as shown in Step 4. At this point the chart has been proven within acceptance limits by phantom testing and is ready for clinical trials.

Clinical Trials

Limited clinical trials are permissible with the new chart. All images should be recorded, with repeated images saved for analysis. When clinical trials are proceeding without excess repeated exposures, the new technique chart can move into the clinical fine-tuning stage.

Clinical Fine-Tuning

The clinical fine-tuning process will adjust and finally validate the entire chart. At this point the new technique chart can be adopted. However, ongoing fine-tuning then begins as a permanent process.

Ongoing Fine-Tuning

Ongoing fine-tuning is the process that maintains the accuracy of the entire exposure system and gives radiographers and radiologists confidence in the exposure and diagnostic processes.

SUMMARY

Technique systems function best when the large number of variables can be held constant while a single factor is permitted to vary. In a fixed kilovoltage system the kVp is held constant for a given range of subject densities and contrasts, while the mAs is varied to achieve an appropriate image receptor exposure.

Fixed kilovoltage technique systems tend to decrease patient dose because the kilovoltage is always at the maximum possible level. In addition, the consistency in kVp levels results in a uniform image contrast and a lengthened exposure latitude. There are also disadvantages to a fixed kilovoltage technique system. These systems tend to provide a lower overall contrast than do variable kilovoltage systems and this is usually perceived by radiologists as less pleasing to the eye. Additionally, small incremental changes in exposure for variations in body part thickness may not be possible with systems that fix kVp and vary mAs, due to less variety in mA stations and exposure times as compared to the kVp settings.

The optimal kVp is the maximum kVp level that will produce images with appropriate contrast that are consistently within acceptance limits. This kVp level must ensure sufficient penetration of the subject as well as provide acceptable image contrast. A number of optimal kVps are established for a fixed kVp system and are specific for a range of subject densities and contrasts. In other words, the so-called fixed kVp is fixed only for a specific range of part thicknesses for a particular procedure.

Establishing a fixed kVp technique chart involves producing phantom images, selecting the optimal phantom image, extrapolating a technique chart, and performing phantom testing, clinical trials, clinical fine-tuning, and ongoing fine-tuning.

REVIEW QUESTIONS

1. What is the principle of a fixed kVp exposure system?

2. What are the basic advantages of a fixed kVp exposure system?

3. What are the basic disadvantages of a fixed kVp exposure system?

4. Define optimal kVp.

5. How is the optimal kVp established?

6. What should be the minimal mAs increments used for variations in part thickness when using a fixed kVp exposure system?

REFERENCES AND RECOMMENDED READING

Bryan, G. J. (1970). *Diagnostic radiography: A manual for radiologic technologists.* Baltimore: Williams & Wilkins.

Cahoon, J. B. (1961). Radiographic technique: Its origin, concept, practical application and evaluation of radiation dosage. *The X-Ray Technician, 32,* 354–364.

Carlstein, C. J. (1971). Radiography of compressed air workers using optimum kilovoltage. *Radiologic Technology, 43*(1), 10–14.

Carroll, Q. B. (2003). *Fuchs's radiographic exposure, processing, and quality control* (7th ed.). Springfield, IL: Charles C Thomas.

Clark, K. C. (1953). An introduction to high-voltage technique. *Radiography, 19,* 21–33.

Compton, S. (1987). Bit conversion of technical factors in vascular procedures. *Radiologic Technology, 58*(5), 413.

Cullinan, A., & Cullinan, J. (1994). *Producing quality radiographs* (2nd ed.). Philadelphia: J. B. Lippincott.

Du Pont, E. I. de Nemours & Co. Medical Products Department, Customer Technology Center. *Bit system of technique conversion.* Wilmington, DE: Author.

Dyke, W. P. (1975). Depth resolution: A mechanism by which high kilovoltage improves visibility in chest films. *Radiology, 117,* 159–164.

Eastman Kodak Company, Health Sciences Markets Division. (1980). *The fundamentals of radiography* (12th ed.). (Kodak Publication M1-18). Rochester, NY: Author.

Eastman, T. R. (1969). Chest technique through body habitus. *Radiologic Technology, 41,* 80–84.

Eastman, T. R. (1971). Automated exposures in contemporary radiography. *Radiologic Technology, 43*(2), 80–83.

Eastman, T. R. (1973). Measurement: The key to exposure with manual techniques. *Radiologic Technology, 45,* 75–78.

Eastman, T. R. (1975). Technique charts: The key to radiographic quality. *Radiologic Technology, 46,* 365–368.

Eastman, T. R. (1978, July/August). A history of radiographic technique. *Applied Radiology* 97–100.

Eastman, T. R. (1979). *Radiographic fundamentals and technique guide.* St. Louis, MO: C. V. Mosby.

Files, G. W. (1952). *Medical radiographic technique.* Springfield, IL: Charles C Thomas.

Fodor, J., & Malott, J. C. (1993). *The art and science of medical radiography* (7th ed.). St. Louis, MO: C. V. Mosby.

Fodor, J., Malott, J. C., Ross, J. A., & Porter, M. (1985). Indications for the use of high kVp in the plain film examination of the abdomen. *Radiologic Technology, 57*(2), 159–161.

Fuchs, A. W. (1934). Radiography of entire body employing one film and a single exposure. *Radiography and Clinical Photography, 10,* 9–14.

Fuchs, A. W. (1938). Higher kilovoltage technic with high-definition screens. *Radiography and Clinical Photography, 14*(3), 2–8.

Fuchs, A. W. (1943). The optimum kilovoltage technique in military roentgenography. *American Journal of Roentgenology, 50,* 358–365.

Fuchs, A. W. (1945). Military photoroentgen technique employing optimum kilovolt (peak) principles. *The American Journal of Roentgenology, 53,* 587–596.

Fuchs, A. W. (1948). Relationship of tissue thickness to kilovoltage. *The X-Ray Technician, 19,* 287–293.

Fuchs, A. W. (1949). Control of radiographic density. *The X-Ray Technician, 20,* 271–273, 291.

Fuchs, A. W. (1950). The rationale of radiographic exposure. *The X-Ray Technician, 22,* 62–68, 76.

Fuchs, A. W. (1958). *Principles of radiographic exposure and processing* (2nd ed.). Springfield, IL: Charles C Thomas.

Funke, T. (1966). Pegged kilovoltage technic. *Radiologic Technology, 37,* 202–213.

Gratale, P., Turner, G. W., & Burns, C. B. (1986). Using the same exposure factors for wet and dry casts. *Radiologic Technology, 57*(4), 325–328.

Hiss, S. S. (1975). Technique management. *Radiologic Technology, 46*(5), 369.

Hiss, S. S. (2003). *Understanding radiography* (4th ed.). Springfield, IL: Charles C Thomas.

Hopper, B. S. (1957). Radiography above 100 peak kilovolts. *The X-Ray Technician, 29*(1), 9.

Jenkins, D. (1980). *Radiographic photography and imaging processes.* Lancaster, England: MTP Press Limited.

Jerman, E. C. (1926a). Extremity technic. *Radiology, 6,* 252–254.

Jerman, E. C. (1926b). Potter-Bucky diaphragm technic. *Radiology, 6,* 336–338.

Jerman, E. C. (1928). *Modern x-ray technic.* St. Paul, MN: Bruce.

Koenig, G. F. (1957). Kilovoltage as a qualitative factor. *The X-Ray Technician, 29,* 1–4, 13.

Koenig, G. F. (1966). Potential. *Radiologic Technology, 37*(4), 184–198.

Kratzer, B. (1973). A technique computer: Scientific approach to radiologic technology. *Radiologic Technology, 42*(4), 142–150.

Lyon, N. J. (1962). Optimum kilovoltage techniques. *The X-Ray Technician, 33,* 398–401.

Mahoney, G. J. (1959). A slide rule for kVp-mAs adjustments facilitating the use of high kilovoltage. *The X-Ray Technician, 31,* 35–38.

McDaniel, C. T. (1965). Tissue absorption theory applied to formulation of radiographic technique resulting in time as the variable factor. *Radiologic Technology, 37*(2), 51–55.

Merrill, H. F. (1960). High kilovoltage radiography. *The X-Ray Technician, 32*(3), 259.

Morgan, J. A. (1977). *The art and science of medical radiography* (5th ed.). St. Louis, MO: Catholic Hospital Association.

Morgan, R. H. (1949). An analysis of the physical factors controlling the diagnostic quality of roentgen images. *American Journal of Roentgenology and Radiation Therapy, 54,* 128; 54, 395; 55, 67; 55, 627.

Morgan, R. H. (1961). Physics of diagnostic radiology. *Physical foundations of radiology* (3rd ed.). New York: Paul Hoeber/Harper & Row.

Ott, T. T. (1963). Extending the range of medical radiography to 150 kilovolts. *The X-Ray Technician, 34*(6), 335–343.

Revesz, G., Shea, F. J., & Kundel, H. L. (1982). The effects of kilovoltage on diagnostic accuracy in chest radiography. *Radiology, 142,* 615–618.

Roderick, J. F. (1950). Photographic contrast in roentgenology. *The X-Ray Technician, 22,* 141–150, 163.

Roderick, J. F. (1952). Latitude in roentgenology. *The X-Ray Technician, 24,* 187–196, 220.

Sante, L. R. (1942). *Manual of roentgenological technique* (9th ed.). Ann Arbor, MI: Edwards Brothers.

Schwarz, G. S. (1958). A simple universal unit system of radiographic exposures suited to departmental, national, and international standardization. *Radiology, 71,* 573–574.

Schwarz, G. S. (1959a). Extended range radiography. *Radiology, 69,* 419–423, 1957.

Schwarz, G. S. (1959b). Kilovoltage and radiographic effect. *Radiology, 73,* 749–760.

Schwarz, G. S. (1960). Kilovoltage conversion in radiography. *The X-Ray Technician, 31,* 373–379, 436.

Schwarz, G. S. (1961). *Unit-step radiography.* Springfield, IL: Charles C Thomas.

Seeman, H. E. (1968). *Physical and photographic principles of medical radiography.* New York: Wiley & Sons.

Thomas, J. B. (1959). High kilovoltage equipment and technique. *The X-Ray Technician, 30*(6), 500.

Trout, E. D., Graves, D. E., & Slauson, D. B. (1949). High kilovoltage radiography. *Radiology, 52,* 669–683.

Tuddenham, W. J., Hale, J., & Pendergrass, E. P. (1953). Supervoltage diagnostic roentgenography. *American Journal of Roentgenology, 70*(5), 759–765.

United States Army. (1955, March). *Principles of radiographic exposure* (TM 8-282). Washington, DC.

United States War Department. (1941, July 3). *Technical manual: Roentgenographic technicians* (TM 8-240). Washington, DC.

van Dijk, D. (1955). Some factors influencing the results in radiography. *Medicamundi, 1,* 27–32.

Williams, W. A. (1960). Standardization of x-ray technique. *The X-Ray Technician, 32*(2), 137.

Wilsey, R. B. (1921). The intensity of scatter x-rays in radiography. *American Journal of Roentgenology, 8,* 328–338.

Wynroe, R. F. (1955). Some observations on kilovoltage variations. *Radiography, 21*(251), 242–243.

Yurcessen, E. H. (1954). Trend for higher kilovoltage for adequate penetration. *The X-Ray Technician, 26*(2), 96.

(Reprinted by permission of Dr. Marion Frank)

The Case of the Last Dinner

Of course this is a snake, but can you tell if the last dinner is still within the GI tract?

Answers to the case studies can be found in Appendix E.

CHAPTER 36

Variable Kilovoltage Systems

The [radiographer] who does his work by the "hunch method" can never successfully compete with one who having mastered the fundamentals is enabled to develop a proper procedure and put into the film any quality that may be desired.

Ed. C. Jerman, the Father of Radiography in the United States

KEY TERM

patient equivalent phantom

OBJECTIVES

Upon completion of this chapter, the student should be able to:

- Describe a variable kilovoltage technique system.

- Discuss the primary advantages and disadvantages of variable kVp technique systems.

- State the 2 kVp rule.

- Explain why more than a single kilovoltage scale is required.

- Calculate new exposure factors from a single satisfactory exposure when mAs ratios are provided.

- Synthesize a stepped variable kVp technique chart from control images.

PRINCIPLES OF A VARIABLE KILOVOLTAGE PEAK EXPOSURE SYSTEM

A variable kilovoltage x-ray exposure technique system is one in which the kilovoltage to be used for a particular projection is varied depending on measured body part thickness. The thicker the body part, the higher the value of kilovoltage assigned. A milliampere-second value is specified for each body part to be examined. Its value depends on image receptor exposure and other parameters.

In use, the radiographer sets the mAs specified for the part and measured part thickness. The value of kVp corresponding to that thickness is found on the chart. For example, in Table 36-1, a 12 cm thick part will require 54 kVp (e.g., an average shoulder).

Advantages and Disadvantages

Technique systems that use variable kilovoltage offer the advantage of permitting small incremental changes in exposure to compensate for variation in body part thickness. These changes in exposure may not be possible with systems that fix kilovoltage and vary milliampere-seconds because of an insufficient number of settings on the exposure timers of many x-ray generators.

A potential disadvantage of the variable kilovoltage technique arises when one considers the complexity of the effect of changing kilovoltage on the way the subject is imaged. Increasing kilovoltage reduces image contrast. Reducing contrast may be helpful if the initial kilovoltage is too low to provide adequate penetration of the part (Figure 36-1A). The reduction in contrast that occurs when kilovoltage is too high can reduce the radiologist's ability to see fine detail in the image (Figure 36-1C). A useful variable kilovoltage system must use values of kilovoltage that provide adequate penetration of the part and result in a level of contrast that is acceptable to the radiologist (Figure 36-1B).

TABLE 36-1.	2 kVp per cm Chart				
cm	10	11	12	13	14
kVp	50	52	54	56	58

The radiation exposure to the patient is strongly dependent on the kilovoltage used for the projection. In general, the higher the kilovoltage, the lower the patient dose. When kilovoltage is at an appropriate level for the body part examined, patient dose considerations are less of a factor when deciding whether to establish an exposure system using fixed or variable kVp.

Historical Development

In the early days of radiography it was common practice to use a change of 2 kVp for every 1 cm of tissue thickness. A kilovoltage progression could be readily computed by taking two times the centimeter measurement. To this value a constant, such as 30 kVp, was added to achieve a kVp value high enough to penetrate the part. This produces a basic variable kVp formula:

$(2 \text{ kVp} \times \text{part cm}) + 30 \text{ kVp} = \text{new kVp}$

> ***EXAMPLE:*** What is the proper kilovoltage for a 20 cm part thickness?
>
> ***Answer:***
>
> $(2 \text{ kVp} \times \text{part cm}) + 30 \text{ kVp} = \text{new kVp}$
> $(2 \text{ kVp} \times 20 \text{ cm}) + 30 \text{ kVp} = \text{new kVp}$
> $(40 \text{ kVp/cm}) + 30 \text{ kVp} = 70 \text{ kVp}$

It was found that multiple kilovoltage scales were needed because the values selected from the progression could be too low to provide adequate penetration of body parts, such as the shoulder or cervical spine, which contain dense bone with little soft tissue (Table 36-2A). Higher kilovoltage scales were created by increasing the base kilovoltage added. For example, if kilovoltage were computed using 40 kVp instead of 30 kVp, the formula would be:

$(2 \text{ kVp} \times \text{part cm}) + 40 \text{ kVp} = \text{new kVp}$

52 kVp	1200 mAs	42" SID
16:1 grid	300 RS	1550 mR

A

70 kVp	160 mAs	42" SID
16:1 grid	300 RS	580 mR

B

115 kVp	10 mAs	42" SID
16:1 grid	400 RS	106 mR

C

FIGURE 36-1 Comparison of contrast produced at three kilovoltage ranges: (A) high contrast at low (52) kilovoltage; (B) ideal contrast produced at approximate (70) kilovoltage; and (C) low contrast produced at high (115) kilovoltage.

TABLE 36-2. Variable Kilovoltage Scales

A 2 kVp/cm + 30		B 2 kVp/cm + 40		C 2 kVp/cm + 50	
cm	kVp	cm	kVp	cm	kVp
2	34	2	44	2	54
3	36	3	46	3	56
4	38	4	48	4	58
5	40	5	50	5	60
6	42	6	52	6	62
7	44	7	54	7	64
8	46	8	56	8	66
9	48	9	58	9	68
10	50	10	60	10	70
11	52	11	62	11	72
12	54	12	64	12	74
13	56	13	66	13	76
14	58	14	68	14	78
15	60	15	70	15	80
16	62	16	72	16	82
17	64	17	74	17	84
18	66	18	76	18	86
19	68	19	78	19	88
20	70	20	80	20	90
21	72	21	82	21	92
22	74	22	84	22	94
23	76	23	86	23	96
24	78	24	88	24	98
25	80	25	90	25	100
26	82	26	92	26	102
27	84	27	94	27	104
28	86	28	96	28	106
29	88	29	98	29	108
30	90	30	100	30	110
31	92	31	102	31	112
32	94	32	104	32	114
33	96	33	106	33	116
34	98	34	108	34	118
35	100	35	110	35	120
36	102	36	112	36	122

EXAMPLE: What is the proper kilovoltage for the same 20 cm part thickness using the new formula?

Answer:

$$(2 \text{ kVp} \times \text{part cm}) + 40 \text{ kVp} = \text{new kVp}$$
$$(2 \text{ kVp} \times 20 \text{ cm}) + 40 \text{ kVp} = \text{new kVp}$$
$$(40 \text{ kVp/cm}) + 40 \text{ kVp} = 80 \text{ kVp}$$

All values would be correspondingly higher with the new formula. For example, the values of shoulder and cervical spine views measuring 12 cm would be 64 kVp instead of the 54 kVp previously obtained. By increasing or decreasing the value of kVp added as a constant, it is possible to create an array of kilovoltage scales. The scales shown in Tables 36-2A–C were computed using 30, 40, and 50 kVp as the constant:

$$(2 \text{ kVp} \times \text{part cm}) + 30 \text{ kVp} = \text{new kVp}$$
$$(2 \text{ kVp} \times \text{part cm}) + 40 \text{ kVp} = \text{new kVp}$$
$$(2 \text{ kVp} \times \text{part cm}) + 50 \text{ kVp} = \text{new kVp}$$

Note that the kilovoltage values for a 20 cm thick body part are shown as 70 kVp, 80 kVp, and 90 kVp, depending on the scale selected.

Changes of 10 kVp in the base number added were used in the belief that a change of ±10 kVp would compensate for doubling and halving mAs. In practice 30, 40, or 50 can be easily added to centimeters doubled by the radiographer mentally and the assigned value of kVp can thus be readily determined when charts are not available. Milliampere-second values were found by trial and error but, once determined, were listed for a particular body part and kilovoltage selected by measuring the part. A useful technique chart was thus created.

It was found in practice that 80 kVp for a 20 cm abdomen using equipment and image receptors of the time was nearly ideal. In 1948, Fuchs suggested that kVp be fixed at 80 for the abdomen, with mAs varied to compensate for the size difference of patients. Fixed kilovoltage techniques, sometimes called optimum techniques, are described in Chapter 35. They are mentioned here to point out that similar results may be obtained regardless of the system employed in order to handle the variables of kVp, mA, and time.

Although the kilovoltage scales shown in Table 36-2A, B, and C were useful in practical pa-tient radiography, and in fact would still be useful, two assumptions used in their computation were found to be false. The notion that a ±10 kVp change will balance a change of double or half mAs has largely given way to the so-called 15 percent rule. This rule suggests decreasing kVp by 15 percent to reduce exposure by half and increasing kVp by 15 percent to double exposure. Although the 15 percent rule better reflects the exponentially nonlinear changes that occur when kilovoltage is altered, it is not totally accurate either. These relationships are among the most complex in radiography and remain difficult to quantify.

When the 15 percent rule is applied, it can be readily seen that a 7.5 kVp change is required at 50 kVp (15 percent × 50 kVp) to balance a 50 percent reduction in mAs, while at 100 kVp, a 15 kVp change (15 percent × 100 kVp) is required. This reflects the fact that at low kilovoltage a small change in kVp can have a large effect on exposure, while at higher kilovoltage a larger change will be required to produce the same effect. A uniform change of 2 kVp per centimeter in tissue thickness will not function satisfactorily over a wide range of tissue thicknesses. At a fixed value of mAs and proper exposure of an average patient, images of thicker patients will become increasingly underexposed as patient size increases.

Early users of variable kilovoltage techniques computed kVp scales using 2 kVp per centimeter plus a constant and ±10 kVp between the scales. They were able to use such charts successfully chiefly because the range of variation in adult body part thicknesses is small (see Table 34-1). Thus, kilovoltage values used for a particular body part are within a relatively narrow range. Since mAs values were found by trial and error using kilovoltage from the scales according to patient measurement, problems due to the use of ±10 kVp change between the scales were minimized, if not entirely eliminated. In addition, a patient whose body habitus varies from the norm is easily recognized by an experienced radiographer, and it was common practice then, as now, to increase or decrease the mAs according to the radiographer's professional judgment in compensation for body habitus and known pathological conditions.

ESTABLISHING A STEPPED VARIABLE KVP SYSTEM

The variable kilovoltage technique systems used today have evolved from the earlier systems. A modern stepped kVp system can be developed in a manner similar to the "pegged kilovoltage technic" system published by Funke in 1966. These systems are based on the concept that straight variable kilovoltage charts are inadequate (such as those shown in Table 36-2A, B, and C). They all recommend kVp settings for extremely small parts that may not provide adequate penetration. These charts also recommend kVp settings for extremely large parts that may produce excessive scatter fog. In other words, unsatisfactory contrast is produced for both small and large part sizes with a straight variable kilovoltage chart.

The kVp Scale

This problem is remedied by establishing a limited variable kilovoltage scale that meets three criteria:

1. All contrast is acceptable to the radiologists.
2. Small part size kVp recommendations provide adequate penetration.
3. Large part size kVp recommendations avoid excessive scatter fog.

Initial Phantom Images

The limited variable kilovoltage scale is determined by producing a series of radiographs according to a straight variable kilovoltage charts such as those shown in Table 36-2A, B, and C. A phantom in a variable depth water bath is used to simulate the various part thicknesses. A variable depth water bath is made by placing a radiographic phantom in a watertight Plexiglas box and then filling it with water to the desired centimeter thickness. A much less complicated, although suboptimal simulation of this procedure, is to simply image a phantom at various kVp levels without changing the part thickness. Both procedures will produce a series of phantom images ranging from very high (or even inadequate penetration) contrast to very low contrast with excessive scatter fog.

Select Optimal Phantom Image

If the resulting image is over or underexposed, a repeat image with an appropriate mAs adjustment is made. This process is continued on subsequent patients until ideal diagnostic quality images are obtained. The kVp should not be altered from the value shown for part thickness in Table 36-3.

The use of a **patient equivalent phantom** can reduce or eliminate the need for patient exposures. The American National Standards Institute (ANSI) patient equivalent phantom (PEP) is recommended for this purpose. Technical factors required to produce a density of OD 1.4 with the PEP are suited for use on a 21 cm AP lumbar spine patient. Use the kVp for a 21 cm patient from the chart and find the mAs required by trial exposures. If an ANSI phantom is not available, a smooth bottom plastic wastebasket filled with tap water to a depth of 17 cm has been used successfully for technique development. Use kVp from the chart for a 21 cm AP lumbar spine, and by trial exposure find the mAs required to produce OD 1.4.

The series of images that are produced will demonstrate a wide range of contrast. They are evaluated by **all** radiologists and those other physicians deemed critical to the image quality process. Each physician indicates those images they are not willing to accept for diagnosis. When this evaluation is complete, the variable kilovoltage scale is reduced to only those kVp levels that are within the acceptable diagnostic range for the physicians who will be diagnosing from the images. This reduction will eliminate some of the part sizes from the chart (see Table 36-3, Step 1).

Extrapolate Technique Chart

Once the range of acceptable diagnostic images has been established, a complete technique chart can be computed. The elimination of suboptimal images leaves only the kVp ranges acceptable to the physicians and forms a limited "step" of acceptable kilovoltage. Steps should be formed in groups of 4–5 cm increments as this makes mAs adjustments much simpler.

TABLE 36-3. Stepped Variable kVp Technique Chart

2 kVp/cm + 40							
Establishing a Limited Variable kVp Scale				Extrapolating kVp Steps		Fine-Tuning of Extrapolated kVp Values	
Step 1				Step 2		Step 3	
cm	kVp	mAs	evaluation	kVp	mAs	kVp	mAs
4	54	20	reject	70	5	70	5
6	56	20	reject	72	5	72	5
8	58	20	reject	74	5	74	5
10	60	20	reject	76	5	76	5
11	62	20	reject	78	5	70	10
12	64	20	reject	80	5	72	10
13	66	20	reject	82	5	74	10
14	68	20	reject	84	5	76	10
15	70	20	acceptable	70	20	70	20
16	72	20	acceptable	72	20	72	20
17	74	20	acceptable	74	20	74	20
18	76	20	acceptable	76	20	76	20
19	78	20	acceptable	78	20	78	20
20	80	20	acceptable	80	20	80	20
21	82	20	acceptable	82	20	82	20
22	84	20	acceptable	84	20	84	20
23	86	20	reject	70	80	78	40
24	88	20	reject	72	80	80	40
25	90	20	reject	74	80	82	40
26	92	20	reject	76	80	84	40
27	94	20	reject	78	80	78	80
28	96	20	reject	80	80	80	80
29	98	20	reject	82	80	82	80
30	100	20	reject	84	80	84	80
31	102	20	reject	70	320	78	160
32	104	20	reject	72	320	80	160
33	106	20	reject	74	320	82	160
34	108	20	reject	76	320	84	160
35	110	20	reject	78	320	78	320
36	112	20	reject	80	320	80	320
37	114	20	reject	82	320	82	320
38	118	20	reject	84	320	84	320

The mAs Scale

Establishing the kVp steps in increments of 4–5 cm permits simple doubling or halving of mAs to maintain image density. Changes of 4–5 cm in tissue thickness require doubling or halving of mAs to maintain approximately the same image receptor exposure. The chart is revised to eliminate the rejected kVp ranges by establishing extrapolated kVp steps for the entire chart (see Table 36-3, Step 2). At this point in the development of the chart it should be obvious that there are a number of inappropriate kVp ranges. For example, a 14 cm part should not be radiographed at 84 kVp, nor should a 31 cm part be radiographed at 70 kVp. Therefore, it is necessary to fine-tune the extrapolated kVp steps to bring these kVp values within appropriate ranges for penetration and scatter control (see Table 36-3, Step 3). This is accomplished by applying the 4–5 cm rule and/or the 15 percent rule to modify the kVp to an appropriate value while maintaining an acceptable exposure. Note that in Table 36-3, Step 3, the kVp steps follow an even 4 cm, doubling or halving of mAs pattern with only the 20 mAs values utilizing the entire accepted range of 70–84 kVp. This is because the fine-tuning process determined that the upper kVp range (78–84 kVp) produced overpenetration of the small part sizes while the lower kVp range (70–78 kVp) did not adequately penetrate the larger part sizes.

Phantom Testing

Phantom testing is recommended prior to performing patient examinations. At the minimum, phantom testing should be done for a median, small, and large part size as a fine-tuning mechanism for the extrapolated chart prior to clinical use.

Clinical Trials

Limited clinical trials are then permissible with the new chart. All images should be recorded with repeated images saved for analysis. When clinical trials are proceeding without excess repeated exposures, the new technique chart can move into the clinical fine-tuning stage.

Clinical Fine-Tuning

The clinical fine-tuning process is designed to adjust and validate the entire chart. At this point the new technique chart can be adapted. However, ongoing fine-tuning then begins as a permanent process.

Ongoing Fine-Tuning

Ongoing fine-tuning is the process that maintains the accuracy of the entire exposure system and is crucial to both radiographers and radiologists developing a confidence in the exposure and diagnostic processes. It is performed by maintaining an accurate record of modifications to existing techniques for review by the person responsible for quality control.

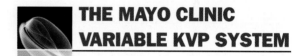

THE MAYO CLINIC VARIABLE KVP SYSTEM

A modern version of a variable kilovoltage chart currently in use in the Mayo Clinic Department of Diagnostic Radiology is shown in Table 36-4. A precursor to this chart was originally established by Raymond Runge of Mayo Clinic about 1925. As was common practice, the first versions were constructed using kilovoltage corresponding to two times the centimeter measurement plus a constant. Runge recognized the deficiencies of this approach and made revisions in his later experiments by using a water phantom, which greatly improved the results. Modifications were made by Winkler to further refine the kilovoltage progressions and, also by Stears and Frank for rare-earth intensifying screens.

The kVp Scale

The kilovoltage versus measured centimeter thickness chart shown in Table 36-4 has the kilovoltage values arranged in seven columns plus one column corresponding to centimeter thickness of the part examined. For a given centimeter thickness, there are up to seven kVp values that may be selected. For a 21 cm patient thickness, these values are 52, 58, 63, 72, 80, 95, and 115 kVp. Note that the kilovoltage columns are labeled Scale 8, Scale 4, Scale 2,

TABLE 36–4. Kilovoltage vs. Measured Centimeter Thickness Chart

SCALE 8	SCALE 4	SCALE 2	SCALE 1	CM	½ SCALE	¼ SCALE	⅛ SCALE
		47	52	6	58	63	72
		48	53	7	59	64	73
		49	54	8	60	66	74
		50	55	9	61	68	76
	SCALE 4	51	56	10	62	70	78
	47	52	58	11	63	72	80
	48	53	59	12	64	73	82
	49	54	60	13	66	74	84
	50	55	61	14	68	76	87
SCALE 8	51	56	62	15	70	78	91
47	52	58	63	16	72	80	95
48	53	59	64	17	73	82	98
49	54	60	66	18	74	84	101
50	55	61	68	19	76	87	105
51	56	62	70	20	78	91	110
52	58	63	72	21	80	95	115
53	59	64	73	22	82	98	120
54	60	66	74	23	84	101	125
55	61	68	76	24	87	105	130
56	61	70	78	25	91	110	135
58	63	72	80	26	95	115	140
59	64	73	82	27	98	120	
60	66	74	84	28	101	125	
61	68	76	87	29	105		
62	70	78	91	30	110		
63	72	80	95	31	115		
64	73	82	98	32	120		
66	74	84	101	33	125		
68	76	87	105	34	130		
70	78	91	110	35	135		
72	80	95	115	36	140		
73	82	98	120	37			
74	84	101	125	38			
76	87	105	130	39			
78	91	110	135	40			
80	95	115	140	41			

EXTREMITY CASSETTE

CM	kVp
1	45
2	47
3	49
4	52
5	55
6	58
7	61
8	64
9	67
10	70

TABLE 36-4.	Kilovoltage vs. Measured Centimeter Thickness Chart (continued)

Extremity—Non-Bucky	TIME	mA	kVp			TFD	CASSETTE
REGULAR CASSETTE				45" (ALL)			
Ankle/Elbow	.016	200	1/4			48"	24 × 30 cm
Tibia–Fibula	.016	200	1/4			48"	14 × 17 in
Calcaneus	.016	200	1/2			48"	8 × 10 in
Wrist–Carpal Tunnel	.033	200	65 kVp			48"	8 × 10 in
Cast–Plaster	.033	200	1/4			48"	
Cast–Fiberglass	.016	200	1/4			48"	
EXTREMITY CASSETTE			SM	MED	LG		
Hand/Wrist PA/OBL	.025	200	58	60	62	48"	24 × 30 cm
Hand/Wrist LAT	.025	200	63	65	67	48"	8 × 10 in
Forearm	.025	200	Extremity Scale			48"	7 × 17 in
Toes	.025	200	58	60	62	48"	24 × 30 cm
Foot	.025	200	63	65	67	48"	24 × 30 cm
Lateral Calcaneus	.025	200	63	65	67	45"	8 × 10 in

Scale 1, 1/2 Scale, 1/4 Scale, and 1/8 Scale. The kilovoltage change from one scale to the next at any given centimeter thickness is that amount that will be equal to reducing mAs by half or doubling it. For example, using kilovoltage values from Scale 1 as a base at the 21 cm level (72 kVp), a shift to 1/2 Scale (80 kVp) will permit reducing mAs by 1/2. A change from Scale 1 to 1/4 Scale allows mAs to be reduced to 1/4 the value for kVp Scale 1, while kVp from the 1/8 Scale would allow use of 1/8 the mAs. Use of the lower kVp values obtained from Scale 2, Scale 4, and Scale 8 would require the use of two times, four times, or eight times the mAs used with the kVp from Scale 1.

Images obtained are similarly exposed but, because of the extreme range of kilovoltage used (52–115), vary widely from too high to too low contrast (see Figure 36-1). In practice, the column from which kilovoltage is selected is specified to produce a level of contrast preferred by radiologists. For a patient 21 cm in thickness, the 1/2 Scale value, 80 kVp, is used if the generator is single phase. Lower kVp from Scale 1 (72 kVp) is chosen to maintain similar image contrast if a three-phase generator is used. Arrangement of the kilovoltage columns such that the kVp changes by moving from any column to its neighbor permits halving or doubling mAs while allowing great flexibility in the use of the scales. This also permits selection of a kVp value to provide adequate penetration of any examined part, and thus produces optimum image contrast.

The kilovoltage change necessary between the scales to balance doubling or halving mAs was initially derived from water phantom experiments. Kilovoltage progression (the increase in kilovoltage needed for each increase of one centimeter of tissue thickness) was obtained by using a doubling increase in kilovoltage for each 5 cm increase in part thickness. For example, in Table 36-4, the kVp value for a 21 cm measurement shown in 1/2 Scale

(80 kVp) is listed in Scale 1 for a 26 cm measurement, and the 1/2 Scale value for 26 cm (95 kVp) is listed in Scale 1 corresponding to 31 cm. All scales have been constructed using a double technique kVp value for each 5 cm change in thickness. Values for centimeters between the technique doubling points are chosen to provide a smooth progression but rounded off to the nearest whole kVp.

Determination of kilovoltage, though important, gives only one of the primary exposure factors. In a variable kVp technique system, kilovoltage selection is made by first measuring the examined part and then selecting a value from the kVp tables, as previously described. Values of distance, milliamperage, and time must also be determined in any useful technique system.

Source-to-Image Receptor Distance

The inverse square relationship between SID and radiation intensity permits a small difference in SID to translate into a large difference in exposure of the image receptor. For this reason, the SID should be specified for each examination.

As a practical matter, and to avoid off focal distance grid cut-off of primary radiation, the focal distance of the x-ray table Bucky should be used. Because some table grids are difficult to examine without dismantling the x-ray table, it may be helpful to know that most equipment manufacturers provide 40″ focal distance grids for most x-ray tables. For this reason, a 40″ SID is often the best choice, unless the particular Bucky grid employed is known to have been manufactured for use at another focal range.

A useful SID selection for most routine radiography would be 40″ (100 cm) for flat Bucky work and extremities, with 72″ (180 cm) used for upright chest work. It is important that whatever SID is selected, the value be noted on the technique chart, and that all users of the chart recognize that an alteration in technique must be made if the specified SID is not used for a particular examination.

mAs. A useful technique system requires determination of the value of mAs that will provide proper

exposure to the image receptor when used in combination with the kilovoltage chosen. During phantom testing, milliamperage-seconds are increased or decreased in doubling or halving increments for sequential radiographs until proper exposure is achieved. The mAs value that has been determined is then recorded in terms of mAs or mA and time use on the technique chart. This method of determining mAs by trial and error was thoroughly described by Fuchs. Kratzer's Supertech™, Trinkle's Du Pont Bit System, the Siemens Point System, and Schwartz's XVS system are examples of other systems and devices that have been designed to assist in the process of x-ray technique development. Although the number of trial and error exposures that must be made can be dramatically reduced with the use of any of the systems mentioned above, the development of an effective x-ray technique system for an individual x-ray department can be successfully accomplished only by that department.

mAs Ratios

In the late 1980s Frank and Winkler presented a method of computing an x-ray exposure technique with the use of mAs ratios. The system of mAs ratios was devised by Winkler, who set up mathematical relationships from trial and error exposure determinations for various body parts that had been made by Runge. Reference to the kilovoltage scales in Table 36-4 is made to select values of kVp for use with mAs values for the examined part, which are computed using the mAs ratios after a base exposure is found. The advantage of the system lies in the radiographer's ability to compute mAs values for all body parts once the mAs value for only one body part has been found by trial and error. The need to examine large numbers of patients with multiple trials is eliminated. Minor changes in computed mAs values found for some views may be desirable following a period of use.

The resulting technique system of mAs ratios combined with kilovoltage varied with part thickness may be categorized as **variable kVp within an optimal range.** For example, the average thickness for an adult shoulder ranges from 12–16 cm.

Kilovoltage for these extremes will be 64–72 kVp (from 1/2 Scale, shown in Table 36-4). Thus, the actual kilovoltage range typically used is narrow for any given body part. The best features of variable kVp techniques (small incremental changes) and fixed kVp techniques (optimal contrast) are obtained.

As previously described, the thickness of the examined part is measured where specified or along the path of the central ray. The value of the kVp corresponding to the thickness of the part is selected from the kVp chart. For example, for a shoulder measuring 14 cm, 1/2 Scale is specified with a three-phase generator and a value of 68 kVp is found, while the mAs is fixed.

The mAs ratios used in technique computation are shown in Table 36-5. Computed mAs values are used with kilovoltage corresponding to part thickness from the chart in Table 36-4. In this system, the AP projection of the lumbar spine is assigned a value of 1.0. Existing exposure techniques, which had been established by Runge using trial and error exposure for each body part, were used in computing the ratios by the following formula:

$$\frac{\text{mAs for body part}}{\text{mAs for AP lumbar}} = \text{mAs ratio for body part}$$

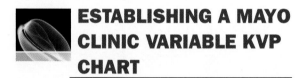

ESTABLISHING A MAYO CLINIC VARIABLE KVP CHART

Initial Phantom Images

When a new technique chart is computed using the mAs ratios, mAs for the AP lumbar spine is first found by patient examination. In the process, the patient's thickness is measured, kVp is selected from the kilovoltage chart found in Table 36-4 and the required mAs is estimated based on previous experience. Only those patients referred for a lumbar spine examination should be involved in the process.

Select Optimal Phantom Image

If the resulting image is over or underexposed, a repeat image with an appropriate mAs adjustment is made. This process is continued on subsequent patients until ideal diagnostic quality images are obtained. The kVp should not be altered from the value shown for part thickness in Table 36-4.

The use of a patient equivalent phantom can reduce or eliminate the need for patient exposures. The American National Standards Institute (ANSI) patient equivalent phantom (PEP) is recommended for this purpose. Technical factors required to produce a density of OD 1.4 with the PEP are suited for use on a 21 cm AP lumbar spine patient. Use the kVp for a 21 cm patient from the chart and find the mAs required by trial exposures.

Extrapolate Technique Chart

Once the mAs value that produces an optimal diagnostic quality image for the AP lumbar spine has been established, a complete technique chart is computed from that value as follows:

1. Values are substituted in the mAs ratio formula. For example, if 66 mAs was found to be a good value for the AP lumbar, it becomes the constant for all further calculations.
2. The mAs ratio for the body part is found in Table 36–5 and the formula is used to calculate the new mAs for the body part.

EXAMPLE: The shoulder has an mAs ratio of 0.30. What is the appropriate mAs value that should be used for a system that produces a satisfactory AP lumbar at 66 mAs?

Answer:

$$\frac{\text{mAs for body part}}{\text{mAs for AP lumbar}} = \text{mAs ratio for body part}$$

$$\frac{\text{mAs for body part}}{66 \text{ mAs}} = 0.30$$

$$\text{mAs for body part} = 66 \text{ mAs} \times 0.30$$

$$\text{mAs for body part} = 19.8 \approx 20 \text{ mAs}$$

TABLE 36-5. mAs Ratios

	Body Parts		
Examination	mAs Ratios	kVp 3-Phase	kVp 1-Phase
Skull AP & LAT Adult	.45	$\frac{1}{2}$ scale	$\frac{1}{4}$ scale
Cervical AP	.60	$\frac{1}{2}$	$\frac{1}{4}$
Lateral (Cross Table)	.15	$\frac{1}{2}$	$\frac{1}{4}$
OBL (Tabletop)	.20	$\frac{1}{2}$	$\frac{1}{4}$
Swimmers	.75	1	$\frac{1}{2}$
Odontoid (30″)	.25	$\frac{1}{2}$	$\frac{1}{4}$
Pillar	1.00	$\frac{1}{4}$	$\frac{1}{8}$
Thoracic AP (Filter)	1.50	1	$\frac{1}{2}$
(without Filter)	.75	1	$\frac{1}{2}$
Thoracic LAT (Filter)	3.04	2	1
(without Filter)	.50	2	1
Thoracic Lower LAT (No Filter)	.60	2	1
Lumbar AP and Abdomen (19–23 cm)	1.00	1	$\frac{1}{2}$
Lumbar OBL (19–23 cm)	1.50	1	$\frac{1}{2}$
Lumbar LAT	1.50	1	$\frac{1}{2}$
Lumbar LOC LAT	1.50	1	$\frac{1}{2}$
Lumbar Graft LAT (L5–S1)	3.04	2	1
Lumbar Flexion/Extension	3.04	2	1
Pelvis & Hip/OBL	1.50	1	$\frac{1}{2}$
Hips LAT	1.50	1	$\frac{1}{2}$
Sacrum AP	1.50	1	$\frac{1}{2}$
Coccyx AP	1.50	1	$\frac{1}{2}$
Sacrum, Coccyx LAT	3.00	2	1
S-I Joints	1.50	1	$\frac{1}{2}$
Shoulder AP	.30	$\frac{1}{2}$	$\frac{1}{4}$
Y or Neer View	.30	$\frac{1}{2}$	$\frac{1}{4}$
Transthoracic Lateral	.13	$\frac{1}{2}$	$\frac{1}{4}$
Axillary (Grid)	.30	$\frac{1}{2}$	$\frac{1}{4}$
Scapula AP & LAT OBL	.39	$\frac{1}{2}$	$\frac{1}{4}$
Clavicle	.30	$\frac{1}{2}$	$\frac{1}{4}$
Humerus	.30	$\frac{1}{2}$	$\frac{1}{4}$
Femur	.60	$\frac{1}{2}$	$\frac{1}{4}$
LAT & OBL fir Vessels	.40	$\frac{1}{2}$	$\frac{1}{4}$
Knee	.19	$\frac{1}{4}$	$\frac{1}{8}$
Intercondylar Notch	.075	$\frac{1}{2}$	$\frac{1}{4}$
Patella (Merchants)	.075	$\frac{1}{4}$	$\frac{1}{8}$
Chest, Lateral Supine (Bucky)	.025	$\frac{1}{2}$	$\frac{1}{4}$
Bucky Chest	.17	$\frac{1}{2}$	$\frac{1}{4}$
Chest, Lateral Supine (Bucky)	.25	1	$\frac{1}{2}$
Chest, Lateral Decubitus (Grid)	.13	$\frac{1}{2}$	$\frac{1}{4}$
Lateral Sternum	1.50	1	$\frac{1}{2}$
Ribs Above Diaphragm	.25	1	$\frac{1}{2}$
Ribs Below Diaphragm (19–23 cm)	1.00	1	$\frac{1}{2}$

TABLE 36-5.	mAs Ratios (continued)		

| Examination | Extremities[1] | | |
	mAs Ratios Extremities[1]	kVp 3–Phase	kVp 1–Phase
Regular cassette: Non–Bucky			
Ankle/Elbow	.075	$\frac{1}{2}$ scale	$\frac{1}{4}$ scale
Tibia–Fibula	.075	$\frac{1}{2}$	$\frac{1}{4}$
Calcaneus	.075	$\frac{1}{4}$	$\frac{1}{8}$
Wrist–Carpal Tunnel	.075	65 kVp	73 kVp (no caliper)
Cast–Plaster	.15	$\frac{1}{2}$	$\frac{1}{4}$
Cast–Fiberglass	.10	$\frac{1}{2}$	$\frac{1}{4}$
Extremity cassette: Non–Bucky			
Hand/Wrist–PA/OBL	.25	58 60 62	
Hand/Wrist–LAT	.25	63 65 67	
Forearm	.25	EXT Scale (use caliper)	
Toes	.25	58 60 62	
Foot	.25	63 65 67	

—mAs ratios are based on: Lumbar AP, 21 cm technique and a density of 1.4 (± 0.10) from the standard phantom.[2] Always use this *base technique* for the calculations.

—All values are for bucky/grid unless specified.

—All values are for adult techniques.

—All values are for 48″ unless specified.

—The following examinations each have three exposure time and kVp values. The mAs ratio is for the *middle measurement* (19–23 cm): Lumbar AP and Abdomen; Lumbar Oblique; Ribs below diaphragm.

[1]May vary depending on tabletop attenuation and speed of system.

[2]Gray, Winkler, Stears, Frank, *Quality Control in Diagnostic Radiology*. Aspen Publishers Incorporated, Rockville, 1983.

The kilovoltage is selected from 1/2 Scale (see Table 36-4), which yields 64 kVp for a shoulder measuring 12 cm. Technical factors for the shoulder are 20 mAs, 64 kVp. An appropriate mA and time selection for 20 mAs might be 200 mA at 0.10 second.

Computed techniques should be entered in a technique chart that is prominently posted in the x-ray control booth for ready reference by the radiographers (Table 36-6).

It is usually most advantageous to list values of mA and time rather than mAs unless only mAs is shown on the control. This approach frees the radiographer from being required to calculate appropriate mA and time values and reduces the likelihood of errors that could cause repeats. Additionally, the use of a single mA setting eliminates the potential for exposure problems caused by variations in x-ray output that may exist between the mA stations available on a generator, and calculations of technical factors are simplified.

TABLE 36-6. Variable Kilovoltage Technique Chart

Examination	Time	mA	kVp	mAs	TFD	Cassette
Skull					45"(ALL)	
SKULL, AP, LAT Adult	.20	200	$1/4$	40	48"	24 × 30 cm
Cervical spine						
Cervical AP 10° ↑	.15	200	$1/4$	30	48"	8 × 10 in
Lateral (Cross-Table) (NON–GRID)	.05	200	$1/4$	10.2	48"	24 × 30 cm
OBL (Table Top)	0.66	200	$1/4$	13.2	48"	24 × 30 cm
Swimmer's	.40	200	$1/2$	80	48"	24 × 30 cm
Odontoid	.20	200	$1/4$	40	30"	8 × 10 in
Piller 30° ↓	.30	200	$1/8$	60	48"	24 × 30 cm
Thoracic spine						
Thoracic AP (Filter)	.40	200	$1/2$	80	48"	24 × 30 cm
Thoracic LAT (Filter)	.60	↓	1	120	48"	24 × 30 cm
	THIN	AVERAGE		PORTLY		
	100 mAs	150 mAs		200 mAs		
Thoracic Lower LAT (Filter)	.30	200	1	60	48"	24 × 30 cm
Lumbar spine/abdomen						
Lumbar AP 5° ↑ and Abdomen						
−18 cm	.15	200	$1/4$	30	48"	24 × 30 cm
19–23 cm	.30	200	$1/2$	60	48"	24 × 30 cm
24 cm	.60	200	1	120	48"	24 × 30 cm
Lumbar OBL 42° 5° ↑						
−18 cm	.10	200	$1/8$	20	48"	24 × 30 cm
19–23 cm	.20	200	$1/4$	40	48"	24 × 30 cm
24 cm	.50	200	$1/2$	100	48"	24 × 30 cm
Lumbar LAT Meas L–2	.40	200	$1/2$	80	48"	30 × 35 cm
Lumbar Loc LAT Meas L–5	.40	200	$1/2$	80	48"	8 × 10 in
Lumbar Graft LAT	.40	200	$1/2$	80	48"	24 × 30 cm
Lumbar Flexion & Extension	.40	200	$1/2$	80	48"	30 × 35 cm
Pelvic region						
Pelvis & Hips AP / OBL 5° ↓	.40	200	$1/2$	80	48"	35 × 43 cm
Hips LAT	.80	200	$1/2$	160	48"	24 × 30 cm
Sacrum AP 5° ↑	.40	200	$1/2$	80	48"	24 × 30 cm
Coccyx AP 10° ↓	.40	200	$1/2$	80	48"	24 × 30 cm
Sacrum, Coccyx LAT	.80	200	1	160	48"	24 × 30 cm
S–I Joints (R & LPO 20°)	.40	200	$1/2$	80	48"	24 × 30 cm

TABLE 36-6. Variable Kilovoltage Technique Chart (continued)

Examination	Time	mA	kVp	mAs	TFD	Cassette
Shoulder						
Shoulder AP	.10	200	$\frac{1}{4}$	20	48″	24 × 30 cm
Neer View	.10	200	$\frac{1}{4}$	20	48″	24 × 30 cm
Transthoracic Lateral	.10	200	$\frac{1}{2}$	20	48″	35 × 43 cm
Axillary Grid	.10	200	$\frac{1}{4}$	20	48″	24 × 30 cm
Scapula AP & LAT OBL	.10	200	$\frac{1}{4}$	20	30″	24 × 30 cm
Clavicle	.10	200	$\frac{1}{4}$	20	48″	24 × 30 cm
Humerus	.10	200	$\frac{1}{4}$	20	48″	35 × 43 cm
Westpoint View (non-grid)	.033	200	$\frac{1}{4}$	6.6		
Femur, knee						
Femur	.10	200	$\frac{1}{4}$	20	48″	35 × 43 cm
LAT & OBL for Vessels	.10	200	$\frac{1}{4}$	20	48″	35 × 43 cm
Knee	.05	200	$\frac{1}{8}$	10	48″	24 × 30 cm
Intercondylar Notch	.025	200	$\frac{1}{4}$	5	48″	Non-Bucky
Patella (Merchants)	.033	200	$\frac{1}{8}$	6.6	48″	Non-Bucky
Ingrowth knee	.066	200	$\frac{1}{8}$	13.2	45″	35 × 43 cm
Chest						
AP Supine, All (non-grid)	.10	200	$\frac{1}{4}$	20	48″	Non-Bucky
Bucky Chest	.05	200	$\frac{1}{4}$	10	45″	
Lateral Supine (Bucky)	.066	200	$\frac{1}{2}$	13.2	48″	35 × 43 cm
Lateral Decubitus (Grid)	.05	200	$\frac{1}{4}$	10	48″	35 × 43 cm
Lateral Sternum	.40	200	$\frac{1}{2}$	80	48″	30 × 35 cm
RAO AP-Sternum	.20	200	1	40	45″	24 × 30 cm
Ribs						
Ribs above diaphragm	.10	↓	$\frac{1}{2}$	varies	48″	24 × 30 cm
	THIN	AVERAGE		PORTLY		
	150 mAs	200 mAs		300 mAs		
Ribs below Diaphragm						
−18 cm	.15	200	$\frac{1}{4}$	30	48″	24 × 30 cm
19−23 cm	.30	200	$\frac{1}{2}$	60	48″	24 × 30 cm
24 cm	.60	200	1	120	48″	24 × 30 cm

EXAMPLE: Assume that 66 mAs was found to be appropriate for the AP lumbar spine and the 200 mA station at 0.33 second was used. If the 200 mA station is chosen as a constant, only the exposure time for the AP lumbar needs to be used with the mAs ratio to compute the exposure time for other body parts. What exposure time should be used for a pelvis when the pelvis ratio is 1.5?

Answer:

$$\frac{\text{mAs for body part}}{\text{mAs for AP lumbar}} = \text{mAs ratio for body part}$$

When the mA station is a constant, only the exposure time needs to be calculated:

$$\frac{\text{sec for body part}}{0.3 \text{ sec}} = 1.5$$

sec for body part = 0.33 sec × 1.5
sec for body part = 0.495 ≈ 0.5 sec

In this example, the technique for the pelvis is found to be 0.5 second at 200 mA, with the kVp measured from kVp Scale 1. Time values for other body parts are computed in the same way and entered in the technique chart. When an exact match between the time value computed cannot be made because of the limited number of time selections available on the x-ray control, the next greater time value should be used.

mA Station Selection. The speed of image receptors currently used, in combination with thermal load capacities of x-ray tubes usually supplied with x-ray equipment, will generally allow the use of the small focal spot at 100 mA single phase and 200 mA three phase for nearly all common procedures. However, reference must be made to the single exposure rating chart for the tube to ensure that exposures computed are indeed within the capacity of the small focal spot. For example, the single-phase tube rating chart that was previously

shown in Figure 6-24 would permit a maximum of 0.2 second at 200 mA and 80 kVp. Thus the exposure computed for the pelvis in the preceding example (0.5 sec, 200 mA, and kVp as measured) would not be allowed with a single-phase generator and this x-ray tube on the small focal spot. Use of the large focal spot would be necessary. However, for a 150 mA small focal spot, a maximum exposure of 4 sec at 80 kVp is permitted. Thus the 150 mA station could be used at the small focal spot. It is important to check the tube's single exposure rating chart and to be certain that the correct chart for the focal spot size, generator type, and rotor speed is used because the tube's ratings are strongly dependent on these factors.

Measurement of Part Thickness

Effective use of a variable kVp technique chart requires precise measurement of part thickness. This is accomplished with a measuring caliper. As a rule, measurement of part thickness along the path of the central x-ray beam is used. For accuracy in measurement, the measuring caliper should be angled if the x-ray beam is angled. However, if the technique chart was constructed by someone using different measuring standards, the same rules used for the chart must be followed by everyone who uses it.

There are two exceptions to this general rule of measuring along the path of the central x-ray beam when the mAs ratio system in Table 36-5 is used. These are the AP projection of the lumbar spine and/or abdomen and the lateral lumbar spine. The AP lumbar or abdomen should be measured just below the tip of the sternum. The lateral lumbar spine should be measured at L2.

Special Considerations. The range of part thickness found in patients is relatively narrow for most body parts, such as the skull, knee, or shoulder (see Table 34-1). For this reason, the use of a single kVp progression can be specified for these examinations without the kVp becoming so low on the thinner patients as to result in underpenetration and such high contrast or so high on the thicker patients as to produce images with insufficient contrast. However, in abdominal examinations patient thickness in the AP dimension varies over an extremely wide range. Though most patients will fall into the range of 19–23 cm, patients who measure as little as 17 cm or as much as 34 cm will frequently be found. Although the kilovoltage range used with a 1ɸ generator for most patients (19–23 cm) will be relatively narrow, 76 to 84 kVp (Table 36-4, 1/2 Scale), extended use of the same variable kVp scale for the 17 cm thick patient would show 73 kVp and for the 34 cm patient 130 kVp. Body part penetration and the resultant image contrast are strongly influenced by kVp level. Should these values be used, it will quickly be noted that 73 kVp is too low and 130 kVp too high for the best results. To avoid this problem in practice, the mAs should be reduced to half and the kVp value increased for the small patients. The mAs should be doubled and the kVp value decreased for the larger patients, resulting in the following modification to the AP lumbar technique chart:

Part thickness	Chart scale to be used with 1ɸ generator	Chart scale to be used with 3ɸ or high frequency generator
18 cm and below	1/4 Scale	1/2 Scale
19–23 cm	1/2 Scale	Scale 1
24	Scale 1	Scale 2

In practice, this maintains kVp within the range of 76–84 kVp for a 1ɸ unit, and image contrast problems attendant with the use of too low or too high kVp are avoided.

Phantom Testing

Phantom testing is recommended prior to performing patient examinations. As a minimum, phantom testing should be done for a small, medium, and large part size as a fine-tuning mechanism for the extrapolated chart prior to clinical use.

Clinical Trials

Limited clinical trials are permissible with the new chart. All images should be recorded, with repeated images saved for analysis. When clinical trials are proceeding without excess repeated exposures, the new technique chart can move into the clinical fine-tuning stage.

Clinical Fine-Tuning

The clinical fine-tuning process will adjust and finally validate the entire chart. At this point the new technique chart can be adopted. However, ongoing fine-tuning then begins as a permanent process.

Ongoing Fine-Tuning

Ongoing fine-tuning is the process that maintains the accuracy of the entire exposure system and gives radiographers and radiologists confidence in the exposure and diagnostic processes.

SUMMARY

A variable kilovoltage x-ray exposure technique system is one in which the kilovoltage to be used for a particular projection is varied depending on measured body part thickness. A milliampere-second value is specified for each body part to be examined.

Technique systems that use variable kilovoltage offer the advantage of permitting small incremental changes in exposure to compensate for variation in body part thickness. A potential disadvantage of the variable kilovoltage technique arises when one considers that the effect of changing kilovoltage on the way the subject is imaged is complex. Increasing kilovoltage reduces image contrast. Reducing contrast may be helpful if the initial kilovoltage is too low to provide adequate penetration of the part. A reduction in contrast that occurs when kilovoltage is too high can reduce the radiologist's ability to see fine detail in the image. A useful variable kilovoltage system must use values of kilovoltage that provide adequate penetration of the part and result in a level of contrast that is acceptable to the radiologist.

Initially, variable kVp systems were established using a 2 kVp change for each centimeter of tissue thickness. A constant was added to this value, such as 30, 40, or 50 kVp, to get the kVp level up to a value that would provide adequate penetration. Application of the 15 percent rule shows that a uniform increase of 2 kVp for each centimeter change will not work satisfactorily over a wide range of tissue thicknesses.

Based on a number of years of field testing, a variable kVp system was established which reflects the need to adjust the kVp level based on the examination being performed. Seven scales were developed with the kVp change from one scale to the next at any given centimeter of thickness being the amount that will balance cutting the mAs in half or doubling it. Once the selected kVp scale is determined, the mAs values are computed using mAs ratios after a base exposure is found. The AP lumbar projection is used for the base exposure. This eliminates the need for multiple trial and error exposures.

The effective use of a variable kVp system requires precise measurement with the use of calipers.

REVIEW QUESTIONS

1. Which exposure factor(s) become constant(s) in a variable kilovoltage technique system?

2. What are the primary advantages and disadvantages of variable kVp technique systems?

3. What is the 2 kVp rule?

4. Why is more than a single kilovoltage scale required?

5. What is a stepped variable kVp chart?

6. What is the formula that is used to calculate new exposure factors from a single satisfactory exposure when mAs ratios are provided?

REFERENCES AND RECOMMENDED READING

Cahoon, J. B. (1961). Radiographic technique: Its origin, concept, practical application and evaluation of radiation dosage. *The X-Ray Technician, 32*, 354–364.

Carroll, Q. B. (1993). *Fuchs's radiographic exposure, processing, and quality control* (5th ed.). Springfield, IL: Charles C Thomas.

Cullinan, A., & Cullinan, J. (1994). *Producing quality radiographs* (2nd ed.). Philadelphia: J. B. Lippincott.

Du Pont, E.SI. de Nemours & Co. Medical Products Department, Customer Technology Center. *Bit system of technique conversion.* Wilmington, DE: Author.

Eastman Kodak Company, Health Sciences Markets Division. (1980). *The fundamentals of radiography* (12th ed.) (Kodak Publication M1-18). Rochester, NY: Author.

Eastman, T. R. (1969). Chest technique through body habitus. *Radiologic Technology, 41*, 80–84.

Eastman, T. R. (1973). Measurement: The key to exposure with manual techniques. *Radiologic Technology, 45*, 75–78.

Eastman, T. R. (1975). Technique charts: The key to radiographic quality. *Radiologic Technology, 46*, 365–368.

Eastman, T. R. (1978, July/August). A history of radiographic technique. *Applied Radiology*, 97–100.

Eastman, T. R. (1979). *Radiographic fundamentals and technique guide.* St. Louis, MO: C. V. Mosby.

Files, G. W. (1952). *Medical radiographic technique.* Springfield, IL: Charles C Thomas.

Fodor, J., & Malott, J. C. (1993). *The art and science of medical radiography* (7th ed.). St. Louis, MO: C. V. Mosby.

Fodor, J., Malott, J. C., Ross, J. A., & Porter, M. (1985). Indications for the use of high kVp in the plain film examination of the abdomen. *Radiologic Technology, 57*(2), 159–161.

Fuchs, A. W. (1934). Radiography of entire body employing one film and a single exposure. *Radiography and Clinical Photography, 10,* 9–14.

Fuchs, A. W. (1948). Relationship of tissue thickness to kilovoltage. *The X-Ray Technician, 19,* 287–293.

Fuchs, A. W. (1949). Control of radiographic density. *The X-Ray Technician, 20,* 271–273, 291.

Fuchs, A. W. (1950). The rationale of radiographic exposure. *The X-Ray Technician, 22,* 62–68, 76.

Fuchs, A. W. (1958). *Principles of radiographic exposure and processing* (2nd ed.). Springfield, IL: Charles C Thomas.

Funke, T. (1966). Pegged kilovoltage technic. *Radiologic Technology, 37,* 202–213.

Gratale, P., Turner, G. W., & Burns, C. B. (1986). Using the same exposure factors for wet and dry casts. *Radiologic Technology, 57*(4), 325–328.

Gray, J. E., Winkler, N. T., Stears, J. G., & Frank, E. D. (1983). *Quality control in diagnostic radiology.* Rockville, MD: Aspen.

Hiss, S. S. (1975). Technique management. *Radiologic Technology, 46*(5), 369.

Hiss, S. S. (2003). *Understanding radiography* (4th ed.). Springfield, IL: Charles C Thomas.

Hopper, B. S. (1957). Radiography above 100 peak kilovolts. *The X-Ray Technician, 29*(1), 9.

Jenkins, D. (1980). *Radiographic photography and imaging processes.* Lancaster, England: MTP Press Limited.

Jerman, E. C. (1926a). Extremity technic. *Radiology. 6,* 252–254.

Jerman, E. C. (1926b). Potter-Bucky diaphragm technic. *Radiology, 6,* 336–338.

Jerman, E. C. (1928). *Modern x-ray technic.* St. Paul, MN: Bruce.

Koenig, G. F. (1957). Kilovoltage as a qualitative factor. *The X-Ray Technician, 29,* 1–4, 13.

Koenig, G. F. (1966). Potential. *Radiologic Technology, 37*(4), 184–198.

Kratzer, B. (1973). A technique computer: Scientific approach to radiologic technology. *Radiologic Technology, 42*(4), 142–150.

Mahoney, G. J. (1959). A slide rule for kVp-mAs adjustments facilitating the use of high kilovoltage. *The X-Ray Technician, 31,* 35–38.

McDaniel, C. T. (1965). Tissue absorption theory applied to formulation of radiographic technique resulting in time as the variable factor. *Radiologic Technology, 37*(2), 51–55.

Morgan, J. A. (1977). *The art and science of medical radiography* (5th ed.). St. Louis, MO: Catholic Hospital Association.

Morgan, R. H. (1949). An analysis of the physical factors controlling the diagnostic quality of roentgen images. *American Journal of Roentgenology and Radiation Therapy, 54,* 128; *54,* 395; *55,* 67; *55,* 627.

Morgan, R. H. (1961). Physics of diagnostic radiology. *Physical foundations of radiology* (3rd ed.). New York: Paul Hoeber/Harper & Row.

Ott, T. T. (1963). Extending the range of medical radiography to 150 kilovolts. *The X-Ray Technician, 34*(6), 335–343.

Revesz, G., Shea, F. J., & Kundel, H. L. (1982). The effects of kilovoltage on diagnostic accuracy in chest radiography. *Radiology, 142,* 615–618.

Roderick, J. F. (1950). Photographic contrast in roentgenology. *The X-Ray Technician, 22,* 141–150, 163.

Roderick, J. F. (1952). Latitude in roentgenology. *The X-Ray Technician, 24,* 187–196, 220.

Sante, L. R. (1942). *Manual of roentgenological technique* (9th ed.). Ann Arbor, MI: Edwards Brothers.

Schwarz, G. S. (1958). A simple universal unit system of radiographic exposures suited to departmental, national, and international standardization. *Radiology, 71,* 573–574.

Schwarz, G. S. (1959a). Extended range radiography. *Radiology, 69,* 419–423, 1957.

Schwarz, G. S. (1959b). Kilovoltage and radiographic effect. *Radiology, 73,* 749–760.

Schwarz, G. S. (1960). Kilovoltage conversion in radiography. *The X-Ray Technician, 31,* 373–379, 436.

Schwarz, G. S. (1961). *Unit-step radiography.* Springfield, IL: Charles C Thomas.

Seeman, H. E. (1968). *Physical and photographic principles of medical radiography.* New York: Wiley & Sons.

United States Army. (1955, March). *Principles of radiographic exposure* (TM 8-282) (Washington, D.C.: United States Army).

United States War Department. (1941, July 3). *Technical manual: Roentgenographic technicians* (TM 8-240) (Washington, D.C.: United States War Department).

van Dijk, D. (1955). Some factors influencing the results in radiography. *Medicamundi, 1,* 27–32.

Williams, W. A. (1960). Standardization of x-ray technique. *The X-Ray Technician, 32*(2), 137.

Wilsey, R. B. (1921). The intensity of scatter x-rays in radiography. *American Journal of Roentgenology, 8,* 328–338.

Wynroe, R. F. (1955). Some observations on kilovoltage variations. *Radiography, 21*(251), 242–243.

CHAPTER 37 | Automatic Exposure Controls

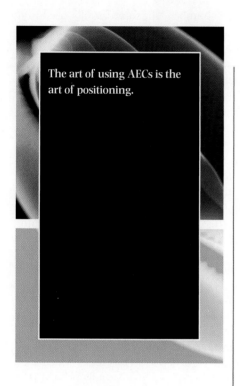

The art of using AECs is the art of positioning.

KEY TERM

minimum response
time

OBJECTIVES

Upon completion of this chapter, the student should be able to:

- Explain why the art of automatic exposure control is the art of positioning.

- Accurately identify configuration size, shape, and position for various brands of ionization chambers.

- Describe how to modify image receptor exposure when using an automatic exposure control.

- Describe various common subject density and subject contrast problems when using AECs.

- Explain the effect of collimation on AEC image quality.

- Provide solutions to minimum response time and backup time problems.

- Explain how to modify the suggested technical factors on an anatomically programmed control unit.

- Discuss the advisability of the creative use of AECs.

The operation of ionization chamber automatic exposure controls (AECs) is discussed in Chapter 5, X-Ray Equipment. It is important to remember that although the term *phototiming* may be used in clinical practice, the generic terms *automatic exposure control* (AEC) and *automatic exposure device* (AED) refer to both antique phototiming devices and the ionization chambers currently in use. Although referred to as phototiming, the term actually refers to the use of ionization chambers. In nearly all instances the principles are applicable to phototimers as well as ionization chambers.

AECs have been popular since their introduction by Russell H. Morgan in 1942. He designed the first phototimer for use with mass chest screening photofluorographic units. It was designed to react to the dominant area of the radiograph that is proportional to the general appearance of the entire image.

The ionization chamber is designed for a single purpose, best illustrated by the proper term for the device—**automatic exposure control.** The single function of an AEC is to eliminate the need for the radiographer to set an exposure **time.** The radiographer loses control over time, and as a result **mAs,** when using an AEC. All other factors, **especially mA and kVp,** must still be set manually.

Radiographers can fall into the habit of depending on AECs to produce diagnostic images in situations for which they were never designed. When using an AEC it is critical that the **location** of the ionization chamber be determined and the precise **positioning** of tissue over that location be achieved. These factors can be remembered by thinking of the use of AECs as another of the radiographic **arts** based on professional expertise and a sound technical understanding.

IONIZATION CHAMBERS

The most critical element in using AECs is the exact position of the **ionization chambers** because positions differ for various brands and models of equipment (Figure 37-1). **Automatic exposure devices provide diagnostic quality exposures only for structures positioned directly above the ionization chambers.** Therefore, the most important

fact to remember when using automatic exposure devices is that **the art of using AECs is the art of positioning.** Experienced radiographers become extremely adept, often to the point of being artistic, in carefully positioning exactly the right amount of tissue over the chambers.

Ionization chamber AECs are usually used in a three-chamber configuration. The most common relationship of the three chambers is with the center chamber at the center of the image receptor with right and left chambers slightly higher. This configuration places the center chamber below the duodenum and transverse colon for most abdominal examinations, thus eliminating problems with gastric and bowel gas being placed over the chamber. This configuration also places the right and left chambers away from the mediastinum and completely within the lobes of the lungs during chest radiography. As long as the exact chamber locations are known, this configuration will not affect phototiming ability during other examinations.

Determining Configurations

Determining the location of the AEC chambers can be a difficult task. Some manufacturers provide plastic inserts for collimators that project an image of the chamber location, size, and shape with the positioning light beam (Figure 37-2). These inserts are accurate for only the specified SID (usually printed in a corner of the insert). When projection inserts are not provided, the radiographer must be capable of determining the location, size, and shape. This can be accomplished by producing an image without a body part as the subject, exposed at very low kVp for maximum contrast (see Figure 37-1).

Controlling Configurations

AEC consoles permit various combinations of the ionization chambers to be activated in order to control the exposure. Most units permit any single cell or all three cells to be activated. Some units permit other combinations to be utilized, for example, right and left chambers together or all three at once. These options provide the radiographer with 7 different combinations of the 3 chambers. In these situations, often termed "averaging," the signals from

52 kVp	4 mAs	72" SID
16:1 grid	200 RS	3.12 mR

40 kVp	5.1 mAs	40" SID
10:1 grid	200 RS	9.66 mR

A

B

FIGURE 37-1 Automatic exposure control ionization chamber configurations. (A) An image of a configuration with square ionization chambers. The middle cell is centered to the image receptor while the outside cells are placed high. (B) An image of a configuration with both square and circular chambers (outlined in pencil). The middle cell is square and centered to the image receptor while the outside cells are round and high. (C) Actual square ionization chamber configuration. The middle cell is centered to the image receptor while the outside cells are high. Note the wire leads to each ionization chamber.

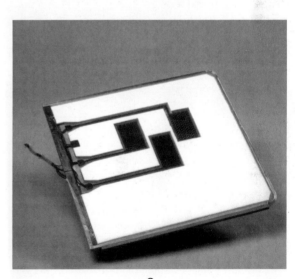

C

the cells are sent to a special operational amplifier, which sums the voltages received from each cell and divides by the number of cells that have been activated. When the appropriate voltage for a diagnostic quality exposure is reached, the exposure is terminated by the operational amplifier. When more than one cell is activated, the cell receiving the most radiation will contribute the greatest electrical signal and therefore have the most influence on overall exposure. For example, if three cells are activated and an abdomen is positioned so that barium is over one cell and normal tissue over the other two cells, the resultant image will be slightly overexposed because the operational amplifier was dividing the incoming voltage by all three cells but only two cells were contributing to the signal. If the cell

FIGURE 37-2 Projection of AEC locations from collimator positioning light.

under the barium was the only one activated, the image would be greatly overexposed, probably to the back-up time limit, because insufficient radiation was received to terminate the exposure. Cell selection is therefore determined by the radiographer based on knowledge of anatomy and positioning.

Density Controls

All AEC systems permit the adjustment of the amount of radiation necessary to send the exposure termination signal. These controls regulate the image receptor exposure but often have different labels, depending on the manufacturer. Typical AEC density control labels are −3, −2, −1, 0, 1, 2, 3, or 1/4, 1/2, N, 1 1/4, 1 1/2. Most labels use the center control as the normal density (0 and N in the two examples) and permit both increases and decreases. Some units use a single density control while others use a major and a minor control. Major controls operate large exposure changes while minor controls operate fine adjustment.

The density controls should not be used to compensate for patient part thickness or kVp changes. The AEC system is designed to calculate this compensation automatically. Proper use of the density controls is accomplished when the configuration of the ionization chamber cells cannot be adapted to the necessary positioning, for example, when an image is produced that is slightly overexposed for the lung fields and a decrease in exposure is desired even though the patient and ionization chambers are properly positioned.

Exposure Technique Charts

Automatic exposure controls require the use of exposure technique charts that specify the technical parameters to be used. The only difference from non-AEC charts is that cell locations are given while time settings are eliminated, as the AEC fulfills that function automatically.

POSITIONING SKILLS

The AEC will produce a diagnostic exposure for whatever tissue is placed directly over the chamber. When the radiographer possesses good positioning skills, the vast majority of AEC exposures will produce diagnostic quality results. Poor positioning skills result in an increased repeat rate when using AECs. There are numerous instances when variables in tissue density and contrast may complicate the precise location of the tissue of interest over the ionization chamber. Knowledge of when these instances are likely to occur and the experience to adequately compensate for them are important. When not enough of the structure of interest is positioned over the activated ionization chamber, the AEC cell will attempt to produce a diagnostic quality exposure for whatever is over it (Figures 37-3 and 37-4).

The skilled radiographer detects the majority of these conditions through careful observation of the patient and consideration of the patient's history. A proper clinical history can reduce the number of repeated images and produce excellent images.

FIGURE 37-3   Improper positioning over AEC cell. Although this lateral cervical spine is underexposed, note that the region at the center of the image receptor, where the AEC cell was activated, is a nearly perfect exposure.

FIGURE 37-4   Improper AEC cell selection. Although this PA chest is overexposed, note that the region at the center of the image receptor, where the AEC cell was activated is a proper exposure for the thoracic spine.

Subject Density and Contrast Problems

AEC problems with subject density and contrast occur whenever an unexpected density is present or when an expected density is lacking. For example, fluid in the lungs causes increased subject density and contrast, for which the AEC would remain on longer, making an aerated lung overexposed for diagnosis. A case of emphysema would produce the opposite result.

Collimation

Collimation of the primary beam is another important consideration when using AECs. Attempts to tightly collimate should be avoided near ionization chamber locations. If the primary beam is collimated from an activated chamber, the chamber operates as if the tissue is extremely dense. The resulting long exposure will create an overexposed image.

The use of wider collimation can also create problems because the full primary beam will produce scatter radiation that may undercut the patient (Figure 37-5). This undercutting scatter will cause the AEC to terminate the exposure while some areas of the image are still underexposed.

Timing Problems

Minimum response time and the proper use of a **backup time** are important considerations when using AECs. The minimum response time is the length of time necessary for the AEC to respond to the ionization and send a signal to terminate the exposure. Modern AECs have a minimum response time in the region of 0.001 second. However, the use of extremely high-speed systems for smaller part sizes can cause problems when AECs need less than 0.001 second to produce a diagnostic quality exposure. In these instances, mA should be decreased to permit longer AEC time.

A

B

FIGURE 37-5 Undercutting scatter. (A) The uncollimated primary beam produces scatter that undercuts the patient and causes the AEC to prematurely terminate the exposure. (B) An image that is overexposed in the upper right quadrant due to undercutting. *(Reprinted with permission from the American Society of Radiologic Technologists from Automatic exposure control: A primer, [1988]. Radiologic Technology, Vol. 59, No. 5, 1988, p. 425. Radiograph courtesy of Seymour Sterling)*

The backup time should be set at 150 percent of the anticipated manual exposure time, although U.S. public law requires that generators automatically terminate AEC exposures at 600 mAs or 60 kilowatt seconds (kWs) (kVp × mA × time) above 50 kVp, and 2,000 mAs below 50 kVp. When the backup time is too short, it will terminate the exposure before the AEC signal, thus producing an underexposed image. In these instances, the backup time should be increased to a level where the AEC is terminating the exposure at the proper time.

Anatomically Programmed Radiography

Anatomically programmed radiography (APR) units combine an AEC system with a technique chart that is computerized to correspond to anatomical procedures. The control console permits the choice of an anatomical region (for example, the chest) and the projection (for example, PA). This choice results in the computer entering the suggested average technique (for example, 120 kVp, 600 mA, with the right and left ionization chambers activated). The radiographer may override the suggested technique when patient condition, pathology or other factors make it desirable to do so.

Creative Positioning

The experienced radiographer often becomes extremely adept at positioning exactly the right amount of tissue over the chambers. Experienced radiographers should remember that **a manual technique will always provide a precisely repeatable exposure,** whereas an AEC exposure leaves the radiographer guessing.

Care must be taken when AEC cells are not completely covered by tissue. The most common compensation in this circumstance is to deactivate the uncovered cell. However, if no cell is covered by normal tissue for the area of interest, deactivation is not the answer. In these instances, creative techniques must be used. For example, if a cell is covered by an appropriate percentage of tissue, it may react with an appropriate exposure. These techniques require much experience and should not be attempted by inexperienced radiographers.

SUMMARY

The ionization chamber is designed for a single purpose, best illustrated by the proper term for the device—automatic exposure control. The single function of an AEC is to eliminate the need for the radiographer to set an exposure time. The radiographer loses control over time, and as a result mAs, when using an AEC. All other factors, especially mA and kVp, must still be set manually.

When using an AEC, it is critical that the location of the ionization chamber be determined and that the precise positioning of tissue over that location be achieved. AEC locations differ for various brands and models of equipment. Automatic exposure devices provide a diagnostic quality exposure only for structures positioned directly above the ionization chambers. AECs are usually used in a three-chamber configuration. The most common relationship of the three chambers is with the center chamber at the center of the image receptor with right and left chambers slightly higher.

AEC consoles permit various combinations of the ionization chambers to be activated in order to control the exposure. When more than one cell is used, the signals from the cells are sent to a special operational amplifier which sums the voltages received from each cell, divides by the number of cells that have been activated, and then terminates the exposure.

All AEC systems permit the adjustment of the amount of radiation necessary to send the exposure termination signal. These controls regulate the density but often have different labels, depending on the manufacturer. Typical AEC density control labels are −3, −2, −1, 0, 1, 2, 3, or 1/4, 1/2, N, 1 1/4, 1 1/2. Some units use a single density control, while others use a major and a minor control.

Problems can result with the use of AEC devices when variations occur in subject density or contrast. Collimation must also be used consistently to ensure proper results. The AEC's minimum response time can also cause exposure problems when very fast systems are used. Backup times should be set at 150 percent of the expected manual technique time.

REVIEW QUESTIONS

1. What is the principal function of the automatic exposure control?

2. What are the typical number and configuration of the ionization chambers?

3. What is the purpose of an operational amplifier?

4. When should the density controls be used?

5. How can changes in subject density result in AEC problems?

6. How can collimation affect AEC image quality?

7. Define minimum response time.

REFERENCES AND RECOMMENDED READING

Bruce, G. (1976). Automatic exposure control: A few notes. *Radiography, 42*(503), 235.

Bushberg, J. T., Seibert, J. A., Leidholdt, E. M., & Boone, J. M. (2003). *The essential physics of medical imaging* (2nd ed.). Philadelphia: Lippincott Williams & Wilkins.

Bushong, S. C. (2004). *Radiologic science for technologists: Physics, biology, and protection* (8th ed.). St. Louis, MO: Elsevier/C. V. Mosby.

Croft, M. J. (1986). Filtration, the answer to the automatic exposure control response problem. *Radiologic Technology, 57*(5), 447.

Cullinan, A., & Cullinan, J. (1994). *Producing quality radiographs* (2nd ed.). Philadelphia: J. B. Lippincott.

Curry, T. S., Dowdey, J. E., & Murry, R. C. (1990). *Christensen's introduction to the physics of diagnostic radiology* (4th ed.). Philadelphia: Lea and Febiger.

Eastman, T. R. (1971). Automated exposures in contemporary radiography. *Radiologic Technology, 43*(2), 80–83.

Fodor, J., & Malott, J. C. (1993). *The art and science of medical radiography* (7th ed.). St. Louis, MO: C. V. Mosby.

Hiss, S. S. (2003). *Understanding radiography* (4th ed.). Springfield, IL: Charles C Thomas.

Jenkins, D. (1980). *Radiographic photography and imaging processes.* Lancaster, England: MTP Press Limited.

Karila, K. T. K. (1989). Manual or automatic exposure controller imaging in mammography. *Radiography Today, 54*(618), 35.

Morel, J. M. (1957). Phototiming. *Radiologic Technology, 29*(3), 165.

Morgan, R. H. (1942). A photoelectric timing mechanism for the automatic control of roentgenographic exposure. *American Journal of Roentgenography and Radium Therapy, 48,* 220–228.

Morgan, R. H. (1943). The automatic control of exposure in photofluorography. *Public Health Reports, 58,* 1533–1541.

Morgan, R. H. (1943). The control of diagnostic quality in roentgenograms of the chest. *American Journal of Roentgenography and Radium Therapy, 50,* 149–161.

Olson, A., & High, M. (1981). Performance of automatic exposure controls when used with rare-earth intensifying screens. *Radiology,* p. 491.

Seeram, E. (1985). *X-ray imaging equipment: An introduction.* Springfield, IL: Charles C Thomas.

Sprawls, P. (1987). *Physical principles of medical imaging.* Rockville, MD: Aspen.

Sprawls, P. (1990). *Principles of radiography for technologists.* Rockville, MD: Aspen.

Stears, J. G., Gray, J. E., & Frank, E. D. (1988). Radiologic exchange (automatic exposure control function). *Radiologic Technology, 59*(6), 521–522.

Sterling, S. (1988). Automatic exposure control: A primer. *Radiologic Technology, 59*(5), 421–427.

Thompson, T. T. (1985). *A practical approach to modern imaging equipment,* (2nd ed.). Boston: Little, Brown.

CHAPTER 38

Exposure Conversion
Problems

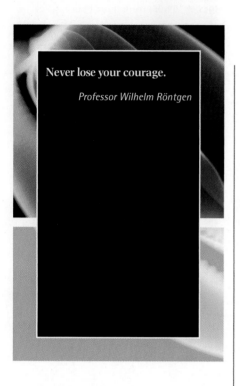

Never lose your courage.

Professor Wilhelm Röntgen

OBJECTIVES

Upon completion of this chapter, the student should be able to:

- Discuss the limitations of standard conversion tables.

- Explain the concept of direct and inverse relationships versus proportions.

- Calculate appropriate new exposure factors for multiple changes in exposure factor variables.

STANDARD CONVERSION RELATIONSHIPS AND TABLES

A primary concern when using conversion tables is their tendency to oversimplify complex exposure problems. It is safer to think of radiographic exposure factors as relationships to one another rather than as direct conversions. The radiographer uses conversion tables as guidelines, with the realization that the great number of variables in any imaging system make all conversion factors variables, not constants. Conversion tables are designed to assist in producing an image within acceptance limits. Production of an image of optimal diagnostic quality usually requires fine-tuning. Conversion tables, like all other factors, require fine-tuning before being integrated into an exposure system.

Most conversion tables are designed to provide a method of maintaining image receptor exposure. It is important to understand the interrelationship between variables and their effects on the four image quality factors: density, contrast, recorded detail, and distortion.

The effect of a particular variable is best described as either a direct relationship, in which an increase in the variable causes an increase in the effect, or an inverse relationship, in which an increase in the variable causes a decrease in the effect, and vice versa. The description of a relationship as direct or inverse does not necessarily indicate that the relationship is **proportionally** direct or inverse. In other words, a proportionally direct relationship would indicate that a linear relationship exists between the variable and the effect, whereas a direct relationship would simply indicate that as the variable changes, the effect changes in the same direction, not necessarily in a linear manner.

Table 38-1 is a master table indicating the relationship of most radiographic image variables on density, contrast, recorded detail, and distortion. Conversion tables are provided for the factors that are commonly considered when converting from one exposure factor or system to another, especially regarding maintaining image receptor exposure (Tables 38-2 through 38-10).

TABLE 38-1. Effects of Radiographic Exposure Variables on the Primary Factors

D = direct relationship (when the variable changes, the effect changes in the same direction).

I = inverse relationship (when the variable changes, the effect changes in the opposite direction).

X = decreases if variable is greater or less than optimal.

0 = no effect

NOTE: Many effects are not linearly proportional.

Variable	Effect On			
	Density	Contrast	Recorded Detail	Distortion
EQUIPMENT				
Generator Phase	D	X	0	0
Kilovoltage	D	X	0	0
Millamperage–seconds	D	0	0	0
SID	I	0	D	I
OID	I	X	I	D
TUBE				
Focal Spot Size	0	0	I	0
Filtration	I	I	0	0
Beam Restriction	I	D	0	0
SUBJECT				
Part Thickness	I	X	I	D
Tissue Type	I	X	0	0
Additive Pathology	I	X	0	0
Destructive Pathology	D	X	0	0
IMAGE RECEPTOR				
Grid Ratio	I	D	0	0
Film/Screen Relative Speed	D	0	I	0
Film Processing				
Developer Time	D	I	0	0
Developer Temperature	D	I	0	0
Developer Replenishment	D	I	0	0

TABLE 38-2. Exposure Maintenance Rules

All these rules help **maintain the same exposure**

• 2KVP/CM RULE

Variable kVp Theory

Maintains exposure by changing kVp for different part sizes.

Changes by 2 kVp for every cm of part size.

EXAMPLE: 60 kVp for 10 cm = 64 kVp for 12 cm

• 4–5 CM RULE

Fixed kVp Theory

Maintains exposure by changing mAs for different part sizes.

Double or halve mAs for every 4–5 cm part size.

EXAMPLE: 10 mAs for 20 cm = 20 mAs for 24 cm

• 15% RULE

Variable and Fixed kVp Theory

Maintains exposure when kVp is changed.

Increase kVp 15% AND decrease mAs to half

EXAMPLE: 60 kVp and 10 mAs = 69 kVp and 5 mAs

Decrease kVp 15% AND increase mAs double

EXAMPLE: 60 kVp and 10 mAs = 51 kVp and 20 mAs

Disclaimer: The above rules are not "Laws of Exposure" by any means. They are simply rules of thumb that have proven useful for generations of radiographers. The actual physical processes that determine exact exposure rates and image quality factors are extremely complex and vary not only from one radiographic unit to another, but over time with the same unit. **These rules may be considered useful with a range of 1–2 densities for part sizes from 10–20 cm and kVp ranges of 60–80.** However, they are often close enough to produce diagnostically useful images throughout the diagnostic radiography range of body part sizes and kVp levels.

TABLE 38-3. Conversion Factors: Effect of Generator Phase on Exposure

When Converting Generator Phase		To Maintain Exposure, Multiply mAs by a
From:	To:	Conversion Factor of:
1ϕ2p	3ϕ6p	0.6
1ϕ2p	3ϕ12p/HF	0.5
3ϕ6p	1ϕ2p	1.6
3ϕ6p	3ϕ12p/HF	0.8
3ϕ12p/HF	1ϕ2p	2.0
3ϕ12p/HF	3ϕ6p	1.2

TABLE 38-4. The Fifteen Percent Rule

To maintain exposure when increasing kVp: increase kVp 15 percent and reduce mAs to half.

To maintain exposure when decreasing kVp: decrease kVp 15 percent and double mAs.

TABLE 38-5. The mAs Formula

$$mA \times seconds = mAs$$

TABLE 38-6. The Exposure Maintenance Formula

$$\frac{mAs_1}{mAs_2} = \frac{D_1^{\,2}}{D_2^{\,2}}$$

where mAs_1 = original mAs

mAs_2 = new mAs

D_1 = original distance

D_2 = new distance

The same formula can be expressed as:

$$mAs_2 = \frac{mAs_1 \times D_2^{\,2}}{D_1^{\,2}}$$

TABLE 38-7. Recommended Compensation for Subject Part Thickness

$$mAs = 2X \text{ or } 0.5X \text{ mAs per 5 cm}$$
$$= 15\% - 20\% \text{ mAs per cm}$$
$$kVp = 2 \text{ kVp per cm}$$

NOTE: Because scatter production varies with total part thickness, these figures are based on 60–80 kVp for a 20 cm part. The recommendations for changes are less accurate further from this average range.

TABLE 38-8. Grid Ratio Conversion Formula

$$\frac{mAs_1}{mAs_2} = \frac{GCF_1}{GCF_2}$$

TABLE 38-9. Grid Ratio Conversions

(Approximate values based on clinical tests of pelvis and skull.)

Grid Ratio	60 kVp	85 kVp	110 kVp
No grid	1	1	1
5:1	3	3	3
8:1	3.75	4	4.25
12:1	4.75	5.5	6.25
16:1	5.75	6.75	8

Adapted with permission from *Characteristics and Applications of X-Ray Grids*, Liebel-Flarsheim division of Sybron Corporation, Cincinnati, Ohio.

TABLE 38-10. Relative Speed Formula

$$\frac{mAs_1}{mAs_2} = \frac{RS_2}{RS_1}$$

SOLVING COMPLEX EXPOSURE PROBLEMS

The most difficult part of developing technique exposure factor skills is learning how to use the information in actual clinical situations. The difficulty lies in the fact that clinical problems usually present complex situations with more than one variable. Now that each variable has been explored in detail, it is necessary to learn how to solve complex exposure problems with many variables.

Methodology

A very simple method can be used to assess a complex exposure problem. Although the analytical decision making process can be used, it is simpler to work through the variables. If the same variables are considered for each problem, it is less likely that a factor will be missed.

Radiographic variables that should be considered when solving a clinical exposure problem can be classified into four major areas: equipment, tube, patient, and image receptor. Each of these four areas has its variables, as shown in Table 38-1. The

variables are easier to remember than it first appears. Equipment is composed of phase plus the four primary factors (kVp, mA, time, and distance). The tube is focal spot, filtration, and field size. The subject consists of part density and contrast. The image receptor includes grid and film/screen variables.

Mistakes in solving complex exposure problems are invariably caused by failure to consider one of these variables. Even when the solution to a problem appears self-evident, a moment taken to consider all the variables may reveal a hidden factor that would have been missed otherwise.

The following problems demonstrate this methodology.

EXAMPLE: A satisfactory image is produced as follows:

1ϕ2p, 80 kVp, 40 mAs, 40″ SID, 8:1 grid, 250 RS

If a new image is to be produced with the following changes—3ϕ6p, 12:1 grid, 400 RS—what changes should be made to maintain the original exposure?

Answer: The following variables must be considered:

Equipment: generator phase from 1ϕ2p to 3ϕ6p
Image receptor: grid from 8:1 to 12:1
Image receptor: film/screen combination from 250 RS to 400 RS
Each variable must be converted for the new exposure:
Equipment: generator phase from 1ϕ2p to 3ϕ6p
The conversion factor for 1ϕ2 to 3ϕ6 = mAs × 0.6

40 mAs × 0.6 = 24 mAs

Image receptor: grid from 8:1 to 12:1
The conversion factor formula for grid changes is

$$\frac{mAs_1}{mAs_2} = \frac{GCF_1}{GCF_2}$$

The conversion factor for an 8:1 grid = 4
The conversion factor for a 12:1 grid = 5.5, so

$$\frac{24 \text{ mAs}}{mAs_2} = \frac{4}{5.5}$$

$$mAs_2 \times 4 = 24 \text{ mAs} \times 5.5$$

$$mAs_2 \times 4 = 132 \text{ mAs}$$
$$mAs_2 = \frac{132 \text{ mAs}}{4}$$
$$mAs_2 = 33 \text{ mAs}$$

Image receptor: film/screen combination from 250 RS to 400 RS
The conversion formula for RS changes is

$$\frac{mAs_1}{mAs_2} = \frac{RS_2}{RS_1}$$

The RS change is from 250 RS to 400 RS, so

$$\frac{33 \text{ mAs}}{mAs_2} = \frac{400}{250}$$

$$mAs_2 \times 400 = 33 \text{ mAs} \times 250$$
$$mAs_2 \times 400 = 8{,}250 \text{ mAs}$$
$$mAs_2 = \frac{8{,}250 \text{ mAs}}{400}$$
$$mAs_2 = 20.63 \text{ mAs}$$

So the new exposure factor conditions require a change to 20.63 mAs to duplicate the original exposure factors.

EXAMPLE: A satisfactory image is produced as follows:

3ϕ6p, 80 kVp, 20 mAs, 72″ SID, 12:1 grid, 400 RS

If a new image is to be produced with the following changes—3ϕ12p, 68 kVp, 100 mA, 10:1 grid, 200 RS—what changes should be made to maintain the original exposure?

Answer: The following variables must be considered:

Equipment: generator phase from 3ϕ6p to 3ϕ12p
Equipment: kVp from 80 to 68
Equipment: mAs = time × 100 mA
Image receptor: grid from 12:1 to 10:1
Image receptor: film/screen combination from 400 RS to 200 RS
Each variable must be converted for the new exposure:
Equipment: generator phase from 3ϕ6p to 3ϕ12p
The conversion factor for 3ϕ6p to 3ϕ12p = mAs × 0.8

$$20 \text{ mAs} \times 0.8 = 16 \text{ mAs}$$

Equipment: kVp from 80 to 68
The conversion when decreasing kVp by 15 percent is doubling the mAs.

$$80 \text{ kVp} \times 15\% = 12 \text{ kVp}$$
$$80 \text{ kVp} - 12 \text{ kVp} = 68 \text{ kVp}$$
$$\text{so, } 16 \text{ mAs} \times 2 = 32 \text{ mAs}$$

Image receptor: grid from 12:1 to 10:1
The conversion factor formula for grid changes is

$$\frac{mAs_1}{mAs_2} = \frac{GCF_1}{GCF_2}$$

The conversion factor for an 8:1 grid = 3.75
The conversion factor for a 12:1 grid = 4.75, so

$$\frac{32 \text{ mAs}}{mAs_2} = \frac{4.75}{3.75}$$

$$mAs_2 \times 4.75 = 32 \text{ mAs} \times 3.75$$
$$mAs_2 \times 4.75 = 120 \text{ mAs}$$
$$mAs_2 = \frac{120 \text{ mAs}}{4.75}$$
$$mAs_2 = 25.3 \text{ mAs}$$

Image receptor: film/screen combination from 400 RS to 200 RS
The conversion formula for RS changes is

$$\frac{mAs_1}{mAs_2} = \frac{RS_2}{RS_1}$$

The RS change is from 400 RS to 200 RS, so

$$\frac{25.3 \text{ mAs}}{mAs_2} = \frac{200}{400}$$

$$mAs_2 \times 200 = 25.3 \text{ mAs} \times 400$$
$$mAs_2 \times 200 = 10{,}120 \text{ mAs}$$
$$mAs_2 = \frac{10{,}120 \text{ mAs}}{200}$$
$$mAs_2 = 50.6 \text{ mAs}$$

Equipment: mAs = time × 100 mA

$$\frac{50.6 \text{ mAs}}{100 \text{ mA}} = \text{time}$$
$$0.51 = \text{time}$$

So the new exposure factor conditions require a change to 50.6 mAs to duplicate the original exposure factors. Using 100 mA, the exposure time would be set at 0.51 second.

SUMMARY

A primary concern when using conversion tables is their tendency to oversimplify complex exposure problems. It is safer to think of radiographic exposure factors as relationships to one another rather than as direct conversions. Conversion tables are designed to assist in producing an image within acceptance limits. Most conversion tables are designed to provide a method of maintaining image receptor exposure. It is important to understand the interrelationships between variables and their effects on the four image quality factors: density, contrast, recorded detail, and distortion.

The effect of a particular variable is best described as either a direct relationship, in which an increase in the variable causes an increase in the effect, or an inverse relationship, in which an increase in the variable causes a decrease in the effect, and vice versa. A proportionally direct relationship would indicate that a linear relationship exists between the variables.

The most difficult part of developing technique exposure factor skills is learning how to use the information in actual clinical situations. It is necessary to learn how to solve complex exposure problems with many variables. A very simple method can be used to assess a complex exposure problem. If the same variables are considered for each problem, it is less likely that a factor will be missed.

Radiographic variables that should be considered when solving a clinical exposure problem can be classified into four major areas: equipment, tube, patient, and image receptor. Mistakes in solving complex exposure problems are invariably caused by failure to consider one of the variables. Even when the solution to a problem appears self-evident, a moment taken to consider all of the variables may reveal a hidden factor that would otherwise have been missed.

REVIEW QUESTIONS

1. What is the primary purpose of conversion tables?

2. When making exposure factor conversions, it is important to consider the effect on which of the image quality factors?

3. What is the meaning of a direct relationship?

4. What is the difference between a relationship and a proportion?

5. When solving complex exposure problems, the variables can be classified into what four major areas?

REFERENCES AND RECOMMENDED READING

Cullinan, A., & Cullinan, J. (1994). *Producing quality radiographs* (2nd ed.). Philadelphia: J. B. Lippincott.

Du Pont, E. I. de Nemours & Co. Medical Products Department, Customer Technology Center. *Bit system of technique conversion.* Wilmington, DE: Author.

Eastman Kodak Company Health Sciences Markets Division. (1980). *The fundamentals of radiography* (12th ed.) (Kodak Publication M1-18). Rochester, NY: Author.

Eastman, T. R. (1979). *Radiographic fundamentals and technique guide.* St. Louis, MO: C. V. Mosby.

Files, G. W. (1952). *Medical radiographic technique.* Springfield, IL: Charles C Thomas.

Fodor, J., & Malott, J. C. (1993). *The art and science of medical radiography* (7th ed.). St. Louis, MO: C. V. Mosby.

Gratale, P., Turner, G. W., & Burns, C. B. (1986). Using the same exposure factors for wet and dry casts. *Radiologic Technology, 57*(4), 325–328.

Hiss, S. S. (2003). *Understanding radiography* (4th ed.). Springfield, IL: Charles C Thomas.

Jenkins, D. (1980). *Radiographic photography and imaging processes.* Lancaster, England: MTP Press Limited.

Jerman, E. C. (1928). *Modern x-ray technic.* St. Paul, MN: Bruce.

Kratzer, B. (1973). A technique computer: Scientific approach to radiologic technology. *Radiologic Technology, 42*(4), 142–150.

Lauer, O. G., Mayes, J. B., & Thurston, R. P. (1990). *Evaluating radiographic quality: The variables and their effects.* Mankato, MN: The Burnell Company.

Morgan, J. A. (1977). *The art and science of medical radiography* (5th ed.). St. Louis, MO: Catholic Hospital Association.

Sante, L. R. (1942). *Manual of roentgenological technique* (9th ed.). Ann Arbor, MI: Edwards Brothers.

Schwarz, G. S. (1961). *Unit-step radiography.* Springfield, IL: Charles C Thomas.

(By permission of Mayo Foundation for Medical Education and Research. All rights reserved)

The Case of the Dripping Film

What caused the horizontal lines and dripping marks on this radiograph?

Answers to the case studies can be found in Appendix E.

UNIT VI Special Imaging Systems

Several special imaging systems deserve consideration to complete a basic foundation in the principles of radiographic imaging. These include the use of specialized diagnostic equipment for **mobile radiography, fluoroscopy,** the oldest and most common dynamic radiographic modality, and radiographic **tomography.**

The specialized systems utilized in the **technical aspects of mammography** and **vascular imaging equipment** are explored as well as the unique design requirements of these fields of radiologic science. Most modern imaging modalities utilize computers to accomplish digital image processing. Those that rely completely on digital processing include **computed tomography (CT)** and **magnetic resonance imaging (MRI),** which, although recognized as specialty areas within radiologic technology, continue to serve as extensions of the radiographer's knowledge.

Although within the scope of departments of radiology, the specialty areas of ultrasound (diagnostic medical sonography), nuclear medicine, and radiation therapy (oncology) are not addressed in this text because they are recognized as separate established professional disciplines with their own accreditation and certification processes. Proper study of these professions generally requires a recognized educational program of one or more years in length encompassing the study of entire subjects beyond the realm of this text.

A thorough study of the six units of this text: **Creating the Beam, Protecting Patients and Personnel, Creating the Image, Analyzing the Image, Comparing Exposure Systems and Special Imaging Systems** provides the thorough physical basis required of the radiologic or imaging sciences professional. Basic physical knowledge must be combined with an equally thorough and correlated knowledge in the anatomical sciences of anatomy, positioning, physiology, and pathology to form the complete basis of radiography knowledge. Only when this basis is added to an elementary understanding of human interactions and combined with clinical experience does the true professional radiographer emerge.

553

CHAPTER 39

Mobile Radiography

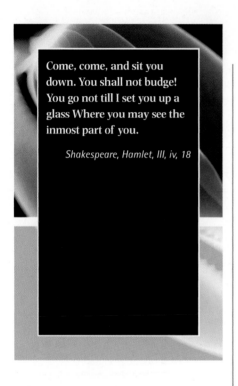

Come, come, and sit you down. You shall not budge! You go not till I set you up a glass Where you may see the inmost part of you.

Shakespeare, Hamlet, III, iv, 18

OBJECTIVES

Upon completion of this chapter, the student should be able to:

- Determine factors that contribute to the difficulty of mobile radiography.

- Explain appropriate communications methods for mobile examinations.

- Describe items that must be considered when arranging a patient room for a mobile examination.

- Recommend methods for accomplishing acceptable variations of standard radiographic projections, especially chest examinations, for air-fluid levels.

- Assess the radiation protection rules for mobile radiography.

- Differentiate light-duty portable x-ray units from full-power mobile units.

- Evaluate the advantages of capacitor-discharge and battery-powered mobile units.

- Explain why technical factor selection is more difficult during mobile radiography.

- Describe the effect of various generator waveforms on kVp.

- Identify advantages of standardizing mobile SID to one of 40″ (100 cm), 56″ (140 cm), or 72″ (180 cm).

- Determine appropriate grids for mobile examinations.

- Appraise various image receptor systems for mobile applications.

The mobile radiographic examination is often the ultimate test of the radiographer's competence and skill. Accomplishing an optimal quality image without stationary equipment on the most difficult patients is a prime achievement. An understanding of the special considerations involved in mobile examinations is important for the radiographer.

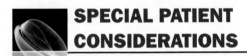

SPECIAL PATIENT CONSIDERATIONS

Mobile examinations are more difficult to accomplish because there are so many additional variables—variables that would be constants with a stationary unit—when manipulating and positioning both patient and equipment. In many instances the reason an examination is requested at the bedside is to avoid transporting the patient because of his physical condition. Special adaptations of routine projections, imaginative equipment manipulation, and innovative technical factor considerations are often required.

In surgery or the emergency unit, the stress of performing in a high-tension environment may be added to the patient problems. These situations often include limitations due to aseptic conditions and the presence of additional critical equipment (e.g., ventilators, multiple intravenous solutions, cardiac lines, etc.).

Communication

Although good communication with the patient is not a special consideration during mobile examinations, it is advisable for the radiographer to park the mobile unit outside a patient's room before entering to establish the proper rapport. The patient's permission must be obtained before proceeding with the examination, an explanation of the procedure should be given, and some rearrangement of equipment and room furnishings must usually be accomplished before bringing the mobile unit into the room.

The unconscious or incognizant patient requires the same explanation that a cognizant patient would receive. In many instances conscious but incognizant patients will be more cooperative if they hear a kindly voice of explanation prior to being touched. In surgery, the attending physician or operating room nurse must be consulted before entering, and this procedure should be followed even in an emergency suite.

Manipulating Equipment

Extreme care must be taken when manipulating equipment in a high-technology environment such as intensive care, surgery, or the emergency unit. The importance of other equipment must be considered, especially when it must be moved to make room for the x-ray unit. Care must be exercised to ensure that power supplies, oxygen tubes, catheters, intravenous lines, and the like, have enough slack to permit movement. Finally, the radiographer must take care not to bump the bed or other equipment when moving the mobile unit out of the way or when driving it into position. Although this seems to be an obvious consideration, it is easily overlooked when one's mind is on the examination. Wall-suspended television units are especially hazardous to both the x-ray tube and the radiographer's head. Neither the radiographer nor the patient can afford to be in a hurry when preparing for a mobile examination. It is the radiographer's duty to return all items to their original locations prior to leaving the area.

Positioning and Pathology

Patients requiring examinations with mobile equipment are often unable to assume standardized positions. Clinical experience and a thorough knowledge of acceptable positioning variants are required for this problem. For example, the inability of the patient to sit on the side of a bed requires an AP projection of the chest instead of the preferred PA projection. A patient in orthopedic traction may not be able to straighten the knee. Thus, a distal knee joint and mid-shaft and proximal hip exposure will be required to avoid gross distortion and to satisfactorily demonstrate the entire femur from a single projection. However, routine positioning practices should still be carried out to the extent possible. For example, during chest radiography most cognizant patients are capable of moving the scapula from the lung fields by rolling their shoulders forward, as they would if the examination were performed on stationary equipment.

Even with difficult or uncooperative patients, chest radiography should be performed with the patient in a semi-erect position in the vast majority of instances. Patients who have been confined to a bed,

especially when pathology is present, are prone to disease processes that cause collections of fluid. Even elevating the thorax to the level of a pillow (perhaps only 10° from supine) may provide an opportunity to demonstrate a fluid level. Ideally, air-fluid level demonstration is best accomplished with the patient in a completely erect position, utilizing a horizontal beam (Figure 39-1). Demonstration of air-fluid levels when a patient is unable to assume an erect position causes gross distortion of anatomical structures (Figure 39-2). This distortion may be great enough to render the image useless for normal chest diagnosis. **When it is determined that air-fluid demonstration is a priority, two projections may be required: one for air-fluid levels and the other for a normal projection of the chest.**

FIGURE 39-1 Demonstration of air–fluid levels. A coconut was used to demonstrate the effect of various positions and tube angles on air–fluid levels. (A) Recumbent AP projection with beam perpendicular to the air–fluid level. (B) Upright AP projection with beam parallel to the air–fluid level. (continues)

The radiographer must not assume that an apparently well patient is able to be transported to stationary equipment. For example, an ambulatory patient on whom a mobile chest examination is requested may in fact be under observation for myocardial infarct and may be susceptible to the sudden onset of potentially serious symptoms.

The radiographer must also not assume that every mobile examination will result in a poorer image quality than examinations performed in the radiology department. The same myocardial infarct patient may be capable of providing a detailed history that makes delineation of the heart shadow the primary image quality goal, of assuming an erect position on the edge of a bed, and of holding a cassette to permit a 72″ (180 cm) PA projection essen-

tially identical in quality to an image produced with a stationary unit.

Because the mobile examination is performed at the patient's bedside, there is an increased possibility of artifacts, such as personal items (e.g., dropped hair pins, jewelry, etc.), layers of coverings (e.g., insulated blankets, several sheets, etc.), and medical equipment (e.g., nasogastric tubes, intravenous lines, catheters, electrocardiographic leads, clamps, etc.). A careful and tactful examination of the area of interest should be performed prior to exposure to locate and remove as many of these artifacts as possible. It is usually possible to carry out this examination during positioning, which also presents an opportunity to check for a necklace, bra, brace, and so on. Clamps holding various tubes and lines should be moved as far from the

C.

D.

FIGURE 39-1   (continued) (C) The cassette was at a 45° angle to the plane of the floor with the beam parallel to the air–fluid level and therefore parallel to the floor. (D) The cassette was at a 45° angle to the plane of the floor and therefore at a 45° angle to the air–fluid level, with the beam perpendicular to the cassette. Note that the central ray must be parallel to the floor to demonstrate distinct air–fluid levels.

FIGURE 39-2 A chest radiograph demonstrating distortion due to improper source-to-image receptor alignment during a mobile examination. The central ray and image receptor were not perpendicular to one another.

area of interest as possible. For example, intensive care unit chest radiography often requires movement of intravenous, respiratory, and cardiac lines from over the lung fields. **A nursing staff member or physician should be consulted before moving any lines, especially venous and arterial.** It is desirable to limit coverings to a single smoothed layer of gown or sheet.

SPECIAL RADIATION PROTECTION CONSIDERATIONS

During a mobile examination the radiographer is bringing a radiation hazard into an area not designed for radiation protection. Professional responsibility for ensuring radiation protection becomes a fundamental operating procedure during all mobile radiography. This is a prime opportunity for radiographers to educate the public, health professionals, physicians, and other patients concerning proper radiation protection practices. A duty exists to protect the patient,

| TABLE 39-1. | Radiation Protection Rules for Mobile Radiography |

1. Recognize a duty to protect your patient, health professionals, physicians, the public, and yourself.

2. Request the public, health professionals, physicians, and other patients to leave the immediate area prior to exposure.

   (Always inform these persons that you will be finished in a moment, request them to remain nearby, and inform them promptly when you are finished.)

3. Announce in a loud voice your intent to make each exposure and permit sufficient time for others to leave.

4. Carry at least two lead aprons: one for yourself, the other for your patient. If you have an assistant, he, too, must have an apron.

5. Never place your hand or any other body part within the primary beam.

6. Provide gonadal protection for your patient.

7. Achieve maximum distance from the patient (not the tube) immediately prior to exposure, in accordance with rules requiring the use of a 6′ cord on mobile units.

8. Label and handle each cassette carefully to avoid repeats.

health workers, the public, and oneself. The rules shown in Table 39-1 should never be violated. The mobile unit should not be used as a portable shield. When standing behind a mobile unit, a lead apron is required to ensure sufficient protection. Radiographers should also move to a maximum distance from the mobile unit by extending the exposure control cord prior to making the exposure. It is not unreasonable to ask others, especially patients sharing a room if they would prefer to leave the area for a few moments while the exposure is made.

TYPES OF EQUIPMENT

X-ray units are available in a wide array of sizes and capabilities, many of which can be classified as mobile. Although often described as portable units (the

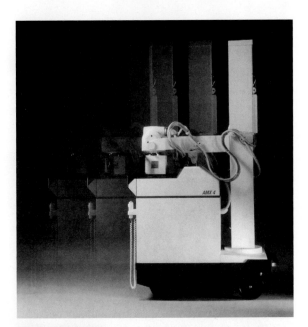

FIGURE 39-3 A typical full-powered mobile radiographic unit. *(Courtesy of GE Healthcare)*

truly portable unit can be hand carried), the proper description is mobile. The need for mobile x-ray equipment has been apparent from the earliest days of radiography; one unit was designed to fit in a suitcase. During World War I, the Picker Corporation developed a mobile unit that has remained popular for bedside radiography in hospitals. Today there are two major classifications of mobile equipment: portable light-duty units and full-power institutional units (Figure 39-3).

Power Supplies

Light-duty mobile units and some full-power units obtain power from wall outlets. Although some older units required 220 volts, modern units are usually designed to use 110 volts. The more advanced full-power units use batteries for a power supply and are capable of greater voltages. Units that are not battery equipped may be susceptible to line voltage fluctuations due to other resistances operating from the same circuit.

When using a mobile unit that is drawing power from a wall outlet, the voltage compensator must be accurately adjusted immediately prior to exposure.

Battery units are usually equipped with circuitry to monitor battery strength, and normal maintenance procedures include periodic replacement of old batteries. However, battery cell failure is a potential cause of erratic exposures.

Generators

Specialized generators have been developed specifically for mobile equipment. Capacitor-discharge units and battery-powered units are the most common. Capacitor-discharge units produce a constant potential output, while battery-operated units produce output that is essentially 3ϕ (Figure 39-4).

Power Drive

An additional advantage of a battery-powered unit is that power is available to drive the unit itself. In large institutions, power-driven units quickly become the radiographer's best friend. The drive switch on a mobile unit should be of the dead-man type so that its release immediately disengages the power drive. The size and weight of a battery-powered mobile x-ray unit are considerable and extreme care must be observed when piloting it. Patients and staff could be seriously injured by careless driving. Radiographers must be cautious in looking ahead, especially at corners and intersections, just as when driving a car.

AUTOMATIC EXPOSURE CONTROL

Automatic exposure control (AEC, AED, or photo-timing) is available for most mobile units in the form of a paddle ionization chamber, the Mobil-AID® Automatic Exposure Control (a registered trademark of Advanced Instrument Development, Inc.) (Figure 39-5). This unit functions exactly as an ionization chamber AEC in a stationary unit except that the chamber is contained within a paddle that can be positioned behind the cassette. The critical element in the use of the Mobil-AID AEC is the accuracy of the positioning of the ionization chamber. All the elements of positioning used with stationary AECs must be applied to the positioning of the paddle and the positioning of the patient.

A.

B.

FIGURE 39-5 Mobil–AID® Automatic Exposure Control for mobile procedures. *(Courtesy of Advanced Instrument Development, Inc.)*

FIGURE 39-4 Mobile unit generator waveforms. (A) A battery-powered unit. (B) A capacitor discharge unit.

SPECIAL TECHNICAL FACTOR SELECTION CONSIDERATIONS

Establishing technical factors for mobile units almost always involves conversion of multiple variables (i.e., generator phase, filtration, grid, etc.) from stationary equipment technique systems. Because multiple conversions increase the risk of error, it is advisable to establish individual technique charts for each mobile unit. There are numerous special considerations when establishing these charts.

Kilovoltage

Most mobile units produce an x-ray beam with an average photon energy that is quite different from that of stationary equipment. Full-power rotary 3ϕ units that are battery powered produce a waveform, as shown in Figure 39-4A. Because this waveform has essentially no ripple, it is actually more efficient and will produce a higher average photon emission than a 3ϕ, 12-pulse unit.

Capacitor discharge units have serious kilovoltage limitations. Careful examination of the waveform in Figure 39-4B illustrates the difference from pulse generators. With a capacitor discharge unit, voltage drops approximately 1 kV/mAs. Therefore, voltage is about 0.5 kV/mAs less than initial kVp. The total voltage drop may be as much as 30 percent. (For example, an exposure at 80 kVp and 40 mAs would end at 56 kVp and average only 68 kV.) The mAs used with a capacitor unit should not exceed 30 percent of the kVp. For example, not more than 24 mAs should be used at 80 kVp.

Milliampere-Seconds

Low-power units may not be capable of the high mAs required for grid radiography and may even require the use of kVp instead of mAs to obtain sufficient image receptor exposure for some examinations. When these problems are present, a motion problem will invariably develop because longer exposure times are used. For a relatively healthy and cooperative patient, a double or even triple exposure may be considered in order to overcome this problem. However, the radiographer must be **extremely** cautious not to overload the tube in this situation.

Distance

A primary cause of repeated mobile exposures is failure to measure distance. **Every mobile procedure must have SID measured.** Radiographers who estimate SID must be within 15 percent to avoid producing a significant exposure difference. A 72″ (180 cm) chest image must be exposed between 61″ (153 cm) and 83″ (208 cm) to produce an optimal exposure using 72″ (180 cm) factors.

Figure 39-6 illustrates common problems encountered in mobile chest radiography. The size of the room and the location of the bed and ancillary equipment may not permit a mobile unit to be manipulated into a position from which a standard 40″ (100 cm) or 72″ (180 cm) projection can be obtained. Position A may be unobtainable because of tube height limitations. Position B is usually obtainable but does not optimize information because at an SID of 40″ (100 cm) it magnifies the heart and, when the patient cannot sit erect, does not provide the geometry to demonstrate air-fluid levels. Positions C and D may be obtainable when air-fluid levels are required, but position C causes magnification.

The most reliable method of eliminating exposure fluctuations due to distance is to use only the two standardized distances, 40″ (100 cm) and 72″ (180 cm), with the addition of 56″ (140 cm) for mobile radiography. The 56″ (140 cm) distance should be employed only when 40″ (100 cm) is undesirable because of magnification, yet 72″ (180 cm) is not possible due to room and/or equipment limitations. As seen earlier in Table 28-3, mAs conversions are provided to maintain exposure at these distances ac-

FIGURE 39-6 Common distance problems during mobile chest radiography.

cording to the rule of doubling or halving mAs with each distance change (i.e., 40″ [100 cm] to 56″ [140 cm] to 72″ [180 cm]).

Grids

Proper alignment to a grid is difficult when the patient is supine but the grid is on a soft bedding surface, which easily permits the grid to tilt, unless the patient's weight is almost exactly distributed around the center of the grid. Proper alignment is even more difficult when the image receptor is at an angle other than parallel or perpendicular.

Figure 39-7 illustrates the problems created by this common situation. The radiographer must attempt to align the central ray and the image receptor perpendicular to one another. Although this is a relatively simple task when the relationships are as shown in Figure 39-7A, it becomes very difficult when the reference points are not parallel or perpendicular.

Most people can draw a simple angle, such as 45°, quite accurately, but accuracy becomes more difficult when the baseline is at an angle. Figure 39-8 demonstrates this difficulty. Angling off-center to a focused grid by as little as 5° can result in sufficient grid cut-off to visibly reduce image receptor exposure.

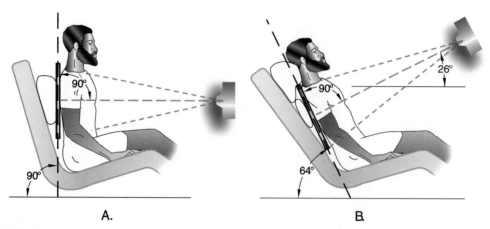

FIGURE 39-7 Alignment problems during mobile chest radiography. (A) A simple alignment problem correctly resolved. (B) A difficult alignment problem correctly resolved.

Grids that permit wide exposure and centering latitude assist in these problems. **Low-ratio grids (5:1 and 6:1) are often preferred for mobile radiography.** Use of a parallel, instead of a focused grid also increases latitude.

Image Receptor Systems

Because there are more variables with mobile radiography, it is appropriate to provide a wider latitude image. Wider-latitude images usually exhibit slower speed, greater resolution, and lower contrast. It is also appropriate to take the opposite position and utilize a faster system to reduce patient dose and overcome the limitations of lower power equipment. However, when rotary 3φ battery-powered units are available, their output capabilities remove equipment limitation rationales.

Other Factors

Other technical factors are not significantly different between mobile and stationary equipment, although the exact specifications for equipment will vary. For example, mobile equipment seldom requires fractional focal spots.

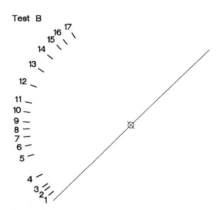

FIGURE 39-8 Difficulty of angle estimation with an angled baseline. If a line is drawn from one of the numbers to the dot, which number would create a 90° angle? A 15° angle? A 37° angle? Record your answers for both tests A and B, and then look on page 564 for the correct answers. Do not tilt your head or the book when completing Test B.

SUMMARY

Mobile examinations are more difficult because there are so many additional variables—variables that would be constants with a stationary unit—when manipulating and positioning both patient and equipment. In many instances the reason an examination is requested at the bedside is to avoid transporting the patient because of his physical condition. Special adaptations of routine projections, imaginative equipment manipulation, and innovative technical factor considerations are often required. Good communication with the patient is a necessary part of all radiographic procedures. The unconscious or incognizant patient requires the same explanation that a cognizant patient would receive.

Extreme care must be taken when manipulating equipment in a high-technology environment such as intensive care, surgery, or the emergency unit. Care must be exercised to ensure that power supplies, oxygen tubes, catheters, intravenous lines, and the like, have enough slack to permit movement.

Patients requiring examinations with mobile equipment are often unable to assume standardized positions. Clinical experience and a thorough knowledge of acceptable positioning variants are required for this problem. Because the mobile examination is performed at the patient's bedside, there is an increased possibility of artifacts, such as personal items, layers of coverings, and medical equipment.

During a mobile examination the radiographer is bringing a radiation hazard into an area not designed for radiation protection. A duty exists to protect the patient, health workers, the public, and oneself.

X-ray units are available in a wide array of sizes and capabilities, many of which can be classified as mobile. There are two major classifications of mobile equipment: portable light-duty units and full-power institutional units. Light-duty mobile units and some full-power units obtain power from wall outlets. The more advanced full-power units use batteries for a power supply and are capable of greater voltages. Specialized generators have been developed specifically for mobile equipment. Capacitor-discharge units and battery-powered units are the most common. Capacitor-discharge units produce a constant potential output, while battery-operated units produce output that is essentially 3ϕ.

Establishing technical factors for mobile units almost always involves conversion of multiple variables (i.e., generator phase, filtration, grid, etc.) from stationary equipment technique systems. Because multiple conversions increase the risk of error, it is advisable to establish individual technique charts for each mobile unit. A number of factors should be considered when establishing mobile technique charts, including kilovoltage, milliamperage, distance, grids, and image receptor systems.

REVIEW QUESTIONS

1. Why are mobile procedures often more difficult than those performed using stationary units?

2. What should the radiographer do before bringing mobile equipment into a patient's room?

3. What must be considered when manipulating mobile equipment in a high-technology environment?

4. What must a radiographer do to adequately visualize air-fluid levels on a chest radiograph?

5. What are the two most common generators used for mobile equipment?

6. What type of generator waveform is produced with a full-powered battery-operated mobile unit?

7. Why is it important to measure distance (SID) for all mobile procedures?

8. What type of grids are preferred for mobile procedures?

REFERENCES AND RECOMMENDED READING

Adler, A., & Carlton, R. R. (2003). *Introduction to radiography and patient care* (3rd ed.) Philadelphia: Elsevier/Saunders.

Ball, J., & Price, T. (1989). *Chesneys' radiographic imaging.* Oxford: Blackwell Scientific.

Barnhard, H. J. (1978). The bedside examination: A time for analysis and appropriate action. *Radiology, 129,* 539–540.

Benbow, M. (1994). The selection of kVp during mobile radiography on the special care baby unit. *Radiography Today, 60(686),* 19–20.

Bushberg, J. T., Seibert, J. A., Leidholdt, E. M., & Boone, J. M. (2003). *The essential physics of medical imaging* (2nd ed.) Philadelphia: Lippincott Williams & Wilkins.

Bushong, S. C. (2004). *Radiologic science for technologists: Physics, biology, and protection* (8th ed.). St. Louis, MO: Elsevier/C. V. Mosby.

Cantwell, K. G., Press, H. C., & Anderson, J. E. (1978). Bedside radiographic examinations: Indications and contraindications. *Radiology, 129,* 383–384.

Cullinan, A., & Cullinan, J. (1994). *Producing quality radiographs* (2nd ed.). Philadelphia: J. B. Lippincott.

A device for improving the quality of bedside decubitus exams. (1979). *Radiologic Technology, 51(1),* 88.

Eisenberg, R. L., Akin, J. R., & Hedgcock, M. W. (1980). Optimal use of portable and stat examination. *The American Journal of Roentgenology, 134,* 523–524.

Evans, S. A., Harris, L., Lawinski, C. P., & Hendra, I. R. F. (1985). Mobile x-ray generators: A review. *Radiography, 51(595),* 89–107.

Floyd, C., Baker, A., Lo, J., & Ravin, C. (1992). Measurement of scatter fractions in clinical bedside radiography. *Radiology, 183(3),* 857–861.

Fry, O. E., & Gianturco, C. (1960). Bedside radiography reduction of patient exposure and orientation of grid cassettes. *Radiologic Technology, 31(4),* 387.

Hasse, R. A. (1991). New trends in portable x-ray batteries and technology. *Radiology Management, 13(3),* 42–44.

MacMahon, H., Yasillo, N., & Carlin, M. (1992). Laser alignment system for high-quality portable radiography. *RadioGraphics, 12,* 111–120.

Marlowe, J. E. (1983). *Surgical radiography.* Baltimore: University Park Press.

O'Donovan, P., Skipper, G., Litchney, J., Salupo, A., & Bortnick, J. (1992). Device for facilitating precise alignment in bedside radiography. *Radiology, 184(1),* 284.

Osborn, R. R. (1960). Improved portable radiographs of the trunk without the use of grids or Bucky. *Radiologic Technology, 32(2),* 145.

Rossi, R., Harnisch, B. D., & Hendee, W. R. (1982, December). Evaluation of an automatic exposure control device for mobile radiography. *Radiology, 823.*

Schaefer, C. (1989, December). Improved control of image optical density with low-dose digital and conventional radiography in bedside imaging. *Radiology, 713.*

Seeram, E. (1985). *X-ray imaging equipment: An introduction.* Springfield, IL: Charles C Thomas.

Thompson, M. A., Hattaway, M. P., Hall, J. D., & Dowd, S. B. (1994). *Principles of imaging science and protection.* Philadelphia: W. B. Saunders.

Trew, D. J. (1970). The 'cordless' mobile x-ray machine. *Radiography, 36(427),* 159–164.

Weaver, K. E., Barone, G. J., & Fewell, T. R. (1978). Selection of technique factors for mobile capacitor energy storage x-ray equipment. *Radiology, 128,* 223–228.

Wolbarst, A. B. (1993). *Physics of radiology.* Norwalk, CT: Appleton & Lange.

Answers to Figure 39-8

Test A	Test B
90° = 15	90° = 15
15° = 3	15° = 4
37° = 8	37° = 7

Fluoroscopy

> . . . in February, 1896, fantastic, vague, and startling reports emanated from the foreign press regarding a wonderful device "invented" by Professor Salvioni of Perugia, Italy, called the cryptoscope, that permitted instantaneous visualization of human, living, and moving bones. . . . At about the same time Professor McGie of Princeton University also developed a . . . skiascope. Edison also constructed a similar device about which extensive publicity soon developed. He named it the fluoroscope.
>
> Arthur W. Fuchs, "Edison and Roentgenology"
> Reprinted with permission from the American Journal of Roentgenology.

KEY TERMS

carriage
fluoroscopic screen
fluoroscopy
flux gain
image intensification
    tube
minification gain
total brightness gain

OBJECTIVES

Upon completion of this chapter, the student should be able to:

- Differentiate fluoroscopic examinations from static diagnostic radiographic examinations.

- Describe a typical basic fluoroscopic image chain.

- Explain the difference between the operation of a fluoroscopic and a diagnostic x-ray tube.

- Describe the advantages of image intensified fluoroscopy over conventional screen fluoroscopy.

- Explain the functions and operation of the image intensification tube input screen, photocathode, electrostatic focusing lenses, and anode and output screen.

- Explain the operation of a multifield magnification image intensification tube.

- Discuss the effects of minification and flux gain on total brightness gain.

- Explain the basic function of a fluoroscopic automatic brightness control.

- Discuss the factors that affect fluoroscopic image contrast, resolution, distortion, and quantum mottle.

- Explain the operation of an optical mirror viewer system, video camera CCD, video camera tube, and video monitor.

- Evaluate the three basic types of fluoroscopic viewing systems.

- Explain the uses of dynamic and static fluoroscopic recording systems.

- Evaluate various types of fluoroscopic recording systems for various clinical situations.

- Explain digital fluoroscopic image acquisition.

- Relate problems with mobile radiographic equipment to mobile fluoroscopic equipment.

- Discuss various methods of reducing dose to the patient, the radiographer, and the radiologist during a fluoroscopic examination.

HISTORICAL DEVELOPMENT

Fluoroscopy (fluoro) is a dynamic radiographic examination, compared to diagnostic radiography, which is static in character. Fluoroscopy involves active diagnosis during an examination. For this reason, fluoroscopy is primarily the domain of the radiologist. The radiographer's role becomes that of an assistant during the examination, although routine post-fluoroscopic radiography is the responsibility of the radiographer. **Radiographers should perform fluoroscopy only for static examinations** where diagnosis is not involved, such as spot imaging the terminal ilium.

The invention of the fluoroscope is credited to Thomas A. Edison in 1896, the year after Röntgen's discovery of x-rays. However, technically speaking, Röntgen discovered x-rays fluoroscopically when he noticed their ability to demonstrate skeletal anatomy as he brought a lead disc into the beam and observed the dynamic movement of his own fingers projected onto a fluorescent screen. Fluoroscopic procedures have, therefore, been a part of diagnostic radiography since its inception.

A fluoroscopic imaging chain consists of a specialized x-ray tube with an image receptor, called the **fluoroscopic screen,** that can be viewed during an x-ray exposure. The first fluoroscopes were held by hand in front of the patient and x-ray tube and included a viewing hood to eliminate extraneous light.

Later units attached the fluoro screen to the x-ray table. In both systems, the radiologist's face and eyes received the full primary beam. A great number of the pioneers in radiology became martyrs of the science because of the design of early fluoro units. Once the biological hazards of radiation became apparent, the design of the fluoroscope was changed to permit viewing by an arrangement of mirrors. This arrangement shielded the primary beam in a leaded enclosure while the mirrors transmitted the optical image to the viewer. **Image intensification tubes** were developed in 1948, and they resulted in video camera and monitor systems (see Figure 5-1) which began to replace mirror viewers. However, there is still a significant loss of detail with a video system, a fact that cannot be appreciated unless an opportunity to view a fluorescent screen through a mirror system arises.

 FLUOROSCOPIC USES

Although the fluoroscopic image was preferred originally, the need to document findings, coupled with immense improvements in the resolution capabilities of diagnostic radiography, not to mention reductions in the dose to the patient, caused fluoroscopy to become less popular. It is currently used only for studies that require observation of dynamic physiological functions, for example, the flow of barium through the gastrointestinal tract, swallowing, the injection of a contrast medium into the heart, etc.

Fluoroscopic Positioning Previewing

Fluoroscopy is not intended to be used as a preview to positioning. Radiographers spend 2 years or more learning how to position the patient properly. There should be no reason for a radiographer to use fluoroscopy as a positioning guide. This procedure would cause unnecessary patient exposure to ionizing radiation. Radiographers should obtain a satisfactory image 95 percent of the time, and this degree of expertise entails not just positioning but technical factors and equipment variations as well.

 ## TYPES OF EQUIPMENT

The fluoroscopic x-ray tube and image receptor are mounted on a C-arm to maintain their alignment at all times (Figure 40-1). In the United States, federal regulations prohibit the use of a fluoroscopic x-ray tube when the entire primary beam is not resulting in an image. The C-arm permits the image receptor to be raised and lowered to vary the beam geometry for maximum resolution while the x-ray tube remains in position. It also permits scanning the length and width of the x-ray table. There are two types of C-arm arrangements, both described by the location of the x-ray tube. Under-table units have the x-ray tube under the table, while over-table units suspend the tube over the patient.

The arm that supports the equipment suspended over the table is called the **carriage.** It typically includes an image intensification tube (on an under-table unit) or the x-ray tube (on an over-table unit), controls for power drive to the carriage, brightness (which regulates the tube mA), spot image selection, tube shutters, spot imaging and/or cine camera, video input tube, and other controls. Although it can be disengaged and pushed away from the table to gain access to the patient, exposure cannot commence until the carriage is returned to a full beam intercept position.

FIGURE 40-1 C-arm alignment of fluoroscopic x-ray tube and image receptor.

FLUOROSCOPIC X-RAY TUBES

Fluoroscopic x-ray tubes are very similar to diagnostic tubes except that they are designed to operate for longer periods of time at much lower mA. Where a typical diagnostic tube operates at 50–1,200 mA, **the fluoroscopic mA range is 0.5–5.0 mA.** The tube target must be fixed to prevent an SOD of less than 15″ (38 cm). The fluoroscopic tube is operated by a foot switch, which permits the fluoroscopist to have both hands free to operate the carriage and position and palpate the patient. Care must be taken to not accidentally activate the foot switch when the unit is in operating mode before or after examinations. Fluoroscopic tubes are equipped with electrically controlled shutters that permit maintenance of close collimation from the fluoro carriage during both fluoroscopy and spot imaging.

IMAGE INTENSIFICATION TUBES

Early fluoroscopic screens were very dim. Dark adaptation, a procedure in which light levels are reduced for a period of at least 10–15 minutes to permit the rods of the eye to become activated, was a time-consuming and irritating part of the radiologist's work routine. The exclusive use of the rod cells constituted a serious threat to diagnostic accuracy because visual acuity is controlled by the cones, which require daylight (photopic) levels of light in order to function. Photopic visual acuity is about 10 times greater than scotopic acuity. The brightness of the fluoro image was not raised to daylight levels until image intensification technology was developed in 1948.

An image intensification tube is designed to electronically amplify the brightness of an image. Modern image intensifiers are capable of increasing image brightness 500–8,000 times. Photopic visual acuity becomes active when the brightness is about 1,000 times that of a fluoroscopic screen. Their primary use is in fluoroscopy equipment, although variations of the design are used in other modalities.

A typical image intensifier is shown in Figure 40-2. The primary x-ray beam exits the patient and strikes the input screen of the image intensifier tube, which is a vacuum tube with a cathode and an anode. The fluorescent screen is built into the image intensifier as its input screen. **The fluorescent screen absorbs the x-ray photons and emits light photons,** which immediately encounter the photocathode (the cathode of the tube) that is in contact with the input screen to prevent divergence of the light beam. **The photocathode absorbs the light photons and emits electrons.** The electrons are then accelerated from the cathode toward the anode and the output screen by the potential difference that exists between the cathode and anode. At the same time the electron beam is focused onto the output screen, which is much smaller than the input screen. **Electrostatic lenses are used to accelerate and focus the electrons. The primary brightness gain occurs from the acceleration and focusing of the electron beam.** The acceleration of the electron beam increases its energy and its ability to emit light at the output screen. The focusing of the electron beam intensifies the image into a smaller area. **The output screen absorbs the electrons and emits light photons,** which are then available for viewing or further electronic processing by a video system. Note the changes in the quantity of photons and electrons in the image at each stage of the intensification process.

The entire image intensification tube is encased in a lead-lined housing that effectively absorbs the primary beam while permitting the intensified light photon image to be transmitted to the viewer. An ion pump device called a getter is used to remove ions produced during operation and to maintain the vacuum within the tube.

Input Screen and Photocathode

The input fluorescent screen consists of a 0.1–0.2 mm layer of sodium-activated cesium iodide (CsI) phosphors coated onto the concave surface of the image intensification tube. This surface may be made of glass, titanium, steel, or aluminum and ranges from 6″ (15 cm) to 23″ (58 cm) in diameter, depending on the manufacturer and use. The screen is concave to maintain the same distance between each point on the input screen and its correspon-

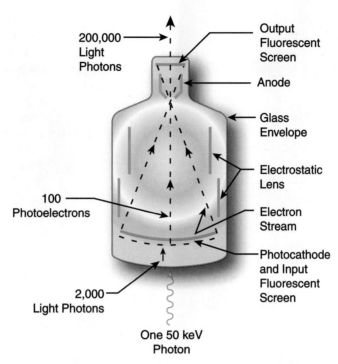

200,000
Light
Photons

Output
Fluorescent
Screen

Anode

Glass
Envelope

Electrostatic
Lens

100
Photoelectrons

Electron
Stream

Photocathode
and Input
Fluorescent
Screen

2,000
Light Photons

One 50 keV
Photon

FIGURE 40-2   An image intensification tube. The quantity of photons and electrons in the image changes at each stage of the intensification process, with the output significantly greater than the input.

ding location on the output screen. Failure to maintain this distance would result in distortion of the image because points farther from the center would be more magnified. The CsI phosphors are packed together very tightly so they absorb about 66 percent of the incident beam, producing a good conversion efficiency, or quantum yield. The phosphors then emit light photons vertically, in proportion to the absorption, thus reducing the lateral spread of light photons that would reduce the image detail. As an example, a single 25 keV incident photon would typically produce over 1,500 light photons. This conversion efficiency permits the fluoro system to function with minimal activation of the phosphors.

An extremely thin protective coating is applied to the input screen to prevent a chemical interaction with the photocathode. The photocathode material is composed of photoemissive metals, usually cesium and antimony compounds, which are applied to the protective coating. The two materials appear to be a single coating when examined. The photoemissive materials absorb the light photons and emit electrons in a process called photoemission. The process is similar to thermionic emission except that the stimulation is light instead of heat.

Electrostatic Lenses

The electrostatic lenses are a series of charged electrodes located inside the glass envelope of the tube. Because the electrons are negative, the charge of the lenses accelerates and focuses the electron stream, which carries the fluoroscopic image. As with an optically focused image, the focal point reverses the image so the output screen image is reversed from the input screen image (right becomes left and superior becomes inferior). The concave input screen reduces distortion by maintaining the same distance between all points on the input screen and their corresponding locations on the output screen, regardless of the position of the focal point.

Magnification Tubes.   The greater the voltage supplied to the electrostatic lenses, the greater the acceleration and the closer the focal point moves toward the input screen. Image intensification tubes can be designed to magnify the image electronically by changing the voltage on the electrostatic lenses. They are often called multifield, dual-field, triple-field, or quad-field intensifiers.

Increased voltage focuses the electrons at a point closer to the input screen and this causes the image to be magnified when it reaches the output screen (Figure 40-3). Magnification image intensifiers are capable of 1.5–4× magnification, which is usually controlled at the fluoro carriage. Some tubes are capable of up to four different magnifications. Resolution can be increased from ≈4 lp/mm to ≈6 lp/mm when the magnification mode is used. The tubes are described according to the diameter of the area of the input screen that will be imaged. For example, a 23/15 dual-focus tube has a 9″ (23 cm) input screen when operating normally and uses a 6″ (15 cm) area when magnifying. The magnification factor is calculated as:

$$\text{magnification} = \frac{\text{input screen diameter}}{\begin{array}{c}\text{diameter of input screen}\\\text{used during magnification}\end{array}}$$

EXAMPLE: What is the magnification for an image viewed with an image intensification tube with an input screen diameter of 9″ (23 cm) that is using a 5″ (13 cm) diameter area during magnification?

Answer:

$$\text{magnification} = \frac{\text{input screen diameter}}{\begin{array}{c}\text{diameter of input screen}\\\text{used during magnification}\end{array}}$$

$$\text{magnification} = \frac{9''}{5''}$$

$$\text{magnification} = 1.8$$

The excess edges of the image are not transmitted by the output screen; therefore, the primary beam field should be collimated to the viewing field when these tubes are operated in magnification mode. Minimal magnification is used for most studies because it reduces contrast problems due to minification and flux gain and permits viewing of the entire primary beam field.

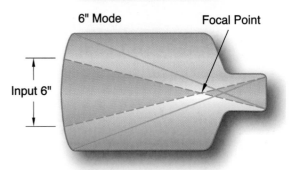

FIGURE 40-3 A magnification image intensification tube. Changes in the focal point produce the magnification.

Anode and Output Screen

The anode is positively charged and is normally supplied with about 25 kV. This charge causes a tremendous attraction of the negative electrons from the photocathode. The anode is positioned inside the glass envelope, immediately in front of the output screen. It has a hole in its center that permits the accelerated electrons to pass through the anode field and onto the output screen.

The output screen is also a glass fluorescent screen. It is a silver-activated zinc-cadmium sulfide phosphor (ZnS-CdS:Ag) that was also used as the input phosphor in early tubes. The phosphor is extremely small (1–2 mm), and the output anode screen is very thin (4–8 mm) to produce high resolution (≈70 lp/mm). The electrons that strike the screen are converted into green light photons that exit the tube. Because all phosphors emit light isotropically, an opaque filter is used under the output phosphor layer to prevent most of the light emitted in that direction from returning to the input screen, where it would degrade the image. Some newer intensifiers use a fiber-optic disc in place of the glass output screen. Fiber optics eliminate the isotropic emission problem and are capable of transmitting the image some distance without loss of resolution.

Total Brightness Gain

Total brightness gain is a measurement of the increase in image intensity achieved by an image intensification tube. It is determined by two factors: minification gain and flux gain.

Minification Gain. Minification gain occurs as a result of the same number of electrons that were produced at the large input screen being compressed into the area of the small output screen. Most image intensification tubes have input screens of 6″ (15 cm) or 9″ (23 cm), although 12″ (30 cm) and larger tubes have been available for special applications. The typical output screen has a diameter of 1″ (2.5 cm). The minification gain is calculated as the ratio between the area of the input and output screens.

$$\text{minification gain} = \frac{\text{input screen diameter}^2}{\text{output screen diameter}^2}$$

EXAMPLE: What is the minification gain for an image intensification tube with an input screen diameter of 6″ (15 cm) and an output diameter of 1″ (2.5 cm)?

Answer:

$$\text{minification gain} = \frac{\text{input screen diameter}^2}{\text{output screen diameter}^2}$$
$$\text{minification gain} = \frac{6^2}{1^2}$$
$$\text{minification gain} = \frac{36}{1}$$
$$\text{minification gain} = 36$$

Minification gain is simply an increase in brightness or intensity, not an improvement in the quality or number of photons making up the image.

Flux Gain. **Flux gain** is a measurement of the increase in light photons due to the conversion efficiency of the output screen. For example, if the output phosphor produces 50 light photons for each electron that strikes it, the flux gain would be 50. Flux gain does not take into account the conversion efficiency of the input screen. It deals only with the gain accomplished by the electron to light conversion at the output screen. Flux gain causes a decrease in image quality exactly as intensifying screens decrease resolution in diagnostic images as a result of the penumbral effect of individual phosphor crystals.

Total Brightness Gain. Total brightness gain can be calculated by several methods. As a function of minification and flux gain, the formula is:

$$\text{brightness gain} = \text{minification gain} \times \text{flux gain}$$

EXAMPLE: What is the total brightness gain for an image intensification tube with a minification gain of 36 and a flux gain of 60?

Answer:

brightness gain = minification gain × flux gain
brightness gain = 36 × 60
brightness gain = 2,160

However, the original formula was:

$$\text{brightness gain} = \frac{\text{intensity of output phosphor}}{\substack{\text{intensity of Patterson B–2} \\ \text{fluoroscopic screen}}}$$

A Patterson B–2 fluoro screen was chosen as the reference point because it was in common use at the time. This formula has lost acceptance because the Patterson B–2 screens would vary from one batch to another and their deterioration was not linear.

Because the Patterson B–2 screen is no longer available, this standard is now obsolete. Although it appears that the term *brightness gain* will continue in use, its measure is a conversion factor that is the ratio of the intensity of the output phosphor to the input exposure rate.

$$\text{conversion factor} = \frac{\text{intensity of output phosphor}}{\text{mR/sec}}$$

Output phosphor intensity is measured in candelas (cd), the unit of luminous intensity.

$$\text{conversion factor} = \frac{\text{cd/m}^2}{\text{mR/sec}}$$

Typical values for modern image intensifier systems are

$$80 - 250 \frac{\text{cd/m}^2}{\text{mR/sec}}$$

This represents a gain of 8,000–25,000 times.

Brightness gain deteriorates as much as 10 percent per year because, just as with intensifying screen phosphors, the input and output screen phosphors age. Although difficult to measure, brightness gain can be evaluated by monitoring the radiation dose required to obtain a diagnostic image from a standard phantom, such as an abdomen or pelvis.

FLUOROSCOPIC GENERATORS

The generators used for static radiography are also used for fluoroscopy. Usually the operator's console includes a control that activates the fluoroscopic system and bypasses the static radiography system.

Brightness Control

A wide variety of systems with different names are used to automatically maintain satisfactory fluoroscopic image density and contrast. Automatic brightness control (ABC) is the most common term although automatic dose control (ADC) and automatic brightness stabilization (ABS) accomplish the same result. They maintain the brightness of the image by automatically adjusting the exposure factors as necessary according to subject density and contrast. Most ABC systems monitor the current flowing between the cathode and anode of the image intensification tube or the intensity of the output screen. In all systems, the primary beam is changed when current and intensity fall below established levels. Regulation of the primary beam can be accomplished by varying kVp, mA, and pulse time. Most ABCs use combinations of these methods in a man-

ner similar to a stepped variable kVp technique system. For example, kVp is gradually increased to the maximum acceptable contrast level, then mA is doubled while kVp is stepped down to the lowest acceptable contrast level and the procedure is started over again. All ABCs have a relatively slow response time, which is noticeable during routine fluoroscopic scanning because the image density adjustment lags a moment behind rapid changes in tissue density. Automatic gain control (AGC) is part of the video camera control system. It responds very quickly but does not change the x-ray exposure factors.

IMAGE QUALITY

Because the imaging chain of a fluoroscopic system is so complex, there are more factors that affect each of the quality elements of the image than in static radiography. In addition to contrast, resolution, and distortion, quantum mottle must also be considered.

Contrast

Contrast is controlled by increasing the amplitude of the video signal, although it is affected by other factors. Image intensified fluoroscopic contrast is not only affected by scattered ionizing radiation but is also affected by penumbral light scatter in the input and output screens, and light scatter within the image intensification tube itself. Scattered ionizing radiation not only produces scatter photons arriving at the input phosphor but also produces some background fog from incident photons that are transmitted through the tube to the output screen or that backscatter from the output to the input screen. Light photons also scatter as they are reflected and refracted within the tube. Since light is emitted isotropically from the output phosphor, some of it will strike the input screen, causing a backscatter effect. All these effects combine to produce a background fog that raises the base density of the image. This affects image contrast exactly as film processing base plus fog affects film contrast. By raising the lowest density value, it decreases the total visible contrast. The overall effect is of reduced contrast. There is also a decrease in image contrast near the edges of the images.

TABLE 40-1.	Typical Limiting Spatial Resolution in Fluoroscopy	
Field of View: cm (inches)	**1,023-Line Video: Line Pairs/mm**	**525-Line Video: Line Pairs/mm**
14 (5.5)	2.7	1.4
20 (7.9)	2.0	1.0
27 (10.6)	1.6	0.7
40 (15.7)	1.3	0.5

Note. From *The Essential Physics of Medical Imaging* (2nd ed.), by J. Bushberg, J. Seibert, E. Leidholdt, and J. Boone, 2002, Philadelphia: Lippincott Williams & Wilkins. Reprinted with permission.

Resolution

The primary limitation on most fluoroscopic resolution is the 525-line raster pattern of the video monitor. For nonvideo recording, such as spot filming or direct optical viewing, the ability to resolve recorded detail in a fluoroscopic system will vary depending on the geometrical factors, just as in static radiography. However, the geometrical factors are different, including minification gain, electrostatic focal point, input and output screen diameter, and viewing system resolution (especially television system resolution), as well as OID and phosphor size and thickness. CsI image intensifiers are capable of ≈ 2 lp/mm. Optical mirror systems that permit indirect viewing of the fluoro screen are capable of ≈ 3 lp/mm. Magnification or multifield image intensifiers are capable of up to ≈ 2.7 lp/mm in the magnification mode (Table 40-1).

Distortion

Size distortion is caused by the same factors that affect static radiographic magnification, primarily OID. Magnification image intensifiers that produce a magnified image by changing the electrostatic focal point within the tube do not significantly affect actual size distortion. Although a magnified image often appears to have more distortion, the distortion is also present in the minified image. It is simply easier to detect when enlarged.

Shape distortion is caused primarily by geometric problems in the shape of the image intensification tube. Although the input screen is concave, it does not completely eliminate edge distortion at the output screen. Electrons at the outer edges of the image tend to flare outward as they are electrostatically focused. Part of this problem is caused by the repulsion of electrons from one another due to their like charges. Figure 33-4 illustrates the edge distortion problem in image intensification tubes. This effect is called vignetting or pincushion distortion and may comprise 8–10 percent of the image area. Some of the vignetting effect is also caused by the effect of the divergence of the primary beam from the x-ray tube focal spot. Vignetting also causes image intensity to be greater at the center of the image and less at the edges. Consequently, distortion is minimized and contrast is improved at the center of the fluoro image.

Quantum Mottle

Quantum mottle is a blotchy or grainy appearance caused by insufficient radiation to create a uniform image. Since the quantity of photons is controlled by the mA and time settings, with static radiography any mA and time combination can be used to accumulate sufficient radiation to create a uniform image. With fluoroscopy, the time factor is controlled by the length of time the eye can integrate, or accumulate, light photons from the fluoro imaging chain. Because this period is 0.2 second, fluoroscopy must provide sufficient photons, through mA, to avoid mottle. Quantum mottle is also a large part of video noise and is a special problem during fluoroscopy because the units operate with the minimum number of photons possible to activate the fluoro screen. The factors that influence mottle are those that affect the total number of photons arriving at the retina of the eye. This includes radiation output, beam attenuation by the subject, the conversion efficiency of the input screen, minification gain, flux gain, total brightness gain, viewing system, and the distance of the eye from the viewing system. Increasing the efficiency of any of these factors can assist in reducing quantum mottle, but the most common solution is to increase the fluoro tube mA.

VIEWING SYSTEMS

A number of viewing systems have been developed to deliver the image from the output screen to the viewer. These include digital, video, cine, and spot imaging systems. Some of these systems permit dynamic real-time viewing, while others are for static images. The viewing time, resolution, and processing time vary.

Video Viewing System

The most commonly used fluoroscopic viewing system is video. Closed circuit video is used with all transmission through cables to avoid broadcast interference. A system includes a video camera attached to the image intensification tube output phosphor and a display monitor for viewing. Fluoroscopic video cameras use a vidicon or Plumbicon™ tube or a charge-coupled device (CCD).

Video Camera Tubes

The vidicon and Plumbicon™ tubes are similar in operation, differing mainly in their target layers. A Plumbicon™ tube has a faster response time than a vidicon tube. The tube consists of a cathode with a control grid, a series of electromagnetic focusing and electrostatic deflecting coils, and an anode with face plate, signal plate and target (Figure 40-4).

Cathode. The cathode consists of a heating assembly that forms an electron gun by thermionically emitting electrons that are shaped into a beam by a control grid. The electron beam is then accelerated toward the target but is decelerated by the anode and a wire mesh in front of the target. This arrangement brings the electrons to a near standstill where they are straightened so the beam strikes the target perpendicularly. At the same time the focusing coils bring the electron beam to a point to maintain resolution. Pairs of deflecting coils serve to cause the electron beam to scan the target in a path known as a raster pattern (Figure 40-5). Commercial television uses a 525 horizontal line raster pattern, but high-resolution video systems now offer 1,050 line systems. The speed of the electron gun movement is difficult to comprehend. The electron beam scans across the screen nearly 1,000,000 times per minute. However, to avoid flicker each scan is divided into two halves, with the first half scanning even-numbered lines and the second half scanning odd-numbered lines. This permits the 30 scans to be projected as 60 half frames per second and flickering is eliminated. (European systems operate at 25 scans for 50 half frames per second to match the 50 Hz current.) The raster pattern significantly reduces the resolution of the image and is the primary disadvantage of a video viewing system.

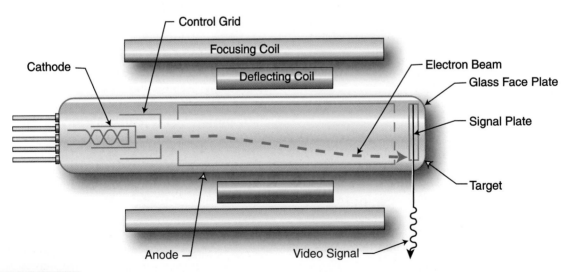

FIGURE 40-4 A video camera tube.

FIGURE 40-5 A video monitor raster scanning pattern. The electron beam scans the diagonal lines as active traces while the horizontal lines are inactive retraces to position for the next active trace. The electron beam scans 262 1/2 alternate lines every 1/60 second and the second set of lines the next 1/60 second. Consequently, the entire 525-line raster pattern is scanned every 1/30 second. This is 30 times per second, which is 15,720 scan lines per second.

Anode. The output phosphor of the image intensification tube is coupled with the face plate of the vidicon tube by fiber optics or optical lenses. This permits the light photons to be transmitted to the signal plate and target. The signal plate consists of a thin film of graphite charged with a positive voltage. It is thin enough to transmit light yet thick enough to conduct the electronic signal out of the tube. The target consists of a thin insulating mica coating in which globules of a light sensitive photoconductive material are suspended in a matrix.

Vidicon tubes use antimony trisulfide (Sb_2S_3), while Plumbicon™ tubes use lead oxide (PbO). The globules are approximately 0.001 inch (0.025 mm) in diameter and their size determines the resolving power of the tube. Each globule is capable of absorbing light photons and then releasing electrons equivalent to the intensity of the absorbed light. The loss of electrons creates a positive charge at the globule, which in turn causes the signal plate to become negatively charged. When the electron gun's beam scans the target, it discharges the globules. This sequential discharging of the globules releases the signal plate's charge as a pulsed signal. This sequential pulsing is the video signal, which can be translated back into an image via the electron gun of the viewing monitor.

The vidicon tube is connected to the output screen of the image intensification tube by either fiber optics or an optical lens system. Fiber optics are bundles of extremely small, light-conducting cable. They are very durable but do not permit the image intensification tube output to be intercepted for spot filming. Spot filming requires an optical lens system similar to the old mirror optical viewing system. The use of beam splitting mirrors permits the image to be recorded by a spot filming device while being viewed. Other systems use a fully silvered mirror to interrupt viewing while deflecting the image for spot filming. Optical lens systems are considerably larger and are easily distinguished by the large size of the housing on top of the image intensification tube. They must be handled gently to avoid trauma to the lenses and mirrors.

Video Camera Charge-Coupled Devices (CCD)

A CCD is a semiconducting device capable of storing a charge from light photons striking a photosensitive surface. When light strikes the photoelectric cathode of the CCD, electrons are released proportionally to the intensity of the incident light. As with all semiconductors, the CCD has the ability to store the freed electrons in a series of P and N holes, thus storing the image in a latent form (see Chapter 4). The video signal is emitted in a raster scanning pattern by moving the stored charges along the P and N holes to the edge of the CCD, where they are discharged as pulses into a conductor. The primary advantage of CCDs is the extremely fast discharge time, which eliminates image lag. This is extremely useful in high-speed imaging applications such as cardiac catheterization. Other advantages are that CCDs are more sensitive than video tubes, they operate at much lower voltages, which prolongs their life, they have acceptable resolution and they are not as susceptible to damage from rough handling.

Video Monitor

A video monitor (or television tube) is a cathode ray tube (CRT) that consists of a vacuum tube with a fluorescent phosphor coated on the inside of the front screen and an electron gun with deflecting and focusing electromagnets (Figure 40-6). The electron gun is the cathode while the anode is plated onto the front screen. The monitor creates an image as the gun sprays the pulsed stream of electrons from the camera onto the screen phosphor. The gun follows the same raster pattern used by the camera. The phosphor crystals emit light when struck by electrons and transmit it as a visual image through the glass of the screen to the viewer. The video monitor

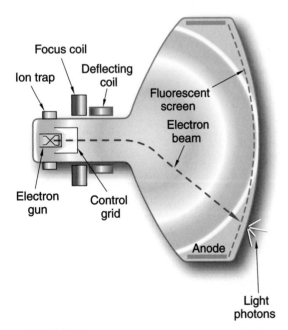

FIGURE 40-6 A video monitor (cathode ray tube [CRT]).

is the most restrictive element in the fluoro imaging chain resolution. A 525-line monitor is capable of displaying between 1–2 lp/mm. Magnification of this image by the video camera or an optical system can increase resolution significantly. Video monitors often operate in the low kilovoltage range and can emit low energy x-rays.

The video monitor viewing conditions change with viewing distance, raster pattern, and screen size. A 525-line pattern on a 9″ monitor has a minimum viewing distance of 37″, while 70″ is suggested for a 17″ monitor. High-resolution patterns (1,050 lines) may be viewed closer; a 9″ monitor has a minimum viewing distance of 17″, while 36″ is suggested for a 17″ monitor. Contrast and brightness can be adjusted with controls on the monitor itself. However, these controls cannot compensate for contrast and brightness problems within the imaging chain. Conversely, the monitor should be checked prior to assuming a problem is in the imaging chain.

DIGITAL FLUOROSCOPY

Digital fluoroscopy is achieved through the use of a thin film transistor (TFT) in contact with the image intensifier (II) output anode screen. The TFT replaces the image intensifier in nondigital fluoro systems. A TFT is a pixelated unit with a photodiode connected to each pixel element. The photodiode converts the light from the II output screen to an electronic signal. A unique feature of TFTs is that they are relatively insensitive to x-ray photons. In fact, some manufacturers add a CsI scintillator element to the image receptor to increase sensitivity by adding back the x-ray photon energy. CsI phosphors absorb x-ray photons and emit light that can be recorded by the TFT. Details on the function of TFTs are part of Chapter 25, Digital Radiography.

Digital fluoroscopy resolution cannot be as high as radiography because the clinical value is outweighed by patient exposure concerns. Consequently, digital fluoro pixels are between 200 μm and 300 μm, as compared to radiography pixels, which are 100–150 μm. Some manufacturers combine up to four radiography pixels into a single image processing pixel for fluoroscopic functions.

RECORDING THE FLUOROSCOPIC IMAGE

Dynamic Systems

Dynamic recording of fluoroscopic images has been limited to cine film and videotape, although laser videodisc would be possible if the recorders were not so expensive.

Cine Film Systems

Cinematic or cine film imaging systems are sometimes referred to as cinefluorography. They consist of a cine (movie) camera positioned to intercept the image produced by the output screen of the image intensification tube. They require about 90 percent of the image intensity for proper exposure levels. Both 16 mm and 35 mm formats are currently in use. Although they dramatically increase resolution when compared to video systems, they also require significantly greater patient dose.

Cine cameras operate by recording a series of static images at high speed. When the images on processed film are projected at the same high speed, the eye becomes incapable of differentiating the separate images and perceives them as a single image in motion. Cine cameras must be synchronized to ensure that the pulses of radiation from the generator coincide with the opening of the shutter to expose the film. This is usually accomplished by operating the camera at either 30 or 60 frames (images) per second to coordinate with the 60 Hz rectified current operating the x-ray tube. Without synchronization, the output screen intensity would vary during the 1 30 or 1 60 second the shutter was open, resulting in some frames being underexposed. To assist in synchronization, the x-ray tube is grid biased or grid pulsed by placing a negatively charged wire across the cathode focusing cup. When the grid wire is turned off and on in pulses, it permits the cathode to pulse electrons to the x-ray tube anode, thus producing a pulse synchronized x-ray beam.

Cineradiographic film is usually viewed as both movie and stop-action film. It must be shown at 16 frames per second if smooth motion is to be perceived. Because the eye can perceive flicker at up to 50 frames

per second, movie projectors operate at 24 frames per second and show each frame twice, thus pulsing the light 48 times per second and eliminating flicker.

The generator and fluoro x-ray tube in a cine system must be able to handle large heat loads. Although individual exposure factors for a single frame are minimal, when multiplied by the 30–60 frames per second required to produce cine, a significant heat load is produced. A 3φ, 12 pulse, 70–80 KW generator and a liquid cooled, 50–60 KW tube with a 0.6 mm focal spot are suggested.

Videotape Recording. Both 1/2″ VHS and high-resolution VHS-S videotape recorders are used to record fluoroscopic images. The VHS-S system requires high-resolution cameras, recorders, tape, and monitors but offers a significant increase in resolution that is highly desirable in fluoroscopic systems. All systems utilize tape cassettes and operate the same as home video systems. Magnetic recording and playback heads produce and read a pattern of magnetic particles on the tape, producing a pulsed video signal. In most medical applications only the video track on the tape is used. The audio and synchronization tracks are left empty.

Static Spot Imaging Systems

Spot imaging systems, although part of the fluoroscopic imaging chain, must be considered separately because they are limited to static images. They are necessary when a permanent record of the fluoroscopic examination is desired to document findings. They are therefore used with nearly every fluoro examination.

Spot imaging permits a permanent static record to be made when information important to diagnosis (either positive or negative) is observed fluoroscopically. It is possible to use spot imaging equipment to rapidly record a series of static images in a manner that functions as a dynamic record. Angiographic procedures that use serial static exposures can use spot imaging when the image resolution is satisfactory.

Spot imaging may be accomplished by several methods. Cassettes (radiographic film and intensifying screens in cassettes), 105 mm chip film, and 70 mm roll film are still common formats. Each has its merits.

Cassettes. Cassette spot imaging uses standard radiographic cassettes equipped with a pair of intensifying screens. Standard sizes are 9″ × 9″ (24 cm × 24 cm) although some units will accept 8″ × 10″ (18 cm × 24 cm) cassettes.

The cassette, stored in a lead-lined compartment in the fluoroscopic carriage, can be moved into the primary beam field via controls located on the fluoro carriage. The x-ray tube current is simultaneously boosted to radiographic levels (100–1,200 mA). The carriage controls permit selection of the area of the cassette to be exposed, automatically collimate the tube and spot image mask shutters to the appropriate size, and position the cassette properly. Common selections are a full frame exposure, known as 1-on-1, two half frame exposures, 2-on-1 vertical and 2-on-1 horizontal, and four exposures, 4-on-1. The radiographer is usually responsible for replacing exposed cassettes when a radiologist is spot filming with them. In these circumstances the radiographer must observe the exposure selections to anticipate when a new cassette will be required. After the exposure is initiated an AEC terminates it and the cassette is automatically returned to the storage compartment. The process is slow because of the time required to move the cassette into place for exposure.

Cassette spot imaging causes the highest dose to the patient. Cassettes may require up to 300 µR per exposure at the entrance to the cassette. This may translate into a 30 mR entrance skin per exposure. It has been estimated that each spot image may be equal to more than a minute of fluoroscopic time. As with any radiographic examination, images should not be produced unless they will contribute significantly to the management of the patient. There is a definite tendency in the United States to overdocument negative findings because of malpractice litigation experiences.

105 mm Chip Film. Chip spot imaging uses 105 mm × 105 mm cut film. The process is relatively fast, up to 12 frames per second, because the only movement necessary prior to exposure is the beam splitting of the mirror.

Digital Fluoroscopy

Digital fluoroscopy units process the image coming from the charge coupled device (CCD) by sending an analog signal through an analog-to-digital converter (ADC) microchip. See Chapter 24 (Digital Image Processing) for a complete discussion of this process.

Once the fluoroscopic image has been converted to a digital signal, it can be manipulated as desired and transferred repeatedly without loss of quality. Display on a monitor permits changes in density (digital window level), contrast (digital window width), magnification, filtration enhancements, and other techniques to be applied to the image.

Digitization also permits storage on computer disk, transfer via electronic means such as teleradiology systems or the Internet, and hard-copy printing via laser dry image processors.

MOBILE FLUOROSCOPIC EQUIPMENT

Mobile C-arm fluoroscopic units are extremely popular for surgical procedures (Figure 40-7). When coupled to a videodisc unit, both static and dynamic imaging can be instantly available. The units operate exactly as do stationary fluoroscopic units, although controls may have different labeling. All the cautions and adaptations for mobile radiography are applicable to mobile fluoroscopy.

RADIATION PROTECTION DURING FLUOROSCOPY

The Patient

Fluoroscopic units operate with the minimum radiation output possible for the efficiency of the imaging system. There is no appreciable difference in the patient dose between an optical mirror viewing system and a video system. The entrance skin exposure for

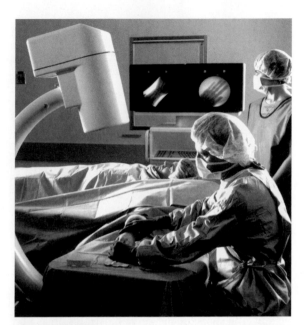

FIGURE 40-7 A mobile C-arm fluoroscopic unit.
(Courtesy of GE Healthcare)

the patient is the surface closest to the source. With an under-table unit the ESE is measured from the surface next to the tabletop. With an over-table unit it is measured from the surface toward the fluoro carriage. The tabletop exposure rate should not exceed 10 R/min and for most units should range from 1 to 3 R/min. The minimum source-to-skin distance is 12″ (30 cm) for mobile fluoroscopic equipment and 15″ (38 cm) for stationary equipment.

In the United States, federal law requires an audible 5-minute timer. Although it can be reset as many times as necessary to complete a procedure, it is intended to serve as a reminder to the radiologist of how much total exposure time is being used. Fluoroscopy is interrupted when the 5 minutes have elapsed and the radiographer must reset the timer to continue the procedure.

Magnification image intensifiers cause increased patient dose because the automatic brightness control (ABC) will increase the tube output to compensate for the loss of electrons within the image intensification tube during magnification. The x-ray tube should have the collimation shutters closed to the viewing image size when in the magnification mode. When magnifying, the output screen of the image intensification tube does not receive the entire image from the input screen so it is possible to irradiate tissue that cannot be viewed. Although these image intensifiers may have interlocks that automatically collimate when magnifying, attention to this detail decreases patient dose.

Patient dose for cinefluorography is significant. The minimum exposure required at the entrance to the image intensification tube is 20 μR per frame. This often translates into an entrance skin exposure of 2,000 μR/frame (2 mR/frame). At 60 frames per second this results in 2 mR/frame × 60 frames/sec = 7,200 mR/min = 7.2 R/min.

Spot image recorders vary in dose to the patient. Cassettes often require 30 mR per exposure while 105 mm film averages about 10 mR per exposure. Of course, these rates may vary with the sensitivity of the image intensification system and the exact mechanics of and film used in the recording system.

The Radiographer and Radiologist

A lead apron of at least 0.25 mm Pb/eq must be worn by all persons (other than the patient) who are present in the fluoroscopic room during exposure. An apron designed to cover the front and sides of the body is usually sufficient, although a wraparound apron for both front and back should be considered if the radiographer is required to turn his or her back to the patient and x-ray tube during the procedure. Radiographers assisting during fluoroscopy must develop the ability to back and sidle around the room during exposures, always keeping the front of the body with its lead apron facing the patient and tube. If the hands must be placed within the primary beam, lead gloves of at least 0.25 mm Pb/eq must be worn.

The primary source of exposure to the radiographer and radiologist is the patient. It is worth noting that the highest energy scatter occurs at a greater than 90° angle to the incident beam (skewed toward the tube) and is greatest at the entrance surface more than at deeper depths because of the lower attenuation of the beam at the surface. It is also worth

FIGURE 40-8 An isodose curve for a typical fluoroscopic unit. The shape of the curve illustrates areas of lesser dose during fluoroscopic procedures. *(Adapted with permission from Wold, G. J., Scheele, R. V., and Agarwal, S. K. [April 1971] Evaluation of Physician Exposure During Cardiac Catheterization, Fig. 3 and 4, p. 189, Vol. 99)*

remembering that according to the inverse square law, a single step back from the patient will decrease the dose exponentially (Figure 40-8). The slot immediately under the tabletop where the Bucky tray is positioned for diagnostic radiography is also at the gonadal level. Fluoroscopic units must have a lead shield to cover this slot. However, it must be brought into position by moving the Bucky tray to the head or foot of the table prior to beginning fluoro. Strips of lead rubber, forming a drape, are positioned between the fluoroscopist and patient to absorb the majority of the patient scatter. The radiographer has one advantage during fluoroscopy in that he or she may position himself or herself behind the radiologist. This not only adds an additional lead apron, but the entire body of the fluoroscopist is there to protect the radiographer.

Fluoroscopy units with cassette spot filming devices are available in front and rear loading models. The front loading models require the fluoroscopist to eject the cassette and lift the arm to permit the radiographer to remove the exposed cassette and insert an unexposed replacement. During this procedure it is difficult to operate the fluoroscopic unit, but if it is operated, the radiographer is protected from scatter by a lead drape, the fluoroscopist, and the fluoroscopist's lead apron as well as his or her own lead apron. Rear-loading models require the radiographer to lift the exposed cassette from the rear of the carriage. This usually requires stepping onto a platform at the rear of the fluoroscopy table and places the radiographer within inches of the patient (the source of scatter radiation). Fluoroscopy units should not be operated during replacement of spot imaging cassettes from rear-loading units.

Others

The radiographer has a duty to require that anyone present in the fluoroscopy room during an examination wear a lead apron. All persons, regardless of rank or authority, should be informed of this requirement. Fluoroscopy should not be initiated until everyone complies.

SUMMARY

Fluoroscopy (fluoro) is a dynamic radiographic examination that involves active diagnosis during the examination. For this reason fluoroscopy is primarily the domain of the radiologist. The radiographer's role becomes that of an assistant during an examination. Fluoroscopy is currently used for studies that require observation of dynamic physiological functions, for example, the flow of barium through the gastrointestinal tract, swallowing, the injection of a contrast medium into the heart, etc.

The fluoroscopic imaging chain consists of a specialized x-ray tube with an image receptor, called the fluoroscopic screen, that can be viewed during an x-ray exposure. The fluoroscopic x-ray tube and image receptor are mounted on a C-arm to maintain their alignment at all times. Fluoroscopic x-ray tubes are very similar to diagnostic tubes except that they are designed to operate for longer periods of time at much lower mA. Where a typical diagnostic tube operates at 50–1,200 mA, the fluoroscopic mA range is 0.5–5.0 mA. An image intensification tube is designed to electronically amplify the brightness of an image. Modern image intensifiers are capable of increasing image brightness 500–8,000 times.

During fluoroscopy, the primary x-ray beam exits the patient and strikes the input screen of the image intensifier tube, which is a vacuum tube with a cathode and an anode. The fluorescent screen is built into the image intensifier as its input screen. The fluorescent screen absorbs the x-ray photons and emits light photons, which immediately encounter the photocathode (the cathode of the tube) that is in contact with the input screen to prevent divergence of the light beam. The photocathode absorbs the light photons and emits electrons. The electrons are then accelerated from the cathode toward the anode and the output screen by the potential difference that exists between the cathode and anode. At the same time, the electron beam is focused onto the output screen, which is much smaller than the input screen. Electrostatic lenses are used to accelerate and focus the electrons. The primary brightness gain occurs from the acceleration and focusing of the electron beam. Brightness gain is a measurement of the increase in image intensity and is determined by minification gain and flux gain. The acceleration of the electron beam increases its energy and its ability to emit light at the output screen. The focusing of the electron beam intensifies the image into a smaller area. The output screen absorbs the electrons and emits light photons, which are then available for viewing or further electronic processing by a video system. The primary factors that affect the quality of the fluoroscopic image include contrast, resolution, distortion, and quantum mottle.

A number of viewing systems have been developed to deliver the image from the output screen to the viewer. These include optical mirror, video, cine, and spot imaging systems. Some of these systems permit dynamic real-time viewing, while others are for static images. The viewing time, resolution, and processing time vary. During fluoroscopy, it is possible to record either a dynamic or a static image. Dynamic imaging systems include cine film systems and videotape recording. Static spot imaging systems include cassettes, 105 mm chip film, and videodisc recorders.

Fluoroscopic units operate with the minimum radiation output possible for the efficiency of the imaging system. The entrance skin exposure for the patient is the surface closest to the source. The tabletop dose rate should not exceed 10 R/min and for most units should range from 1 to 3 R/min.

A lead apron of at least 0.25 mm Pb/eq must be worn by all persons (other than the patient) who are present in the fluoroscopic room during exposure. The primary source of exposure to the radiographer and radiologist is the patient, with the highest energy scatter occurring at a 90° angle to the incident beam. The radiographer has a duty to require that anyone present in the fluoroscopy room during an examination wear a lead apron.

REVIEW QUESTIONS

1. Why is fluoroscopy the domain of the radiologist?

2. What is the typical basic fluoroscopic imaging chain?

3. How does a fluoroscopic x-ray tube differ from a diagnostic x-ray tube?

4. Why is an image intensification system a significant advantage over the conventional screen fluoroscopy?

5. What is the basic function of the fluorescent screen, the photocathode, the electrostatic lenses, and the output screen?

6. What is the formula used for determining brightness gain?

7. What is the purpose of the automatic brightness control?

8. What is the primary limitation of resolution of the fluoroscopic image?

9. What are the basic components of the tube used in a video camera?

10. What are the types of dynamic and static filming systems used to record the fluoroscopic image?

11. What radiation protection practices should be adhered to by the radiographer during fluoroscopy?

REFERENCES AND RECOMMENDED READING

American Association of Physicists in Medicine. (1998). *Managing the use of fluoroscopy in medical institutions (Report of Task Group 6, AAPM Report 58).* College Park, MD: Medical Physics.

Barnes, G. T., & Tishler, J. M. (1981). Fluoroscopic image quality and its implications regarding equipment selection and use. In C. M. Coulam, J. J. Erickson, F. D. Rollo, & A. E. James. (Eds.), The physical basis of medical imaging. New York: Appleton-Century-Crofts.

Beekmans, A. G. (1982). Image quality aspects of x-ray image intensifiers. *Medicamundi, 27,* 25.

Birken, H., & Bejczy, C. I. (1978). A new generation of x-ray image intensifiers. *Medicamundi, 18*(3), 120.

Brink, G. S. (1973). Fundamentals of image intensification: Design and application. *Radiologic Technology, 44*(5), 317.

Bushberg, J., Seibert, J., Leidholdt, E., & Boone, J. (2002). *The essential physics of medical imaging* (2nd ed.) Philadelphia: Lippincott Williams & Wilkins.

Bushong, S. C. (2004). *Radiologic science for technologists: Physics, biology, and protection* (8th ed.). St. Louis, MO: Elsevier/C. V. Mosby.

Curry, T. S., Dowdey, J. E., & Murry, R. C. (1990). *Christensen's introduction to the physics of diagnostic radiology* (4th ed.). Philadelphia: Lea and Febiger.

De Voss, D. (1985). *Basic principles of radiographic exposure.* (2nd ed.). Baltimore: Williams & Wilkins.

Fuchs, A. W. (1947). Edison and roentgenology. *The American Journal of Roentgenology, 57*(2), 145–156.

Gough, L. (1987). Remote-controlled fluoroscopy in a pediatric hospital. *The Canadian Journal of Medical Radiation Technology, 18*(3), 93.

Gray, J. E., Stears, J. G., Lopez, F., & Wondraw, M. A. (1984, February). Fluoroscopic imaging: Quantitation of image lag or smearing. *Radiology,* 563.

Gray, J. E., Winkler, N. T., Stears, J. G., & Frank, E. D. (1983). *Quality control in diagnostic imaging: A quality control cookbook.* Baltimore: University Park Press.

Hynes, D. M., Edmonds, E. W., & Baranoski, D. (1981). Reducing fluoroscopic dosage and cause. *Diagnostic Imaging, 3,* 32–37.

Image intensification systems. (1974). *Radiologic Technology, 46*(3), 196.

Morgan, D. (1990). Applying 100 millimetre and digital technology to general radiography. *Radiography Today, 56*(642), 11–13.

Rich, J. E. (1970). *The theory and clinical application of intensified fluoroscopy in the radiology department.* Milwaukee, WI: General Electric Company Medical Systems Division.

Seeram, E. (1978). Some characteristics of the cesium iodide x-ray image intensifier. *The Canadian Journal of Radiography, Radiotherapy, and Nuclear Medicine, 9*(1), 42–43.

Seeram, E. (1985). *X-ray imaging equipment: An introduction.* Springfield, IL: Charles C Thomas.

Siedband, M. P. (1981). Fluoroscopic imaging. In C. M. Coulam, J. J. Erickson, F. D. Rollo, & A. E. James, (Eds.), *The physical basis of medical imaging.* New York: Appleton-Century-Crofts.

Skucas, J., & Gorski, J. W. (1976). Comparison of image quality of 105mm film with conventional film. *Radiology, 118,* 433–437.

Stears, J., Gray, J. E., & Frank, E. D. (1989). Radiologic exchange (dose reduction with 105mm spot films). *Radiologic Technology, 60*(6), 515–516.

Thompson, M. A., Hattaway, M. P., Hall, J. D., & Dowd, S. B. (1994). *Principles of imaging science and protection.* Philadelphia: W. B. Saunders.

Wesenberg, R. L., & Amundson, G. M. (1984). Fluoroscopy in children: Low exposure technology. *Radiology, 153*(1), 243–247.

Wolbarst, A. B. (1993). *Physics of radiology.* Norwalk, CT: Appleton & Lange.

CHAPTER 41

Radiographic Tomography

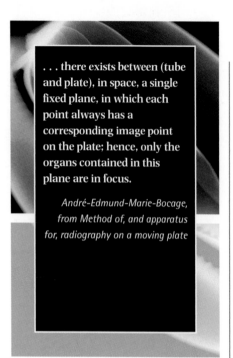

> . . . there exists between (tube and plate), in space, a single fixed plane, in which each point always has a corresponding image point on the plate; hence, only the organs contained in this plane are in focus.
>
> *André-Edmund-Marie-Bocage, from Method of, and apparatus for, radiography on a moving plate*

KEY TERMS

blur
digital tomosynthesis
exposure amplitude
focal plane
fulcrum
pantomography
section interval
section thickness
tomographic
  amplitude
tomography
zonography

OBJECTIVES

Upon completion of this chapter, the student should be able to:

- Define tomography.

- Explain the tomographic principle.

- Explain the relationship of tomographic amplitude to exposure amplitude.

- Describe the effects of tomographic amplitude, distance from the fulcrum, distance from the image receptor, and the orientation of tube motion on image blur.

- Explain the causes of tomographic phantom images.

- Explain the function of the fulcrum.

- Describe the dimensions of the focal plane.

- Correlate changes in exposure amplitude with their effect on section thickness.

- Describe a section interval.

- Evaluate linear tomographic quality parameters.

- Compare various types of linear, circular, and complex tomographic motions.

- Establish a tomographic procedure, including section thickness and interval, for a clinical problem.
- Describe the specialized tomographic techniques.

- Select appropriate exposure factors for a tomographic examination after a satisfactory preliminary scout radiograph has been produced.
- Explain the process of acquiring a digital tomosynthetic image.

Tomography is a radiographic technique that employs motion to show anatomical structures lying in a plane of tissue while blurring or eliminating the detail in images of structures above and below the plane of interest. It primarily demonstrates coronal sections, although sagittal sections of most body parts and transverse sections of the head may be accomplished through positioning.

First developed in 1921, and long the premier investigative procedure for removing superimposing structures, tomography is now used in only a few limited areas. Since the advent of modern computerized sectional imaging techniques (i.e., computed tomography and magnetic resonance imaging), its use has declined rapidly, although it is still considered of value for routine examination of the kidneys during intravenous pyelography. Tomography has also been found useful when computerized modalities are too costly or unavailable and digital tomosynthesis is establishing its value as a routine diagnostic modality.

Although many have claimed credit for the development of tomography, only nine investigators actually had a part in its development, beginning with André Edmund Bocage (French dermatologist 1892–1953) and including the American radiographer Jean Kieffer. Tomography has been called planigraphy, stratigraphy, and laminography over the years, and it is still sometimes called body section radiography.

THE TOMOGRAPHIC PRINCIPLE

The principle of tomography is based on synchronous movement of two of the three elements in a tomographic system: the x-ray tube, the object, and the image receptor. Most tomographic units synchronize the movements of the x-ray tube and the image receptor in opposite directions around a stationary **fulcrum** (pivot point) during the exposure. Their alignment is maintained by a rigid attachment, such as a metal rod. The object to be examined is placed at the fulcrum (Figure 41-1). The result is a tomographic image in which the area located at the fulcrum is sharp because it has not moved in its relationship to the tube and the image receptor during the exposure (Figure 41-2). However, structures above and below, which would have been superimposed, are now blurred due to the motion. The reduced exposure permits visualization of

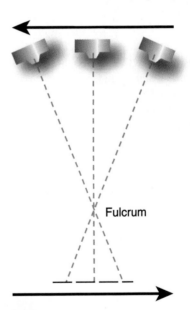

Fulcrum

FIGURE 41-1 The tomographic principle—the interrelationships. The x-ray tube and image receptor are attached so they move in opposite directions while maintaining their alignment. The fulcrum, as the point around which the movement occurs, remains the single unmoving point. Objects placed at the fulcrum are imaged sharply, while all other objects are blurred.

A   B   C

FIGURE 41-2 A tomogram of the maxillary sinuses in an AP projection with the fulcrum (A) 19 cm from the table; (B) 20 cm; and (C) 21 cm. The structures that are sharp are located within the fulcrum focal plane. Structures above and below the focal plane are blurred. Note the opacification of the right maxillary sinus and the thickening of the mucosal wall in the inferior left sinus.

the sharp details of the area of interest through their blurred images.

Although tomography is a dynamic process, it can be understood by careful consideration of the tomographic concept. Oblique projections or tube angle projections are used to project objects away from one another. Tomography builds on this geometry in a dynamic manner (Figure 41-3). As the tube proceeds through the tomographic motion, the projected images are first at a severe tube angle, which gradually decreases to a perpendicular beam, which then increases to a severe tube angle in the opposite direction. The resulting projection of superimposed objects first to one side, then to the other, causes their projected image to be streaked, or blurred, across the length of the image receptor. The longer the blurring, the less opportunity to create a sharp image. The shorter the blurring, the sharper the image. Therefore, there is a direct relationship between distance from the fulcrum and blurring. The greater the distance from the fulcrum, the greater the blurring and vice versa.

Those images that lie in the plane of the fulcrum will be projected onto exactly the same location on the image receptor because the image receptor is moving at exactly the proper rate to maintain their location. Objects located above and below the fulcrum will be projected onto varying locations on the image receptor as it moves, thus blurring their images. The further the object is from the fulcrum, the

Tube travel

Fulcrum

Image receptor travel

FIGURE 41-3 The tomographic concept. The ball is projected to the right of the triangle as the exposure begins but is blurred completely across the triangle to appear at the left by the end of the exposure. Also note that the box goes through the same blurring, but in the opposite direction.

greater the difference between its projected motion and the motion of the image receptor. This causes its image to be projected at various locations. The more its image is blurred, the easier it is to visualize sharp, unblurred structures through the blurring.

Because the creation of a section of sharply defined tissue is similar to cutting slices out of the body for examination, terms such as *cuts* and *slices* have evolved. Because these phrases can easily cause immense distress when overheard by patients, the radiographer should strive to adhere to the term *section*, avoiding *cut* and *slice*.

TOMOGRAPHIC QUALITY

Tomographic Amplitude

The **tomographic amplitude,** arc or angle is the total distance the tube travels (Figure 41-4). The x-ray tube does not have to be engaged in an exposure for the entire tomographic angle. However, the tomographic amplitude is always greater than or equal to the exposure amplitude. There is an inverse relationship between the tomographic amplitude and the section thickness, as discussed later.

Exposure Amplitude

The **exposure amplitude,** arc, or angle is the total distance the tube travels during the exposure (see Figure 41-4). The x-ray tube is engaged in an exposure for the entire exposure angle. The exposure amplitude is always equal to or less than the tomographic amplitude.

Blur

Blur is the streaking or smearing that results in the loss of nearly all recorded detail of objects outside the focal plane. There is an inverse relationship between blurring and the image receptor exposure of objects. Increased blurring causes decreased exposure, thus making an object more transparent. This permits objects within the focal plane to be seen through the blurring. Blur is affected by the tomographic amplitude, distance from the fulcrum, distance from the image receptor, and orientation of tube motion.

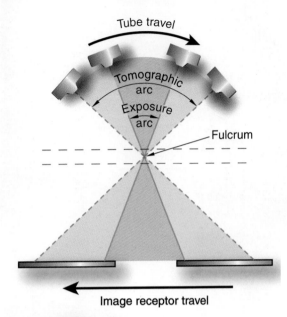

FIGURE 41-4   Tomographic and exposure amplitude, arc, or angle.

Tomographic Amplitude. The tomographic amplitude has a direct linear relationship to blur width. As the tomographic amplitude increases, blur increases in direct proportion. For example, doubling the tomographic amplitude will double image blur.

Distance from the Fulcrum. The distance from the fulcrum has a direct relationship to blur width. As the distance of an object from the fulcrum increases, blur increases.

Distance from the Image Receptor. The distance from the image receptor has a direct relationship to blur width. As the distance of an object from the image receptor increases, blur increases. For example, blurring of superimposed structures around a pulmonary lesion is greater when the affected side is positioned down for lateral decubitus tomograms because this positions the unaffected lung farther from the image receptor.

Orientation of Tube Motion. The orientation of tube travel has a direct relationship to blur width. As the orientation of tube travel approaches perpendicularity, blur increases. Figure 41-5 shows the

FIGURE 41-5 The effect of the orientation of tube motion on the long axis of the object. The tomographic phantom has a star pattern of wires. When the fulcrum is 1 cm below the wires, blurring occurs. This image was produced with a linear motion from the top to the bottom of the radiograph. Arrows illustrate where the wire perpendicular to the direction of motion is projected with maximum blurring. The wire parallel to the direction of motion is projected with no lateral blurring. (The linear motion causes blurring only as elongation at the ends of the wire.) The wires at 45° are projected with intermediate amounts of blurring. *(Courtesy of Philips Medical Systems, N. A.)*

difference between an image of a structure that is perpendicular to a linear tomographic motion and one that is parallel.

Phantoms

Phantoms are sometimes called blur edges or blur margins. They are images that do not correspond to existing structures. They are false images and, as such, are dangerous to the diagnostic process. Phantoms are produced during complex tomographic motions, especially circular, when the tube motion is parallel to the long axis of the structure

FIGURE 41-6 Phantoms caused by circular tomographic motion. Although the top and bottom of the circle produce motion that is perpendicular to the long axis of the object, the sides produce parallel motion. During the time the parallel motion occurs, the image blurring is decreased, thus producing a sharper and more dense image. This sharper and more dense image is the phantom, blur edge, or blur margin.

(Figure 41-6). They are also caused by blur overlap (Figure 41-7) and displacement of blur margins due to the tomographic motion. For example, a dense bony structure may have its blur margin projected into a soft tissue area. Especially in cranial and chest tomography, the decreased blur density may simulate a pathological soft tissue condition. Reduced section thickness and increased exposure amplitude decrease phantom images.

Fulcrum

The fulcrum is the pivot point around which the motions of the tube and the image receptor are centered. It determines the focal plane and thereby controls the section level. The fulcrum may be fixed so that the patient is moved up and down to change the section level (the Grossman principle). More commonly, the fulcrum is adjustable so that it moves up and down while the patient remains stationary.

Focal Plane

The **focal plane** is often referred to as the section, although the terms *section level, layer height, object*

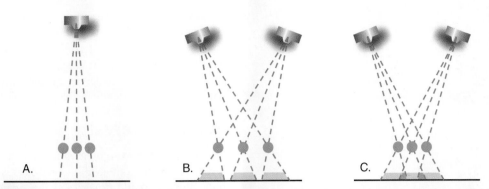

FIGURE 41-7 Tomographic blur overlap phantoms. (A) The sharp image of three wires produced by a static radiograph. (B) The blurred image of three wires produced by a small exposure amplitude. (C) The blur overlap that produces two phantom images from three wires imaged with a large exposure amplitude.

FIGURE 41-8 The effect of exposure angle on section thickness. *(Courtesy of Railfare Enterprises Limited)*

plane, and *depth of focus* have also been used. It is the region within which the image exhibits satisfactory recorded detail and is controlled by the level of the fulcrum. The focal plane is not an exactly defined region. Objects located near the fulcrum are less blurred, while objects located further from the fulcrum are more blurred. Consequently, gradually in-

creasing recorded detail eventually reaches a point where it is considered of diagnostic sharpness. This point defines the margins of the focal plane.

Section Thickness

Section thickness is the width of the focal plane and is controlled by the exposure angle (Figure 41-8).

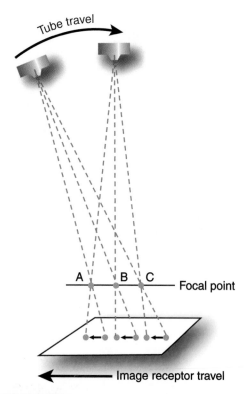

FIGURE 41-9 The effect of tomographic movement on magnification of objects in the focal plane.

Exposure angle is inversely proportional to section thickness. As the exposure angle increases, section thickness decreases. Conversely, as the exposure angle decreases, section thickness increases.

Section thickness occurs in a plane parallel to the image receptor (Figure 41-9). Although there is an increase in magnification due to the increased OID of object C as the x-ray tube moves to the left, there is also a corresponding increase in the SOD and SID. The ratio of SID to SOD, the magnification ratio, remains the same, as do the ratios for objects A and B. Therefore, although magnification has an effect on the detail and sharpness of tomographed objects, tomographic motion does not change the total effect from that seen in a static radiograph of the same area.

Most tomographic images exhibit less contrast than static images of the same regions because of the decreased tissue density that is being imaged with a single section. The decreased difference in subject density also constitutes decreased subject contrast. Additionally, the blurring of structures above and below the fulcrum increases the base density of the image. Increased base density decreases contrast because fewer densities remain within the diagnostically visible range of densities.

Section Interval

The distance between fulcrum levels is the **section interval.** During tomographic procedures, the section interval should not exceed the section thickness. Tomographing an object with section intervals greater than the section thickness creates gaps of unexamined tissue that may permit misdiagnosis.

A procedure must be planned to establish appropriate section intervals. At least one full section above and below the area of interest is required to prove completion of the sectioning. Careful consideration of section thickness permits the use of section intervals that create a slight overlapping of sections. For example, an exposure amplitude that produces a 0.5 mm section thickness should be used with fulcrum changes of 0.4 mm to permit a 0.1 mm overlap (0.05 mm at the top and bottom of each section).

 TYPES OF MOTION

Tomography was first achieved with a linear motion. However, numerous types of complex or pluridirectional tube motions have been developed, which provide a total distance of tube travel up to nearly five times that of a linear motion although, to avoid excessive shape distortion, their amplitude does not exceed 48°. In addition, they provide motion significantly different from the shape of the subject, thus increasing perpendicular movement and reducing phantom images. Essentially, these motions add a second dimension to linear tomography (Figure 41-10B–G). Tomographic motion can be visualized by quality assurance pinhole tracings.

Complex motions require equipment that counter-rotates the grid as the tube moves. The image receptor is moved but is not counter-rotated since it must remain aligned to the anatomical structures of the patient. Counter-rotation of the grid eliminates the need for a reciprocating mechanism to blur the grid lines.

Linear

Linear tomography occurs when the movement of the tube and image receptor are along a straight line (Figure 41-10A). Linear motion has a major quality problem because the SID and OID change as the tube moves. Both SID and OID are greater at the extreme left and right positions than at the center position.

During the tomographic motion the distances are in constant fluctuation.

Linear tomography also has a significant decrease in image quality because blurring is dependent on the orientation of the structure to the linear motion. Structures that are parallel to the motion are not so much blurred as they are streaked. Figure 41-5 illustrates the blurring of lines perpendicular to linear motion and the streaking (elongating) of parallel lines. Linear streaking causes sharp images from structures as much as several centimeters away from the fulcrum. Elongated linear streaking is not a phantom image; it is the image of structural margins that were not blurred.

Linear motion places severe limitations on the total tomographic amplitude. Because the angle of the tube to the object and the image receptor has limits beyond which shape distortion is objectionable, the thinness of the tomographic section is also limited (Figure 41-11). Total tomographic arc is limited to 48°. The only method of decreasing section thickness is to develop complex tomographic motions that permit greater amplitude.

Linear tomography remains popular because it is an inexpensive addition to a diagnostic x-ray unit. It requires a rod to attach the x-ray tube and the Bucky tray, an adjustable fulcrum through which the rod may pivot, and a motor to drive the x-ray tube stand. All other tomographic motions require specialized units designed to provide the desired motion through complicated tracks, gears, pivots, etc.

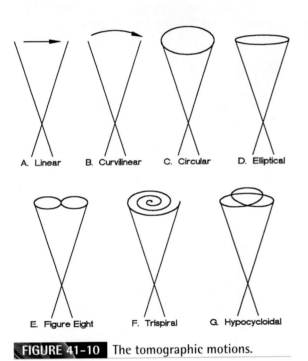

A. Linear   B. Curvilinear   C. Circular   D. Elliptical

E. Figure Eight   F. Trispiral   G. Hypocycloidal

FIGURE 41-10 The tomographic motions.

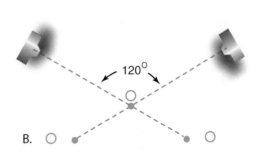

A.   B.

FIGURE 41-11 Limitations to total linear tube amplitude due to excessive distortion produced at the extreme edges of large angles such as 120°.

Because the motion of the tomographic unit creates the tomographic sectional image, it is critical to maximize the motion. This is accomplished by aligning the long axis of the part of interest to the direction of the tube motion. For example, tomograms of the sternum should be done with the long axis of the patient's body perpendicular to the length of the x-ray table. Inability to accomplish this type of positioning for numerous areas of the body is a disadvantage of linear tomography.

Curvilinear

Curvilinear tomography improves on the linear motion by maintaining SID and OID and reducing magnification differences (see Figure 41-10B). It is still of limited value due to the single, linear direction of the motion.

Circular

Circular tomographic motions (see Figure 41-10C), although a vast improvement over linear motions, do not eliminate edge phantoms (see Figure 41-6). They require specialized equipment and exposure times of 3–6 seconds. Consequently, they are seldom used because most units capable of circular motions are also capable of more complex motions, as discussed below.

Elliptical

Elliptical tomographic motions (see Figure 41-10D) eliminate some of the edge phantoms of circular motions, especially when the long axis of the ellipse is perpendicular to the long axis of the object of interest. As with circular motions, they are seldom used because most units capable of elliptical motions are also capable of more complex motions.

Figure Eight

Some tomographic units provide a motion that forms a figure eight (see Figure 41-10E) while others are more random in nature. These motions eliminate most phantom images, although their total tomographic amplitude is not as great as that of trispiral or hypocycloidal motions.

Trispiral

The trispiral motion (see Figure 41-10F) provides maximum tomographic amplitude, thus producing the thinnest possible section.

Hypocycloidal

The hypocycloidal motion (see Figure 41-10G) also provides maximum tomographic amplitude, thus producing the thinnest possible section.

DIGITAL TOMOSYNTHESIS

Digital radiographic tomography is called **digital tomosynthesis** because the computed radiographic images are manipulated by a post-acquisition algorithm to simulate tomographic exposures instead of actually producing additional images. Tomosynthetic processing requires about 10 exposures to establish an adequate image base from which reprocessing can be done. The primary advantage over traditional film/screen tomography is that the resulting images can be manipulated as well as re-created in various planes without reexposing the patient. Figure 41-12 explains the tomosynthetic process in detail.

Flat panel image receptors (as used in direct computed radiography) are best for tomosynthetic systems because they provide rapid readout. The image dataset is acquired by making about 10 static exposures at slightly different central ray angles through the region of interest (ROI). Post-acquisition image processing permits reconstruction of any desired plane through the exposed area. In addition, post-acquisition algorithms for modifying blur, density/brightness, contrast, and other quality factors can be used as necessary.

TOMOGRAPHIC PROCEDURES

Tomography is most often used to localize objects that are difficult to see due to superimposed structures. Because the section thickness determines

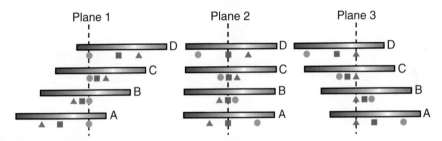

FIGURE 41-12 **Digital Tomosynthesis.** *(Note. From The Essential Physics of Medical Imaging [2nd ed.], by J. Bushberg, J. Seibert, E. Leidholdt, and J. Boone, 2003, Philadelphia: Lippincott Williams & Wilkins. Reprinted with permission)*

how much tissue is visualized for each section, each examination must be evaluated to determine an appropriate series of tomographic sections. Routine procedures often begin with a preliminary scout exposure for diagnostic comparisons. This image is also useful in establishing exact structural locations and verifying exposure factors.

Exposure Factors

Choosing proper technique exposure factors for tomography requires special attention to compensate for the time needed for the tomographic amplitude.

Time. It is critical that the time be set first. The exposure time must match the length of time required for the x-ray tube to complete the tomographic amplitude. An exposure time that is less than the amplitude will not permit full blurring

and will project erratic phantoms. An exposure time that is greater than the amplitude will increase the density of the image at the final tube position, thus increasing the recorded detail while decreasing the blurring of structures outside the focal plane. Complex tomographic motions often require 3 or 6 second exposures.

Milliamperage. Dedicated tomography unit generators provide special stations below 100 mA to permit appropriate mAs to be set with the long times required for complex tomographic motions. Stations of 10, 15, 20, 25, 30, 40, and 50 mA are extremely helpful in these situations. Approximately 30 percent more mAs is required for a wide angle tomogram due to the loss of scatter density caused by the air gap at the extremes of the tomographic motion. Zonographic tomograms usually require the same mAs as static images.

Kilovoltage. All fine exposure adjustments must be accomplished by variations of kVp because of the limitations imposed by the fixed time settings. The 15 percent rule is a critical tool in determining these adjustments. It is also useful to recall that a 5 percent change in kVp is required to produce a visible exposure difference in most images. Because these adjustments tend to increase kVp to the point where contrast may become a problem, every possible device that will eliminate scatter radiation should be employed. These include maximum collimation (to the exact area of interest), lead masks at the tabletop, high ratio grids, and compression bands.

Specialized Techniques

Narrow-Angle Tomography or Zonography. **Zonography** or narrow-angle tomography (exposure amplitudes of less than 10°) is used when localization is necessary because the exact location of a structure is unknown or when a survey is being performed, for example, on a lesion of the lung or on the kidneys. A small exposure amplitude is used to produce a thick section (Figure 41-13A). Zonography has reasonable contrast but poor recorded detail because of the thick section.

Wide-Angle Tomography. Wide-angle tomography is used when a lesion has been localized or a specific structure has been determined to require a more detailed examination. A series of thinner sections may then be used (see Figure 41-13B). Wide-angle tomography has inherently low contrast but a reasonable amount of recorded detail because of the thin section. It is useful in the examination of small bone structures, such as the inner ear, although computed tomography now has much to offer in this area of diagnosis.

Panoramic Tomography. Specialized equipment has been developed to permit slit scan radiography of the curved surfaces of the face and head, especially of the mandible (Figure 41-14). The terms **pantomography,** *orthopantomography,* and *panoramic tomography* have been used to describe this type of

FIGURE 41-13 The effect of exposure amplitude on section thickness. (A) A small exposure amplitude to produce a thick section for localization or as a survey examination. (B) A larger exposure amplitude to produce thin sections for detailed examination. *(Reprinted with permission from Littleton, J. T. [1976]. Tomography: Physical principles and clinical applications. Baltimore, MD: The Williams & Wilkins Co.)*

FIGURE 41-14 A panoramic projection of the mandible.

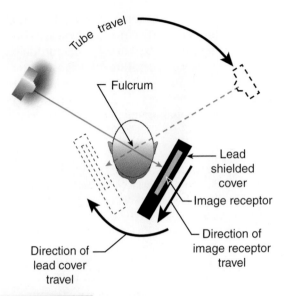

FIGURE 41-15 Panoramic tomographic equipment.

x-ray unit. Slit scan radiography uses only the perpendicular photons of the primary beam by using a lead mask to collimate the beam to a narrow slit. Both the x-ray tube and the image receptor rotate past the slit during the exposure to lay out the structure of interest, much like rolling paint from a roller onto a wall (Figure 41-15).

SUMMARY

Tomography is a radiographic technique employing motion to show structures lying in a plane of tissue while blurring or eliminating the detail in images of structures in other planes. It primarily demonstrates coronal sections, although sagittal sections of most body parts and transverse sections of the head may be accomplished through positioning.

The principle of tomography is based on synchronous movement of two of the three elements in a tomographic system: the x-ray tube, the object, and the image receptor. Most tomographic units synchronize the movements of the x-ray tube and the image receptor in opposite directions around a stationary fulcrum during the exposure. Those images that lie in the plane of the fulcrum will be projected onto exactly the same location on the image receptor because the image receptor is moving at exactly the proper rate to maintain their location. Objects located above and below the fulcrum will be projected onto varying locations on the image receptor as it moves, thus blurring their images.

The tomographic amplitude, arc, or angle is the total distance the tube travels. The exposure amplitude, arc or angle is the total distance the tube travels during the exposure. The exposure amplitude is always equal to or less than the tomographic amplitude. Blur is the streaking or smearing that results in the loss of nearly all recorded detail of objects outside the focal plane and is affected by the tomographic amplitude, distance from the fulcrum, distance from the image receptor, and orientation of tube motion. Blur edges and blur margins are called phantoms.

The focal plane is often referred to as the section, although the terms section level, layer height, object plane, and depth of focus have also been used. It is the region within which the image exhibits satisfactory recorded detail and is controlled by the level of the fulcrum. Section thickness is the width of the focal plane and is controlled by the exposure angle. The distance between fulcrum levels is the section interval. During tomographic procedures, the section interval should not exceed the section thickness.

Tomography was first achieved with a linear motion. Complex or pluridirectional tube motions have been developed, which include circular, elliptical, figure eight, trispiral, and hypocycloidal.

Choosing proper exposure factors for tomography requires consideration of exposure time, milliamperage, and kilovoltage. Specialized tomographic techniques include narrow-angle, wide-angle, and panoramic tomography.

REVIEW QUESTIONS

1. Define tomography.

2. How does a basic tomographic system operate?

3. What is the difference between tomographic amplitude and exposure amplitude?

4. What factors affect tomographic blur?

5. What is the function of the fulcrum?

6. How is section thickness controlled?

7. Which of the tomographic motions alters distance during the exposure arc?

8. What are the advantages of complex tomographic motions?

9. Why is it important to establish the exposure time prior to setting the other exposure factors for a tomogram?

10. Differentiate between the uses of narrow-angle and wide-angle tomography.

REFERENCES AND RECOMMENDED READING

Ball, J., & Price, T. (1989). *Chesneys' radiographic imaging.* Oxford: Blackwell Scientific.

Barnes, G. T., & Moreland, R. F. (1981, October). A linear tomographic alignment test object. *Radiology, 247.*

Bushberg, J. T., Seibert, J. A., Leidholdt, E. M., & Boone, J. M. (2003). *The essential physics of medical imaging* (2nd ed.). Philadelphia: Lippincott Williams & Wilkins.

Bushong, S. C. (2004). *Radiologic science for technologists: Physics, biology, and protection* (8th ed.). St. Louis, MO: Elsevier/C. V. Mosby.

Coulam, C. M., Erickson, J. J., & Gibbs, S. J. (1981). Image and equipment considerations in conventional tomography. In C. M. Coulam, J. J. Erickson, F. D. Rollo, & A. E. James, (Eds.), *The physical basis of medical imaging.* New York: Appleton-Century-Crofts.

Cullinan, A., & Cullinan, J. (1994). *Producing quality radiographs,* (2nd ed.). Philadelphia: J. B. Lippincott.

Curry, T. S., Dowdey, J. E., & Murry, R. C. (1990). *Christensen's introduction to the physics of diagnostic radiology* (4th ed.). Philadelphia: Lea and Febiger.

Dowdell, L. C. (1984). *The joy of sectioning.* Toronto: Railfare.

Durzich, M. L. (1978). *Technical aspects of tomography.* Baltimore: Williams & Wilkins.

Forster, E. (1985). *Equipment for diagnostic radiography.* Lancaster: MTP Press.

Littleton, J. T. (1976). *Tomography: Physical principles and clinical applications.* Baltimore: Williams & Wilkins.

Littleton, J. T., & Durizch, M. L. (1983). *Sectional imaging methods: A comparison.* Baltimore: University Park Press.

Lockery, R. M. (1971). Principles of body-section radiography. *Radiologic Technology, 42*(5), 335.

Marlowe, N. A. (1983). The application of blurred undersubtraction in polytomography. *Radiologic Technology, 54*(6), 455.

Milner, S. C., & Case, J. (1984). Tomographic exposure angle: A comparison of two tests. *Radiography, 50*(592), 177.

Moore, C. J., Hopewell, R., Moores, B. M., & Eddleston, B. (1979). Test procedures for conventional tomographic x-ray equipment. *Radiography, 45*(540), 284.

Ramthun, B. (1988). Tomography of the posterior cervical spine fusion: A new concept. *Radiologic Technology, 60*(1), 27–31.

Smith, W. V. J. (1971). A review of tomography and zonography. *Radiography, 37*(433), 5.

Soni, V. P. (1977). A review of tomography. *Canadian Journal of Radiography, Radiotherapy, and Nuclear Medicine, 8*(4), 172–189.

Tomographic exposure angle. (1984). *Radiography, 50*(594), 291.

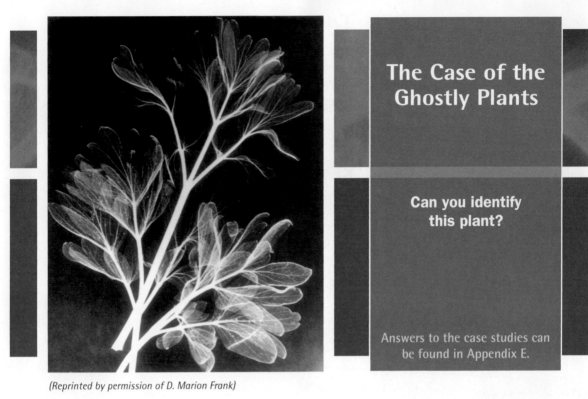

(Reprinted by permission of D. Marion Frank)

The Case of the Ghostly Plants

Can you identify this plant?

Answers to the case studies can be found in Appendix E.

CHAPTER 42

Technical Aspects of Mammography

Eugene D. Frank, M.A., R.T.(R), FASRT, FAERS

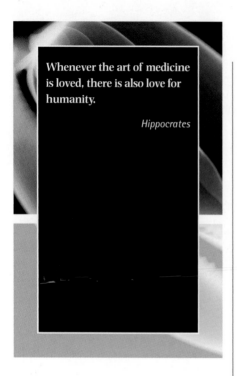

Whenever the art of medicine is loved, there is also love for humanity.

Hippocrates

KEY TERMS

bias focusing
digital mammography
  unit
effective target angle

extended cycle
molybdenum
reciprocity law failure
reference axis

reference axis target
  angle
rhodium

OBJECTIVES

Upon completion of this chapter, the student should be able to:

- Explain the development of the regulations and guidelines underlying the performance of mammography.

- Describe the unique aspects of the mammography x-ray generator.

- Describe the distinctive design and application of the mammography x-ray tube and its associated components.

- Specify the accessory components of the mammography machine, detailing their unique design and function in producing quality images.

- Assess the critical importance of specialized equipment in producing breast images.

- Explain the basic elements of digital mammography.

HISTORICAL DEVELOPMENT

Mammography, today, has evolved into one of the most critical and demanding x-ray examinations performed. Every aspect of the examination has to be carried out with the utmost precision. The technical and clinical aspects of the procedure today are guided by strict regulations and specific guidelines. **Mammography is presently the only radiography examination fully regulated by the federal government.** Mammography today requires a team approach. Several professionals, including the radiologist, medical physicist, and, most importantly, an ARRT registered radiographer, preferably with credentials in mammography.

There is much attention and regulation placed on the technical and clinical aspects of mammography due to the following. The American Cancer Society estimates that 216,000 women will be diagnosed with breast cancer annually and that 40,000 women will die of this disease (about 1,600 men will be diagnosed also). Approximately 1 out of 8 women will develop breast cancer over a lifetime. Until recently, breast cancer was the leading cause of death from cancer among women. Lung cancer has now become the leader. Breast cancer is the leading cause of cancer deaths in females between the ages of 15 and 54. Most notably, the incidence of breast cancer, as a result of participation in screening, has increased 3 to 4 percent annually since 1982. The overall age-adjusted incidence rates are higher in white women compared with African American women. However, for African American women under age 50, the incidence is nearly three times higher. The size of the population at risk for developing breast cancer is also growing every year.

It is well known that mortality from breast cancer can be reduced significantly through widespread participation in breast screening. For women whose cancers are detected when they are small and confined to the breast, the vast majority are alive and well 10 years later. The diagnosis of breast cancer is not easily made. **The highest resolution and contrast** attainable has to be brought out in the breast image—more than any other x-ray examination.

Remember, from previous chapter readings, that very high resolution and contrast cannot occur in the x-ray image without a corresponding increase in radiation exposure. The risk from ionizing radiation, therefore, is always of concern in mammography.

Although radiation exposures in mammography are relatively safe today as a result of improvements in technology, and certainly due to stringent regulations, one has to recognize that patient exposure is still an important consideration, and the exposure is relatively high in comparison to x-ray examinations of other body parts. The entrance skin exposure (ESE) for a 5 cm compressed breast is approximately 1,000 mR, and the ESE for a 21 cm lumbar spine AP projection is 220 mR.

1900s

Mammography has been performed since the early 1900s. In those early years, it was not a technologically well-developed examination. The results were unpredictable, and the technical quality of the images was very poor. Dr. Raul Leborgne of Uruguay was one of the first physicians to perform extended research on mammography, and he published the first textbook on the topic in 1953.

1960

Research into mammography continued at a very low level until about 1960 when Dr. Robert Eagan, then at M. D. Anderson Hospital in Houston, first described the use of a high mA, low kVp exposure technique with direct exposure industrial x-ray film. He introduced the technique of removing the aluminum filter from the port of the x-ray tube so the low-energy x-rays could exit. He also introduced the use of a cylindrical extension cone to reduce scatter radiation. Mammography in the 1960s was performed using a conventional x-ray machine. The x-ray tube at that time had a tungsten anode and a large 2 mm focal spot was common. Typical exposure techniques utilized 28 kVp and 300 mA, with exposure times up to 6 seconds (1,800 mAs). Direct exposure x-ray film was used without a grid. Unfortunately, the exposure to the patient was extremely high. Exposures during this era were between **50 to 100x higher** than exposures applied today. Early mammographers reported exposures greater than **50 R** per projection. If repeat radiographs were performed, erythema of the skin would often occur. Eagan's development of a special technique to optimize the x-ray equipment to image the breast prompted the beginning of widespread research into the use of mammography.

1967

In 1967, CGR (France) introduced the first **dedicated** mammography machine (Figure 42-1). The production model of this machine featured a molybdenum anode, 0.7 mm focal spot, and a beryllium window port. In addition, the unit had a built-in device to compress the breast. As a result of these technical improvements, contrast and resolution in the breast image were greatly enhanced. However, exposure to the patient increased compared to Eagan's technique because of the continued use of direct exposures on industrial x-ray film and a higher mAs was required due to the reduced x-ray output of the molybdenum anode. The radiography community during this time was discovering an uncomfortable tradeoff. High-resolution and high-contrast breast images could not be produced without introducing high exposure to the patient. It was during this time that the **benefit-versus-risk debates** about mammography practice ensued.

Research continued, and in the early 1970s, Siemens (Germany), Philips (Netherlands), and Picker and General Electric (USA), also introduced dedicated mammography machines. During the early 1970s, nearly every large radiology department in the world was performing mammography.

1971

In 1971, Xerox (USA) introduced a commercially available system of imaging the breast known as xeromammography. The Xerox **dry process** system utilized a conventional overhead x-ray tube with a tungsten anode. However, the filter had to be removed from the port and a low kVp of 40–50, set on the generator. The x-ray exposure was made on an electrically charged imaging plate instead of using screen and film. The imaging plate was then placed in a special development unit and the breast image

FIGURE 42-1 A 1967 Senograph, produced by CGR (France), became the first commercially available dedicated mammography machine. The unit contained the first molybdenum anode, 0.7 mm focal spot, beryllium window port, and compression device. *(Courtesy of GE Healthcare)*

came out on heavy paper in shades of blue. No film processors or viewboxes were needed. Although a dedicated x-ray machine did not have to be purchased, a special processing machine was needed. Xeromammography was extensively used until the mid-1980s because it produced high contrast images and high resolution (Figure 42-2). Radiation exposures to the patient were lower than Eagan's technique. However, the exposure, which ranged from 2 R to 4 R per projection, was still relatively high. Continued research led to significant improvements in screen/film mammography and lower exposures. Major changes in the design and use of the dedicated mammography machine prompted a major decline in the use of xeromammography for breast imaging by the late 1980s.

1972

In 1972, during the intensive growth and research period in mammography, Du Pont (USA) introduced the first dedicated screen/film system for mammog-

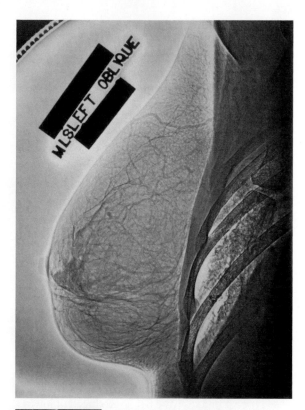

FIGURE 42-2 A 1978 xeroradiographic breast image. Xeromammography produced high contrast and high resolution at doses lower than direct x-ray film exposure. Images were obtained with conventional radiographic equipment, tungsten target, aluminum filter, and 45 kVp.

FIGURE 42-3 A 1975 Kodak mammography cassette, the first cassette developed especially for mammography. It contained a Min-R rare-earth phosphor single emulsion screen (black arrow) and green sensitive Min-R single emulsion (white arrow) film. Design of the cassette allowed the screen and film to be placed close to the breast. Top of cassette is indicated by double arrows.

raphy, **Lo Dose I.** The system utilized a single emulsion film and a single emulsion calcium tungstate screen that was placed in a light-safe polyethylene bag and vacuum sealed. Utilizing a screen for the first time in mammography prompted a major reduction in exposure time and a corresponding reduction in radiation exposure to the patient of nearly **20×.** Use of a screen increased the very low inherent subject contrast of the breast in the image. Unfortunately, there was also a corresponding reduction in resolution when compared to direct x-ray exposure and xeromammography. However, the combined effects of a dramatic increase in contrast, reduced motion unsharpness, and corresponding exposure reduction was so significant that screen/film mammography

gradually became commonplace. During the 1970s, radiologists debated whether to use the Xerox process or screen/film imaging, and many departments chose to use both.

1975

In 1975, a significant event occurred when Kodak (USA) introduced its specially designed for mammography **Min-R** screen, film, and cassette system. The Min-R single emulsion screen, which used the new green emitting rare-earth phosphor, gadolinium oxysulfide, was paired with an orthochromatic (green and blue sensitive) single-emulsion film also called Min-R. The increased screen speed prompted an exposure reduction and there was very negligible loss of resolution. The screen was mounted in a specially designed low-absorption cassette and the screen and film placed so they were as close to the breast as possible (Figure 42-3). Using the cassette saved darkroom time and problems associated with the polyethylene bags. Also during this time, Du Pont introduced an increased speed version of their screen/film—**Lo Dose II.**

1978

The most recent and technologically significant event in mammography occurred in 1978 when Philips (Netherlands) introduced a new generation of dedicated mammography machines (Figure 42-4). This new machine contained the first reciprocating grid. It was also equipped with a foot-pedal; power-driven, breast compression device; aluminum and molybdenum filter selection; automatic exposure control (AEC); a microfocus focal spot; magnification capability; and a high-output generator. Although the introduction of the grid increased the radiation exposure by a factor of **2 to 3×,** the high contrast image that resulted from the reduction in scattered x-rays, in particular for large and dense breasts, was a dramatic improvement in image quality. Fortunately, at this very

FIGURE 42-4 A 1978 Philips (Netherlands) dedicated mammography machine containing the first reciprocating grid. Introduction of this generation of mammography machines ushered in the modern era of utilizing dedicated machines for mammography. *(Courtesy Philips Medical Systems)*

same time, Kodak introduced an increased speed version of its Min-R film, Ortho-M, which reduced the radiation exposure by 50 percent, entirely offsetting the increase in exposure from the use of the grid. The modern era of mammography had begun.

1985–1990

In 1985, a nationwide evaluation of x-ray trends (NEXT) study discovered a wide variation in mammographic image quality and in radiation exposures to the patient. Independent studies done later supported the NEXT data and found similar and additional unacceptable variations in image quality. Citations found in the studies included poor processor performance, inexperienced operators of the equipment, improper physician interpretation, poor exposure techniques, and a general inability to perform the examination in a consistent manner.

Concern about the quality of mammography led to the development of the American College of Radiology (ACR) accreditation program in 1987. This voluntary program required mammography sites to meet quality standards to ensure that optimally exposed breast images were being produced at low radiation exposures to the patient. Components of the ACR program included an assessment of both mammographic phantom and actual clinical images for optimal resolution and contrast, measurement of the average glandular dose to the breast, and processor performance. In 1990, additional standards were set forth, which included specific aspects of the equipment and accessory devices, personnel, and the documentation of an effective quality control program. By June 1994, 66 percent of the mammography machines in the United States had passed the ACR voluntary accreditation. Of those that failed, the three most common reasons for failure in descending order were: poor clinical images, failure of the phantom image to demonstrate appropriate contrast and resolution, and poor processor performance.

1991

In 1991, the American Registry of Radiologic Technologists (ARRT) implemented its first **advanced-level** examination specifically for mammography.

The examination was designed to ensure that the radiographers who perform mammography have appropriate comprehension of exact positioning techniques, have knowledge of the broad spectrum of mammography projections, understand technical factor selection, and know other specific technical, clinical, and affective aspects related to the performance of the examination. Radiographers who pass the advanced-level mammography examination are formally recognized to perform mammography and use the initial (M) after their radiography credential RT(R).

1992–1994

In 1992, as a result of the American Cancer Society's high visibility public relations campaign that all women over 40 undergo screening mammography, and also because of federal legislation that provided reimbursement for screening mammography in women eligible for Medicare, the federal government enacted the Mammography Quality Standards Act (MQSA). The act was written because of lobbying from the ACR due to the great concern about the poor quality mammography being performed. The act went into effect on October 1, 1994, and requires all sites (except VA facilities) that provide mammography service to meet quality standards and become certified for operation by the secretary of the Department of Health and Human Services (DHHS). Enactment of the MQSA marks the first time the use of an x-ray machine and a specific x-ray examination are regulated by the federal government.

1999

On April 28, 1999, the Final Rule of the MQSA went into effect after several years of public comments. MQSA is now officially known as Public Law 105-248. Today, dedicated mammography machines are produced by a variety of manufacturers. These machines are mechanically and electronically designed to meet the stringent radiographic and positioning requirements of breast imaging, and they are used with specially designed screens, film, and cassettes. There are no xeromammography systems in use today. Mammography equipment is presently capable of producing extremely high-contrast images with very high resolution, and the radiation exposures to the patient are reasonably low. However, researchers continue to seek higher contrast and resolution for breast images and methods for lowering the exposure.

2000

In February 2000, the first **digital mammography unit** was approved for sale in the United States. The machine was the General Electric Senographe 2000 D. At the time of this writing in 2004, four manufacturers are providing approved digital mammography systems. The U.S. Congress has passed legislation authorizing increased Medicare reimbursement for this new technology. Digital mammography holds great promise; however, research continues to ensure that it produces results of equivalent diagnostic accuracy to screen/film mammography. Many trials using digital mammography are currently underway. It is expected that by 2006 the results of these trials will be completed.

This chapter discusses the current technical aspects of screen/film mammography. The reader should note that every component in the mammography system is modified from conventional radiology. Each component is designed specifically to maximize contrast and resolution while at the same time engineered to keep the radiation exposure to the patient at minimal levels. Table 42-1 illustrates the primary technical differences between mammography and conventional x-ray machines. The light-weight (some weigh only 500 lbs.) entirely self-contained mammography unit, which can easily be pushed around a room and simply plugged in, is a relatively sophisticated x-ray machine. Its sole design and purpose is to image the human breast.

 GENERATOR CHARACTERISTICS

Manufacturers of dedicated mammography machines use the new **high-frequency** generators (see Chapter 5) which were introduced by Siemens (Germany) in 1987. There are several reasons for using high-frequency generators in mammography. These

TABLE 42-1. Technical Differences between Mammography and Conventional Radiography		
	Mammography	Conventional
Generator*	1φ high frequency	1φ, 3φ, Capacitor discharge, Falling load
Voltage frequency*	>10,000 Hz	60 Hz
Voltage ripple	<4%	4–100%
kVp†	25–28	50–130
mA†	20–160	100–1000
Exposure time (s)†	0.4–4.0	0.01–2.0
Power rating	3–10 kW	50–200 kW
AEC	1 detector	3 detectors
Film density (OD)††	>1.30	1.10
Backup timer (mAs)	600 grid, 300 non-grid	600
Focal spot size (mm)	0.1 or 0.3	0.6 or 1.2
SID (cm)	60–65	102–122
X-ray beam utilized	Anode side only	Anode and cathode side equally
Effective target angle‡	22°–24°	7°–17°
Reference target angle**	7.5°–12°	7°–17°
Anode	Molybdenum or Rhodium	Tungsten
Tube port	Beryllium	Glass
Filter	Molybdenum or Rhodium	Aluminum
HVL (mm AL)	0.3 (30 kVp)	2.3 (80 kVp)
Grid	4:1 or 5:1	6:1–16:1
Screen–film speeds†‡	100–320	100–1,200
Resolution (lp/mm)	12–20	5–10

* Some high-frequency generators are being introduced in conventional radiology.
† Range used in clinical practice.
†† Mammography density measured on the ACR Plexiglas™ phantom.
Conventional density measured on 21 cm Plexiglas™ phantom.
‡ Measured from the vertical central ray.
** Measured from the reference axis/center of image receptor.
†‡ Relative speeds of mammography screens are slower than conventional screens with same number.

generators virtually eliminate voltage regulation problems and allow very precise control of kVp, mA, and exposure time—important considerations in breast imaging. The linearity and reproducibility of the x-ray exposures are excellent. High-frequency x-ray output waveform ripple is much lower than three-phase, 6-pulse ripple at usually less than 4 percent. The high frequency (100 kHz) allows more efficient x-ray production and, therefore, produces a higher effective energy x-ray beam. The result is higher x-ray output for a given kVp and mA setting.

High-frequency generators do not require an autotransformer, line compensation circuit, or space-charge compensation circuit. This greatly reduces equipment bulk, cost, and space requirements. The high-frequency generator system is uniquely housed within the single-standing mammography unit (Figure 42-5). These new generators operate

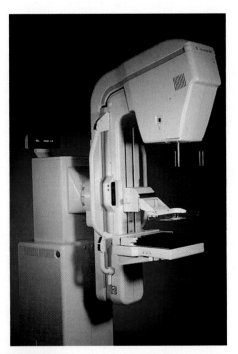

FIGURE 42-5 A 1995 Bennett (USA) current generation mammography machine containing a high-frequency generator, uniquely housed within the standing unit. Operates on single-phase incoming line power. *(Courtesy Bennett Technologies)*

on single-phase incoming line power, which simplifies installation and greatly reduces cost. High-frequency generators can also be designed to operate from batteries for use in mobile mammography vans. Several manufacturers have designed the high-frequency generator and x-ray tube within the same housing.

kVp

A significant difference between mammography and conventional x-ray machines is the low kVp utilized. The kVp selections on the generator will range from 22 to 40 kVp. The kVp commonly used in clinical practice varies between **25 and 28 kVp.** The advantage of using low kVp is its ability to produce a very low-energy (soft) x-ray beam that produces high radiographic contrast. High contrast is desirable in breast images because the radiologist must be able to delineate clearly the normal and diseased structures of the breast tissue. Breast tissue is considered **soft tissue** and it is entirely made up of glands, fibers, and fat, which have very low inherent subject contrast (Figure 42-6). The radiologist must have sufficient contrast available in the image to visualize microcalcifications as small as 0.1 to 0.3 mm, and other subtle parenchymal structures. The major disadvantage of using kVp in the 20s range is that there is a high absorption of the low-energy x-rays in the breast, which contributes significantly to patient dose.

Exposure Time, mA, mAs

Mammography generators also utilize low mA settings. Depending on the manufacturer, the mA can vary from about 2 to as high as 180. Generators typically will have a variable mA selection from **20 to 100,** and many manufacturers design a single mA setting for the small focal spot (e.g., 20 mA) and one for the large focal spot (e.g., 80 mA). Low mA settings are necessary because of the power rating limitations placed on the smaller sized anode and the small focal spot sizes. The power ratings of mammography generators vary between 3 and 10 kilowatts (kW) compared to 50 to 1,200 kW on conventional x-ray generators.

In clinical practice, the specific mA selected is determined based on the principle of keeping exposure times short enough to decrease patient motion. However, the time should not be extremely short, which would cause grid artifacts (textured or structured patterns) to appear in the image. Because the mammography system produces a high-resolution image, grid lines have the potential of being prominently shown and will degrade image quality. Conversely, exposure times that exceed **1 second** will result in **reciprocity law failure.** Typical exposure times in clinical practice will vary from **0.4 to over 1 second** for standard projections. Exposure times for projections using the magnification technique are much longer, varying from **2 to 4 seconds** due to the low mA used with the 0.1 mm focal spot. When performing magnification studies, mammographers

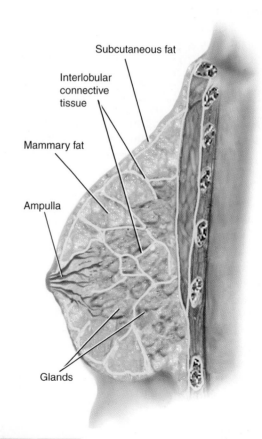

Subcutaneous fat

Interlobular connective tissue

Mammary fat

Ampulla

Glands

FIGURE 42-6 Female breast made up entirely of glands, fibrous tissues, and fat. Creates low inherent subject contrast in the mammographic image.

must be very cautious, and explicit instructions must be given to the patient so motion is kept to a minimum during these longer exposures. Unfortunately, the screen response to the long exposure times that occur during magnification studies prompts reciprocity law failure, for which the radiographer must compensate. Additional exposure times from **10 to 30 percent** are required to maintain optimal density at these long exposure times. Fortunately, high-quality mammography machines have sophisticated built-in circuitry that will automatically compensate for reciprocity law failure so that repeat radiographs are kept to a minimum.

Automatic Exposure Control

Automatic Exposure Control (AEC) is an integral component on every dedicated mammography generator. Like the AEC circuitry used on conventional radiography equipment, its design and purpose is to provide consistent image receptor exposure for the various thickness and density compositions of breast tissues and for the range of kVp used. Because of the high-contrast imaging environment in mammography, there is minimal exposure latitude in terms of film density. Small variations in film density will affect the contrast required to visualize the subtle breast tissue and to diagnose cancer.

Automatic control of exposure techniques is crucial in breast imaging because of the wide range of breast thicknesses and density compositions. A 4 cm compressed breast on a number of similarly aged women can cause a range of x-ray exposure times from **0.05 ms to over 1 second**! It is virtually impossible for the radiographer to determine the exact density composition of breast tissues; therefore, it is difficult to determine the exact exposure time required if AEC were not used. The introduction of AEC on dedicated mammography machines, in particular the current generation machines, prompted a significant reduction in repeat rates for mammography.

The AEC system on most mammography machines utilizes a single radiation-sensitive detector located **behind** the cassette. The detector is capable of moving toward the nipple, from its primary position at the chest wall, to allow for maximum variations in breast size and for critical magnification

FIGURE 42-7 General design of a mammography machine and its accessory components. Note vertical alignment of the chest wall edge of cassette and compression paddle, straight portion of extension cone, and angle of the anode.

work (Figure 42-7). Most detectors will have 10 stops between the chest wall and the nipple. The AEC system should be capable of being calibrated for two different screen/film systems and also for non-grid, grid, and magnification options.

The optical density (OD) of the ACR Plexiglas™ mammographic phantom image should not be less than **1.20** and preferably about **1.30 OD**. The film density, as measured using the ACR standardized exposure technique, should be within ±0.15 OD for the range of kVps used and for phantom Plexiglas™ thicknesses from 2 to 6 cm. The generator must contain a **density compensation circuit** that contains at least two + and two − settings. Each setting, or step, should result in a 12% to 15% change in mAs, or approximately a 0.15 change in optical film density to allow maximum flexibility for all imaging requirements. Mammography generators have a **backup timer** similar to conventional AEC systems. The backup timer for grid techniques must be set at **600 mAs,** and for non-grid and magnification techniques, **300 mAs.** If the backup time is reached during a breast exposure, the radiographer should select a **higher kVp** setting for the repeat radiograph. The density compensation circuit should not be increased as is typically done in conventional AEC imaging. The primary reason backup time is reached in breast imaging is because of the inability of the low-energy photons to penetrate the breast. (This will usually occur on large or dense breasts.) A density compensation circuit increase will only prompt the backup timer to be reached again because the energy of the x-ray beam did not change; therefore, penetration of the breast will not occur. If the AEC system is left on during imaging of a breast with an implant in place, the backup time will also be reached. (Only **manual** exposure techniques should be used for implant imaging.)

Quality mammography generators have highly sophisticated microprocessor controlled circuits that provide accurate and reproducible film densities over the entire range of kVp settings required and for the different thicknesses and densities of breast tissue. Well-designed AEC circuitry can automatically compensate for reciprocity law failure during long exposures. Current machines may also contain circuits that can automatically adjust the kVp to a higher level during the actual exposure. This allows the film to be properly exposed and the backup time will not be reached if the breast is large or dense. The circuit adjusts the kVp by sensing the radiation intensity during the first 100 milliseconds of the exposure. If the current is too low, the kVp is automatically increased. When purchasing a new mammography machine, the AEC nomenclature should be carefully checked and tested to ensure that it has accurate density tracking and, therefore, will reproduce film densities for all requirements within ±0.10 OD.

X-RAY TUBE

Design

The most distinctive aspect of the mammography machine is the design and application of its x-ray tube and peripheral components. Each component described in this section has a very novel design compared to its counterpart in conventional radiology. The specific design or use of some components will increase contrast, resolution, or radiation exposure. Other components counteract this and cause a decrease in contrast, resolution, or exposure. The production of a high-quality breast image involves many tradeoffs. Taken altogether, however, the x-ray tube design and the components are capable of achieving high resolution and high contrast at moderate radiation exposure levels. First and foremost, the mammography equipment must be engineered to provide the high contrast and resolution required to visualize microcalcifications and the subtle parenchymal structures of the breast. Achieving the right balance of contrast, resolution, and low radiation exposures is a formidable challenge in breast imaging.

Heel Effect

The anode configuration in a mammography x-ray tube produces a prominent heel effect due to the short source-to-image receptor distance (SID) and the use of a narrow target angle. Because the x-ray tube is aligned with the cathode placed directly over the chest wall area and the anode outward toward the nipple end, the heel effect fortunately can be used to maximum advantage (Figure 42-8). Recall that the cathode side of the x-ray beam has a significantly greater intensity of x-rays compared to the anode side. A more uniform-density breast image can be produced because the more intense x-rays are at the chest wall where there is greater tissue thickness (Figure 42-9). The primary reason the cathode end of the x-ray tube is placed directly over the chest wall edge of the image is to take advantage of the prominent heel effect of the anode.

Cathode

The cathode in a mammography x-ray tube consists of standard helical-shaped tungsten filaments in a focusing cup. Mammography tubes typically utilize a single filament wire for both the large and small focal spots. When the small focal spot is engaged, a negative voltage is applied to the focusing cup, which acts to reduce the size of the electron stream creating the smaller focal spot. This is called **bias focusing** (see

FIGURE 42-8 Patient positioned on a mammography machine. Note short SID of 60 cm, which produces a prominent heel effect. Cathode side of the x-ray tube is placed over patient's head and anode side outward toward nipple. This orientation allows the bulk of the x-ray tube housing to be placed away from the patient's head for ease of positioning.

Chest wall

FIGURE 42-9 Mammography x-ray tube oriented with the cathode side placed over the chest wall area and the anode side placed outward toward the nipple end. Heel effect is used to maximum advantage with this orientation. Greater intensity x-rays are placed over the chest wall area where the breast is thicker, producing a more uniform density image.

Chapter 6). Some machines utilize two separate filaments for the small and large focal spots.

The high resolution needed in mammography requires substantially smaller effective focal spot sizes than those used in conventional radiography. In addition, the majority of mammography machines utilize a relatively short SID of only **60 to 76 cm** (24 to 30 inches), which necessitates the use of microsized focal spots to diminish the increased geometric unsharpness. A nominal **0.3 mm large** focal spot is used for the routine contact images and a nominal **0.1 mm small** focal spot is used for magnification images.

In all x-ray tubes, the effective focal spot size varies in length along the cathode-anode axis at the plane of the film due to the line-focus principle. As a result, a larger focal spot size is always projected on the cathode side (Figure 42-10A). Because mam-

mography tubes are oriented with the cathode side placed over the chest wall, the focal spot shape and size phenomenon creates a serious dilemma: resolution is substantially decreased at the chest wall where many lesions are found. The phenomenon is more pronounced for magnification techniques. Another phenomenon that can complicate breast imaging occurs if the actual focal spot and central ray are positioned over the center of the image as in conventional radiology. Due to the short SID, several millimeters of posterosuperior breast tissue will not be imaged (Figure 42-10B). These two negative geometric properties associated with the focal spot in mammography are diminished via the **off-center placement** of the glass x-ray tube unit within the tube housing. The glass tube is moved maximally to-

FIGURE 42-10   (A) Conventional radiography x-ray tube with focal spot and vertical central ray positioned over center of the cassette. Note focal spot length is projected larger in size toward the cathode end due to the line-focus principle. (B) Conventional focal spot and vertical central ray positioned over center of cassette prompting posterosuperior breast tissue to be missed on the image.

ward the chest wall so the focal spot on the anode and vertical central ray are positioned **directly over the chest wall** (Figure 42-11A and B). The geometric dilemma is diminished by **eliminating** the entire cathode side of the x-ray beam. Although the effective focal spot size remains larger at the chest wall, utilizing the anode half of the beam provides slightly greater resolution because the projected focal spot sizes at the image plane are smaller on this side. Therefore, a smaller effective focal spot is projected at the important chest wall area (see Figure 42-11A). Placing the x-ray tube off center also enables the vertical central ray to enter **straight in** at the chest wall eliminating the possibility of missing the posterosuperior breast tissue in the image (see Figure 42-11B). The heel effect continues to be advantageous because there does remain greater intensity at the vertical central ray point than at the anode end. Recall that the x-ray intensity decreases gradually from the cathode toward the anode.

This unique design prompts a change in the orientation of the mammography x-ray beam. Because the vertical central ray is positioned at the chest wall (edge of the film), the x-ray directed to the center of the cassette is actually the mid-portion of the anode half of the x-ray beam. This new **angled** central ray is termed the **reference axis** in mammography (see Figure 42-11B).

The physical size of the focal spot in mammography is determined and measured by the manufacturers at the **reference axis** point on the image receptor plane, not at the vertical central ray point as in conventional radiography. The target angle will measure smaller from the reference axis perspective, and, therefore, the focal spot will also measure smaller. The nominal 0.30 mm large and nominal 0.10 mm small focal spots measure this size in the center of the film at the reference axis point. Therefore, the projected **length** and overall size of the effective focal spot at the vertical central ray point and chest wall will be at least **2× larger.**

FIGURE 42-11 Off-center placement of the x-ray tube within the tube housing. Cathode side of x-ray beam eliminated. (A) Focal spot and vertical central ray placed directly over the chest wall. (B) Vertical central ray placed directly over chest wall structure allows the posterosuperior breast tissue to be imaged. Note new central ray is termed the reference axis. Nominal focal spot size is measured at the reference axis point on the image receptor.

This geometric phenomenon results from the line focus principle and cannot be overcome. The high resolution in the image is maintained, in part, via the use of very small focal spot sizes. This may appear to not be an ideal engineering design, however, a tradeoff must be made. Overall, it is more advantageous to have the cathode end over the more dense chest wall structures to take advantage of the **heel effect.** In addition, this orientation allows the bulk of the x-ray tube housing to be placed away from the patient's head for ease of positioning (see Figure 42-8).

Anode Configuration

Mammography tubes use rotating anodes to take advantage of the increased tube loading. This is particularly important because it enables the use of a higher mA and allows exposure times to be maintained under 1 second.

The **effective target angle** (measured from the vertical central ray point) is **greater** in a mammography tube, varying from **22° to 24°.** The larger effective angle is necessary so the x-ray beam will cover a 24 × 30 cm cassette at the 60–65 cm SID (Figure 42-12A and B). However, the **reference axis target angle** (measured from the center of the x-ray beam as in conventional radiography) is **smaller** varying from **7.5° to 12°.** The reference axis target angle is specified in mammography tubes because it defines the size of the focal spot as measured in the center of the image.

Most manufacturers prefer to use a narrow target angle, as measured from the vertical filament, because it allows greater anode heat capacity for a given effective focal spot size. However, to utilize a narrower angle and maintain x-ray coverage on the cassette, the x-ray tube must be **tilted** (see Figure 42-12B). One manufacturer utilizes a unique design in which the anode is oriented with the stem placed in a ver-

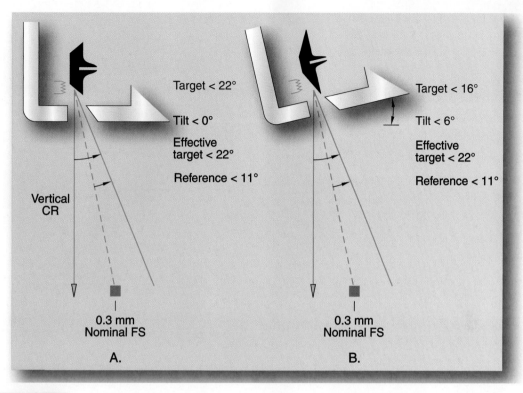

Target < 22°

Tilt < 0°

Effective
target < 22°

Reference < 11°

Vertical
CR

0.3 mm
Nominal FS

A.

Target < 16°

Tilt < 6°

Effective
target < 22°

Reference < 11°

0.3 mm
Nominal FS

B.

FIGURE 42-12   Mammography x-ray tube configurations. (A) Horizontal tube placement and 22° target angle. Large **effective** target angle of 22° allows x-ray coverage of cassette at a short SID. **Reference axis** target angle of 11° creates a 0.3 mm focal spot size in the center of the image. (B) Tilting the tube 6° allows use of a smaller target angle of 16° and prompts the same **effective** angle of 22° and **reference axis** angle of 11° as horizontal tube. Tilting allows greater anode heat capacity due to the smaller target angle.

tical position and the x-ray tube steeply tilted. This allows the **edge** of the anode disk to be used as the actual target rather than the face of the anode (Figure 42-13A and B). The anode edge is designed with two distinct surfaces, one for each focal spot. This design allows radiation coverage of the film with the large focal spot, achievement of maximum anode heat capacity, capability of producing a small effective focal spot, and placement of the effective small focal spot closer to the chest wall, allowing greater resolution. Designing the anode configuration to achieve a small effective focal spot size, allowing maximum x-ray coverage of the cassette, and producing optimal resolution at a short SID are engineering challenges.

Anode Material

The anode in mammography x-ray tubes is made of **molybdenum.** Some manufacturers use a solid molybdenum disk and others design the molybdenum anode with graphite backing similar to conventional radiography. In order to prevent anode surface roughness and pitting, which could ultimately decrease x-ray output, the molybdenum may be doped with about 3 percent vanadium. Like tungsten, molybdenum has a high melting point, and conducts heat well.

Molybdenum is used as the anode material of choice over tungsten for several reasons. Studies indicate that x-ray energies ranging between 17 keV

FIGURE 42-13 Anode oriented with stem placed in a vertical position, a biangular anode disk **end** used as the target, and the tube steeply tilted. Circled inset shows anode end in true vertical position with 0° lower edge and −9° upper edge. (A) Lower edge of anode disk used for large focal spot. Steep 22.5° tube tilt produces a 22.5° **effective** target angle to allow x-ray coverage of the cassette and a 12° **reference axis** angle creates a 0.30 nominal focal spot. (B) Upper edge of anode disk used for small focal spot and magnification studies. The 22.5° tilt produces a 13.5° **effective** target angle, which allows adequate coverage for magnification images. The 7.5° **reference axis** angle creates a 0.10 nominal small focal spot. The small focal spot is projected closer to the chest wall structure, allowing greater resolution.

and 25 keV are required to differentiate the inherent low contrast structures of all types of breasts. Specifically, x-ray energies between the narrow range of **17–20** are preferred. These specific x-ray energies must be present in the mammography x-ray beam to maximize subject contrast and visualize microcalcifications. If the x-ray beam contains energies higher than this narrow range, the x-rays will overpenetrate, scatter, and decrease radiographic contrast. A relatively large number of **photoelectric absorption** interactions is needed to produce the high radiographic contrast that will improve the visibility of detail in the image. Low kVp is necessary to produce the 17–20 keV range of

x-ray photons that will create the photoelectric interactions. Unfortunately, this will introduce a higher radiation exposure to the patient. As in all areas of mammography, a tradeoff must be made. Without low kVp x-rays and high photoelectric absorption, radiographic detail of the breast structures cannot occur.

The three primary breast tissues—adipose, fibrous, and glandular—have very low atomic numbers ranging from 6 to 8. Approximately 40 percent of cancers in the breast contain microcalcifications that have an atomic number of 20. Therefore, kVp settings around 25 are necessary. One must set the generator kVp slightly higher than the atomic num-

FIGURE 42-14   X-ray emission spectrums produced at 26 kVp. (A) Conventional tungsten target with aluminum filter. High volume of photons produced above the preferred mammography range of 17 to 20 keV and high volume below this range. Note entire x-ray beam is bremsstrahlung photons. (B) Mammography molybdenum target and molybdenum filter producing prominent characteristic photons at 17 and 20 keV in the preferred energy range. Very few photons produced above this range. (C) Mammography rhodium target and rhodium filter. Spectrum shape is identical to B but produces a **higher** average energy x-ray beam than molybdenum. Note prominent characteristic photons at 20 and 23 keV, which provide better penetration for larger or more dense breasts at a lower dose to the patient.

ber of the tissues being imaged so there is adequate penetration. Figures 42-14A and 42–14B illustrate an x-ray emission spectrum for a conventional tungsten anode x-ray tube and a molybdenum anode mammography tube operating at 26 kVp. Note that the tungsten anode will produce x-ray photons with energies in the preferred 17–20 keV range. It also produces a high volume of photons above this range and a relatively large number below the range. The x-ray photons above the preferred mammography range will produce Compton interactions that decrease contrast, and the x-ray photons below this range will be virtually all absorbed via the photoelectric process and only contribute to patient dose. The entire tungsten produced x-ray beam consists of bremsstrahlung x-rays.

TABLE 42-2.   Characteristic X-Rays from Mammography X-Ray Targets

Electron Shells	Molybdenum (Z-42)	Rhodium (Z-45)
	keV*	
L to K	17	20
M to K	20	23

The x-ray emission spectrum produced from the molybdenum anode has a drastically different shape. Note that the most prominent x-ray photons are **characteristic.** The characteristic x-rays are created from displacement of the K-shell binding electrons in the molybdenum atom (Table 42-2).

Characteristic x-rays will account for approximately 30 percent of the total x-rays in the molybdenum beam at 30 kVp. Most importantly, there is an increased volume of characteristic x-ray photons produced at exactly 17 and 20 keV in the preferred range, which creates a nearly perfect x-ray beam for breast imaging. When properly filtered, the molybdenum anode produces very few x-ray photons above the preferred mammographic energy range. The x-ray photons below this range are photoelectrically absorbed and aid in producing high subject contrast. Unfortunately, they also contribute to dose. Many textbooks refer to the molybdenum x-ray emission spectrum as being essentially homogeneous due to the high concentration of x-rays in a very narrow range.

The advantages of using molybdenum for the anode material in mammography tubes are:

- **Increased number of low-energy photons** are produced.
- **High radiographic contrast** is achieved in the image.
- **Production of specific x-ray energies** required for breast imaging.

The disadvantages of molybdenum are:

- **Less x-ray photon output** due a to lower atomic number—42.
- **Increased mAs required** to maintain image receptor exposure.
- **Increased dose** to the patient.

The higher contrast image produced by the molybdenum target is illustrated in Figure 42-15.

Recently, a new anode material, **rhodium,** was introduced for use in mammography. The slightly higher atomic number of rhodium, 45, creates higher energy x-ray photons (see Table 42-2). The primary advantage of using rhodium is that the characteristic x-rays it produces have energies that are **2–3 keV higher** than molybdenum. In the rhodium x-ray emission spectrum, the x-ray photon energies shift slightly to the right and the characteristic x-rays are prominent at **20 and 23 keV** (Figure 42–14C). This provides better penetration of large breasts or those breasts that are very dense. Of significance also is that rhodium's higher average

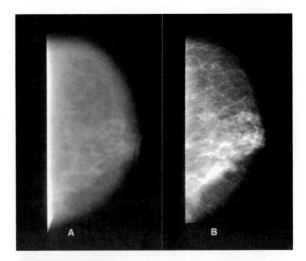

FIGURE 42-15 Craniocaudal projection of the same patient's breast produced at 30 kVp showing effect of molybdenum anode on radiographic contrast. (A) Tungsten anode produces suboptimal radiographic contrast. (B) Molybdenum anode produces significantly higher contrast and greater visibility of detail. *(Images courtesy of C. Vyborny, M.D., Ph.D.)*

energy x-ray beam prompts a reduction in exposure time of approximately 25 percent. When used with the appropriate filter, use of a rhodium anode can decrease x-ray exposure by 50 percent or more. The primary disadvantage of rhodium as an anode material is that its higher energy beam is not appropriate for use on small to regular sized breasts, or those breasts that are not dense. Therefore, it cannot be the sole anode material. To take advantage of the inherent properties of rhodium, one manufacturer has designed a **biangular** anode, similar to Figure 42-13, in which the same disk contains a track for molybdenum and a separate track for rhodium, selectable by the operator. The x-ray tube can be moved in one of two positions, one for each of the two focal spots. This allows both focal spot sizes to be available for each track. Interestingly, another manufacturer has recently introduced a dual-track anode that contains molybdenum and **tungsten,** selectable by the operator also. The tungsten anode is used with a rhodium filter and, like the rhodium anode, is designed to be used on the larger or more dense breasts at a significantly reduced exposure.

While molybdenum is the primary anode material used, all machines will have either rhodium or tungsten as an alternate choice.

Filtration

The port of the x-ray tube in mammography is specially designed. **Beryllium,** with an atomic number of 4, is used in the port of all mammography x-ray tubes to allow the low-energy x-rays to exit. Glass cannot be used because it would attenuate most of the low-energy x-rays needed to produce the breast image.

Filtration must be used at the tube port on all mammography machines. As in conventional radiography, the primary purpose of filtration is to attenuate the very low-energy x-rays that are not needed to produce the breast image. Without filtration, a relatively large number of 5–10 keV x-rays would exit the tube. In addition, a larger number of 20–30 keV x-rays at the higher energy end of the spectrum would also exit. The 5–10 keV x-rays would all be absorbed in the breast and drastically increase the dose. The 20–30 keV x-rays would degrade image quality by decreasing radiographic contrast. A specific function of the filter in mammography, therefore, is to decrease most of the low and some high-energy bremsstrahlung x-rays to maximize subject contrast. To accomplish this, mammography filters are made of the **same element** as the anode material. For a molybdenum anode the filter is **0.03 mm molybdenum** and for the rhodium target, **0.025 mm rhodium.** The x-ray emission spectrums for molybdenum and rhodium in Figure 42-14 show the effect of this filtration. Eliminating much of the high 20–30 keV photons provides a nearly perfect x-ray beam for breast imaging.

Many mammography machines provide a selectable molybdenum or rhodium filter that can be used with the molybdenum anode. Selection of the rhodium filter with the molybdenum anode will produce an emission spectrum that lies halfway between the molybdenum and the rhodium configurations. The rhodium filter used with the molybdenum anode will produce a higher energy x-ray beam that is more desirable for larger or dense breasts. Use of the rhodium filter will also reduce

radiation exposure by about 38 percent. Caution must be exercised to ensure that the rhodium filter is not used with small and regular sized breasts or non-dense breasts, because it will produce a lower contrast image that would not provide the appropriate visibility of detail.

The half-value-layer (HVL) is an indirect measurement of the total filtration in the path of the x-ray beam. It is expressed in millimeters of aluminum (mm Al). In a mammography machine, the HVL will include the attenuation properties of the beryllium window, molybdenum filter, mirror, and the plastic compression paddle. The minimum HVL is specified by government regulations and should not measure less than **0.30 mm Al** at 30 kVp or **0.25 mm Al** at 25 kVp. This will ensure that adequate filtration is present in the x-ray beam, and the patient will not receive excessive radiation exposure. If the HVL is too high, image quality can be degraded. Excessive filtration, although it would reduce exposure, will decrease overall radiographic image contrast. Therefore, the HVL should not exceed **0.40 mm Al** at 30 kVp. It is recommended that the HVL be maintained as close as possible to the minimal level to ensure that image contrast is maintained at a high level.

Magnification

Magnified projections of the breast are additionally requested when the visibility of detail in very small breast structures and when microcalcifications need to be enhanced. They are also requested when breast structures that lie close together and overlap have to be separated. As many as 10 percent of patients require additional projections using the magnification technique.

The magnification factor on the mammography machine varies slightly among manufacturers and is standardized between 1.5× and 1.8×. Some manufacturers design their equipment with two magnification selections—the second may be as high as 2.0×. To magnify the breast, a raised platform is placed on the cassette holder unit and the breast is placed on top of the platform for the exposure (Figure 42-16).

Magnified projections of the breast provide the following enhancements:

$$\text{Magnification} = \frac{60 \text{ cm}}{40 \text{ cm}} = 1.5x$$

FIGURE 42-16 Breast in position on a raised platform to produce a 1.5× magnification image. There is greater intensity of radiation at the breast when placed closer to the x-ray tube. Magnification technique requires the use of a 0.10 focal spot to maintain resolution.

- **Increased resolution** due to the small focal spot and reduced quantum mottle
- **Reduction in scatter radiation** reaching the film due to the air gap
- **Improved visibility of detail** due to the larger field of view.

Magnifying the breast will technically reduce resolution in the image due to an increase in geometric unsharpness. A magnification of 1.5× will reduce resolution by at least 50 percent from about 20 lp/mm to 10 lp/mm. To regain the lost resolution, a very small 0.10-mm focal spot is utilized, which returns the resolution to the 20 lp/mm level. This is the smallest focal spot size employed anywhere in radiology. Effective resolution may even be improved in magnified images due to a **reduction in noise.** Recall that noise is primarily a product of the

FIGURE 42-17 (A) Magnification image of calcifications in a Plexiglas™ breasts phantom at 1.5× and 26 kVp. (B) Nonmagnified image of same phantom as A.

screen/film combination (quantum mottle). The screen/film combination typically is not changed for magnification techniques. Noise is, therefore, reduced by about 30 percent for 1.5× magnification because significantly more x-ray photons are used per unit volume of tissue to produce the image. This is due to the breast being placed closer to the x-ray tube where there is a higher volume of x-rays available to form the image. For 1.5× magnification, a given square of tissue covers approximately 2.25× more area on the film compared to the contact image, and many more screen phosphors are utilized to form the image.

Scattered radiation is reduced somewhat as a result of the air-gap between the cassette and breast. The reduced scatter increases radiographic contrast and, fortunately, a grid does not have to be used. The breast structures are seen much better when the magnification technique is used due to a combination of the microsized focal spot, the reduction in noise, and the reduction in scatter radiation. When the breast structures are magnified, they are spread apart and the anatomical field of view is enhanced (Figure 42-17A and B).

Radiation exposure to the patient is a major concern in magnification radiography of the breast. Radiation to the breast can increase **2–3X** during a single exposure, even without the use of a grid. This results from the breast being placed much closer to the x-ray source where the radiation intensity is greater. The exact exposure increase will vary among different manufacturers' units depending upon their specific design and magnification factor. The increase in radiation is due also to the additional exposure required because of reciprocity law failure. Use of the 0.10 focal spot requires that the mA be reduced considerably (e.g., 100 mA to 25 mA) due to tube loading. The reduction in mA will prompt exposure times to be increased to **2–4 seconds.** The long exposure time will require the mammographer to explain the procedure carefully and to watch the patient during the exposure so motion does not degrade image quality.

 ACCESSORIES

Grids

Scatter control plays an important role in the production of a high-quality mammographic image. Scatter radiation is produced from the breast during the exposure which contributes to the overall image receptor exposure, and the effect is a reduction in radiographic contrast. Scatter increases significantly for larger and more dense breasts and with higher kVp settings. With the introduction of the grid on dedicated mammography machines in 1978, scatter and secondary radiation reaching the image receptor has been reduced and high contrast maintained in the image. The grid will remove about 80–90 percent of the scatter. Use of a grid in mammography greatly improves radiographic quality and today grids are used for all mammographic images. The use of a grid will, however, increase radiation exposure to the patient by a factor of **2–3x.**

Mammography grids are the linear type with a very low ratio of 4:1 or 5:1. The grid frequency will range from 30 to 50 lines/cm. The grid strips are made of lead as in conventional radiography. However, wood or carbon-fiber are used as the inner space material instead of aluminum in order to keep the bucky factor as low as possible. All mammography grids in use today are a moving type—moving in one direction only. They do not reciprocate. A separate grid device is used for each of the two image receptor sizes used.

Grids are capable of producing artifacts in the image. Typically this occurs with the use of ultra-short exposure times which can be controlled by using an appropriate mA setting that will prevent short exposure times. Grids can also contain inherent artifacts. Upon purchase, mammography grids should be carefully checked before use to ensure they are free of artifacts. A basic quality control check can be performed by making a lighter density film exposure with the grid stationary and another lighter density exposure with the grid moving. If artifacts appear on the image made with the moving grid, the grid should probably be replaced.

Compression Device

All mammography machines contain a compression device that is used to compress the breast (see Figures 42-7 and 42-8). Improvements in breast compression technology in recent years has greatly improved the visibility of detail in breast images. Appropriately applied compression is one of the critical components in the production of a high-quality mammogram. The overall function of compression is to decrease the thickness of the breast, bring the breast structures as close to the image receptor as possible, and increase radiographic contrast (Figure 42-18). The specific advantages of this technique are:

- **Reduced magnification** lessens geometric unsharpness and increases resolution.

- **Reduced tissue thickness** requires less kVp prompting a reduction in scattered radiation and an increase in radiographic contrast.

- **Reduced radiation exposure** because less exposure time is required due to the decreased tissue thickness.

- **Reduced motion unsharpness** occurs because the breast is completely immobilized.

- **Improved visualization** of breast structures because the structures are spread out over a larger area. There is also less superimposition of overlying structures.

- **More uniform image receptor exposure** occurs due to the flattening effect of compression permitting optimal exposure of the entire breast.

FIGURE 42-18 Effect of compression on the breast image. Spot compression on half of the breast (arrow) shows excellent contrast and resolution. Noncompressed side (double arrows) shows decreased density due to a thicker breast when no compression is applied. Significantly increased technical factors would be required to penetrate and achieve appropriate image receptor exposure if compression were not applied and dose would be considerably higher.

Breast Compression

Uncompressed

Scatter to primary ratio
0.8

A.

Compressed

Scatter to primary ratio
0.4

B.

FIGURE 42-19 Breast compression. (A) No compression and scatter to primary ratio of 0.8. Note location of microcalcifications and lesion. (B) Compression decreases scatter to primary ratio to 0.4, breast structures are brought closer to the film and spread out. Decreased tissue thickness and reduction in scatter radiation prompts greater radiographic contrast. Decreased magnification of structures creates greater resolution.

The effect of scatter and contrast is dramatic. A 6 cm thick breast measuring 9 cm in diameter will have a scatter-to-primary ratio of about 0.8, or 80 percent of the exposure results from scatter. If the breast thickness is reduced to 3 cm with the breast area increased to 12 cm due to vigorous compression, the scatter-to-primary ratio is reduced to 0.4, or only 40 percent of the image receptor exposure results from scatter. Radiographic contrast would increase two-fold (Figures 42-19A and B).

The compression device is made of a plastic that allows transmission of the low energy x-rays. The device should have a straight chest wall edge to allow the compression to grasp the breast tissues close to the chest wall edge. Compression is controlled by the radiographer and must be capable of being applied at 25–45 lb. of force. In addition to the standard compression devise, a smaller "spot" device is used to compress localized areas. The device should be checked regularly to ensure that it is working properly and applying the correct amount of pressure.

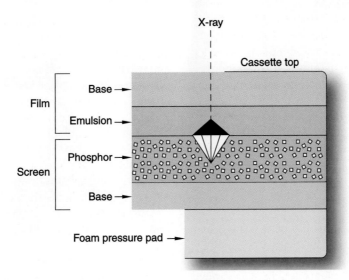

Cross-section of mammography screen and film in cassette. Single screen is placed behind film as a back screen. Single-emulsion film is placed in contact with single-emulsion screen. Design allows high absorption of x-rays in the screen phosphors closest to the film emulsion, which reduces diffusion of light emitted from the screen.

Cassettes

Like many of the previously described components of the mammography unit, the cassettes and screen/film combination used are also designed specifically to image the breast. The use of direct exposure x-ray film for mammography ended in the early 1970s because of the high exposure involved, and intensifying screens have been used ever since. Today, specially designed cassettes containing a single-emulsion screen and used with a single-emulsion film are the standard.

Mammography cassettes are manufactured of plastic or low attenuation carbon-fiber. Carbon-fiber enables the maximum number of x-rays to reach the intensifying screen, thereby keeping exposures at minimum levels. The screen is mounted on a foam pressure pad, and when closed, is placed at the extreme top of the cassette as close to the breast as possible (see Figure 42-3). The single screen is placed **behind** the film so there is high x-ray absorption of the screen phosphors closest to the film emulsion, thereby reducing the diffusion of light emitted from the screen (line-spread function). This arrangement prompts less image noise

and greater resolution (Figure 42-20). The x-ray photons that exit the breast enter the top of the cassette and go through the film before reaching the screen phosphor.

Screens

Mammography screens are manufactured by a variety of companies and they are all very similar in design. Each company offers at least two different screen speeds—typically one screen will be twice as fast as the other. The majority of manufacturers use green emitting **gadolinium oxysulfide** as the screen phosphor material. Mammography screens are much slower than those used in conventional radiography. A slow screen offers reduced noise and increased resolution. Using a screen in mammography instead of direct x-ray exposure offers two distinct advantages—a major reduction in radiation exposure to the patient and a dramatic increase in radiographic contrast. The disadvantage of using a screen is the decrease in resolution and increased image noise. However, a tradeoff must once again be made due to the unacceptably high radiation exposure from the direct exposure technique. Recall that direct exposure required from 50 to 100 times more radiation than screen technique. Fortunately, the overall design of the dedicated mammography machine and its specially engineered components allows high resolution to be maintained despite the use of a screen.

Uniformity of the speed of all the screens used is important. The difference between the minimum and maximum optical densities in all the screens shall not exceed 0.30 OD.

Film

Mammography film is designed to be very high in contrast and resolution. When used with a mammography screen, it is the highest contrast and highest resolution imaging system used in diagnostic radiology. Because the breast structures contain very low inherent subject contrast, a high contrast film is needed to enhance the anatomical structures. Mammography film, like the screen, is single emulsion and designed to be slow in speed. The slow speed prompts low image noise and high resolution. Mam-

mography film is green sensitive to match the spectral characteristics of the green emitting screen. Manufacturers offer at least two different film speeds and two films with different contrast levels. An anti-halation coating is placed on the nonemulsion side of the film. The coating prevents screen light from going through the film and scattering back to the film, which would decrease resolution. Caution must be exercised so the nonemulsion side of the film (shiny side) is not placed in contact with the screen. The screen and film emulsions must always be in direct contact with each other.

Most manufacturers also offer a special film, referred to as "extended film," which is designed to provide the same results as using standard mammography film and **extended cycle** processing. Extended cycle processing is a technique whereby the speed of a standard film can be increased up to 35 percent and radiographic contrast increased measurably, by **doubling the time the film is in the developer solution** (Figure 42-21). With some extended cycle techniques, the developer temperature is increased along with the immersion time. The in-

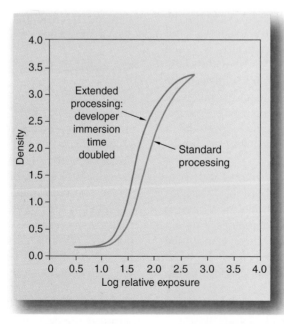

FIGURE 42-21 H and D curve showing effect of extended processing with standard mammography films. Speed and contrast of mammography film is increased when developer immersion time is doubled.

tent of extending the development portion of the processing cycle is to allow the developer solution more time to fully process the silver halide crystals. Single-emulsion film contains a thicker emulsion layer and can benefit from increased development. The advantages of extended film processing are increased radiographic contrast and reduced radiation exposure to the patient. The disadvantage of extended processing is that the increased speed of the film increases radiographic noise and resolution is decreased. In addition, the longer development time also decreases film throughput in high-volume mammography departments. The special "extended look" film described earlier was designed specifically to provide the faster speed and higher contrast without increasing the developer time and without reducing film throughput. Mammographers should exercise caution and use the correct film with the appropriate processor set-up.

Screen/Film Combination

The relative speed of a mammography screen/film combination should not be associated directly with a conventional screen/film system. A **100-speed** mammography system will typically be **50 to 75**

percent slower than a 100-speed conventional system. The stated speed will depend primarily upon the specific speed of the screen, the type and specific speed of film, and whether extended or regular 90-second processing is used. The mammography speed of 100 was arbitrarily assigned to the original Kodak Min-R screen and film developed in 1975. Today mammography screen/film systems range in relative speed from 100 to as high as 320 (Table 42-3).

Researchers continue to work on improving screen/film systems in an effort to keep radiation exposures low and resolution high. Recently, a dual-screen and dual-emulsion film was introduced by Kodak. The back screen is standard thickness and the front screen is one-half the thickness of the back screen. The quantity of light reaching the film emulsion is equal from both screens. The film has anti-crossover light properties, which helps to maintain resolution. The primary advantage of this dual-emulsion system is that the effective speed is doubled compared to using a single screen and film. The disadvantage is that the increased speed produces an increase in image noise thereby decreasing resolution which may be unacceptable for routine mammography images. In addition, it may be difficult to pass the ACR accreditation phantom test

TABLE 42-3.   Screen/Film Characteristics*

Screen	Film (Min–R)	Process	Relative Speed	Mean Glandular Dose (mrad)	Contrast[++]	Resolution[+] lp/mm	Noise
Min–R	M	Standard	100	250[+]	2.95	21	Low
Min–R	E	Extended	140	175	3.25	21	
Min–R Medium	M	Standard	170	150	2.95	19	
Min–R	H	Standard	180	150	3.20	21	
Min–R Medium	E	Extended	240	100	3.25	19	
Min–R Fast	T	Standard	280	125	2.90	18	
Min–R Medium	H	Standard	320	75	3.20	19	High

*   Screens and Film are Eastman Kodak. From Haus, A. G., *Screen-Film Processing Characteristics and Quality Control in Mammography* (KODAK Publication #N-314)

[+]   Average two-view dose from ACR accreditation program data. Measured on RMI 156 phantom.

[++]   Contrast—measured as the average gradient between densities 0.25 and 2.00 above base + fog.

[+]   Limiting resolution—based on 5 percent value of modular transfer function.

with reduced resolution. The shorter exposure time and reduced radiation exposure achieved from this system may, however, be an advantage for magnification techniques.

RESOLUTION

Dedicated mammography systems are capable of producing very high-image resolution compared to conventional radiography. In conventional radiography, limiting resolution will range from a low of about 2 lp/mm in fluoroscopy, to 5 lp/mm for a 300 speed screen/film system, and as high as 10 lp/mm for a 100-speed extremity system. Current mammography systems are capable of producing limiting resolutions as high as 22 lp/mm. Few mammography systems are set up to produce the maximum resolution that is capable in the system in order to keep radiation exposures at minimal levels. The mammography system must provide a minimum of **11 to 13 lp/mm.** Many components, used altogether, play a role in achieving this high resolution, most notably, the microsized focal spots, compression, low kVp, and the slow speed screen/film system. Radiologists are relatively comfortable with the current levels of resolution. Cancer and other pathology can be identified although a magnifying glass is often required to view the small structures in the images and to actually see the high resolution.

Mammography images today are the best ever produced (Figure 42-22). Federal government regulation has mandated that consistent high-quality images be produced wherever mammography machines have met the MQSA standards. Mean glandular dose (MGD) provides the best indicator of risk to the patient instead of ESE. According to the federal government's MQSA program, in 1997 the average MGD for a single screen/film/grid study was 160 mrads (1.6 mGy). The risk from mammography at these levels is low when compared to the decreased deaths that result through screening. The lifetime risk of death from mammography is 5 in 1 million. With doses at their current levels, image noise and resolution are greater considerations than dose.

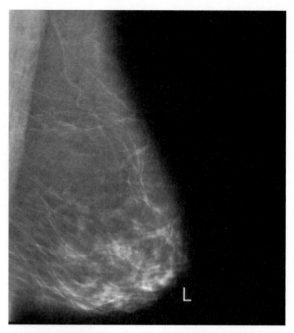

FIGURE 42-22 Mediolateral oblique projection of the breast produced on a current generation mammography machine. High-quality image demonstrates optimal resolution and contrast. Radiation dose is low.

DIGITAL MAMMOGRAPHY

Leaders in clinical mammography feel that screen/film mammography can be improved to increase accuracy. Many palpable or sonographically evident lesions cannot be detected by mammography. A recent prominent study found that the risk of a false-positive image to a 40-year-old is 50 percent. Thus, beginning with National Institutes of Health (NIH) financial support, many universities and research companies are currently involved in extensive design and clinical testing of digital mammography.

The principal advantages of digital mammography include the following:

- The capacity to manipulate the image's contrast and density
- The capacity to transmit images for consultation, teaching, etc.
- Archiving (PACS) for simplified storage and ready access of images

One of the goals in mammography is to provide a high level of contrast between the lesion and the surrounding tissue. Unfortunately, because the breast tissue has similar densities, the attenuation differences between normal breast tissue and cancer are small. In digital mammography, the screen/film system is replaced by a detector, which produces an electric signal that is digitized and stored. This is very similar to computed radiography (CR) and direct radiography (DR) described in Chapter 25.

Various types of detectors are currently used by the current manufacturers of digital equipment. A **phosphor flat panel** system consists of a large-area plate that contains phosphors of thallium-activated cesium iodide (CsI) deposited onto photodiodes. In this system, the photodiodes detect the light emitted by the phosphor and create an electrical signal that is sent to the computer. A **phosphor CCD** system is a second type of detector that also uses the CsI phosphor. Rather than using a large-area plate, the detector is a narrow 1 cm × 24 cm in size. The x-ray beam is collimated to match this detector and both are then scanned over the breast. With this design, the light of the phosphor is sent to a charge-coupled device (CCD), which converts the light into an electric signal. A third system is the **selenium flat panel**. This system does not use a phosphor; instead, the x-ray absorber is amorphous selenium. X-rays absorbed by this material are converted into an electrical charge by a system of electrode pads (Figure 42-23). With these digital detector systems, except CR, it is no longer necessary to have AEC sensors under the plate. The digital detector device acts as a multielement sensor. The traditional **computed radiography** (CR) system is also used in digital mammography as a fourth type of digital system. With CR, removable imaging plates are used with the bucky tray. After exposure, the plates have to be

FIGURE 42-23 A digital direct conversion detector replaces the bucky and film device. This digital detector is 24 cm × 29 cm and contains an amorphous selenium detector. Note the absence of the bucky/IR opening. *(Courtesy of Hologic)*

transported to a reader device where the photostimulable phosphor in the plate is read by a laser light and converted into an electrical signal.

Images produced with digital mammography can be printed out in hard copy; however, one of the advantages of digital systems is that the images can be stored in a picture and archiving communication system (PACS). For maximum efficiency and cost reduction, digital images should be read on the computer monitor in a specially designed viewing station. Storage of digital images continues to be a challenge. A four-view exam will require as much as 240 megabytes of space. A major advantage of using digital mammography is that the images can easily be sent electronically to other physicians for interpretation, to other health care institutions the patient may go to, and to efficiently call back for comparison purposes.

QUALITY CONTROL

The production of an optimal quality breast image may be the most technically challenging of all radiographic examinations. Quality control tests are required under the rules of the MQSA to ensure that high standards of image quality are achieved daily. Some states may require additional tests. The ACR provides a quality control manual for medical physicists that contains a section for radiographers. The manual describes the quality control tests that should be carried out along with their frequency (Table 42-4). The tests must be carried out accurately and at the **minimum** frequency stated. If problems occur in the production of images, the tests may need to be done more frequently. Regular quality control testing is the only means of ensuring that high image quality is always maintained. Slight changes in equipment performance, in particular the film processor and the accessory devices, can affect the contrast, resolution, or radiation exposure.

TABLE 42-4. Mammography Quality Control Minimum Test Frequencies*

Test	Minimum Frequency
Darkroom cleanliness	Daily
Processor quality control	Daily
Screen cleanliness	Weekly
Viewboxes and viewing conditions	Weekly
Phantom images	Weekly
Visual check list	Monthly
Repeat analysis	Quarterly
Analysis of fixer retention in film	Quarterly
Darkroom fog	Semiannually
Screen/film contact	Semiannually
Compression	Semiannually

Hendrick, RE, Bassett, L, Bostco, MA, et al. Mammography Quality Control Manual. Reston, VA. Amercian College of Radiology; 1999. *(Reprinted with permission of the American College of Radiology. No other representaion of this material is authorized without expressed, written permission from the American College of Radiology.)*

SUMMARY

Early detection of breast cancer depends on consistently reliable high-quality images. Image quality standards have been set forth by the American College of Radiology and the federal government's Mammography Quality Standards Act. The imaging requirements needed for mammography are more demanding than for other x-ray examinations. Mammography requires very high radiographic contrast and resolution so microcalcifications as small as 0.1 mm or less can be visualized along with the inherently low-contrast breast tissues. It is essential to use an imaging system that produces low noise. The radiation exposures associated with the examination must be sufficiently low to ensure that there is minimal risk to the patient.

The high subject contrast needed for effective mammography requires the use of low kVp techniques along with a molybdenum anode and a molybdenum filter. The low x-ray energy range will enhance the breast structures and improve the visibility of detail. Two new options for imaging large and dense breasts have recently been introduced. These include the use of rhodium anodes with rhodium filtration and tungsten anodes with rhodium filtration.

Geometric unsharpness is minimized and resolution increased during mammography by using micro-focus focal spots, uniquely designed x-ray tube configurations, the heel effect to advantage, low magnification, and firm breast compression. Although the breast structure is small and low energy is utilized, there is still a significant component of scatter radiation that can obscure contrast. Therefore, low ratio grids are required, along with breast compression, to reduce scattered radiation.

Slow-speed single-emulsion screens and film, along with special cassettes, are required in mammography. Resolution in a mammography system is typically 11 to 13 lp/mm.

REVIEW QUESTIONS

1. What advantage did xeromammography have over direct exposure mammography?

2. List three advantages screen/film mammography has over direct exposure mammography?

3. List at least two reasons why high-frequency generators are used in mammography.

4. What is the kVp range for mammography?

5. What is the AEC backup time for a grid technique?

6. Which end of the mammography tube is placed over the chest wall area?

7. What are two focal spot sizes used in mammography tubes?

8. Which half of the x-ray beam, anode or cathode, is eliminated in mammography?

9. What is the most common anode material used in mammography?

10. List two reasons why x-ray tubes are tilted.

11. Of what material is the port of the x-ray tube in mammography made?

12. List two advantages of producing magnified images of the breast.

13. State the two common grid ratios used in mammography.

14. List three advantages of using breast compression in mammography.

15. Why is the single-emulsion film placed behind the single-emulsion screen in a mammography cassette?

16. Describe extended processing.

17. List three advanages of using digital mammographic systems.

REFERENCES AND RECOMMENDED READING

American Cancer Society. (2003). *Cancer facts and figures—2003.* Atlanta: Author.

American College of Radiology. (1999a). *Mammography quality control for medical physicists.* Reston, VA: Author.

American College of Radiology. (1999b). *Mammography quality control for technologists.* Reston, VA: Author.

Barnes, G. T., & Brezovich, I. A. (1978). The intensity of scattered radiation in mammography. *Radiology, 126,* 243–247.

Barnes, G. T., Wu, X., Wagner, A. J., & Rubin, E. (1989). Scatter control in mammography: Past, present and future [abstract]. *Radiology, 173,* 472.

Buchanan, R. A., Finkelstein, S. I., & Wickersheim, K. A. (1976). X-ray exposure reduction using rare earth oxysulfide intensifying screens. *Radiology, 118,* 183–188.

Bushberg, J. T., Seibert, J. A., Leidholdt, E. M., & Boone, J. M. (2002). *The essential physics of medical imaging* (2nd ed.) Philadelphia: Lippincott Williams & Wilkins.

Egan, R. L. (1964). *Mammography.* Springfield, IL: Charles C Thomas.

Egan, R. L., McSweeney, M. B., & Sprawls, P. (1983). Grids in mammography. *Radiology, 146,* 359–362.

Elmore, J. G., Barton, M. B., Mocert, V. M., et al. (1998). Ten-year risk of false-positive screening mammograms and clinical breast examinations. *New England Journal of Medicine, 338,* 1089–1096.

Feig, S. D., & Ehrlich, S. M. (1990). Estimation of radiation risk from screening mammography: Recent trends and comparison with expected benefits. *Radiology, 174,* 638–647.

Gray, J. E., Winkler, N. T., Stears, J. G., & Frank, E. D. (1983). *Quality control in diagnostic imaging: A quality control cookbook.* Baltimore: University Park Press.

Haus, A. G., Metz, C. E., Chiles, J. T., & Rossmann, K. (1976). The effect of x-ray spectra from molybdenum and tungsten target tubes on image quality in mammography. *Radiology, 118,* 705–709.

Haus, A. G., Paulus, D. D., Dodd, G. D., Cowart, R. W., & Bencomo, J. (1979). Magnification mammography: Evaluation of screen film and xeroradiographic techniques. *Radiology, 133,* 223–226.

Hendrick, R. E. (1990). Standardization of image quality and radiation dose in mammography. *Radiology, 174,* 648–656.

Hendrick, R. E. (1992). Quality assurance in mammography: Accreditation, legislation, and compliance with quality assurance standards. *Radiological Clinics of North America, 3,* 243–255.

Kimme-Smith, C., Bassett, L. W., Gold, R. H., Roe, D., & Orr, J. (1987). Mammographic dual screen, dual emulsion film combination: Visibility of simulated microcalcifications and effect on image contrast. *Radiology, 165,* 313–318.

Kimme-Smith, C., Rothchild, P. A., Bassett, L. W., Gold, R. H., & Moler, C. (1989). Mammographic film processor temperature, development time, and chemistry: Effect on dose, contrast and noise. *American Journal of Roentgenology, 173*, 65–69.

Kimme-Smith, C., Wang, J., Debruhl, N., Basic, M., & Bassett, L. W. (1994). Mammograms obtained with rhodium vs molybdenum anodes: Contrast and dose differences. *American Journal of Roentology, 162.* 1313–1317.

Logan, W. W., & Norlund, A. W. (1979). Screen-film mammography technique: Compression and other factors. In W. W. Logan and E. P. Muntz, (Eds.), *Reduced dose mammography* (pp. 415–431). New York: Masson.

National Council of Radiation Protection and Measurements. (1988). *Quality assurance for diagnostic imaging.* (NCRP Report No. 99), Bethesda, MD: Author.

Pisano, E. D. (2000). Current status of full-field digital mammography. *Radiology, 214*, 26-28.

Sickles, E. A., & Feig, S. A. (1993). American College of Radiology statement on screening mammography for women 40–49. *ACR Bulletin, 49*, 5.

Tabar, L., & Haus, A. G. (1989). Processing mammographic films: Technical and clinical considerations. *Radiology, 173*, 65–69.

Vyborny, C. J., & Schmidt, R. A. (1992). Technical image quality and the visibility of mammographic detail. In A. G. Haus, M. J. Yagge, (Eds.), *Syllabus: A categorical course in physics: Technical aspects of breast imaging* (pp. 85–93). Oak Brook, IL: Radiological Society of North America.

Yaffee, M. F., and Rowlands, J. A. (1997). X-ray detectors for digital radiography. *Physics in Medicine and Biology 42.* 1–39.

Yaffe, M. J. (1990). Physics of mammography: Image recording process. *RadioGraphics, 10*, 341–363.

CHAPTER 43

Vascular Imaging Equipment

Bradley C. Johnson B.S.R.T. (R) and
Robin Jones M.S.R.T. (R)

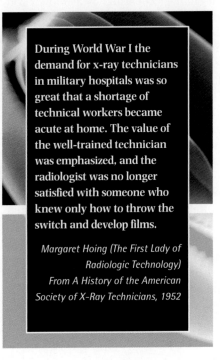

During World War I the demand for x-ray technicians in military hospitals was so great that a shortage of technical workers became acute at home. The value of the well-trained technician was emphasized, and the radiologist was no longer satisfied with someone who knew only how to throw the switch and develop films.

Margaret Hoing (The First Lady of Radiologic Technology)
From A History of the American Society of X-Ray Technicians, 1952

KEY TERMS

contrast media
 injection device
digital angiography
digital cineradiography
digital subtraction
 angiography

OBJECTIVES

Upon completion of this chapter, the student should be able to:

- Differentiate among the different types of historic image recording devices.

- Describe the components of digital image acquisition.

- Differentiate among the modes of digital image acquisition.

- Identify various image post-processing functions.

- Describe the structure and function of the C-arm assembly.

- Describe the structure and function of the angiographic table.

- Describe the structure and operation of contrast medium injection devices.

- Explain the various quality control measures taken with vascular imaging equipment.

The equipment in the vascular imaging laboratory is very unique in nature. The imaging equipment must accommodate for rapid image acquisition while withstanding high amounts of heat. In order for this to occur, special generators and x-ray tubes are required. The generators should offer high-performance capabilities to produce optimal images while reducing patient exposure. The x-ray tubes must work with the image intensifier and computer system to produce quality digital images for each particular exam. The x-rays tubes have to accommodate for different modes of digital image acquisition. Once the images are acquired, they should be able to be manipulated using a computer system. Additional equipment, such as a contrast medium injector, is required to assist in the diagnostic process. A quality control program is implemented and maintained in order for high-quality image production to continue. This chapter highlights these key points as they pertain to vascular imaging equipment and vascular imaging procedures.

HISTORY OF
VASCULAR IMAGING

Image recording in the vascular imaging laboratory has changed quite drastically over the years. Historically, images were recorded on radiographic film using various devices that allowed for rapid sequence filming. Today, however, radiographic film is almost obsolete with the use of digital imaging.

There were three main types of rapid sequence filming devices used: the roll film changer, the cut film changer, and the cineangiographic camera. The roll film changer consisted of a 60-foot continuous roll of radiographic film that allowed for approximately 60 exposures. This rapid film changer consisted of a grid, upper and lower intensifying screens, pressure plate, film cutter, and supply and receiving bins (Figure 43-1). The grid, which was located between the upper intensifying screen and the patient, was used to absorb scatter radiation generated in the patient before it reached the film and degraded image quality. The upper and lower intensifying screens enhanced the ability of the x-ray beam to produce a diagnostic image on the film. The pressure plate helped in this process by compressing the upper and lower intensifying screens against the film, ensuring uniform film/screen contact. Unexposed film was contained in the supply bin until it was exposed. After exposure, the film was housed in the receiving bin until it could be developed. A film cutter near the receiving bin was used to manually cut the exposed images away from the rest of the unexposed roll of radiographic film.

FIGURE 43-1 The roll film changer. This diagram demonstrates how film travels from the supply magazine (ready position) between the intensifying screens (expose position) into the receiving magazine (park position).

The cut film changer assembly resembles the roll film changer, except the radiographic film was pre-cut to a size, usually 14" × 14". In addition, the supply magazine only allowed for a maximum of 30 unexposed films to be held (Figure 43-2).

Cineangiographic cameras, which resembled movie cameras, replaced the television camera tube to record images on film for later playback. These cameras were generally used during cardiac catheterizations where detailed images of fast-moving anatomic structures were needed. Cine cameras provided better spatial image detail than electronically acquired images but with an increased radiation dose to the patient. Cine cameras were available in 16 mm or 35 mm film format. The 35 mm film format increased patient radiation exposure compared to 16 mm but produced larger images.

Cineangiographic systems consisted of a camera and x-ray tube which were synchronized. This means that the x-ray tube was energized only during the cineangiographic film exposure and not during film advancement. This synchronization, which prevents any unnecessary exposure to the patient, was accomplished through the work of the synchronous motors.

The cineangiographic imaging system consisted of three very important components: automatic brightness control, beam-splitting mirror, and cine camera. The automatic brightness control, or ABC, was used to compensate the beam quality and/or quantity for differences in anatomic thickness or density by adjusting the kVp, mA, or both. The beam-splitting mirror permitted simultaneous filming and viewing of the images during the procedure. This mirror would direct 10 percent of the image to the television monitor and the other 90 percent to the cine camera. The cine camera, which resembles a movie camera, was a complex device that allowed for the filming of the cineangiographic images.

The cine camera consisted of a lens, iris diaphragm, shutter, aperture, pressure plate, transport mechanism, film supply, and take-up reels (Figure 43-3). The optical lens would focus light from the output phosphor of the image intensifier tube onto the cine film. The iris diaphragm, which was located between the lens and the shutter, restricted the divergence of the light from the lens. The shutter was a rotating half-disk situated in front of the aperture that interrupted the flow of light to the film as it rotated. The shutter opening was approximately 160° to 180°. The aperture was a rectangular opening that further restricted the amount of light entering the camera. The pressure plate, which was located behind the aperture in the cine camera, functioned in maintaining a firm contact between the film and the aperture. The transport mechanism

FIGURE 43-2   The cut film changer. This diagram demonstrates how film travels from the supply magazine (ready position) between the intensifying screens (expose position) into the receiving magazine (park position).

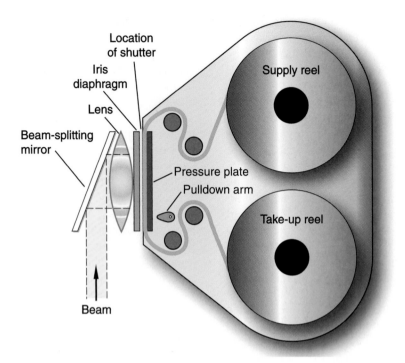

Location of shutter

Iris diaphragm

Lens

Beam-splitting mirror

Supply reel

Pressure plate

Pulldown arm

Take-up reel

Beam

FIGURE 43-3 The cine camera.

transported the unexposed film from the supply reel to the aperture for exposure and finally to the take-up reel until it could be developed.

Exposures in a cine camera could be made by either the action of the shutter or the action of the x-ray beam. In shutter exposure, the shutter opens for exposure to the film and closes for advancement of the cineangiographic film. In x-ray beam exposure, constant potential generators allowed for the pulsating of the x-ray beam. The pulsating beam not only allowed for the advancement of the film after the exposure but also eliminated the need for the shutter.

DIGITAL IMAGE ACQUISITION

The invention of digital image acquisition has improved the imaging ability of the angiographic suite. Digital image acquisition involves using computers in conjunction with the imaging equipment to produce quality diagnostic digital images. These

computers have increased the resolution of the image while reducing radiation dose to the patient. In addition, there is a reduction in cost to the patient and institution. Digital images can be manipulated after acquisition, therefore decreasing the need for repeat exposures. For example, the contrast can be adjusted on an image that is too light. Digital images are easier to store than conventional images because they take up less space and are easier to obtain when they are needed. These images can be stored in an archive system that can be accessed at any time. Digital image acquisition requires the use of specialized equipment in order to produce a digital image. This specialized equipment includes a high-frequency generator, an x-ray tube, an image intensifier, and an image processor (Figure 43-4).

Generator

High-frequency generators, usually in the multiphasic or three-phase format while offering 12 pulses

FIGURE 43-4   A vascular imaging laboratory.

per second, are selected for vascular imaging laboratories because of their high-performance capabilities. These generators allow for high mA stations, usually 800–1000 mA, with relatively low kVp settings, usually 50–100 kVp. A high mA station with a low kVp setting will improve the visibility of the contrast medium against the surrounding soft tissue structures. In addition, using high mA stations allows for short exposure times.

The x-ray tube in the vascular imaging laboratory operates in the radiographic mode even during digital fluoroscopy. To prevent the x-ray tube from overheating, the high-frequency generator is switched off and on very rapidly, causing pulsing of the x-ray beam. This pulsing is known as pulse-progressive fluoroscopy. Interrogation time is the time required to prepare the x-ray tube for exposure; in other words, the time needed for the x-ray tube to be switched on and reach the selected kVp and mA stations. Extinction time is the time required to stop the exposure or shut off the x-ray tube. Vascular imaging requires high-frequency generators that allow for interrogation and extinction times of less than 1 ms.

X-Ray Tube

Vascular imaging x-ray tubes vary slightly from general imaging x-ray tubes in their ability to withstand

high amounts of heat while providing optimal images. High heat amounts are produced by extended periods of fluoroscopy and rapid sequences of exposures made over a short period of time. Since heat production occurs at the anode, this will determine heat tolerance. Short-term loading ability is the amount of heat an anode can tolerate for a sequence of exposures. Continuous heat-loading ability is the amount of heat the anode can tolerate during a fluoroscopic exposure. Overall, the heat-loading ability is determined by the size and construction of the anode disk. Larger diameter anode disks, usually 15 cm or greater, are combined with a large target angle or focal spot size to accommodate for the increased heat production. A thicker anode disk, usually 5 cm or greater, constructed of molybdenum with a graphite backing improves the heat loading capacity of the vascular x-ray tube.

The heat capacity ability of the vascular x-ray tube is measured by the calculation of heat units generated at the anode. Heat units are calculated by multiplying the peak kilovoltage, milliamperage, time in seconds, rectification constant, and number of consecutive exposures together. The rectification constant is determined by the type of generator being used. A single-phase generator has a rectification constant of 1, while the three-phase and multiphasic generators have a rectification constant of 1.35 and 1.40, respectively. Vascular imaging requires an x-ray tube with a 1 MHU (mega heat unit) heat capacity in order to keep up with the daily imaging requirements.

Image Intensifier

The image intensifier can either be analog or digital in nature. An analog image intensifier requires the use of charge-coupled devices (CCD) and analog-to-digital converter to produce a digital image. The CCD replaces the television camera in the vascular imaging system. The CCD consists of crystalline silicon that is located on the output phosphor of the image intensifier. Digital images are obtained when the silicon is illuminated, causing generation of an electrical charge. This electrical charge is then sent as a signal to the analog-to-digital converter. The analog-to-digital converter digitizes the signal from the CCD by converting the signal into pixels or picture elements. On the other hand, a digital image intensifier acquires the images digitally so no special conversion equipment is needed. Digital image intensifiers are composed of silicon pixel detectors and are known as flat panel or digital detectors.

Image Processor

The last part of the digital image acquisition system is the image processor. The image processor consists of image-processing hardware and a computer. The image-processing hardware controls the speed of the imaging equipment. This hardware allows for real-time viewing of the images, meaning images are seen as they are acquired. The computer controls the various components of the imaging system, including the generator, x-ray tube, image-processing hardware, and image storage device. This computer allows for the different modes of digital image acquisition. In addition, the computer allows for manipulation of the digital images. Once manipulated, these images are stored as part of a picture archiving and communication system (PACS) or network system. These images can also be printed using a laser printer or transferred to a compact disk or videotape.

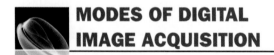

MODES OF DIGITAL IMAGE ACQUISITION

Digital image acquisition can occur in three different modes: **digital angiography** (DA), **digital subtraction angiography** (DSA), and **digital cineradiography** (cine). Once images are acquired, the image processor can manipulate, export, or store these images (Table 43-1).

Digital Angiography

Digital angiography, also known as spot filming, replaced traditional spot-film devices in the vascular imaging laboratory. Digital angiography involves the production of one image, similar to the last fluoroscopy hold image. This mode of acquisition is generally used when only a few images are needed for a procedure. For example, a spot film is taken post insertion of a peripherally inserted central catheter (PICC) to check tip placement and as a record of the procedure.

Digital Subtraction Angiography

Digital subtraction angiography involves eliminating bone and soft tissue structures from an image so that only the contrast-filled vessels remain. In order for DSA acquisition to occur, three steps must be accomplished. First, a scout or mask image must be obtained. The scout image contains all of the anatomy of interest prior to the injection. Next, the injection process must occur. The resulting image, known as the native image, displays all of the anatomy, including the contrast-filled vessels. Finally, the mask image is laid over the native image. The computer then subtracts all of the like structures, leaving only the contrast-filled vessels in the image (Figure 43-5). However, if patient motion (voluntary or involuntary) occurs between the scout image and the injection, an artifact will appear on the resulting image. DSA is normally used when imaging vessels of the head, chest, and extremities.

TABLE 43-1. Modes of Digital Image Acquisition		
Mode	Number of Images	Use
Digital Angiography	Single image	When only a few images are needed for the procedure (e.g., interventional radiology procedures)
Digital Subtraction Angiography	Numerous frames per second	Carotid and cerebral angiography Abdominal and peripheral angiography
Digital Cineradiography	Numerous frames per second	Cardiac catheterization

FIGURE 43-5 Digital subtraction angiography. This figure depicts the stages involved in digital subtraction angiography: (A) scout image; (B) injection image; and (C) resulting subtracted image.

Digital Cineradiography

The last mode of digital image acquisition, digital cineradiography, is used primarily for cardiac catheterization. This type of acquisition involves taking numerous exposures, known as frames, in a second of time. Typically, cardiac catheterization involves exposure rates of 15, 30, or 60 frames per second. These high frame rates provide higher resolution images as compared to general fluoroscopy. In fact, cineradiography can demonstrate events that are normally too fast or cannot be seen by general fluoroscopy. However, as the number of frames per second increases, the patient dose also increases.

IMAGE POST-PROCESSING

After image acquisition occurs, digital images are manipulated or post-processed before they are permanently stored. Manipulating the images before they are stored helps eliminate the need for repeat exposures. The type of post-processing depends on the mode of digital image acquisition.

Windowing, annotation, zoom, and analytic functions can be used on any type of digital image acquisition. Window-level involves adjusting the density, while window-width adjusts the contrast or brightness of an image. Images that are too light or too dark can be adjusted to make them diagnostic quality providing the image has had adequate but not excessive exposure. The annotation function allows the user to dictate on the image itself. This allows the user to identify right or left sides for future viewers. In addition, the user can add comments to the image such as the size and type of a particular catheter. Zoom allows the user to zone in on and magnify a particular area of interest. This function is useful when locating smaller structures such as aneurysms. The final function, analytic tools, involves using various methods to quantitate distances, calculate degree of stenosis, and measure blood flow. These tools can be extremely helpful to vascular imaging personnel during and after the procedure.

The post-processing functions—remasking, pixel shifting, view tracing, and edge enhancement—pertain only to digital subtraction angiography. Re-masking involves selecting another mask image in order to obtain the best subtracted image of the anatomy of interest. This function is used when there is a significant amount of patient motion after the initial mask image. Another post-processing function that compensates for patient motion is called pixel shifting. This function is used when the patient moves slightly from the mask image to the injection image. Pixel shifting allows the user to move the mask image to correspond to the patient movement. The next function, view tracing, involves combining numerous frames into one image to demonstrate a completely filled contrast structure. For example, this function may be used to demonstrate a contrast-filled abdominal aorta from the celiac axis to the iliac bifurcation. The final function, edge enhancement, is used to accentuate the edges of vessels or small structures so they can be seen (Figure 43-6). However, too much edge enhancement can cause distortion of the image.

C-ARM ASSEMBLY

The design of equipment in the vascular imaging laboratory is similar to the design of the portable radiographic equipment used during surgical procedures known as the C-arm assembly. Vascular imaging equipment, however, is much larger in size and is not portable.

A typical C-arm assembly consists of four parts: the x-ray tube, the image intensifier, the gantry, and the point of attachment (Figures 43-7 and 43-8). The x-ray tube is similar in construction to that of a tube found in a digital fluoroscopy room. The x-ray tube is mounted on the bottom of the C-arm assembly.

The image intensifier can be either analog or digital in nature. An analog image intensifier requires the use of a CCD and an analog-to-digital converter to digitize the image. A digital intensifier acquires the image digitally so no special conversion equipment is needed. The image intensifier is mounted on the top of the C-arm assembly.

The final two parts of the C-arm work together to allow manipulation of the assembly. The gantry mounts the C-arm assembly to the floor or ceiling of the vascular imaging laboratory. The point of at-

A

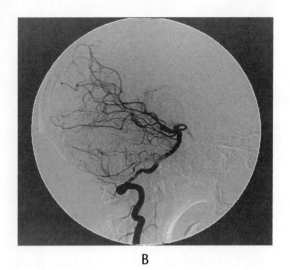

B

FIGURE 43-6   Demonstration of edge enhancement (A) normal image and (B) edge enhanced image.

FIGURE 43-7   C-arm assembly.

FIGURE 43-8   C-arm assembly.

tachment connects the C-arm assembly to the gantry. The point of attachment allows for 180° rotation of the C-arm assembly. This attachment also allows for craniocaudal and oblique angulations needed to image the required anatomy for cardiac or vascular imaging procedures. Therefore, the patient never has to be moved during the procedure.

The most important feature of the C-arm assembly is the relationship of the x-ray tube and image intensifier. In this design, the central ray of the x-ray tube is always perpendicular to the image intensifier and therefore at right angles to the body part.

ANGIOGRAPHIC TABLES

Tables used in vascular imaging laboratories must meet three requirements. First, angiographic tables must be easy to use and convenient for the vascular imaging laboratory personnel. It must be able to provide support and comfort for the patient. Finally, the angiographic table must not degrade the diagnostic quality of the image.

A typical design of an angiographic table involves a table base and a table plate (Figures 43-9 and 43-10). The table base attaches to the floor while the table plate rests on the top of the table base. This design allows for the capability of free floating of the table plate in all directions. In addition, table plate has the potential to be raised or lowered as needed. Sometimes the table plates can be interchanged according to the procedure being performed. For example, a cerebral angiogram may require a table plate that is narrower at the head end to accommodate for lateral projections. The table

plate allows for the attachment of various equipment needed for the procedure such as manual controls, IV poles, restraining devices, contrast medium injection devices, lead shields, and hemodynamic monitoring devices.

Angiographic tables are equipped with a foam pad for patient comfort. This foam pad should be thin enough so image quality is not degraded but thick enough for patient comfort. In addition to the foam pad, arm boards are attached to the angiographic table to support the patient's extremities during the angiographic procedure.

The design material for the angiographic table should not degrade image quality. A low radiation-absorbing plastic and carbon fiber material is the preferred material of composition. A low attenuation table prevents degradation of the image quality, but it also lowers radiation levels to the patient and the vascular imaging laboratory personnel.

CONTRAST MEDIUM INJECTION DEVICES

Contrast medium injector devices allow for a safe delivery of a preset amount of contrast. These devices allow for large bolus injections that are to difficult to be performed by hand. Newer devices even allow for smaller bolus injections that previously could only be performed manually.

FIGURE 43-9 Table assembly.

FIGURE 43-10 Table assembly.

A typical contrast medium injection device consists of the control panel, syringe, warming device, and pressure mechanism (Figure 43-11). The control panel displays the injection parameters, which are manipulated by the cardiovascular interventional technologist. The injection parameters include flow rate, rise, total volume, pressure, and delay. The flow rate is the rate at which the contrast medium is going to be injected. It is measured in cubic centimeters per second (cc/sec.) and is dependent on factors such as catheter length, inner catheter diameter, number of catheter side holes, injection pressure, and viscosity of the contrast medium (Table 43-2). The rise, also known as linear rise, is the time it takes to reach the desired flow rate. Rise is measured in seconds. The total volume is the desired amount of contrast to be delivered. Total volume can be calculated by multiplying the flow rate by the injection duration (V = cc/sec. × s). Total volume is measured in cubic centimeters. The injection pressure is the force needed for a specific dose of contrast medium. Injection pressure is dependent on the size of the vascular structure and the type of catheter used for the injection. Typically, smaller vessels require lower injection pressures. Manufacturer insert information should be consulted for determining safe pressure limits for each specific catheter. Injection pressure is measured in pounds per square inch (psi). The range for injection pressures is 100 to 1200 psi. The last injection parameter, delay, can be either injection or x-ray in nature. An injection delay allows for image acquisition to begin before the injection occurs. This is useful in digital subtraction angiography where a mask image is required. An x-ray delay allows for the injection to occur before image acquisition occurs. This is useful when performing lower extremity arteriography via a catheter in the abdominal aorta and only the vessels distal to the knee need to be visualized.

The contrast medium injector syringe is removable and disposable. The contrast syringe capacity can range from 40 to 260 cc. A new sterile syringe is loaded in the syringe-loading assembly prior to each case.

FIGURE 43-11 Contrast medium injection device.

TABLE 43-2.	Factors Affecting Flow Rate
Viscosity	Lower viscosity permits higher flow rates.
Catheter Length	Shorter catheters permit higher flow rates.
Catheter Internal Diameter	Larger internal diameters permit higher flow rates.
Injection Pressure	Higher psi permits higher flow rates.
Catheter Sideholes	The presence of sideholes in the catheter permits higher flow rates.

The warming device is a thermal sleeve placed over a preloaded syringe to maintain the contrast medium temperature at or near body temperature (37°C, 98.6°F). The warming device maintains temperature but does not increase it from room temperature to body temperature. Therefore, the contrast medium should be warmed prior to the syringe being filled.

The pressure mechanism is an electromechanical motor attached to a jackscrew that drives the piston into or out of the syringe. This piston movement causes the syringe plunger to move forward or backward as needed.

Contrast medium injectors are equipped with numerous safety mechanisms to prevent damage to the catheter and danger to the patient (Table 43-3). Function-monitoring devices, such as a flashing light, audible tone, or written message, are used to notify the cardiovascular interventional technologist of any problems. The problem may be an injector malfunction or operational error such as an omission of an injection parameter. A volume-limiting device prevents excessive amounts of contrast from being delivered to the patient. A pressure-limiting device prevents the injection pressure from exceeding a maximum pressure set prior to the injection. Acceleration regulators allow the electromechanical drive motor to accelerate over an exact duration of time to prevent whiplash of the catheter. Finally, the rate-rise control prevents an instant surge of injection pressure by gradually increasing the psi to the preset limit.

QUALITY CONTROL

Quality control programs in the vascular imaging laboratory are established by the organization to ensure that the angiographic equipment is operating properly and safely. In addition, they are established to ensure that the highest quality image is produced while limiting the radiation exposure to the patient and ultimately lower the cost to both the patient and the organization.

Components of the quality control program should include periodic monitoring of the x-ray viewing and image storage stations, evaluation of

TABLE 43-3.	Safety Mechanisms for Contrast Medium Injectors
Function-Monitoring Device	A flashing light, audible tone, or written message used to notify personnel of any problems
Volume-Limiting Device	Prevents excessive amounts of contrast from being delivered to the patient
Pressure-Limiting Device	Prevents the injection pressure from exceeding a maximum pressure set prior to the injection
Acceleration Regulators	Allow the electromechanical drive motor to accelerate over an exact duration of time to prevent whiplash of the catheter
Rate-Rise Control	Prevents an instant surge of injection pressure by gradually increasing the psi to the preset limit

the x-ray beam, and assessment of the ancillary equipment. X-ray viewing and image storage systems should be tested regularly for their effectiveness. X-ray equipment should be monitored to maintain high-quality images and prevent equipment malfunction. Ancillary equipment, such as the contrast medium injectors and cardiac monitoring device, should be inspected regularly to prevent malfunctions during a procedure. In order for this to occur, scheduled maintenance should be established between the equipment manufacturer and the organization.

In addition to contracts for preventative maintenance and service with the manufacturer, the organization should have members of the biomedical instrumentation department trained to monitor or correct faulty equipment in case of an emergency. By utilizing the biomedical instrumentation department, the vascular imaging laboratory can produce high-quality images while reducing patient dose and lowering cost.

SUMMARY

The vascular imaging laboratory contains specialized radiographic equipment that produces high-quality images of contrast-filled structures within the body. Special high-frequency generators permit the use of high mA settings, short exposure times, and relatively low kVp settings. The high mA stations allow for short exposure times, which reduce patient exposure. In addition to the high-frequency generators, specialized x-ray tubes are required for high-quality digital images. These x-ray tubes must work in conjunction with the image intensifier and computer system for image acquisition. The x-ray tubes should allow for the different modes of digital image acquisition. Image acquisition can be either analog or digital in nature. Once the images have been acquired, the computer system allows the images to be manipulated as needed.

The vascular imaging laboratory also contains specialized ancillary equipment needed to produce high-quality images of contrast-filled structures within the body. The most commonly used device is the contrast medium pressure injector. This equipment allows for large bolus injections that are too difficult to be performed by hand. Newer devices also allow for smaller bolus injections that were previously performed by hand.

For a vascular imaging laboratory to run successfully, it is very important that a quality control program be established and implemented. This program should include scheduled maintenance of the x-ray tube and image acquisition system, image manipulation and viewing systems, and ancillary equipment. The quality control program should be used to maintain safe and successful operation of the equipment, produce the highest image quality, and reduce exposure to the patient and imaging staff.

REVIEW QUESTIONS

1. Describe the parts of a rapid film changer.
2. What is the purpose of the automatic brightness control in a cineangiographic imaging system?
3. Describe pulse-progressive fluoroscopy.
4. What determines the heat-loading ability of a vascular x-ray tube?
5. What are the total heat units generated by a vascular x-ray tube for a series of 12 exposures using 600 mA, 0.5 second, 89 kVp on a multiphasic unit?
6. When using an analog image intensifier, what two devices are required to produce a digital image?
7. What is the purpose of the image processor in a digital image acquisition system?
8. Describe the process of digital subtraction angiography.
9. Which image post-processing function is used when there is a significant amount of motion in a digital subtraction angiography acquisition?
10. What is the most important design feature in the C-arm assembly?
11. What are the three requirements that an angiography table must meet in order to be used in a vascular imaging laboratory?
12. What is the total volume for an injection that has a flow rate of 15 cc/sec. and injection duration of 2 seconds?
13. List the safety mechanisms that contrast medium injection devices are equipped with.
14. List the components of a vascular imaging laboratory quality control program.

REFERENCES AND RECOMMENDED READING

Bushong, S. C. (2004). *Radiologic science for technologists: Physics, biology, and protection* (8th ed.) St. Louis, MO: Elsevier/C. V. Mosby.

Cullinan, A., & Cullinan, J. (1994). *Producing quality radiographs* (2nd ed.). Philadelphia: J. B. Lippincott.

Curry, T. S., Dowdey, J. E., & Murry, R. C. (1990). *Christensen's introduction to the physics of diagnostic radiology* (4th ed.). Philadelphia: Lea & Febiger.

Laudicina, P., & Wean, D. (1994). *Applied angiography for radiographers.* Philadelphia: W. B. Saunders.

Snopek, A. M. (1999). *Fundamentals of special radiographic procedures* (4th ed.). Philadelphia: W. B. Saunders.

Tortorici, M. R., & Apfel, P. J. (1995). *Advanced radiographic and angiographic procedures: With an introduction to specialized imaging.* Philadelphia: F. A. Davis.

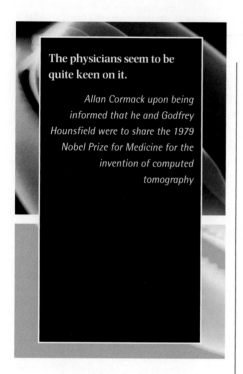

The physicians seem to be quite keen on it.

Allan Cormack upon being informed that he and Godfrey Hounsfield were to share the 1979 Nobel Prize for Medicine for the invention of computed tomography

CHAPTER 44   Computed Tomography

KEY TERMS

collimator pitch'
convolution
deconvolution
gantry

mask
pitch
targeting

OBJECTIVES

Upon completion of this chapter, the student should be able to:

- Relate the invention of computed tomography.

- Describe typical gantry components.

- Explain the basic features of each generation of CT scanners, especially multidetector (MDCT) units.

- Explain why CT tabletops have patient weight limits.

- Compare the requirements for a CT x-ray tube with those of a routine diagnostic tube.

- Explain the operation of a scintillation crystal and photomultiplier tube CT detector.

- Explain the operation of a xenon gas-filled ionization chamber CT detector.

- Discuss the importance of detector alignment and calibration.

- Discuss the use of a CT computer menu or index.

- Describe the major display features possible with advanced software.

- Describe the calculation and use of Hounsfield units.

- Explain reformatting image reconstruction.

- Explain how CT display image density and contrast are controlled.

- Describe the factors affecting resolution, including voxel, pixel, and matrix size.

- Discuss methods of reducing CT image noise and motion.

- Illustrate section shape, partial volume effect, and scan arc to scanning procedures.

- Explain a variety of common CT artifacts.

- Discuss radiation protection of the patient and others during CT examinations.

Computed tomography (CT) produces a digital tomographic image from diagnostic x-rays. The basic principle of CT involves digitizing an image received from a slit scan projection of the patient's body and then back-projecting the image through mathematical algorithms.

Although CT scanning is usually performed transversely, digital processing of information can produce sagittal and coronal sections (Figure 44-1). Because the CT x-ray beam is confined to a slit, much scatter radiation is eliminated from the image. The combination of the transverse sectioning procedure with slit scanning produces an image of significantly better quality than that available with other imaging methods. Primarily the image differentiates various types of soft tissues (e.g., gray matter, white matter, blood, tumor, cerebrospinal fluid, etc.). When digital image data manipulation is added, CT provides more diagnostic information than any other ionizing radiation imaging modality.

As with other tomographic modalities, the terms *cut* and *slice* are used in clinical practice. Because these phrases can easily cause distress when overheard by a patient, the radiographer should strive to adhere to the term *section*, avoiding *cut* and *slice*.

THE INVENTION OF COMPUTED TOMOGRAPHY

The invention of computed tomography has been credited to Godfrey N. Hounsfield for his work in 1970–71, although preliminary work was done by Oldendorf in 1961 and Cormack in 1963, and all three based their work on the investigations of the Austrian mathematician J. Radon, who proved in

1917 that an image of a three-dimensional object could be produced from its mathematical projections. Hounsfield was a research engineer with Electro-Musical Instruments Ltd. (EMI), the English firm that gained international renown as the Beatles' music publishers during the 1960s. His original scanner was built on a lathe bed and required 9 days to produce a single section image. Although the company sold its CT business, it continues to operate American and British EMI. Hounsfield and Cormack were awarded the 1979 Nobel Prize for Medicine. Hounsfield's invention parallels Röntgen's discovery of x-rays as the two most outstanding contributions to medical imaging.

Early CT units were capable of only axial tomography, and the term *computerized axial tomography* (CAT) scanning became a popular acronym. Modern CT units are capable of diverse modes much more complex than simple axial scanning. However, the term *CAT scanning* may endure, as have other antiquated radiologic terms (e.g., flat plate and wet reading). A modern CT unit includes a gantry, table, x-ray tube, detectors, computer, display console and image storage units (Figure 44-2).

SCANNER GENERATIONS

Computed tomography technology advanced very rapidly after Hounsfield's discovery. Scanners are sometimes described by their generation, with the original EMI head scanner considered to be the first. Descriptions of various computed tomography equipment refer to both rays and projections (also called views). A **ray** is a pencil thin beam of radiation that strikes a single detector. A **projection** (or

FIGURE 44-1 Computed tomography sections: (A) sagittal; (B) transverse; and (C) coronal.

FIGURE 44-2 A computed tomography unit. *(Courtesy of GE Healthcare)*

view) is composed of a set of rays striking a detector array (a group of detectors). Although there are no distinct lines between the generations, Table 44-1 illustrates the major characteristics of each.

First Generation

First-generation CT scanners were single ray systems designed for examination of the head only (Figure 44-3). The head was surrounded by a water bag to eliminate air interfaces. A single x-ray tube and a pair of detectors were aligned on a fixed C-arm. The detectors were sodium iodide scintillation crystals with photomultiplier tubes. A pencil-thin slit field, 3 mm $\times$ 26 mm, scanned a 180° arc around the patient's head. Each detector was exposed to a 3 mm $\times$ 13 mm field. First-generation units used a rotating scan and index system that scanned the head linearly (from one side to the other), indexed 1°, repeated the scanning process, indexed another 1°, and so on, for the entire 180° (Figure 44-4). This is also called a translate (scan) and rotate (index) system. The x-ray tube was on during scanning and off during indexing. Although the pair of detectors did not decrease the 180° scanning time, they permitted two anatomical sections to be scanned simultaneously, thus reducing the total examination time by half.

TABLE 44-1.	Major Characteristics of CT Unit Generations
First generation	head only linear scan and rotate (180 scans, 1° rotations) paired detectors (160 measurements per scan) 4.5–5 minute scan time single ray pencil beam single detector
Second generation	single projection fan-shaped beam (permitting whole body scanning) up to 30 detectors 10–90 second scan time linear scan and rotate (6 scans, 30° rotations)
Third generation	single projection fan-shaped beam up to 300 detectors 2–10 second scan time 360° rotation of x-ray tube and detectors crude dynamic capabilities
Fourth generation	single projection fan-shaped beam 360° ring of stationary detectors 2–10 second scan time 360° rotation of x-ray tube dynamic capabilities
Fifth Generation	electron beam scanners stationary tube annular targets cardiac imaging 50 msec imaging
Sixth Generation Helical/Spiral	multiple projection fan-shaped beam 360° ring of stationary detectors 360° rotation of x-ray tube computer controlled table movement through gantry bore continuous scanning throughout entire examination
Seventh Generation	Multidetector CT (MDCT) >10K detector elements 0.5 mm section thickness >20 simultaneous contiguous detectors ≈12–15 sec procedure time (body region scan time)

FIGURE 44-3 A first-generation CT head scanner.

The detectors measured the attenuation coefficient of the exit radiation beam at overlapping 1.7 mm intervals 240 times during each scan. The unit required 4.5 minutes to complete a pair of full 180° scans and 5 minutes to reconstruct the images. Each section was derived from 43,200 measurements (180° × 240) and was displayed on an 80 × 80 matrix. Each display pixel represented a voxel of tissue 3 mm × 3 mm × 13 mm although a 1.5 mm pixel display became available. A common examination routine for the head consisted of 10–12 sections, which required 25–35 minutes to obtain.

Second Generation

Second-generation CT units used a single-projection fan-shaped beam instead of a pencil slit and a linear array of as many as 30 detectors (Figure 44-5). They too are no longer available. The fan-shaped beam

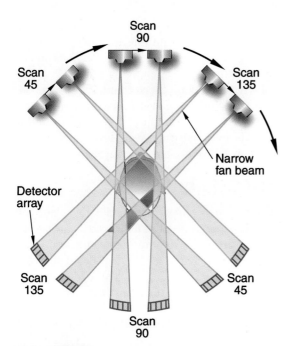

FIGURE 44-4 First-generation CT scan and rotate system. Only three scans (the 45th, 90th, and 135th) are shown to simplify the illustration. A single scan and rotate required 180 scans, each 1° apart.

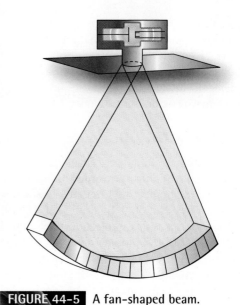

FIGURE 44-5 A fan-shaped beam.

and increased number of detectors permitted scanning and rotation with fewer linear movements. For example, a 30-detector unit could complete the 180° linear movement in only six rotations of 30° each. However, the loss of collimation increased the amount of scatter radiation detected. This is a major disadvantage of all fan beam scanners. A lead mask was added to the detectors to assist in reducing the scatter reaching the detectors. Scan time was reduced to between 10 and 90 seconds, a reasonable respiratory suspension time, thus permitting examination of the whole body.

Third Generation

Third-generation CT units used a wider fan-shaped beam and a curved array of 250–750 detectors to achieve a single projection (Figure 44-6). The fan-shaped beam was wide enough to include the entire body in a single exposure and rotated 360° within the gantry, thus eliminating the linear scan and ro-

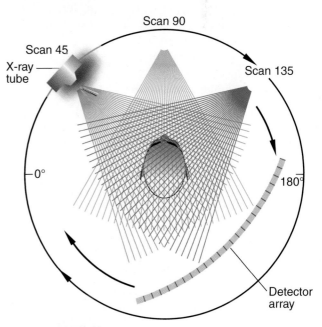

FIGURE 44-6 A third-generation CT scanner.

tate system. A typical third-generation scanner might produce 700,000 measurements per section. Various scanning arcs were usually possible, for example 220° or 360°. Scan time was reduced to between 1 and 12 seconds, permitting sequential images to crudely approximate dynamic functions.

Third-generation units that featured dynamic scanning usually performed at about four scans per minute, which equals the routine scanning time of a fourth generation unit. Because they had only a single detector array, third-generation scanners were prone to ring artifacts (see Figure 44-34c).

Fourth Generation

Fourth-generation CT units were developed as a result of a competitive contract awarded to the American Science and Engineering Company (AS&E) by the United States National Institutes of Health (NIH). They use a single-projection fan-shaped beam with 600–2,000 stationary detectors arrayed in a 360° ring (Figure 44-7). The ring of detectors eliminates movement of detectors, thereby decreasing calibration requirements. As many as 1,200,000 measurements may be processed per section. A wider range of scan arcs, including arcs over 360°, are usually possible with scan times ranging from 0.5 to 10 seconds.

Some fourth-generation scanners are capable of dynamic scanning rates in the range of 15 scans per minute. The limiting factor is the interscan time and the computer processing time, not the actual scanning time. Dynamic scanning is usually achieved by reducing the interscan time to 1–2 seconds and not indexing the gantry. Scanning occurs first in a clockwise direction, then counterclockwise, etc. Another technique, called overscan, may also be available. Overscanning uses a scan of more than 360°. The overscan may be displayed as segmented data from 2, 3 or 4 scans as a single image.

Fifth Generation

The fifth generation of scanners is represented by the technology utilized in a dedicated cardiac unit designed around a rotating electron beam. This is sometimes referred to as Electron Beam Tomography (EBT) or Cardiac Cine CT. The x-ray tube is replaced with a huge electron gun that uses a deflection coil to direct a 30° beam of electrons in a 210° arc around a 360° anode ring (Figure 44-8).

A

B

FIGURE 44-8 Fifth-Generation—Electron Beam Tomography (EBT) or Cardiac Cine CT. (A) Scanner components; (B) Multidetector operation with contrast media injection triggered by patient ECG. *(Courtesy of GE Healthcare)*

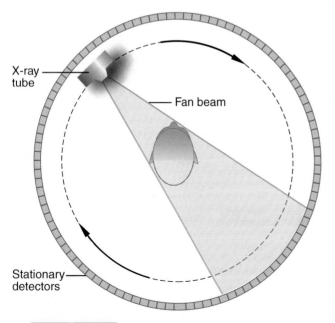

X-ray tube

Fan beam

Stationary detectors

FIGURE 44-7 A fourth-generation CT scanner.

The fan beam that is produced is intercepted by a 360° detector array. Because the electron beam rotates around the anode ring, there is no moving gantry in this design. The patient is placed within the anode ring, somewhat akin to being inside the x-ray tube itself. This unit is a dynamic scanner because it can produce four sections simultaneously within 50 msec. It is also capable of multisection sequencing of injected contrast media triggered by the patient's ECG. This is fast enough to provide real-time dynamic sectional images of the beating heart. Because these images are essentially anatomical movies (or cine) the examination is sometimes referred to as cine CT.

Sixth Generation— Helical/Spiral CT

Helical (spiral) scanners were made possible by advances in slip ring connection technology. Slip rings consist of brushes that fit into grooves to permit the current and voltage to the x-ray tube to be supplied while the tube is in continuous rotation around the gantry (Figure 44-9). This permits scanning of the entire body in a helical pattern without stopping the tube. When the patient table is moved slowly during the x-ray exposure while the tube is in continuous rotation, data comprising a continuous helical scan of the patient is acquired. Both low- and high-voltage slip rings have been developed by different manufacturers.

The term *spiral* is a misnomer. A spiral is a circular motion with a decreasing or increasing diameter. The actual scanning motion has a set circular diameter, which is a helix. The data is acquired in a helical, not a spiral, motion (Figure 44-10).

The primary advantage of helical scanning is a much shorter total scan time (30–40 sec. for the entire abdomen). This in turn permits the use of less contrast media. Not only are patients at less risk of contrast media reaction, the throughput of patients is greatly increased. Another advantage is that for many patients the entire examination can be completed in one breath hold, eliminating overlaps and missed areas due to variations in the amount of air in the lungs between scan sections. This also reduces the possibility of motion artifacts.

FIGURE 44-9   A helical computed tomography scanner slip ring. The brushes are contained in the large unit at the center of the photograph. They fit into grooves in the ring underneath. As the x-ray tube rotates, the necessary electrical connections are maintained without interruption. *(Courtesy of Philips Medical System, Inc. All rights reserved.)*

A   Pitch = 2

B   Pitch´ = 1

FIGURE 44-10   Helical and MSCT/MDCT Scan and Pitch. (A) A single helical scan motion with a pitch of 2. (B) MSCT/MDCT collimator pitch´ of 1.

TABLE 44-2.	Advantages and Disadvantages of Helical (Spiral) Computed Tomography

Advantages
Requires less contrast media resulting in decreased patient risk of contrast media reactions.
Eliminates overlap and missed areas due to variations in breathing for some patients and examinations where the entire scan can be completed in one breath hold.
Motion artifacts are reduced.
Faster scan time increases patient throughput.
Pitch settings can be set to oversample sections of interest.
Reconstruction section thickness can be smaller than the acquisition section thickness.

Disadvantages
Full 360° projection data is not acquired for each section.
Sections are reconstructed to represent approximate acquisition of planar data.

The primary disadvantage is that a full 360° set of data is not acquired for each section because the patient is continuously advancing through the gantry bore during the exposure. The sectional image is created from computer reconstructions of planar sections that approximate the acquisition of planar reconstruction data. Both the advantages and disadvantages are detailed in Table 44-2.

Pitch. Because the patient table moves during the exposure a method to measure and reproduce this motion must be established. **Pitch** is the term that is used to define this extension or contraction of the helix. Pitch is simply the ratio of the distance the table moves (feed) during one 360° tube rotation to the total beam collimation (Figure 44-10). The formula for pitch is:

$$P = \frac{I}{B}$$

where   P = pitch
         I = table increment per 360°
         B = beam width in mm

EXAMPLE: If the table is moving at 15 mm/sec. and a section thickness of 10 mm is being acquired, what is the pitch?

Answer:

$$P = \frac{I}{S}$$

$$P = \frac{15}{10} = 1.5$$

EXAMPLE: If a pitch of 0.8 is being used and a section thickness of 8 mm is being acquired, what is the proper table speed?

Answer:

$$P = \frac{I}{S} \text{ or } I = PB$$

$$I = 0.8 \times 8$$

$$I = 6.4 \text{ mm/sec.}$$

EXAMPLE: If the table is moving at 5 mm/sec. and a pitch of 1.0 is being used, what is the section thickness?

Answer:

$$P = \frac{I}{B} \text{ or } B = \frac{I}{P}$$

$$B = \frac{5}{1.0}$$

$$B = 5 \text{ mm}$$

Collimator Pitch´. Multidetector CT changes the way pitch is calculated because the beam is intercepted and acquired by multiple detectors instead of a single detector receiving the entire beam. The term **collimator pitch´** ("pitch prime") refers to the pitch of a single detector within a MDCT array of image receptors, not the total beam collimation. Table 44-3 includes both pitch formulas.

Increasing the pitch value permits a greater field of view (FOV) to be imaged in a shorter time. However, it is important to understand that **pitch values less than 1.0 imply data oversampling. Pitch values greater than 1.0 imply that some data is being missed.** The ability to set the pitch less than 1.0 and produce oversampling of areas of interest is also an advantage of helical scanning.

TABLE 44-3.	CT Pitch Formulas			
Single Section Pitch or Multiple Section Pitch (Beam Width)	$P = I/B$	where:	P = pitch	
			I = table increment per 360°	
			B = beam width in mm	
Multiple Section Pitch' (Section Width)	$CP' = I/S$	where:	CP' = collimator pitch'	
			I = table increment per 360°	
			S = section width in mm	

FIGURE 44-11   Image resolution in helical and MSCT/MDCT scanner is improved in all three planes. Resolution is increased in the x and y planes by decreasing detector size. Resolution is increased in the z plane by using the smallest detector size and a pitch ≤1.

Another major advantage is that image reconstruction can be set for smaller section thicknesses than those that were acquired.

Resolution. Image resolution in helical scanners (which includes multisection scanners as well) is vastly improved over older models. Resolution issues must be considered from two perspectives: the image matrix pixel size in both the x and y planes and the helical pitch (which forms the z axis) as shown in Figure 44-11.

Increased resolution in the x and y planes is accomplished by technologies that decrease the size of the detectors. Both computer processing and display resolution far exceeds current detector acquisition technology.

Increased resolution in the z plane is accomplished by using the smallest detector size combined with a pitch ≤1.

Seventh Generation—MSCT

Computed tomography units with multiple detectors are known by several terms. **Multisection or multislice computed tomography** (MSCT), **multidetector computed tomography** (MDCT), and **multiple detector array scanners** (MDA) have all appeared in the literature to date. The most appropriate term to use is **multisection computed tomography** (MSCT) because the term *slice* is professional slang and just because a scanner has multiple detectors does not necessarily indicate that multiple sections of data are being collected simultaneously.

Multisection CT units represent a major change in CT technology in that multiple detectors are exposed simultaneously (Figure 44-12). At the turn of the century there were major advancements in detector technology that permitted an array of thousands of parallel bands of detectors to operate simultaneously instead of the single bands of detectors that had been in use up until then. This permitted a single beam exposure to produce multiple sets of image receptor data. When this technology is combined with helical scanning, total examination time is reduced dramatically, with an entire chest or abdomen procedure completed in 15–20 sec.

Because section thickness can be reduced with MSCT, resolution can be increased remarkably.

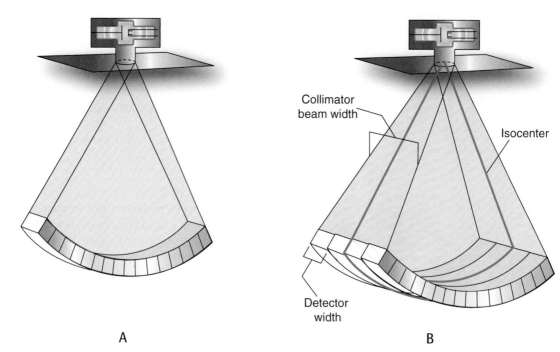

Collimator
beam width

Isocenter

Detector
width

A

B

FIGURE 44-12 Multisection computed tomography (MSCT) resolution. (A) Single section CT resolution is determined by the width of the collimator beam. (B) Multisection CT resolution is determined by the width of the detector.

Section thickness with single section CT scanners is determined by the collimator size, not the width of the detector. Because MSCT scanners are exposing multiple detectors simultaneously, section thickness is determined by the width of the detector, even though the collimation of the beam is wide enough to expose several other bands of detectors (see Figure 44–12). For this reason, resolution in MSCT scanners is determined by the width of the detector, not the width of the collimator.

The MSCT design is more efficient, reduces patient exposure, increases image resolution, and allows post-acquisition reconstruction at new levels as well. For example, a 20 mm collimated beam width can be used to simultaneously expose an array of four 5 mm detector bands (as shown in Figure 44-12). The dataset that is acquired from this exposure can be displayed as four 5 mm sections, two 10 mm sections, or one 20 mm section. Nearly unlimited choices in section thickness become available to the interpreting physician or radiologist assistant.

Some MSCT scanners allow users to set the pitch <1 in order to increase the mAs/section available. This increases the quantity of data to each detector without overloading the x-ray tube. Some manufacturers only allow preset pitch.

All MSCT units use a helical scan system that produces extremely rapid scanning time while maintaining the advantages of higher resolution and reconstruction flexibility. Figure 44-12 illustrates how a four-detector row, single beam helical scan sequence would appear. MSCT units are rated according to the number of detector rows that can be exposed from a single beam collimation. The figure illustrates only four rows to demonstrate the concept. There are 16, 20, and 24 section units in clinical use, and one manufacturer is promoting a 256-section scanner that is under development. These scanners produce thousands of images for each procedure and have created considerable concern over radiologist liability because questions have not yet been answered regarding reasonable standards for how many of these images should be viewed to provide an adequate diagnosis. In the United Kingdom, graduate degree programs for radiographers have been developed to assist in screening huge quantities of images in collaboration with radiologists, and there is now development of radiologist assistant programs in the United States that may provide some relief for this responsibility as well as additional career opportunities for highly qualified and motivated radiographers.

THE COMPONENTS OF A CT UNIT

The Gantry

The **gantry** is the movable frame of the CT unit. It contains the x-ray tube and detectors and is the most visible part of the unit. The gantry frame maintains the alignment of the tube and detectors and contains the equipment necessary to perform the scanning movements. The gantry includes a 50–85 cm (20″–34″) aperture for the patient. Obese patients who exceed the tabletop weight limits must never be forced into the aperture. They may become stuck.

Most gantrys can be angled up to 30° to permit positioning for partial coronal images. This is especially desirable in obtaining transverse scans perpendicular to the vertebral column. Table angulation can sometimes be used in place of gantry angulation. Scanners with the x-ray beam placed near the table side of the aperture permit more comfortable positioning of the patient and may permit coronal or sagittal scanning of some body parts, especially of the head. Both magnetic resonance imaging and CT reconfiguration software may be used in place of positions designed to achieve coronal or sagittal sections.

Positioning lights are usually mounted on the gantry as well. Intense white halogen lights and low-power red laser lights are used for positioning. The body part of interest must be properly centered to the aperture because the extreme edge of the scanning field produces a severely degraded image. There are often three positioning lights for accurate sagittal, coronal, and transverse centering.

Table

The CT table may be either flat or curved. It is usually made of carbon graphite fiber to decrease beam attenuation. Because the top must extend beyond the table to move the patient into the gantry aperture, it must be capable of supporting the entire weight of the patient without sagging when fully extended. Tabletops are rated for maximum weight and it is critical that the radiographer make sure that this weight is not exceeded. Extensive damage to the table may result when attempts are made to examine very large patients who exceed the tabletop weight limit. Physicians must be informed if the CT unit cannot move obese patients into the aperture for examination. Examinations of patients over the weight limit may remove the CT unit from clinical use for all patients for a considerable time while the top is replaced. The top is motor-driven to permit the patient to be moved the exact desired distance between sections. Section intervals may be controlled automatically by a program initiated at the control console. The table must also be capable of vertical movement, both for positioning within the aperture and for ease of patient transfer.

X-Ray Tubes

The rapid sequential exposures required to produce CT images produce massive amounts of heat in the x-ray tube. Most CT x-ray tube difficulties have revolved around attempts to solve this problem. The early scanners used a stationary anode with a 2 mm × 16 mm focal spot operating at 120 kVp and 30 mA. This reduced image resolution significantly. However, since first-generation images were usually displayed on an 80 × 80 matrix, the x-ray tube was not the problem in this system.

As matrix size increased to 512 × 512, rotating anode tubes with focal spots as small as 0.6 mm × 1.2 mm came into use. Small focal-spot scanners use a pulsed beam to reduce the heat load. Modern pulsed scanner tubes operate at 120 kVp, 1–5 msec pulses, and up to 1,000 mA. Some units permit 80 and 140 kVp to be selected, sometimes in alternate pulses, for dual-energy scanning in which comparisons can be made between images at different kVp values. In addition, 0.5–5.0 million heat unit anodes of layered alloys, cylindrical anodes and liquid-cooled and air-cooled tube housing designs have been developed. A CT tube may produce 30 exposures per examination. Because most CT units are scheduled for 10–20 examinations per day, a tube may accumulate 10,000 exposures in a single month. It is not unusual for a CT tube to fail after several months. Only a few last a full year.

The radiation beam is double collimated, once at the tube exit and again at the detector entrance. This assists in eliminating scatter information. Collimation controls the voxel length. Collimation is variable from 1 mm to 13 mm and is usually controlled by the software program. The dimension of the collimation width determines the voxel length, or section thickness.

Detectors

Detectors must be capable of responding with extreme speed to a signal, without lag, must quickly discard the signal, and prepare for the next. They must also respond consistently and be small in size. They are usually placed with a source-to-image receptor distance of 44″ (110 cm).

CT detectors should have high **capture efficiency,** high **absorption efficiency,** and high **conversion efficiency.** These three parameters are called the **detector dose efficiency.**

$$
\begin{array}{r}
\text{capture efficiency} \\
\text{absorption efficiency} \\
+ \text{ conversion efficiency} \\
\hline
\text{dose efficiency}
\end{array}
$$

The capture efficiency is how well the detectors receive photons from the patient. It is controlled primarily by detector size and the distance between detectors. Absorption efficiency is how well the detectors convert incoming x-ray photons. It is determined primarily by the materials used (for example, the scintillation crystal or the gas) as well as the size and thickness of the detector. Conversion efficiency is determined by how well the detector converts the absorbed photon information to a digital signal for the computer.

CT detectors should also have high **stability,** fast **response time,** and a wide **dynamic range.** Stability is controlled by how often the detectors must be recalibrated to meet quality control standards. Response time is the speed with which the detector can react to recognize an incoming photon and recover for the next input. The dynamic range is the ratio of the largest signal that can be measured to the smallest. Typical modern scanners are capable of dynamic ranges of 1,000,000 to 1.

Scintillation Crystals and Photomultiplier Tubes. Early detectors consisted of a scintillation crystal in contact with a photomultiplier tube (Figure 44-13). This system was used in nuclear medicine for many years prior to the advent of CT. A sodium iodide (NaI) crystal absorbs an x-ray photon and produces light flashes (scintillations) in proportion to the energy of the photon and at the exact location where the photon struck within the crystal. This light (photo) is then amplified (multiplied) by the photomultiplier (PM) tube. The light photon strikes the cathode of the PM tube, where it is converted into electrons. The electrons are then amplified by a series of dynodes as they move through the tube. Each dynode has a higher voltage, thereby increasing the number and voltage of the electrons as they move toward the anode. Upon striking the anode, the electrons are converted into a digital signal which can be processed by the computer.

Although sodium iodide scintillation crystals are nearly 100 percent efficient within the diagnostic x-ray range, they exhibit phosphorescent afterglow,

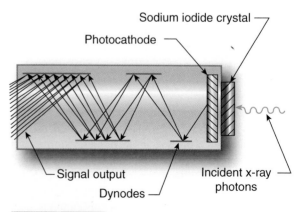

Sodium iodide crystal

Photocathode

Signal output

Dynodes

Incident x-ray photons

FIGURE 44-13 A scintillation crystal and photomultiplier tube detector.

or lag. This makes them useless with the rapid sequential exposures in the later generation scanners. Some units were produced using calcium fluoride (CaF_2), bismuth germinate ($Bi_4Ge_3O_{12}$), cesium iodine (CsI), gadolinium ceramics, and cadmium tungstate ($CdWO_4$) scintillation crystals, which, although less efficient (90 percent), have minimal afterglow. These materials are often bonded directly to the photocathode. A major disadvantage of scintillation-PM detectors was their size and interspace material, which prohibited packing them closer in the detector array. This reduced their total detection efficiency to less than 50 percent.

Xenon Ionization Chambers. Inexpensive CT scanners may use xenon gas-filled ionization chamber detectors (Figure 44-14). They operate on the same principle as an ionization chamber. Essentially, they measure ionization in air by attracting to an electrode the ions created by x-ray photons in the air. The electrodes are usually thin tungsten plates spaced 1.5 mm apart. This spacing determines the maximum detector (and therefore display pixel size) resolution. The electrodes are alternately charged with positive and negative voltages. The quantity of ionic charge at the electrode is proportional to the energy of the photons detected between the elec-

trodes. The detected energy comprises a digital signal that is sent to the computer.

Gas detectors range in efficiency from 60 to 90 percent but exhibit no lag. Ion chamber detectors were not used in the original EMI scanner because they were not sensitive enough. This disadvantage was overcome by using a long ion chamber and filling it with krypton or xenon, the heaviest inert gas, at high compression (20–30 atmospheres).

Although gas-ion detector efficiency may be only 60 percent, these detectors can be packed extremely close in the detector array, permitting a detection efficiency of slightly less than 50 percent, which is similar to that of scintillation-PM detectors.

Xenon detectors are highly directional. In other words, they must be set in a fixed position oriented to the x-ray source. This is why helical scanners do not use xenon detectors.

Solid State. Solid-state detectors are used in all helical and MSCT scanners. They are similar to the detectors used in digital radiography systems but with different performance requirements.

FIGURE 44-14 (A) A xenon gas–filled ionization chamber CT detector. The tungsten plate electrodes are alternately charged with positive and negative voltages. (B) A detector ring in a helical CT unit. *(Courtesy of Philips Medical Systems, Inc. All rights reserved.)*

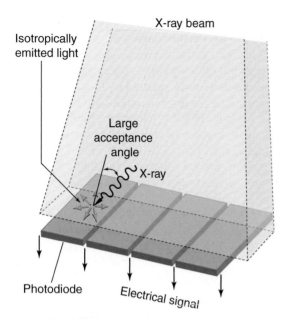

X-ray beam

Isotropically
emitted light

Large
acceptance
angle

X-ray

Photodiode

Electrical signal

FIGURE 44-15 Solid-state detector. A scintillator is bonded to the top of the photodiode. When the incoming x-ray beam activates the scintillator, light photons are emitted, which are detected by the photodiode and converted into an electrical signal. Note the large acceptance angle of the scintillator. This accounts for the vastly increased sensitivity of solid-state detectors and permits the incoming x-ray beam to be a diverging fan shape.

Solid-state detectors combine a calcium tungstate ($CdWO_4$), yttrium, or gadolinium ceramic scintillator with a photodetector (Figure 44-15). The scintillator is bonded to the top of the photodiode to assure accurate pickup of the emitted photons. When the incoming x-ray beam photon activates the scintillator, light photons are emitted isotropically in proportion to the intensity of the incoming light. A major advantage of the scintillator is that it has a large acceptance angle for incoming x-ray photons. This greatly increases the sensitivity of the detector by allowing the incoming x-ray beam to be a diverging fan shape. In other words, the detector does not have to be positioned directly under the perpendicular central ray of the x-ray beam. This allows the entire array of bands of detectors to operate simultaneously. The photodiode detects the light photons emit-

ted by the scintillator and converts them into an electrical signal. However, they require a small gap between adjacent detectors to avoid crosstalk between one another. This limits how close together the detectors can be placed and this impacts the resolution of the scanner.

CT solid-state detectors used in MSCT scanners are typically 1.0 mm × 1.5–15 mm. Digital radiography systems use detectors that are much smaller (typically 0.1–0.2 mm on each side). One reason CT detectors are so much larger is because the CT signal must be very low noise in order to achieve the 20-bit grayscale depth necessary for effective diagnosis.

Because the crosstalk between adjacent detectors is related to the angle of the incoming x-ray beam, some scanners are designed with more narrow detectors at the isocenter of the x-ray beam where the incoming x-ray photons arrive at near 90° angles (Figure 44-16). A typical setup might include 1.0 mm wide detectors at the isocenter with gradually increasing widths of 1.5, 2.0, or 2.5–5.0 mm wide detectors at the outer edges of the collimated beam. Back illumination of photodiodes has allowed closer placement of detector cells at the isocenter. Together these innovations have allowed manufacturers to achieve submillimeter detection widths at the center of the beam. It must be remembered that submillimeter resolution is not available across the entire MSCT helically scanned beam. It is possible only at the isocenter.

Additional techniques for decreasing detector crosstalk include both pre- and post-patient collimation. The post-patient collimator is a set of lead shields immediately in front of the detectors. Septal collimators are also being used as high-resolution collimators between detector rows in multiarray MSCT scanners (Figure 44-17).

There are also innovative post-acquisition algorithms that show promise of additional increases in resolution by correlating information from overlapping sets of binned detectors.

Detector Calibration. Tube and detector alignment is critical in CT because of the tight collimation of the tube and the collimator mask at the detector. The slightest misalignment may produce a concentric ring artifact image that completely overrides clinical information.

FIGURE 44-17   Solid-state detector septal and post-patient collimators. A single row of detectors makes up an array as shown. The gray plates on each side represent the post-patient collimator. The gray strips down the length of the detector row represent the thin septal collimators that divide each row of detectors in order to reduce crosstalk and increase resolution.

Rotating anode tubes are aligned with their long axis perpendicular to the scanning plane. This prevents the anode heel effect within the useful beam while eliminating the gyroscopic effect on the rotating anode.

Detectors must remain in close calibration at all times. Scanner software does this automatically during scanning operations. Detectors that are out of calibration may cause artifacts that destroy image quality.

Computer

The CT computer is designed to control data acquisition, processing, display, and storage. The CT console provides the radiographer with access to the software program that controls data acquisition, processing, and display. Remote consoles may also be linked to the system to permit display and storage functions. Control of data storage may be available at the control console, remote workstations, or at the storage units themselves.

A systems program is used to start up the CT unit. This program turns on and performs quality assurance checks on numerous components in both the x-ray equipment and computer hardware systems, warms up the x-ray tube, etc. It also permits the radiographer to record various problems that need the attention of the service engineer. One of its main functions is to perform calibration checks on the detectors, although this may be an ongoing process during scanning. A diagnostics program with specific quality assurance tests is used by service engineers to troubleshoot the systems.

The CT console operates from a menu or index directory of operations. The radiographer simply uses a keyboard, mouse trackball, or other input device to indicate the desired operation. At the beginning of each examination, patient information, such as identification, history, and the like, is entered or input via a radiology (RIS) or hospital (HIS) data system. This information permits retrieval of the images at a later date and will also be displayed adjacent to each image.

The data acquisition program controls a variety of operations, including tube and detector collimation (pixel size), matrix size, gantry angle, tabletop entrance into the gantry aperture, section increment movements of the tabletop, x-ray tube voltage and amperage, scan speed, pitch, detector/resolution, and the direction of detector signals to the digital image processing section of the computer.

Display Console

The processing and display program controls the digital image production process, including the series of mathematical formulas (algorithms) that compile the image and the display parameters, such as window level and width, reconstructions, and enhancements.

The display console is often part of the main console and appears as a separate CRT with controls (Figure 44-18). Also available are separate reporting workstations that permit radiologists to display images and electronically report the results, and in-

FIGURE 44-18 CT main console with display CRT. *(Courtesy of Siemens Medical Systems, Inc.)*

dependent consoles that contain their own CPU to retrieve and display images from the memory storage units and to receive images from examinations in progress.

Most CT display units permit a wide range of display features to enhance diagnosis. These vary by manufacturer but often include the following.

Scanogram/Sinogram. A localization image **scanogram** or **sinogram** is often displayed as the first image of an examination. It is displayed prior to the examination by slit scanning as the tabletop moves the patient through the tightly collimated primary beam. The resolution of the image is affected by the speed of the scan and the exposure output of the tube. The poorer the scan, the less the patient dose. Because these images are used primarily for localization, image quality is seldom important. The radiographer should advocate the highest-speed scan and the lowest exposure output possible. The addition to the slit scan of dotted lines corresponding to the section intervals provides a convenient reference guide when viewing the sectional images. The scanogram can serve as a diagnostic tool in radiation therapy treatment planning by using a cursor to delineate the margins of a tumor on a series of transverse sections. The scanogram can then compile the cursor delineations to provide a coronal and sagittal outline of the tumor. The scanogram is sometimes called by one of a number of trademark names.

Grid Application. A grid pattern may be added to any image. Radiographers use the grid to confirm exact centering of the patient; radiologists use the grid pattern to describe precise structural locations.

Cursor. A cursor can be used to outline an area of interest. The area can be recorded on film and the Hounsfield unit mean or standard deviation can be displayed for the tissue within the marked area. Hounsfield units (HU) are discussed next. A line can be drawn between any two cursor locations, displaying the area's measurement within the patient. A cursor can also be used by itself to mark an area of interest. Mapping and volume estimates are achieved through cursor guidance as well.

Density contouring software is available that permits selection of a single point by a cursor, with the program highlighting all pixels of matching HU. This feature can be used to outline a tumor or other object to compile volume estimates.

Special software is also available to facilitate **radiation therapy treatment planning** through the use of cursors and integration with dosimetric data from a dosimetry computer.

Reverse Display. Reverse display is available to reverse the image from left to right and/or reverse the density display so that blacks appear white and whites appear black.

Magnification. Although nearly unlimited magnification may be accomplished, distortion usually becomes objectionable beyond $3\times$.

Suppression. Originally designed to suppress the information from surgical clips, this feature permits a problem area, such as a surgical clip, to be outlined and then deleted from the reconstruction data.

Annotation. Text may be added to images for descriptions or anatomical labeling.

Histograms. A histogram is a bar graph which may provide useful diagnostic data in some instances. Software is available to produce these graphs by Hounsfield units and by time versus motion. Volumetric analysis is possible with some histographic data.

A histogram of the Hounsfield units along a line drawn between two cursor points may be useful in some diagnoses. Histograms of various motions versus time may also be displayed for diagnosis of vascular flow or heart motion. These histograms are of limited value in CT because other modalities, especially ultrasonography and nuclear medicine, produce more accurate information.

Three-Dimensional Imaging. Software and separate image processing units are available that will reconstruct CT data into a three-dimensional image (Figure 44–19) that can be manipulated in a manner similar to a draftsman's CAD/CAM computer graphics system. The image can be rotated, tumbled or tilted to demonstrate structures that would otherwise be hidden. Images can be adjusted to various degrees of translucency and can be divided. For example, an image of the head may have soft tissue density reduced to 25 percent, bone density reduced to 50 percent, and the right half of the image removed to permit viewing of the left side of the sella turcica.

CT NUMBERS (HOUNSFIELD UNITS)

The true linear attenuation coefficients of the tissue voxels are not exactly represented by the data received by the CT computer. Therefore, a series of tissue density values has evolved for CT measurements. Originally named computed tomography numbers, they were renamed Hounsfield units (HU) after the Nobel Prize was awarded to Godfrey Hounsfield in 1979. These numbers are calculated by comparing the linear attenuation coefficient of each pixel to the linear attenuation coefficient of water, according to the following formula:

$$\text{CT Number} = 1{,}000\frac{\mu_p - \mu_w}{\mu_w}$$

where: μ_p = linear attenuation coefficient of measured pixel, and
μ_w = linear attenuation coefficient of water.

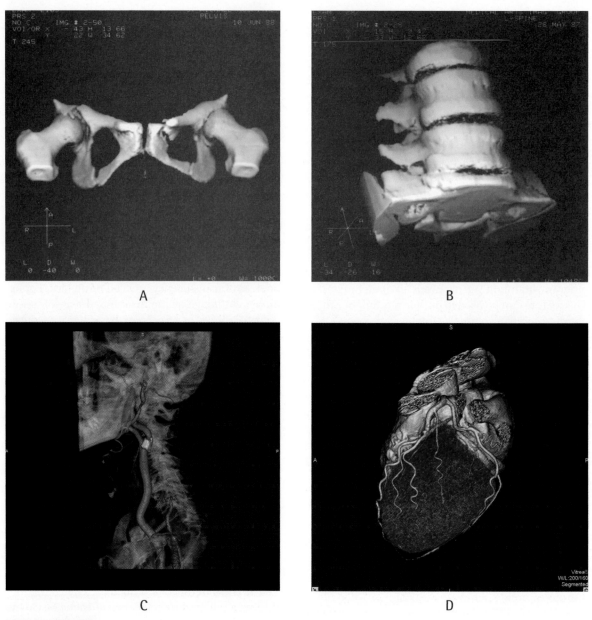

FIGURE 44-19 Three-dimensional CT reconstructions. (A) pelvis, (B) spine, (C) carotid arteries, and (D) coronary arteries. *(Courtesy of Toshiba America Medical Systems, Inc.)*

Therefore, the HU of water is always 0, average bone +1,000, and air −1,000. Table 44-4 illustrates the HU of other tissues. The CT unit can display the HU of any given volume of tissue. Most units use a cursor to delineate the pixels to be measured and then display the HU on the CRT next to the image. Radiologists may use HUs occasionally to assist in diagnosis even though the original hope of defining HUs for specific pathologies has not been realized. The attenuation data received by CT detectors is accurate ± 0.2 percent; therefore, HUs are accurate ±2.

TABLE 44-4.	Hounsfield Units (HU) (CT Numbers) of Various Tissues	
Bone, petrous	+	3,000
Bone, average	+	1,000
Bone, cortical	+	800
Blood, clotted	+	55–75
Spleen	+	50–70
Liver	+	40–70
Pancreas	+	40–60
Kidney	+	40–60
Aorta	+	35–50
Muscle	+	35–50
Brain, white matter	+	36–46
Cerebellum	+	30
Brain, gray matter	+	20–40
Blood	+	13–18
Cerebrospinal fluid	+	15
Tumors	+	5–35
Gallbladder	+	5–30
Water		0
Orbits	−	25
Fat	−	100
Lungs	−	150–400
Air	−	1,000

IMAGE RECONSTRUCTION

The detectors send information proportional to the attenuation coefficient of the voxel of tissue lying between the detector and the x-ray tube. The CT image is then reconstructed using a mathematical algorithm (usually based on Fourier transformation or a combination of convolution and back-projection) of the digitized information received by the computer.

The programs used by CT scanners compensate for numerous intrinsic and extrinsic factors, includ-

ing the emission spectrum of the beam, and weighting factors for the geometrical aberrations caused by beam divergence and semicircular detector arrangement. Reconstruction often requires up to 30 seconds. However, when an array processor is used, reconstruction time can be decreased to less than one second, which is desirable for dynamic studies.

Fourier Transformation and Back-Projection

The primary mathematical method used in the creation of computerized medical images is the Fourier transformation. Transformations are simply conversions of data to more useful forms, as when radiation doses are changed from rems to mSv. Visual transformations can also be useful, as when a decubitus abdomen radiograph is viewed horizontally to facilitate detection of air-fluid levels.

Fourier's mathematics accomplishes transformations of extremely complex functions into separate but simpler functions. For example, a Fourier transform can be applied to separate music into functions of varying amplitudes, frequencies, and timing phases. This data can then be recorded for use in a magnetic tape player or CD-ROM. The Fourier transform permits the reconstruction of portions of the data when the other portions and their relationships are known. It is also possible to use the inverse Fourier transform to change back to the original data.

In digital imaging, the Fourier transform is used on data representing image intensities at specific locations. For example, Figure 44-20 demonstrates different attenuation coefficients at specific image receptor locations.

The information received by the image receptors can be processed through a variety of mathematical formulas (often referred to as algorithms or kernels). The Fourier algorithm is a fundamental formula used in image reconstruction.

It is based on algebraically adding several sets of incoming data from the image receptor. For example, in Figure 44-21, the top two waveforms have been combined to produce the bottom wave. Figure 44-22 illustrates how several different additions would change to combined waveform. Finally, Figure 44-23

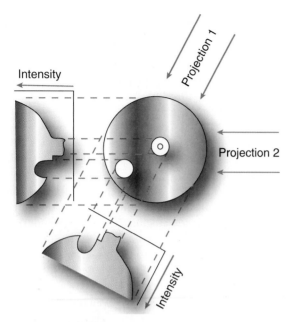

FIGURE 44-20 Image receptor data correlated to specific spatial locations. *(Reprinted from* Computers in radiology, *Greenfield, G. B. & Hubbard, L. [1984] with permission form Elsevier)*

FIGURE 44-21 Basic Fourier algorithm. The top two waveforms have been combined to produce the bottom wave. *(Used by permission from Hedrick, W. R. & Hykes, D. L. [1992]. A simplified explanation of Fourier analysis,* Journal of Diagnostic Medical Sonography, *J. B. Lippincott, Philadelphia, PA, 8[6], 302–303)*

shows how numerous additions would produce a square waveform. Various mathematical algorithms can change or transform the amplitude and time domain to the frequency domain and vice versa. This transformation process is called a Fourier transform or fast Fourier transform (FFT).

The inverse Fourier transformation can be used to mathematically back-project an image of the structures that produced the attenuation coefficients as demonstrated in Figure 44-24.

Convolution and Deconvolution

It is sometimes useful to modify the value of each pixel to enhance or suppress a visual characteristic of the image. This process is actually mathematical filtering. **Convolution is the process of modifying pixel values by a mathematical formula.** It is sometimes called a **mask** because a set of mathematical operations is placed over each pixel, the pixel value is changed, the mask is then applied to the next pixel and so on. The total process is one of

sliding the mask over all the pixel data and then displaying the modified image. **Deconvolution is the process of returning the pixel values to their original level by a reverse process.**

Helical Interpolation

Helical scanning occurs in a pattern that is at an angle to the perpendicular plane that is desired for imaging. To "straighten up" the sectional image, it is necessary to apply post-acquisition algorithms to the dataset. This process is called interpolation. Figure 44-25 shows how these algorithms function. Essentially, the raw dataset is projected, or interpolated, forward or backward into a theoretical per-

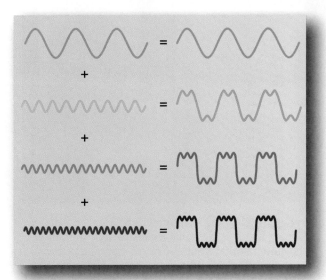

FIGURE 44-22 Basic Fourier algorithm. Several different additions changed to a combined waveform. *(Used by permission from Hedrick, W. R. & Hykes, D. L. [1992]. A simplified explanation of Fourier analysis,* Journal of Diagnostic Medical Sonography. *J. B. Lippincott, Philadelphia, PA 8[6], 302–303)*

FIGURE 44-23 Basic Fourier algorithm. Numerous additions producing a square waveform. *(Used by permission from Hedrick, W. R. & Hykes, D. L. [1992]. A simplified explanation of Fourier analysis,* Journal of Diagnostic Medical Sonography. *J. B. Lippincott, Philadelphia, PA, 8[6], 302–303)*

FIGURE 44-24 Image receptor data correlated to specific spatial locations. *(Reprinted with permission from Greenfield, G. B & Hubbard L [1984].* Computers in radiology, *New York: Churchill Livingstone)*

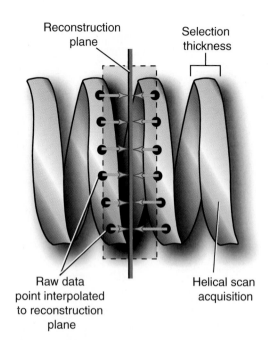

FIGURE 44-25 Helical scanning interpolation. The red line represents the theoretical perpendicular section into which the true helical raw data set is projected (either forward or backward). This theoretical perpendicular section forms the image that is displayed. The section thickness is controlled by the pitch of the raw helical scan acquisition.

pendicular section. It is possible to use these algorithms to create a wide variety of sections that are reconstructions of data, not additional radiation exposure to the patient.

Reformatting

Reconstruction software is available that permits reformatting the information from a series of sectional images to produce an image of a section not actually scanned. For example, the extracted coronal image could be formed by reconstruction of only the appropriate voxels from each of the transverse sections. A typical reformatted CT image is shown in Figure 44-26.

Reformatting may also be used for a magnification technique called **targeting,** which permits an area of interest to be selected for reformatting. The

FIGURE 44-26 A reformatted CT image. The upper image is a coronal reconstruction from data acquired during axial transverse scanning of the cervical spine. Note the square bone fragment from the fracture. It is against the left side of the circular dens of C-2 at the center of the image. *(Courtesy of Barbara Imber and St. Rita's Medical Center, Lima, OH)*

reformatting process reconstructs the image data in a smaller pixel size to permit magnification with less distortion. This technique is used for regions in which extremely fine detail is necessary, such as the inner ear.

IMAGE QUALITY

Computed tomography image quality is primarily controlled by resolution and noise considerations. Density and contrast, as with any digitized image, can be manipulated by the computer. The prime consideration of the radiographer when making decisions regarding how to perform a particular CT examination must involve obtaining the necessary resolution while limiting noise.

Density and Contrast

Display density and contrast differences are varied with window level and width controls. Most CT images can demonstrate contrast differences of as little as 0.4 percent (4 HU), as compared to a minimum of 10 percent for a diagnostic radiograph. Appropriate CT window widths are shown in Table 44-5.

TABLE 44-5.	Appropriate Computed Tomography Window Widths

Area of Interest	Window Width (HU)
Head	70–200
Spine	350–750
Orbits	350–700
Heart	250–350
Abdomen	250–450
Thorax for lungs	1,200–1,400
Inner ear	2,000–4,000

Resolution

The resolution of the CT image depends on pixel, voxel and matrix size. High contrast objects 1.5 times the pixel size or larger can be imaged reliably. For example, a pixel size of 0.5 mm can resolve an object 0.75 mm in size. Low contrast objects may require a larger pixel size to permit the detectors to provide sufficient data to reach a visible difference between the attenuation coefficients. Therefore low contrast objects may actually be seen better with a larger pixel size, although the total resolution is reduced. The current spatial resolution possible is about 0.35 mm, as compared to 0.25 mm and better with diagnostic radiography. However, this resolution is not possible under routine scanning conditions.

Voxel, Pixel, and Matrix Size. Discussion of CT imaging detail must consider voxel, pixel and matrix size. It is possible to have pixels and matrix size equal yet the voxel width may have a considerable effect on image quality. Matrix sizes offered on CT units have included 256×256, 320×320, 360×360, and 512×512. Because most CT images are processed and displayed with a circular field, the actual number of image pixels is less than if the matrix were square. For example, a 512×512 circular field matrix has slightly over 200,000 pixels.

Voxel width may be varied between 8 mm and 13 mm. A common voxel size might be 1 mm $\times$ 1 mm $\times$ 10 mm with 10 mm representing the voxel width. The 20 percent additional tissue volume of a 13 mm voxel requires 60 percent more radiation exposure to produce an image of comparable quality. Therefore, patient dose considerations in CT are similar to those in diagnostic radiography.

Interface Artifacts. Depending on the mathematical algorithm used, imaging aberrations displayed as density differences may occur when two objects have more than a 60 percent difference in attenuation coefficients. These artifacts are called undershoot and overshoot. Any object of greatly different contrast, such as metallic surgical clips, bullets, an old contrast medium and air, is likely to cause a star pattern artifact. The effect can be somewhat modified by using a larger matrix. However, different reconstruction algorithms that mathematically filter or compensate for the effect have been designed for various body parts. For example, a soft tissue algorithm is useless during examination of the inner ear. A special bone algorithm is required to produce useful information when a number of small bony structures are in close proximity to one another.

Magnification. The display or **reconstruction field of view** (FOV) is different from the scan field of view. True CT magnification is achieved by choosing a smaller display field of view. This produces an image with less tissue per voxel, which in turn provides higher resolution and a larger image of a smaller area of interest. Magnification of the matrix field size has no effect on image resolution. When a CT image matrix is magnified it may be possible to perceive individual pixels. This causes the image to appear less sharp. Therefore, most radiologists prefer to diagnose from images of a smaller size that are sharp.

Noise. All digital images have noise problems. **Noise** on a CT image is directly related to the amount of data collected by the detector. It appears as quantum mottle (best seen in an image of a water phantom) and normally comprises 3–5 percent of the image. Most CT image noise is a result of statistical fluctuation in the information recorded by the detector, not a result of computer reconstruction mathematics. **The amount of noise controls the low contrast resolving ability of the CT unit.** A standard CT quality assurance measurement is a daily noise evaluation that is done by imaging a phantom and using a cursor to read the HUs for control areas. Each reading should average at least 100 pixels (10×10 matrix).

A

B

C

FIGURE 44-27 Computer correction of motion: (A) motion artifacts obscuring information; (B) separate images for each third of the scan time reveal all the motion that occurred during the final third of the scan; and (C) reconstruction using only the first two-thirds of the scan time produces a diagnostic quality image.

Motion. Motion on a CT image is a function of exposure time, just as in diagnostic radiography. The exposure time in CT is controlled by the quantity of data detected. Because insufficient data results in a poor quality image, motion during a CT scan is displayed as a series of very poor quality images. For example, a rib that moves is recorded in a series of locations due to the movement instead of in a stationary location if respiration had been suspended. Each of the movement images is of poor quality because the detector received too little data to permit reconstruction of a normal quality image (Figure 44-27). Helical and MSCT scanners can perform interrupted or skip-scanning to compensate for patient breathing motion.

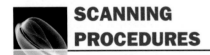 **SCANNING PROCEDURES**

Section Interval and Thickness

The section interval is the distance between scan sections. The section thickness is the width of the volume of tissue being examined (the voxel). Section thickness is usually slightly less than voxel width because of the divergence of the beam. Both the section interval and the thickness are affected by the section shape.

Although section thickness is equivalent to voxel width, or slightly less, a section does not have parallel sides due to the divergence of the x-ray beam. Figure 44-28 illustrates the section shape problem that either overlaps or excludes tissue between sections. One author has described the total scan volume as more like a stack of frisbees than a stack of coins (Figure 44-29). The scanning procedure must take this geometry into account. Overlapping, which occurs with section intervals equal to voxel width, is desirable. For example, a voxel width of 13 mm should use section intervals of 13 mm. In most procedures it is important that no sections of tissue miss examination. Overlap and exclusions must be considered when designing the section interval sequence for the scanning procedure. Most CT unit programs have standardized scanning procedures for the various examinations, although they can be modified to fit specific circumstances and institutional requirements.

Exposure Factors

Most CT scanning is performed at a set kVp. Time is not a factor, as it must be controlled by the scanning program to provide sufficient exposure to the detectors. The CT radiographer can vary the mA to control the primary beam. However, dual energy scanning units require scanning with different kVp values, usually 80 kVp or 140 kVp.

Algorithms

As discussed earlier under image reconstruction techniques, the proper reconstruction algorithm

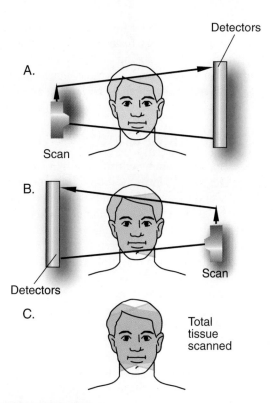

Detectors

A.

Scan

B.

Detectors

Scan

C.

Total tissue scanned

FIGURE 44-28 Section shape due to divergent beam geometry. (A and B) The first scan produces a wedge-shaped volume of scanned tissue. (C) The final scan produces a concave volume of double-scanned tissue with a convex volume of single-scanned tissue at the edges.

must be used to mathematically filter unwanted artifacts. The CT console often combines the proper algorithm with the scanning procedure. High-pass and low-pass filters and other mathematical manipulations can also be performed to improve image quality.

Scan Field Size

The scan field size, or field of view, is set to accommodate the size of the part under examination. The smaller the scan field size, the better the image resolution and the faster the scan time. Common field sizes are 25 cm for the head and magnification of the spine, 35 cm for small bodies and 48 cm for large bodies.

 ARTIFACTS

Motion

Motion is a problem in CT because it produces streak artifacts through the image (Figure 44-30). The algorithm faults when it receives the changes in attenuation that occur at the edges of the moving part. This produces blank pixels, which appear as streaks in these regions.

FIGURE 44-29 The total scan volume is more like a stack of frisbees than a stack of coins.

FIGURE 44-30 A typical computed tomography motion artifact. *(Courtesy of Wil Reddinger, Lima Technical College, Lima, OH)*

Metal or Star

The presence of metallic materials in the patient also cause streak artifacts but may also produce star artifacts (Figure 44-31). The metal objects attenuate nearly 100 percent of the primary beam, which produces an incomplete projection. This may produce a star artifact if the reconstruction algorithm has been unable to create a full set of surrounding projections to smooth the edges of the object. Some CT units have software algorithms designed to reduce and partially correct for these artifacts.

Beam Hardening

Beam hardening artifacts are a result of the attenuation of the beam as it passes through the patient. The CT number of a posterior structure may be much different from a similar anterior structure because the beam reaching the posterior structure has already been significantly attenuated. Beam hardening artifacts are often described as broad dark bands or streaks known as cupping artifacts (Figure 44-32). A capping artifact occurs when the algorithm overcompensates for the beam hardening artifact. Cupping artifacts have lower CT numbers than expected while capping artifacts have higher CT numbers than expected. Software algorithms are available to reduce or partially correct for their effect on the image.

Partial Volume Effect

Because the data from an entire section thickness is averaged together to form the image, the exact location of a section may cause small structures or portions of large structures to be hidden when they comprise only a small percentage of the total section. This is a common concern during CT of the vertebral column when a section interval happens to produce a section where an intervertebral disc comprises a small percentage of the total section volume (Figure 44-33). This is called the partial volume effect. It may obscure any object that is smaller than the voxel width (section thickness) when that object is scanned by two sections. Compensation for the partial volume effect may be overcome in some instances by slightly overlapping sections.

FIGURE 44-31 A typical computed tomography metal or star artifact. *(Courtesy of Wil Reddinger, Lima Technical College, Lima, OH)*

FIGURE 44-32 A typical computed tomography cupping or beam hardening artifact. *(Courtesy of Wil Reddinger, Lima Technical College, Lima, OH)*

A

B

FIGURE 44-33 **(A) A typical computed tomography out of field artifact demonstrating a severe partial volume averaging effect.** *(Courtesy of Wil Reddinger, Lima Technical College, Lima, OH).* **(B) A graphic illustration of the partial volume effect.**

Ring Artifacts

When a single detector goes out of calibration and does not properly record incoming attenuation data the projection (or view) includes a detector error as shown in Figure 44-34A. When this error is multiplied during the scan, an annular or ring artifact, such as that illustrated in Figures 44-34B and C, is produced.

A number of artifacts are unique to computed tomography. The more common include motion, metal, beam hardening, partial volume effect, and ring artifacts.

 RADIATION PROTECTION

Patient Dose

Patient dose during computed tomography was originally measured according to the concepts of diagnostic radiology. Because the CT scan irradiates tissue via a tightly collimated beam that is moved over the patient, it became necessary to find a new method to measure patient dose during CT examinations. In 1981 the U.S. Food and Drug Administration (FDA) Bureau of Radiological Health (BRH), now known as the Center for Devices and Radiological Health (CDRH), developed the computed tomography **dose** index (CTDI) and the multiple scan average dose (MSAD). The CTDI measures the radiation dose to the patient measured within the primary beam of the CT scanner. The MSAD represents the average dose a patient receives during an examination, which would include numerous individual scans (or in the case of a helical scanner, a moving scan). These are actual tissue doses, not the entrance skin exposure that is often used to describe diagnostic radiography examinations.

Example MSAD readings for a head scan vary from 4–8 rads (4–8 cGy). This is very much greater than the typical entrance skin exposure for a single skull radiograph, which may range from 0.105–0.24 rad (0.105–0.24 cGy). Of course, the comparisons are somewhat absurd as the CT examination provides vastly more information than a single radiograph, or even the entire skull series of exposures, which would comprise a full skull examination.

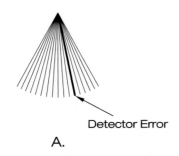

Detector Error

A.

Ring Artifact

B.

C

FIGURE 44-34 A typical tomography ring artifact. (A) The effect of a defective detector cell on a single projection. (B) The sum effect of the multiple projections that comprise the entire image. (C) An example scan with a ring artifact. *(Courtesy of Wil Reddinger, Lima Technical College, Lima, OH)*

Filtration is used in CT in a manner similar to that in diagnostic radiography, although CT uses much greater amounts of filter. A special "bow tie" filter has been developed for CT that matches the beam divergence and shape of the patient's body in transverse section (Figure 44-35).

Dose to Others

Dose to other persons in the scanning room results primarily from scatter from the patient, as during fluoroscopy. Lead aprons and other appropriate protective equipment should be used by anyone in the scanning room during examinations. A routine

Filter
configuration

Detectors

FIGURE 44-35   A CT bow tie filter.

scan might produce a scatter dose of 2 to 5 mrads per section at one meter from the patient. Unless absolutely necessary, no one should be present in the scanning room while the unit is in operation. When someone must be present, he or she should remain as far from the patient as possible to take best advantage of the inverse square law. Standard radiation protection procedures should be followed. The most desirable person to stay with a patient is a relative, then a nonradiology staff member. A radiology department member is the last to be considered. Although use of a remotely controlled power injector is preferred, persons who must manually inject a contrast medium during scanning procedures should stand behind a lead shield, as far from the gantry as possible.

SUMMARY

Computed tomography (CT) produces a digital tomographic image from diagnostic x-rays. The basic principle of CT involves digitizing an image received from a slit scan projection of the patient's body and then back-projecting it through mathematical algorithms.

A modern CT unit includes a gantry, table, x-ray tube, detectors, computer, display console, and image storage units. The gantry is the movable frame of the CT unit. It contains the x-ray tube and detectors and is the most visible part of the unit. The gantry frame maintains the alignment of the tube and detectors and contains the equipment necessary to perform the scanning movements. CT tables are usually made of carbon graphite fiber to decrease beam attenuation and must support the entire weight of the patient without sagging when fully extended. They are rated for maximum weight. Modern pulsed scanner x-ray tubes operate at 120 kVp, 1–5 msec pulses, and up to 1,000 mA. CT detectors include

xenon gas-filled ionization chambers which measures ionization in air by attracting to an electrode the ions created by x-ray photons in the air and solid state detectors.

The CT computer is designed to control data acquisition, process and display, and storage. The CT console operates from a "menu" or index directory of operations. The radiographer uses a keyboard, light pen or other input device to indicate the desired operation. The data acquisition program controls a variety of operations, including tube and detector collimation (pixel size), matrix size, gantry angle, tabletop entrance into the gantry aperture, section increment movements of the tabletop, x-ray tube voltage and amperage, scan speed, and direction of detector signals to the digital image processing section of the computer. The processing and display program controls the digital image production process. The display console permits a wide range of display features, including the scanogram, grid pattern, cursor, density contouring, radiation therapy planning, reverse display, magnification, suppression, annotation, histograms, and three-dimensional imaging. Hounsfield units (HU), or CT numbers, represent the tissue density values for each pixel.

Computed tomography image quality is primarily controlled by resolution and noise considerations. Density and contrast, as with any digitized image, can be manipulated by the computer and are varied with window level and width controls. The resolution of the CT image depends on pixel, voxel, and matrix size. Imaging aberrations (artifacts) displayed as density differences may occur when two objects have more than a 60 percent difference in attenuation coefficients. Noise on a CT image is directly related to the amount of data collected by the detector. Motion on a CT image is a function of exposure time, just as in diagnostic radiography.

The section interval is the distance between scan sections. Its determination is effected by the section shape and the partial volume effect. Section thickness is equivalent to voxel width, or slightly less. Because the data from an entire section thickness is averaged together to form the image, the exact location of a section may cause small structures or portions of large structures to be hidden when they comprise only a small percentage of the total section. This is called the partial volume effect.

A number of artifacts are unique to computer tomography. The more common include motion, metal, beam hardening, partial volume effect, and ring artifacts.

Because of the strictly collimated primary beam, most CT examinations have a patient dose much greater than that of the same part in diagnostic radiography examinations. Filtration is used in CT in a manner similar to that in diagnostic radiography. Dose to other persons in the scanning room results primarily from scatter from the patient, as during fluoroscopy. Lead aprons and other appropriate protective equipment should be used by anyone in the scanning room during examinations.

REVIEW QUESTIONS

1. What are the major components of a modern MSCT unit?

2. What is the gantry?

3. Why are tabletops rated for maximum weight?

4. What is the purpose of the detectors in a CT unit?

5. What operations are controlled by the data acquisition program?

6. What is a scanogram?

7. How are Hounsfield units (HU) (CT numbers) calculated?

8. What controls the density, contrast and resolution of the CT image?

9. Explain the partial volume effect.

10. Explain how a ring artifact is produced.

11. How does patient dose in CT compare to the doses for routine radiography?

REFERENCES AND RECOMMENDED READING

Ambrose, J., & Hounsfield, G. (1973). Computerized transverse axial tomography. *British Journal of Radiology, 46*(148), 1023–1047.

Berland, L. L. (1987). *Practical CT technology and techniques.* New York: Raven Press.

Brooker, M. J. (1986). *Computed tomography for radiographers.* Lancaster U.K.: MTP Press Limited.

Brooks, R. A., & DiChiro, G. (1975). Theory of image reconstruction in computed tomography. *Radiology, 117,* 561.

Brooks, R. A., & DiChiro, G. (1977). Slice geometry in computer assisted tomography. *Journal of Computer Assisted Tomography. 1*(2), 191–199.

Bushberg, J. T., Seibert, J. A., Leidholdt, E. M., & Boone, J. M. (2002). *The essential physics of medical imaging* (2nd ed.) Philadelphia: Lippincott Williams & Wilkins.

Bushong, S. C. (2004). *Radiologic science for technologists: Physics, biology, and protection* (8th ed.). St. Louis, MO: Elsevier/C. V. Mosby.

Chiu, L. C., Lipcamon, J. D., & Yiu-Chiu, V. S. (1995). *Clinical computed tomography for the technologist* (2nd ed.). New York: Raven.

Coulam, C. M., Erickson, J. J., Rollo, F. D., & James, A. E. (1981). *The physical basis of medical imaging.* New York: Appleton-Century-Crofts.

Curry, T. S., Dowdey, J. E., & Murry, R. C. (1990). *Christensen's introduction to the physics of diagnostic radiology* (4th ed.). Philadelphia: Lea and Febiger.

Forster, E. (1985). *Equipment for diagnostic radiography.* Lancaster U.K.: MTP Press.

General Electric. (1976). *Introduction to computed tomography* (Publication 4691). Milwaukee, WI: General Electric Company, Medical Systems Division.

Harper, C. (1979). CT scanners: The industry behind the science. *Radiologic Technology, 51*(2), 199–202.

Hendee, W. R. (1983). *The physical principles of computed tomography.* Boston: Little, Brown and Co.

Hounsfield, G. N. (1973). Computerized transverse axial scanning (tomography): Part I. Description of system. *British Journal of Radiology, 46,* 1016–1022.

Hounsfield, G. N. (1979). Computed tomography: Past, present, and future. In L. Kreel, & R. E. Steiner (Eds.), *Medical Imaging.* Chicago: Year Book.

Kalender, W. A., Arkadiusz, P., & Christoph, S. (1994). A comparison of conventional and spiral CT: An experimental study on the detection of spherical lesions. *Journal of Computer Assisted Tomography, 18*(2), 167–176.

Knapp, R. H., Vannier, M. W., & Marsh, J. L. (1985). Generation of 3-D images from CT scans: Technological perspective. *Radiologic Technology, 56*(6), 391–398.

Kreel, L., & Steiner, R. E. (Eds.) (1979). *Medical imaging.* Chicago: Year Book.

Kuni, C. C. (1988). *Introduction to computers and digital processing in medical imaging.* Chicago: Year Book.

Lee, J. K., Sagel, S. S., & Stanley, R. J. (1990). *Computed body tomography* (2nd ed.). New York: Raven Press.

McCullough, E. C., & Payne, J. T. (1977). X-ray transmission computed tomography. *Medical Physics, 4,* 85.

Morgan, C. L. (1983). *Basic principles of computed tomography.* Baltimore: University Park Press.

Moss, A. A., Gamsu, G., & Genant, H. K. (1984). *Computed tomography of the body.* Philadelphia: W. B. Saunders.

Nagel, H. (2005). *Multislice CT technology.* www.multislice-ct.com/www/page.php?guide=en_introduction_36 retrieved 7-29-05.

Parker, J. A. (1990). *Image reconstruction in radiology.* Boca Raton, FL: CRC Press.

Parkinson, L. (1991). Assessment of dose in computerized tomography. *Radiography Today, 57*(650), 23–28.

Reiser, M., Taskahashi, M., Modic, M., & Becker, C. (2004). *Multislice CT* (2nd ed.). New York: Springer.

Ritman, E. L., Kinsey, J. H., Robb, R. A., Harris, L. D., & Gilbert, B. K. (1980). Physical and technical considerations in the design of the DSR: A high temporal resolution volume scanner. *American Journal of Roentgenology, 134,* 369–374.

Romans, L. E. (1995). *Introduction to computed tomography.* Baltimore: Williams & Wilkins.

Seeram, E. (1978). Computed tomography: An overview. *Radiologic Technology, 49*(4), 491–496.

Seeram, E. (1983). A course on CT for radiologic technologists: A conceptual framework. *The Canadian Journal of Medical Radiation Technology, 14*(1), 11.

Seeram, E. (1989). *Computers in diagnostic radiology.* Springfield, IL: Charles C Thomas.

Seeram, E. (1994). *Computed tomography: Physical principles, clinical applications, and quality control.* Philadelphia: W. B. Saunders.

Short, A. J. (1981). Reconstructions in computerized transverse axial radiography. *Radiography, 47*(557), 119.

Shrimpton, P. (1994). Patient dose in CT and recommendations for reduction. *Radiography Today, 60*(683), 9–11.

Ter-Pogossian, M. M. (1983). Physical principles and instrumentation. In J. K. T. Lee, S. S. Sagel, & R. J. Stanley (Eds.). *Computed body tomography.* New York: Raven.

Whitmore, R. C., Bushong, S., Archer, B., & Glaze, S. A. (1979). Radiation dose in neurological computed tomography scanning. *Radiologic Technology, 51*(1), 21–26.

Wolbarst, A. B. (1993). *Physics of radiology.* Norwalk, CT: Appleton & Lange.

Yaffe, M., Fenster, A., & Johns, H. E. (1977). Xenon ionization detectors for fan beam computed tomography scanners. *Journal of Computer Assisted Tomography, 1*(2), 419–428.

Yoshizumi, T. T., Suneja, S. K., & Teal, J. S. (1989). Practical CT dosimetry. *Radiologic Technology, 60*(6), 505.

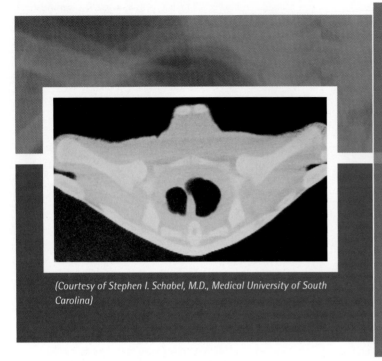

(Courtesy of Stephen I. Schabel, M.D., Medical University of South Carolina)

The Case of the Mysterious Mammal

This computed tomography is of an animal found on the roadside near Jolly Beach, South Carolina. Look carefully at the bone structure to determine what it is.

Answers to the case studies can be found in Appendix E.

CHAPTER 45

Magnetic Resonance Imaging

We are dealing not merely with a new tool but with a new subject, a subject I have called simply nuclear magnetism . . . the history of ordinary magnetism . . . has been rich in difficult and provocative problems, and full of surprises. Nuclear Magnetism . . . is like that too.

Edward M. Purcell from his Nobel Lecture, December 11, 1952 Reprinted from Edelman (1990). Clinical Magnetic Resonance Imaging with permission from Elsevier.

KEY TERMS

cryogen
echo time (TE)
flip angle
free induction decay (FID)
gyromagnetic ratio
inversion time (TI)
Larmor frequency
magnetic resonance
nuclear magnetic moment

precession
proton (spin) density
proton spin density image
quenching
ramping
rate of precession
repetition time (TR)
shim coils
specific absorption rate (SAR)

spin-lattice relaxation time (T_1)
spin–spin relaxation time (T_2)
surface coil
thermal noise

OBJECTIVES

Upon completion of this chapter, the student should be able to:

- Describe the source of the magnetic fields within the body that are used during MRI.
- Describe the properties of proton precession as used in MRI.
- Define T_1, T_2, p, TR, TE, and TI.
- Explain the functions of x, y, and z gradient coils in selecting an image section by the use of the Larmor equation and a gradient magnetic field.
- Describe the use of RF pulses in the various MRI pulse sequences.

- Analyze the various events during a spin-echo pulse sequence.
- Describe the components of an MRI unit, including the stationary magnet, gradient and RF coils, table, and computer consoles.
- Explain how MRI image contrast is controlled.
- Describe the use of paramagnetic contrast agents.
- Discuss methods of reducing MRI image noise.
- Discuss safety measures for protection of all persons who approach the MRI unit magnetic field.

FIGURE 45-1 A sagittal MR image of the head.
(Courtesy of GE Healthcare)

The typical magnetic resonance imaging (MRI) unit looks similar to a CT unit. It has a computer, console, gantry, and table. However, because MRI uses magnetism and radio frequencies (RF) to create diagnostic sectional images of the body (Figure 45-1), the internal construction is quite different. The phenomena that permit MRI are based on magnetism and radio frequencies applied according to the principles of nuclear physics and quantum mechanics. For this reason the imaging process was originally called nuclear magnetic resonance (NMR). Also for this reason, it is critical to understand new physical concepts in order to comprehend how MR images are created and viewed.

THE PHYSICS OF MAGNETIC RESONANCE

In 1924 Wolfgang Pauli suggested that some nuclei spin. It was not until 1946 that nuclear magnetic resonance was first reported by Swiss physicist Felix Bloch (1905–1983) at Stanford and American physicist Edward Purcell (1912–1997) at Harvard. These men shared the 1952 Nobel Prize in physics

for their work. In the late 1960s and early 1970s the basis for diagnostic MRI was developed by several researchers. In 1967 Jasper Jackson produced the first MR signals from a live animal, in 1971 Raymond Damadian reported NMR differences between normal tissue and tumors, in 1972 Paul Lauterbur produced the first magnetic resonance image, in 1975 Damadian produced the first live animal MR images, and by 1977 the first diagnostic human images had been obtained.

Nuclear Magnetism

The nucleus of an atom is a tiny but highly charged piece of matter. The spinning nucleus has angular momentum, or **nuclear magnetic moment.** This rotating charge acts as a current loop and produces a magnetic field, thus causing the nucleus to behave as a microscopic spinning bar magnet; it rotates and flips within the atom like a tiny gyroscope on perfect bearings. When nuclei having magnetic moments are placed in a magnetic field, they tend to align with the field, as does any magnet.

In addition to having a charge, a nucleus also has mass. The spinning mass has a moment of inertia as well as a magnetic moment. The moment of inertia resists changes to angular momentum, thus inhibiting the nucleus from aligning in a magnetic field. This inhibiting factor is measured as the ratio of the magnetic moment to the moment of inertia and is called the **gyromagnetic** (or magnetogyric) **ratio.** It is represented by the Greek letter gamma (γ) and is measured in units of **megahertz per tesla (MHz/T).** Recall from Chapter 4 that the tesla and the gauss are the units of magnetic flux density. One tesla equals 10,000 gauss. Each isotope has a specific gyromagnetic ratio, which allows it to be differentiated during MR imaging (Table 45–1).

Variations in gyromagnetic ratios and in the length of relaxation time after the application of an RF pulse permit the differentiation of various metabolites. This is the general basis of spectroscopy, which, when coupled with static MR images, may provide additional diagnostic information.

Precession of Nuclei. Although the dynamics of rapidly rotating objects are quite complex, several of their properties are easily understood. The most

TABLE 45-1.	Magnetic Resonance Properties of Diagnostically Important Nuclei	
Nucleus	**Gyromagnetic Ratio (MHz/T)**	
^{1}H	42.6	
^{14}H	3.1	
^{13}C	10.7	
^{19}F	40.0	
^{23}Na	11.3	
^{31}P	17.2	
^{39}K	2.0	

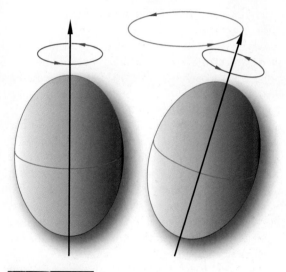

FIGURE 45-2   Precession.

important property is that of a rapidly spinning nucleus when it is subjected to a magnetic field; not only will the nucleus's magnetic field align with the external magnetic field, but it will also begin to wobble. This wobbling, like that of a spinning top when it begins to lose momentum, is actually a rotation of the axis of rotation, or **precession** (Figure 45-2). The rotational precession of the nucleus causes the magnetic field itself to precess. Therefore, the direction of precession indicated in Figure 45-2 also represents the precession of the rotational magnetic field. MR imaging is accomplished through various measurements of this movement of the nuclear magnetic field.

The nuclear magnetic field is continually changing direction as it rotates around the axis of the external magnetic field's lines of flux. The **rate of precession** is indicated by the Greek letter omega (ω) and is calculated as:

$$\omega = \gamma B_{O}$$

where: ω = rate of precession
γ = gyromagnetic ratio
B_{O} = static magnetic field strength

The rate of precession (ω) is also known as the angular velocity of the nuclear magnetic field.

Larmor Frequencies. The gyromagnetic ratio (γ) is fixed for each element. Therefore, the precessional frequency is fixed for a given magnetic field strength. This means that in a static homogeneous magnetic field, all protons in a nucleus of a given

type element will rotate with exactly the same frequency. This frequency is called the **Larmor frequency** and is critical to MR imaging. Only those elements with nuclear angular momentum have nuclear magnetic moments and are capable of producing nuclear magnetic resonance signals. The most important of those that do is the proton, which is also the major isotope of hydrogen (^{1}H), because it is abundant in the human body and has a high gyromagnetic ratio (γ). **The precessional frequency is the Larmor frequency. It is the RF that induces magnetic resonance as well as the RF of the emitted nuclear magnetic resonance signal.**

Production of the Nuclear Magnetic Resonance Signal

The laws of quantum mechanics permit protons to align either with the external magnetic field or against it. This creates two populations of proton orientations relative to the main magnetic field: parallel and antiparallel. When an electromagnetic RF field that is alternating, or resonating, at the Larmor frequency is applied in addition to the static field, protons will alternate from parallel to antiparallel. This phenomenon is called **magnetic resonance.** Protons that are antiparallel have excessive energy, which they emit as electromagnetic radiation in the **radio frequency (RF)** range.

Magnetic resonance imaging data is accumulated by measuring detection differences of only one millionth of a percent (0.000001 percent). When a large number of protons are subjected to a magnetic field, the nuclear magnetic moments immediately begin lining up with the field; some line up in the same direction as the magnetic field while others line up in the opposite direction. For every 200,000,000 hydrogen atoms, about two more will align themselves *with* the predominate external magnetic field. In other words, 100,000,001 atoms will align with the field while 99,999,999 will align against it. This means that the body tissue has become almost imperceptibly magnetized.

The Larmor equation predicts the exact RF that will be emitted by a specific element. When the RF is detected with an antenna and a radio receiver that is tuned to the proper frequency, magnetic resonance imaging is possible.

Production of the nuclear magnetic resonance signal requires applying a Larmor frequency RF and then listening to the RF emissions from the protons. Digital imaging reconstruction techniques are then used to create sectional and three-dimensional images.

MRI Parameters. The primary parameters controlling the MRI process include **proton spin density (N(H) or ρ), spin-lattice or longitudinal relaxation time (T_1), spin-spin or transverse relaxation time (T_2), repetition time (TR), echo time (TE), inversion time (TI), and flip angle.** The parameters that are used vary depending on the pulse sequence used.

Proton (spin) density (ρ or N(H)) is the quantity of resonating spins in a tissue. It is expressed as a percentage of the proton density of water and determines the MR signal strength (sometimes called image brightness) (Table 45-2). Various authors refer to it as proton density (N(H) or PD), spin density (SD), or by the Greek letter rho (ρ). Proton density weighted images are achieved by using a long repetition time (TR) between pulses. This permits the RF signal from a larger number of protons to be detected, thus creating the image from a greater number, or density, of spinning protons. Proton density

TABLE 45-2. Effect of Parameter Variation on MR Image Density (Brightness)

Image Weighting	TR	TE	ρ Increased	Longer T_1	Longer T_2
Proton Spin Density (ρ)	long	short	+	−*	+*
T_1	short	short	+	−	+*
T_2	long	long	+	−*	+

* = some tissues only

images have relatively low contrast due to the slight differences between the percentages of hydrogen present in various tissues (see Table 45-2).

Spin-lattice relaxation time (T_1) is the time required for precessing spins to align with the constant external magnetic field to 63 percent of the maximum possible strength. It is also known as longitudinal relaxation time and is sometimes called thermal relaxation time.

T_1 is the time required for the sum of the magnetic moments, or M_0, to regain its original orientation following a 90° RF pulse. It varies depending on thermal interactions between resonating protons and other nuclear magnetic fields in the atomic lattice. The value of T_1 increases with the strength of the magnetic field. The term longitudinal was originally applied in reference to the time required for precessing to cease and the proton spin to reorient with the original "longitudinal" magnetic field.

The T_1 of hydrogen is approximately three seconds in water but this time varies considerably for hydrogen in different types of tissues. This phenomenon provides the contrast necessary for the MR image. T_1 relaxation characteristics for various body tissues are shown in Table 45-3. Relaxation times vary with the amount of water available. In fact, dehydrated tissues will demonstrate significantly different relaxation times.

When a magnetic field is applied, almost all the proton spins will have aligned after several T_1 times have passed. Magnetic resonance imaging uses only those spins that have not been cancelled out by a corresponding spin in the opposite direction. Although these protons occur in only one out of

TABLE 45-3.   Example T_1 and T_2 Relaxation Times in a 0.15 Tesla Field

Relaxation times vary considerably depending on numerous factors, including the specific conditions surrounding the tissue and external magnetic field strength.

Tissue	T_1	T_2	T_1/T_2	Proton Density (Percent ρ Water)
Fat	170 ms	80 ms	2.1	9.6
Muscle	580 ms	40 ms	14.5	9.3
Brain, white matter	350 ms	80 ms	4.4	10.6
Brain, gray matter	500 ms	100 ms	5.0	10.6
Blood	720 ms	175 ms	4.1	
Cerebrospinal fluid	1,500 ms	260 ms	5.8	10.8
Water	2,500 ms	2,500 ms	0.0	11.0

T_1/T_2 is an indication of contrast differences between T_1 and T_2 weighted images. (Adapted with permission from *Magnetic Resonance Imaging: A Reference Guide and Atlas,* by Allen D. Elster, Philadelphia: J. B. Lippincott Company, 1986.)

100,000,000 atoms, the vast quantity of atoms in even a small voxel of tissue produce a large number of eligible protons. Only these protons are capable of producing an RF when subjected to a magnetic field at the appropriate Larmor frequency.

The mechanism by which protons emit RF is especially complex because it occurs in three dimensions. However, careful consideration of a few simple illustrations will reveal that once the three-dimensional aspect is understood, the basic principle is not so difficult. The sum of the magnetic moments, or M_O, is always in the same direction as B_O (the static magnetic field strength) when the body is within the static external magnetic field. When M_O precesses, it produces a rotating magnetic field which is perpendicular to the original direction of M_O (Figures 45-3A, B). To cause protons to emit an RF, another magnetic field (B_1) must be applied for a brief moment. In Figure 45–3B the magnetic field in the x^1–y^1 plane is precessing synchronously with M_O (at the same angular speed). This precessing magnetic field is stationary in its relationship with M_O. This relationship is more easily understood by comparing it to riding on a carousel. Although the carousel is spinning (like M_O), when one rides on one of the horses the other horses appear to be stationary (x^1–y^1) while objects outside the carousel appear to be spinning around (x–y). If an alternating magnetic field (B_1) is applied in the direction of

x, it will simply cause M_O to rotate further away from z toward y (Figure 45-3C). In order to apply B_1 in the direction of the moving x axis, it is simply pulsed so that it is applied only during the moment that x is aligned with x^1 during every rotation (Figure 45-3C). The concept of T_1 as M_O returns to equilibrium after an RF pulse is shown graphically in Figure 45-9. Because x is rotating at the Larmor frequency with M_O, **the applied magnetic field must be pulsed at the Larmor frequency.**

The Larmor frequency is very high, usually in the MHz range, for the 0.2–4.0 Tesla fields used in MR imaging. For example, the Larmor frequency for hydrogen in a 1.5 T field is 64 MHz, which is within RF bands of the electromagnetic spectrum (see Figure 2-10). The MHz frequency magnetic field for MRI is produced by a properly tuned radio transmitter coil, very similar to the coil used to receive UHF frequency television signals.

Spin-spin relaxation time (T_2) is the time required, after precessing spins have aligned at an angle to the external magnetic field due to an RF pulse, for them to lose 63 percent of their coherence (alignment with each other) due to interactions between the spins. It varies depending on the tissue. It is also known as transverse relaxation time. T_2 is always shorter than T_1. The symbol T_2^* is used to indicate T_2 due to inhomogeneities in the magnetic field and due to spin-spin relaxation. T_2^* is always shorter than

FIGURE 45-3 Proton emission of radio frequencies (RF). (A) B_0 is the direction of the static external magnetic field. M_0 is the direction of the sum of the predominant proton magnetic moments. (B) When M_0 is tipped slightly off the z axis, it immediately begins precessing around the z axis at its Larmor frequency. This causes a perpendicular magnetic field to rotate in the x–y plane, also at the Larmor frequency. (C) If an alternating magnetic field (B_1) is applied in the direction of x, it causes M_0 to rotate further away from z toward y. B_1 is pulsed so it is applied only during the moment x is aligned with x^1 during every rotation. Because x is precessing at the Larmor frequency, the applied magnetic field must also be pulsed at the Larmor frequency.

T2. Of all the parameters described, PD, T_1, and T_2 are intrinsic. The others are extrinsic or controllable by the operator.

Repetition time (TR) is the time interval between pulse sequences. It is usually between 300 and 3,000 ms but is highly variable, always being the longest of the parameters used to describe the sequence.

Echo time (TE) is the time between a 90° pulse and the echo during a spin-echo pulse sequence. It is usually between 10 and 100 ms but is always the shortest time used for a sequence. When more than one echo is recorded, the TE is designated as TE_1, TE_2, etc.

Inversion time (TI) is the time between a 180° pulse and a 90° inversion pulse in an inversion recovery pulse sequence. It is usually between 200 and 2,000 ms.

Flip angle is in gradient echo imaging, increasing flip angle will increase T_1 weighting (Figure 45-4).

Nuclear Magnetic Resonance Pulses. The distance that M_0 precesses from the z axis is determined by the strength of B_1 and by the duration of the pulse. It is measured by the angle of the precession. For example, a 45° pulse tips the rotational axis of M_0 45° away from the z axis. The most common MRI pulses are 90° and 180°. A 180° pulse aligns M_0 with the z axis or, in other words, aligns it perfectly in

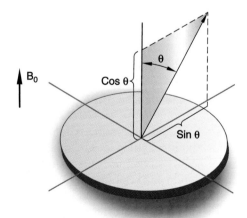

FIGURE 45-4 Gradient echo imaging preserves longitudinal magnetization by utilizing a flip angle of less than 90°.

the opposite direction. A 360° pulse would return the rotational axis to its original position and therefore have no effect. During all pulsing only the protons spinning at the Larmor frequency that matches the pulse frequency will respond. The actual response of proton spin to an RF pulse is to change M_O in a precessing corkscrew motion (Figure 45-5).

A 90° pulse is used to tip the rotational axis of the protons so that they are spinning around the z axis in the x–y plane. Because the protons are functioning as spinning magnets, an electromagnetic force is produced when a coil of wire is positioned within the lines of flux. **The voltage that is detected from this arrangement is the magnetic resonance imaging signal.** The coil is aligned to detect only precession in the x^1–y^1 plane. The frequency of the voltage matches the Larmor frequency of the precessing protons, thus making it possible to detect which element emitted the signal.

Nuclear Magnetic Resonance Decay. The signal that is emitted by the precessing protons decays exponentially. This occurs because the protons' magnetic fields are not exactly the same, even though they are all within the Larmor frequency range. Just as individual atoms of the same element have slight differences, precessional rates also differ slightly. For example, if a hydrogen proton is spinning at its Larmor frequency of 64,000,000 rota-

tions per second and a second proton is spinning at 64,000,001 rotations per second, in 0.5 second the two protons will be exactly opposite one another. When this occurs, their magnetic fields cancel one another. The millions of protons that comprise M_O quickly become out of phase with each other by this process, which is called dephasing. **When a tissue sample has dephased, M_O ceases to exist and the magnetic resonance signal disappears.** **Free induction decay (FID)** is the simplest example of this process. It produces the most basic type of MRI signal, as shown in Figure 45-6. Because an FID signal will vary depending on how many protons are spinning in the tissue volume, it is known as a **proton spin density (ρ) image.** Because proton density does not vary much in soft tissue, this imaging technique produces an extremely low contrast image.

PRODUCTION OF THE MAGNETIC RESONANCE IMAGE

The localization of information for the MR image occurs very differently from computed tomography or any other digital imaging modality, although the final computerized digital image reconstruction algorithms are very similar. Three electromagnetic coils are required to produce magnetic field gradients corresponding to the x, y, or z axis to be imaged. The RF that are detected from these gradient coils, as they are called, can then be analyzed to determine not only the type of atom they came from but also the atom's precise location within the imaging matrix.

Gradient Coils

Data localization in MRI is accomplished through the use of a gradient magnetic field that is superimposed on the static external magnetic field. The gradient coil field system was developed by the American physicist Paul Lauterbur in 1972 at the State University of New York (SUNY) at Stony Brook. Gradient coils can be resistive or superconducting and are located within the bore of the stationary

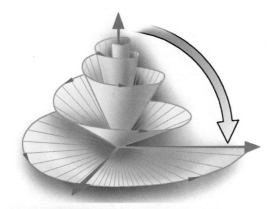

FIGURE 45-5   The precessing corkscrew motion of proton spin to an RF pulse. *(Edelman, R. R., Hesselink, J. R. [1990]. Clinical Magnetic Resonance Imaging with permission from Elsevier)*

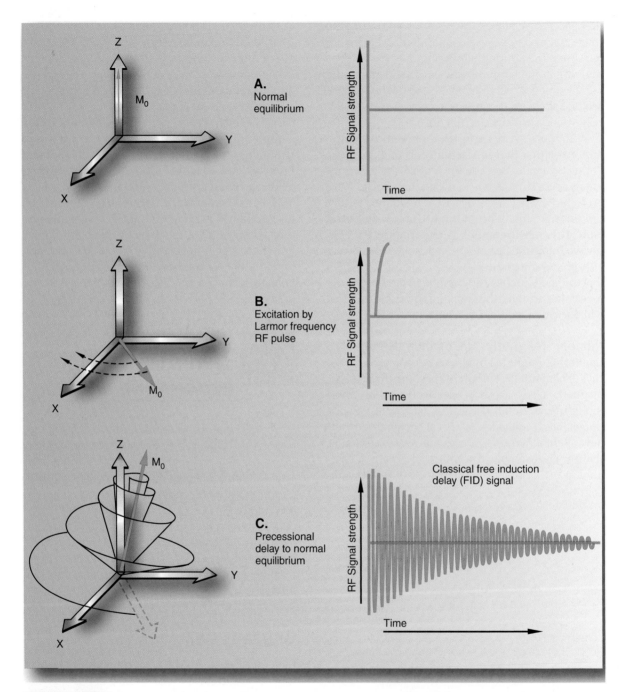

FIGURE 45-6 Classical free induction decay (FID). (A) Normal spin equilibrium. (B) When a Larmor frequency RF pulse is applied, M_0 precesses 90° into the x–y plane, thus producing a maximum strength MR signal. (C) As M_0 emits RF, it loses energy and precesses in a corkscrew back to normal equilibrium while emitting a gradually decaying RF signal.

magnet. They superimpose their magnetic fields on the uniform magnetic field produced by the stationary magnet. A gradient field coil produces a magnetic field somewhat like a magnetic penetrometer in that it grows in strength from one end to the other, varying the field strength in proportion to distance.

Since the strength of the magnetic field affects the precessional frequency of the proton spins, the result is different precessional frequencies according to location along the gradient field. This technique permits the MRI computer to determine the location of an RF signal with digital imaging calculations. It also permits the calculation of T_1 and T_2 as a function of distance along the axis of the magnetic field. Changing the x axis permits detection from an opposite direction and the use of many of the digital reconstruction algorithms employed in computed tomography (see Chapter 44). Other variations between the three gradient coils also permit various oblique sections to be constructed. The basic algorithm in MRI is a two-dimensional Fourier transform (2DFT) method. It is often expanded to a 3DFT to permit faster data acquisition.

Magnetic resonance imaging requires the use of three gradient coils, one each for the x, y, and z axes (see Figure 45-13B). Each coil must be linear and uniform to within a few percentage points. **The gradient coils determine the section thickness as well as the resolution and plane of the image.**

The z axis coil is perpendicular to the imaging plane. It is called the slice selection gradient because it determines the exact location of the section and its thickness. A thicker section is produced by increasing the RF bandwidth or by increasing the magnitude (or slope) of the gradient. The z axis coil can be set to produce transverse, coronal, or sagittal sections by varying the orientation of the z axis so it is replaced by the x or y axis.

The y axis coil is called the phase encoding gradient because it selectively precesses the protons to define the x–y coordinates within the section. This phase gradient must be repeated for each x coordinate in the matrix array. For example, a 256×256 matrix requires the phase gradient to be repeated 256 times to collect data for the entire matrix. This is the basic process of a two-dimensional Fourier transform (2DFT) data projection method.

The x axis coil is called the frequency encoding gradient or the readout gradient because it is applied for each value of the y axis coil. Three-dimensional MR imaging uses the z axis coil to cause a large volume of tissue to begin precessing. X and y encoding gradients are then compared and the collected data is reconstructed in three dimensions.

Although these phasing methods are not always applied to the x and y axes in the order described, spatial location is achieved by phase encoding for one axis while frequency encoding for the other. Variations in the use of all three gradient coils permit the acquisition of various oblique sections through the subject.

Magnetic Resonance Imaging Operations Sequence

The production of MR imaging data varies depending on the pulsing sequence used and on the manufacturer. As an example, a spin-echo pulse sequence of operations might include the following steps to produce an MR image:

1. A gradient is applied along the z axis. A 90° pulse is applied at a desired Larmor frequency. The z gradient selects an x–y plane (section selection). The z gradient is turned off. This produces a precessing M_O in the selected plane. The M_O in the other planes are still aligned along the z axis (Figure 45-7A).

2. A gradient is applied along the y axis for a short time. This produces precessing M_O at various rates depending on their location along the y axis gradient. The phasing of the precessing spins now indicates their location in the y–z plane (phase encoding) (Figure 45-7B).

3. A gradient is applied along the z axis again and a 180° pulse is applied with a frequency that will affect only the x–y plane that is being imaged. The z gradient is then turned off.

4. A gradient is applied along the x axis. This causes the precessing M_O to return a spin-echo at differing frequencies that will indicate their positions along the x axis (readout frequency encoding) (Figure 45-7C). The RF receiver is then turned on and the signals received are sent to the MRI computer for digital image reconstruction.

FIGURE 45-7 Spatial location by gradient fields. (A) Application of the z gradient field produces precession within the selected section (the z axis). (B) Application of the y gradient field produces phase encoding along the y axis. Note that there is still no differentiation of spatial location along the x axis. (C) Application of the x gradient field produces frequency encoding along the x axis. Note that each voxel now has a different precession rate, thus permitting spatial location in the x, y, and z axes.

Radio Frequency Pulse Sequences

The primary variable in the data collection procedure during MRI is the sequence of RF pulses that are used to cause the protons to precess. There is a dramatic difference in the information that becomes visible with the various sequences. The operator must select the appropriate pulsing sequence as well as the proper intervals for the specific examination.

Similar to many computed tomography units, the MRI control console includes programmed selections of sequences for various examinations. However, the knowledgeable MRI technologist can increase the quantity and quality of diagnostic in-

formation by understanding which sequences and intervals are best for specific tissues. The sequences are a series of various magnetic fields from the x, y, and z gradients, RF pulses, flip angles applied at various angles, repetition times (TR), inversion times (TI), and echo times (TE).

Partial Saturation. Partial saturation is also referred to as saturation recovery (SR) or repeated free induction decay (repeated FID). The pulse sequence is a series of 90° RF pulses with the signal measured after each (Figure 45-8A). Note that the y gradient is changed for each pulse sequence to record data from a different anatomical section. The TR is set according to the tissue of interest.

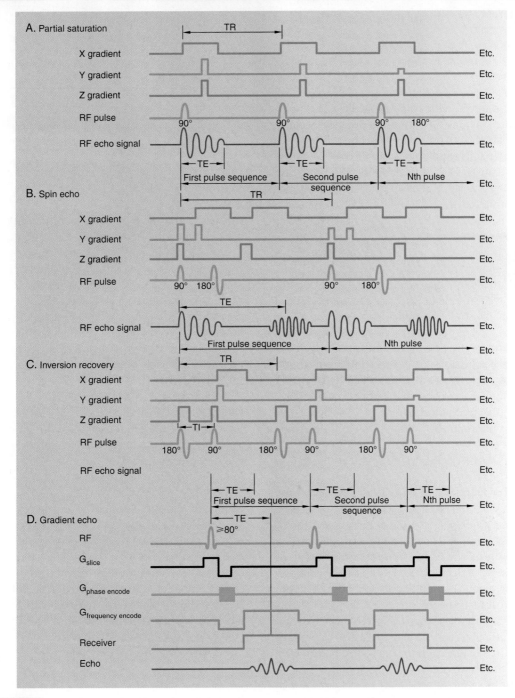

FIGURE 45-8 Magnetic resonance pulse sequences. (A) Partial saturation is a simple series of 90° RF pulses sequenced with short y and z gradient pulses and a long x gradient pulse. The RF signal is classical free induction decay. (B) Spin-echo uses a partial saturation sequence followed by a 180° (refocusing) RF pulse sequenced with an x and z gradient pulse but without a second y gradient pulse. The refocusing pulse flips the proton precession and produces the spin-echo RF signal. The RF signals that are received are a free induction decay followed by the spin-echo that begins faintly, increases to maximum strength , then fades away. TE is measured between the first and the echo RF signals. (C) Inversion recovery uses a 180° RF pulse sequenced with a z gradient pulse prior to a partial saturation sequence. The RF signal is a classical free induction decay that occurs with the 90° pulse. TI is measured between the two RF pulses. Gradient echo imaging uses gradients rather than RF to produce flip angles of less than 90° and low TRs. (D) Gradient echo imaging uses a flip angle other than 90° with a gradient refocusing pulse (rather than a 180° refocusing RF pulse), which takes less time to generate an echo that is sampled at time TE.

If a 90° pulse is repeated before M_O is fully re-established along the z axis, the angle of M_O precession will depend on the first time interval (T_1). Images produced with data collected at this point are known as partial saturation images because they vary with both proton density and the length of T_1. Because different tissues have different T_1 values, contrast can be varied by changing the repetition time (TR). However, when very short recovery times are encountered, the M_O is weak and this produces a very weak RF signal. When long recovery times are encountered, the M_O has time to recover and the T_1 contrast is lost. For this reason partial saturation is not used for most MR imaging. However, short TR T_1 partial saturation sequencing is useful in demonstrating cysts and subdural fluids and has been used for blood flow studies as well.

Spin-Echo. Spin-echo is the most popular pulse sequence because it reduces scan time significantly (Figure 45-8B). It was first described by Carr and Purcell and is therefore also known as the Carr-Purcell (CP) sequence. The basic spin-echo sequence consists of a 90° pulse which initiates a partial saturation sequence. However, it is followed by a 180° pulse (the refocusing pulse) at 50 percent of the TE. The refocusing pulse flips the proton precession and produces a spin-echo RF signal that grows, then fades in intensity. The y gradient is changed for each pulse sequence to record data from a different anatomical section. The TR and TE are set according to the tissue of interest.

The decay or dephasing process is used to advantage in spin-echo imaging by allowing dephasing to continue until it is nearly undetectable. This permits the faster spinning protons to precess further and further out of synch. When the 180° refocusing pulse is used to flip M_O in the opposite direction, the protons that have precessed faster and are the furthest out of synch now begin precessing back into synchrony with those that were slower. At an equal time after the 180° pulse, all the precessions will again be equal. This has the effect of an echo and produces the spin-echo signal. The process operates exactly as if the Indianapolis 500 auto race were begun and allowed to run for one hour. If each car were stopped at the end of the hour, turned around and run for a second hour at exactly the same speed,

TABLE 45-4.	Example T_1 and T_2 Relaxation Times	
Tissue	T_1	T_2
Fat	170 ms	80 ms
Example tumor	580 ms	80 ms
Muscle	580 ms	40 ms

the race would end with all the cars crossing the finish line together. Although this would be a very boring race, in MRI it provides enough time to measure the differences between the precessional rates.

The T_2 term is used during spin-echo MRI to describe where the data collection occurs after the second time interval when 63 percent of the spins have lost their alignment with each other as they decay back toward equilibrium. The T_2 relaxation characteristics for various body tissues are shown in Table 45-4.

Spin-echo pulses are weighted for T_1 by using short TR and TE (see Figure 45-16B). Although a T_1 image is valuable when used in conjunction with a T_2 image, it is not considered useful information by itself. Spin-echo pulses are weighted for T_2 by using long TR and TE (see Figure 45-16C).

Gradient Echo. Gradient echo sequences use a single RF pulse of less than 90°. The signal of the echo is produced by using gradient pulses, rather than RF pulses. Because the RF pulse only slightly decreases the longitudinal magnetization, the recovery time is much quicker. This allows for shorter TR and, therefore, more rapid imaging. Image contrast in gradient echo imaging is controlled largely by flip angle. Gradient echo imaging is used in a wide variety of neuro, body, and orthopedic applications.

Inversion Recovery. Inversion recovery is a three pulse sequence. It consists of a 180° pulse followed by a spin-echo sequence (Figure 45-8C). Because of the time required to accumulate data, it is seldom used in current clinical imaging. Note that the y gradient is changed for each pulse sequence to record data from a different anatomical section. The TR and TI are set according to the tissue of interest.

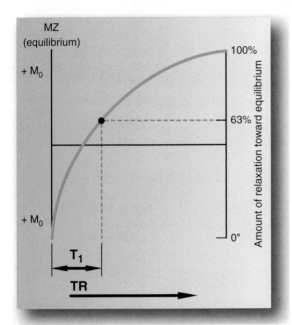

FIGURE 45-9 Relaxation after reversal of M_0 during an inversion recovery pulse. Although the precession is decaying back toward equilibrium, it flips from the $-z$ axis to $+z$ at the solid horizontal line. By definition, T_1 occurs when 63 percent of the return to the maximum field strength (equilibrium) has been attained.

The first pulse is an inverting pulse to invert M_0 into the $-z$ axis. TI is an interpulse time delay that permits M_0 to begin to recover, becoming less and less negative, then rising along the $+z$ axis. No signal is generated during this process because M_0 is not in the x–y plane. However, at a set interval a 90° pulse rotates M_0 into the x–y plane, producing precession and an RF signal. The strength of this signal at the time of the 90° pulse will depend on the TI recovery time that was allowed. Because this is different for each tissue, useful MRI data can be collected. Inversion recovery provides good anatomical contrast because T_1 values for normal tissues vary considerably. Finally, a 180° pulse is used to create the signal.

Because of the reversal of M_0, the RF signal decreases with a short TI, then flips and increases as TI increases (Figure 45-9). The MR unit is usually programmed to display the reversed (negative) range of M_0 so that it is shown to be returning to its original

equilibrium. This permits the image to be displayed lighter as the negative signal decreases and then to continue lighter as the positive signal increases. Short TI inversion recovery techniques are sometimes called STIR imaging.

Other Pulse Sequences. Numerous other pulse sequences have been developed to increase the amount of data collected or to decrease the scanning time. These include various gradient refocused echo (GRE) techniques, including steady-state free precession (SSFP), fast low-angle shot (FLASH), fast-imaging steady-state precession (FISP), and gradient-recalled acquisition steady state (GRASS). Short TI inversion recovery (STIR) and fluid attenuated inversion recovery (FLAIR) are variations of the IR pulse sequence. Echo planar imaging (EPI) is a very efficient sequence for many applications and is the sequence used for diffusion and perfusion imaging.

By using the special contrast properties of blood flow during pulse sequences, magnetic resonance angiography (MRA) is rapidly becoming a routine study. Cardiac gating is often used to trigger each pulse sequence from the electrical signals of the heart, thus decreasing phase mismapping produced from heart motion. Methods used in dynamic MR for cardiac and blood flow studies include gradient motion rephasing (GMR), gradient motion nulling (GMN), motion artifact suppression technique (MAST), presaturation (dark blood sequence), and spatial modulation of magnetization (SPAMM).

Special Acquisition (Fast Spin Echo Techniques)

Because many T_1 relaxation times are relatively long, most MRI units begin to acquire data from additional sections while the first section is still proceeding through the pulse sequence. The TR interval between pulses is used to begin the pulse sequencing of other sections.

K-Space. Fast spin echo (FSE) can be achieved by generating two or more echoes within a single repetition of a sequence. This is accomplished by applying multiple 180° pulses (echo train length) following the first echo. This is done within a single-phase encoding gradient at the beginning of the sequence. The incoming data is then filed in multiple lines of **k-space.** The process continues until all lines are full. Although there are some signal-to-noise ratio (S/N) problems the computer must resolve, FSE sequences can reduce scan time by a factor of the ETL without changing the repetition time (TR), resolution matrix, or the number of acquisitions (NEX), thus significantly reducing overall scan time.

Spiral k-space acquisition is a vastly more complex method that involves simultaneous sampling of data points during out-of-phase oscillation of echo sequences. The collection of the data points represents a spiral as it fills the k-space. The process provides significantly higher contrast for T_2 images.

MAGNETIC RESONANCE IMAGING EQUIPMENT

The typical MRI unit looks similar to a CT unit (Figure 45-10A, B). However, its internal construction is unique, consisting of a stationary magnet within which are fitted gradient and radio frequency (RF) coils (Figure 45-11). The stationary magnet must be extremely strong; field strengths for clinical imaging range from 0.10–7.0 T. A table for the patient and a large computer for image processing, display, and storage complete the MRI system.

Stationary Magnet

Magnetic resonance imaging has been achieved with resistive, permanent, and superconducting magnets. Each has significant differences in potential field strength, stability, uniformity, and cost.

Resistive. Resistive magnets produce a strong field in the range of 0.02–0.4 T from the flow of current in large numbers of turns of wire or conducting ribbons. These magnets are called resistive because of the large amount of resistance produced by this type of wiring configuration. The heat produced by the resistance is so great that resistive magnets are severely limited by their cooling requirements.

A

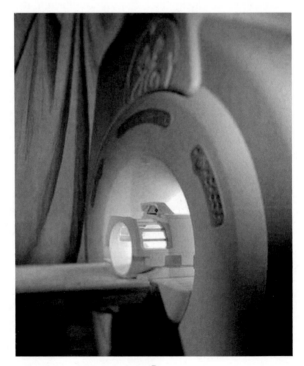

B

FIGURE 45-10 (A) A typical MRI unit. (B) Birdcage headcoil. *(Courtesy of GE Healthcare)*

Resistive magnets provide good uniformity of magnetic field and are relatively inexpensive. However, their field strength is limited and somewhat unstable, they often exhibit longitudinal fringe field problems, and they consume a large amount of electrical power.

Permanent. Permanent magnets of up to 0.3 T have been produced by inducing a strong magnetic field in ferromagnetic materials during manufacturing. These magnets are extremely heavy and may weigh up to 200,000 pounds (100 tons). Attempts have been made to use rare earth alloys to reduce the total magnet weight.

Permanent magnets are inexpensive to maintain and offer transverse field imaging. They also exhibit minimal fringe field problems. Because the strength of permanent magnets is limited by the number of magnetic domains available in the material, they have been used only for relatively low field strength MRI units. Their weight and temperature sensitivity can be a problem.

Superconductive. Superconductive magnets may produce field strengths of up to 4 T or more. They use liquid cryogens to produce extremely low temperatures that permit some conductors to become superconductive. Much effort is currently being devoted to the development of room temperature superconductors. If these efforts are successful, MRI will become much less expensive and much more important as a diagnostic imaging tool.

Strong magnetic fields require enormous quantities of wire loops. For example, a 1.5 T magnet might require 1,000 loops, each carrying 1,000 A. This amperage in so many loops in the same circuit would produce a large quantity of heat and consume a great deal of power. In fact, a resistive magnet of this

RF coil

Gradient coils

Stationary magnet

FIGURE 45-11   A typical MRI unit, with the relationship of the stationary magnet, gradient coil, and RF coil to the patient illustrated.

Liquid helium

Superconducting coil

RF coil

Liquid nitrogen

Gradient coils

Shim coils

Dewar vacuum

FIGURE 45-12 Cross-sectional image of a superconducting MRI unit gantry showing the relationship of the cryogenic dewars to the MR and RF coils.

strength cannot be produced because of these physical limits. The heat would melt the conducting wire and destroy the circuit.

At temperatures near absolute zero (0° Kelvin) some conductors lose nearly all resistance, thus becoming superconductors. This permits the construction of magnets with the strength necessary to permit MRI at 1 T and higher field strengths. Superconduction has been observed as a basic property of atoms, where electrons have been spinning in tiny electromagnetic fields, apparently since the creation of the universe, without losing rotational energy as heat and slowing down.

Special cooling agents, called **cryogens,** must be used to achieve the extremely low temperatures necessary for superconductive magnets. The electromagnetic coils are placed in an insulated chamber called a **dewar,** or **cryostat,** which contains **liquid helium** (Figure 45-12). A dewar is con-

structed much like an insulated Thermos bottle, with the electromagnet inside. Liquid helium has a boiling point of 4°K (−269°C or −452°F) and is used to maintain the coil temperature below 9.5°K (−264°C or −443°F). The liquid helium is then surrounded by another dewar, this one containing **liquid nitrogen,** which has a boiling point of 77°K (−196°C or −320°F). The nitrogen serves as another insulator to help maintain the temperature necessary for the helium to remain liquid. The process of bringing the superconducting magnet to the necessary temperature by using cryogens is called **ramping.**

Superconductive magnets are capable of very high field strengths. They typically produce very stable and uniform fields. However, they are expensive and require expensive site preparation and maintenance. In addition, the high field strengths may cause fringe field problems.

A.   B.

FIGURE 45-13   (A) Shim coils and (B) gradient coils, both surrounding the bore of the stationary magnet.

If the temperature of the cryogens rises to the boiling point of helium, both liquids will vaporize into gases. Neither gas can maintain the necessary environment for superconduction and the electromagnetic coil will rapidly overheat. This process is known as **quenching** and is a serious hazard to the electromagnet, the patient, and personnel during superconductive MRI. The rapid vaporization of the gases can replace the oxygen in areas around the MRI unit. Although safety release valves are designed to vent these gases outside the unit, audible oxygen monitors are required to warn personnel in the event of quenching. Although helium and nitrogen are not poisonous, if the gases displace the air in the examination areas asphyxiation becomes a danger and an explosion is also possible. A patient or technologist would lose consciousness quickly and could die within minutes. A mask and nonmagnetic O_2 tank are required to permit the technologist to remove a patient from the unit as rapidly as possible if the alarms sound. The technologist must put on an oxygen mask before attempting to help a patient or anyone else. If the technologist were to lose consciousness there might be no one else to help others.

In addition to these hazards, the heat buildup that occurs in the electromagnet during a quench usually does severe damage to the coil windings and requires extensive repairs or replacement of the entire coil. Quenching is therefore not only dangerous but also prohibitively expensive. Failure to maintain sufficient cryogenic pressures through regular replacement of natural evaporation is the most likely

cause of a quench. Therefore, the dependability of the cryogenic supply company to the MRI unit is of critical importance.

Shim Coils. All stationary magnets have irregularities in their fields due to the shape and construction of the magnets themselves, the location of ferromagnetic materials near the MRI unit, and the materials used in the construction of the MRI room. These irregularities are compensated for by adding a series of corrective magnetic coils, called **shim coils,** inside the bore of the main stationary magnet. Shim coils can be resistive or superconducting and are custom fitted for each unit by adjusting the current to each (Figure 45-13A).

Magnetic Field Strength. Magnetic field strength decreases inversely with the cube of the distance. This is much faster than the effect of distance (the inverse square law) that is so important in diagnostic radiography. The inverse cube law is complex but is based on the fact that both magnetic north and south poles are always present. The two poles affect each other with increasing significance as distance increases, the result being that the poles begin to cancel each other. This has the effect of reducing the magnetic field strength exponentially, as compared to the inverse square law.

This rapid fall-off of magnetic field strength makes it difficult to establish and maintain a homogeneous field for imaging. Because distance has such a dramatic effect on field strength, it becomes extremely difficult to perform MRI over a large area, even one the size and thickness of the human body.

The basic principles of magnetism are directly involved in determining magnetic field strength (see Chapter 3). The degree of alignment of induced magnetic domains in a material depends on the strength of the magnetic field that is inducing them and the inverse cube of the distance between them. This is expressed as:

$$M_I = \frac{M_O}{D^3}$$

where: M_I = induced magnetic field
M_O = original magnetic field
D = distance

This is of critical importance in understanding how magnetic attraction occurs. Not only does the attraction increase by the inverse cube with distance, but the number of magnetic domains also increases by the inverse cube. These two factors function mathematically so that their product represents the total attraction. In other words, the actual increase is not the inverse cube of the distance but rather the inverse cube of the distance times the inverse cube of the number of magnetic domains. Therefore, attraction occurs by the inverse sixth power. Moving 10 times closer to the magnet actually causes the magnetic field strength attraction to increase by 1,000,000 times.

A free magnet will move to align itself in a magnetic field. For example, the needle of a compass aligns itself on a north-south axis because it experiences the torque of the earth's magnetic field. Torque can be a powerful force in a strong magnetic field. For example, this principle of inducing torque is used to activate the motors that move trains and lift elevators. However, torque also acts on the nucleus of an atom and can cause a nucleus to align with a magnetic field. This is a basic principle in MRI.

Gradient Coils

There are three sets of gradient coils, one each for the x, y, and z axes (Figure 45-13B). They can be operated as required to achieve the appropriate pulse sequence and spatial localization within the anatomical section.

Radiofrequency Coils

Radiofrequency (RF) coils may serve as both the transmitter and the receiver of the MRI signal (although some units use separate RF coils for each function). Because it is desirable to position RF coils as close as possible to the body part to be imaged, they are often sized and shaped to fit specific body parts. This type of coil is known as a **surface coil. Head, neck, and extremity** surface coils are commonly used in either saddle or solenoid shapes (a solenoid head coil is shown in Figure 45-10B). **Solenoid (or birdcage) coils are used in a transverse magnetic field.** A solenoid extremity coil is shown in Figure 45-14A. **Saddle coils are used in a longitudinal magnetic field. However, the best images are produced with surface (or local) coils that are placed directly on the patient, as close to the region of interest as possible.** Body coils permit resolution to the depth of the entire body section but decreased signal-to-noise ratio (SNR) can be a problem. Surface coils permit thinner sections and increased SNR, but they are limited to a depth of resolution of half their diameter (usually 5–6 cm).

It is important to select the RF coil appropriate to the structure being examined. For example, a birdcage coil (Figure 45-14B) would image the entire head quite well but a small surface coil would produce the best image of the TMJ (Figure 45-14C).

Table

The MRI table is usually slightly curved for patient comfort and to conform to the circular shape of the bore of the magnet. As with CT units, tabletops are rated for maximum weight and it is critical that this weight not be exceeded. Extensive damage to the table may result when attempts are made to examine very large patients who exceed the limit. Most tables are driven by hydraulics to move the patient smoothly into the bore of the magnet.

Computer

Data acquisition sequences are complex in most MRI units. The computer must precisely control the gradient and RF coils and their pulsing sequences,

A

B

C

FIGURE 45-14 (A) Extremity coil. (B) Head coil. (C) 3-inch general purpose coils positioned very close to the temporomandibular joint in a dual-array offer increased SNR. *(Courtesy of GE Healthcare)*

as well as collect and process the received RF data. Most data is collected by sampling the received signal during a series of RF windows. All data and images can be stored electronically on magnetic or optical tape or disk. The operator can access the computer through two consoles, one for operating the MRI unit to acquire data, the other for manipulation of images for which data has been collected although some units use a single console.

Operating Console. The MRI unit operator controls the scanning procedure by specifying the radio frequency, RF pulse sequence, pulsing time intervals, matrix size, number of excitations (NEX) or acquisitions, field of view, and section parameters.

The radio frequency is adjusted by tuning the system to the proper Larmor frequency for the tissue to be examined and by tuning the RF coils to receive the desired RF signal that will be emitted from the tissues.

The RF pulse sequences are classified as partial saturation, inversion recovery, spin-echo, or one of the other fast data sequences discussed previously. The MRI computer is programmed to initiate the RF and magnetic field pulses to accomplish the selected sequence. These sequences are usually extremely complex as they commonly use multisection and multiecho techniques to reduce scan time by acquiring data for numerous sections simultaneously. Although the operator does not have to initiate the various pulses, an appropriate sequencing method for the particular examination must be selected.

The most common variable in operating an MRI unit is the time interval (TI, TE, and TR) used to enhance image quality. Appropriate intervals determine how tissue characteristics (such as T_1, T_2, T_2^*, or ρ) are demonstrated on MR images. T_1 and T_2 can vary depending on the tissue of interest, suspected pathology, and clinical experience (see Table 45-3). The time interval (TR) directly affects the total scan time.

As in all digital imaging, the matrix size controls the resolution of the image. The matrix size that is selected also has a direct effect on the total scan time, with a larger matrix producing higher resolution but requiring longer scan times. This is often set as the number of phase encoding steps, with 256 or 512 being common selections. Interpolation schemes can also be implemented to enhance apparent resolution.

The quantity of protons precessing and emitting RF determines the proton density (ρ). The longer the TR, the more time is available for RF emission. The larger the tissue sample or the greater the number of precessing protons in the tissue, the greater is the proton spin density. These factors determine the strength of the RF signal and therefore the intensity (brightness) of the image.

The number of signals used to create the image also has a linear effect on the total scan time. Several terms are used to represent this parameter. These include number of excitations (NEX), number of signal averages (NSA), and number of acquisitions. It also determines the strength of the RF signal.

The field of view (FOV) also affects resolution. A larger FOV decreases resolution.

The section, the interval between sections, and the section thickness can all be controlled by the operator.

Display Console. The image reconstruction algorithms used for MRI are similar to those used in CT. However, there are differences because of the increased data that is collected during the MRI pulse sequences. Depending on the pulse sequence and quantity of data collected, this permits oblique sections as well as routine sagittal, coronal, and even 3D reconstructions.

Most display consoles also permit the addition of software **filters.** Smoothing filters average pixel values but decrease resolution. Noise reduction filters eliminate image densities below a selected level. Edge (contour) enhancement filters accentuate the differences between pixels when those differences exceed a selected value. Other filters for special uses may be created with custom algorithms.

MRI display consoles permit density level windows and contrast widths to be set as with any digital image processing technology. However, MRI units collect significantly more data than CT units and they have the ability to perform more complex data analysis as well. MR angiograms can be projected into multiple planes or rotated about an axis. Reformatting of data to display transverse, sagittal, and coronal images, as well as oblique and three-dimensional images, is also possible without additional data collection (Figure 45-15). Region of interest (ROI) controls permit calculations of pixel values, histograms, and highlighting of specific re-

FIGURE 45-15 A coronal projection image from a 3D Time-of-Flight MR angiogram. *(Courtesy of GE Healthcare)*

gions. Scanograms for anatomical reference, grid application, reverse display, annotation, and simultaneous image display (collaging) are all possible. Electronic magnification of the field of view (FOV) is often used when filming MRI studies.

IMAGE QUALITY

Numerous factors directly affect image quality. The primary visual factor is often called brightness, which is actually the density of the MR image. The RF signal strength determines brightness, although other factors affect it.

Field Strength

Higher strength magnetic fields produce a stronger RF signal. There is a dramatic difference between the imaging parameters and the resultant image for the same tissues when examined under different strength magnets. Although the most efficient field strength has not yet been determined, it most likely is between 1 and 3 T.

Section Thickness

Section thickness is determined by the size (or depth) of the tissue voxel. It is the primary factor of image quality because all signals from a single voxel are mathematically combined to give a single image value for the voxel. Therefore the voxel size determines the smallest tissue differences that can be imaged.

The dimension of a voxel is determined by dividing the size of the field of view by the matrix size:

$$d = \frac{F}{M}$$

where: d = voxel dimension
F = field of view
M = matrix size

EXAMPLE: What is the voxel dimension for a 256 × 256 matrix showing a field of view of 22 cm?

Answer:

$$d = \frac{F}{M}$$

$$d = \frac{22 \text{ cm}}{256}$$

$$d = 0.0859 \text{ cm} = 8.59 \text{ mm}$$

This formula must be applied in both directions (x and y) as many matrices have different x and y sizes.

Effect of MRI Parameters

The effects of the major MRI parameters, proton spin density (ρ), repetition time (TR), echo time (TE), inversion time (TI), spin-lattice relaxation time (T_1), and spin-spin relaxation time (T_2) are summed in Table 45-2.

The present state of MRI diagnosis demands that each examination include at least one T_1 weighted image and at least one T_2 weighted image. This is because proton precession (and therefore the frequency of the RF signal emitted) varies depending on adjacent tissues. As an example, a tumor might have a T_1 and T_2 as shown in Table 45-4. If the tumor were imbedded in fat, a T_1 weighted image would provide the contrast to permit its detection; the tumor would be hidden in a T_2 image because the T_2 relaxation times of the tumor and of fat are

identical, making them appear at the same image density. However, if the same tumor were imbedded in muscle, a T_2 weighted image would be required to provide contrast; the tumor would be hidden in a T_1 image because the T_1 of the tumor and of muscle are identical. Chemical saturation techniques can also be employed to minimize signal from certain structures containing fat or water.

Motion

Motion (temporal resolution) is a special problem in MRI because of the extremely long scan times that must be used. Good communication with the patient is the best method of assuring cooperation in reducing motion artifacts. Much has been written about patient claustrophobia due to the small diameter and long length of the bore of most MRI units. However, only about 5 percent of all patients cannot be examined due to claustrophobia. Cardiac gating procedures that use an electrocardiographic wave to trigger scanning pulses have proven effective in reducing motion in thoracic, cardiac, and cervical spine imaging. Some patients can be led through a breath holding technique in which the technologist activates the pulse sequence at expiration to eliminate diaphragmatic motion. This technique is most effective with pulse sequences of 30 seconds or less.

Spatial Resolution

Resolution is the ability to distinguish one structure from another. Spatial resolution is determined by the homogeneity of the static external magnetic field, the steepness of the gradient fields, and the scan time. Its quality is limited by noise, or the signal-to-noise ratio; when this ratio becomes low, image quality begins to decrease. Current MRI units are capable of resolving objects as small as 0.1 mm.

Signal-to-Noise Ratio

Noise, or extraneous visual information, is measured as the signal-to-noise ratio (S/N). It is determined by the voxel size and detection volume, the quantity of precessing protons, the pulse sequence, and the field strength. It is undesirable because it reduces the visibility of low contrast structures. **The S/N is enhanced by reducing TE and using**

optimal TR. It can also be enhanced by **averaging** a series of RF signals and by the use of a **stronger magnetic field.**

RF coils are sensitive enough that they can detect the tiny electrical currents produced by normal Brownian motion of body electrolytes. Because the quantity of Brownian motion increases with body temperature, it is referred to as **thermal noise.**

Scan Time

As with all digital imaging methods, scan time depends on the quantity of data that must be processed by the computer. In MRI it depends on the pulse sequences, the number of phase encoding steps, and the number of excitations. For example, a 256×256 matrix with a TR of 2 seconds for 2 excitations requires a 17-minute scan time. For three-dimensional MRI, the scan time is usually much greater. Multisection and multiecho pulse sequences are the prime methods of reducing scan time.

Image Contrast

Contrast resolution is dependent upon image contrast, which in turn is determined by the tissue characteristics (T_1 and T_2) and the pulse sequence variables (especially TR and TE). By using knowledge of these parameters, a technologist can produce images to maximize the contrast between tissues. In spin-echo sequences, this relates to the appropriately named T_1 weighted, T_2 weighted, and proton density weighted images. As MRI continues to develop, new techniques are constantly being researched to improve contrast as well as spatial resolution. It is the responsibility of the MR technologist to apply the proper sequences and algorithms to maximize the visualization of both anatomy and pathology.

Image contrast can be controlled to a great extent by the manipulation of the sequence of radio frequency pulses, ρ, TI, TR, and TE. Maximum contrast is obtained when the RF signal strength is at its greatest difference between two tissues. For example, in Figure 45-16A, the T_1 relaxation curves become further apart as time increases. Therefore, the contrast increases with increasing time.

A **T_1 weighted image** is usually produced with a short TR (300–800 ms) to maximize T_1 and a short TE

to minimize T_2 (Figure 45-16B). A **T_2 weighted image** is usually produced with a **long TR** (2–3 sec.) to minimize T_1 and a **long TE** to maximize T_2 (Figure 45-16C). However, there are some situations in which image density actually reverses (Figure 45-16C). In these instances a short TE produces greater T_1 contrast while a long TE produces greater T_2 contrast. When TE is set at the crossover point, no contrast is produced. This is most common in proton density images produced by a moderate length TR. The subject contrast of a T_1 image varies with the magnetic field strength, while T_2 values remain essentially constant.

Whereas CT uses Hounsfield units, there are no standardized units for tissue measurements in MRI because subject contrast depends on the differences between the signals received from the tissues. There are so many different pulse and frequency sequences and algorithms in use that no unit system is yet feasible.

Most pathologies increase both T_1 and T_2. This produces a black, negative contrast image on a T_1 weighted image and a white, positive contrast image on a T_2 weighted image. This contrast disappears when images are not weighted toward either T_1 or T_2. Consequently, efforts should be made to produce weighted images when pathological conditions are to be demonstrated.

The effects of the most common parameter weighting, proton spin density (ρ), T_1, and T_2, on image density (brightness) are shown in Table 45-2.

Chemical Shift Artifact

The chemical shift is the slight difference between the resonating frequencies of similar protons. The differences are so slight that they are expressed in parts per million (ppm). For example, hydrogen in fat resonates at a slightly higher frequency than hydrogen in water (about 3 ppm). This produces a bright band next to a dark band on the MR image at water-fat interfaces and is considered an imaging artifact, although some studies have indicated that proper manipulation of the RF spectrum data can produce useful information from chemical shift. Chemical shift artifacts can be reduced or eliminated by increasing the strength of the gradient fields, although this may also increase the visible noise in the image.

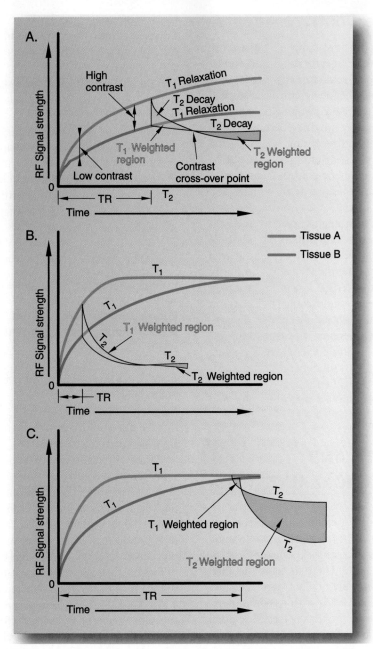

FIGURE 45-16   Obtaining contrast by T_1 and T_2 weighting during spin-echo imaging. The T_1 curves demonstrate recovery back toward equilibrium after the first pulse. The T_2 curves demonstrate decay from the refocusing pulse back toward equilibrium. (A) Relatively equal T_1 and T_2 weighting with a medium TR. Note the contrast crossover point. A short TE after the TR would produce a T_1 weighted image. A long TE after the TR would produce a T_2 weighted image. (B) T_1 weighting occurs with a short TR. The shorter the TE after the TR, the greater the signal difference (contrast) between the tissues. (C) T_2 weighting occurs with a long TR. The longer the TE before the TR, the greater the signal difference (contrast) between the tissues.

(Adapted by permission from Friedman, B. R., Chaves-Munoz, G., & Merritt, C. R. B. [1989]. Principles of MRI. New York: McGraw-Hill, Inc.)

Paramagnetic Contrast Agents

Magnetic resonance imaging contrast agents are primarily **paramagnetic agents designed to enhance the T_1 and T_2 relaxation times of adjacent hydrogen nuclei.** Some agents are classified as T_1 active or T_2 active. They produce complex effects that vary depending on the RF pulsing sequence. For example, T_1 shortening increases the RF signal intensity but T_2 shortening decreases it. In many instances paramagnetic contrast agents permit the visualization of lesions with shorter TR, thus decreasing scan time.

Paramagnetic contrast agents have been developed for oral, intravenous, and inhalation administration, and although this is an active research area in MRI, at the present time the IV agents have predominated. Gadolinium^{+3} (Gd^{+3}), which has seven unpaired electrons, has the strongest relaxation rate properties and has proven effective in demonstrating various types of lesions. However, alone it is extremely toxic and is administered in a chelate with DTPA (diethylenetriaminepentaacetic acid) (Gd-DTPA) to ensure detoxification. IV administration is common, especially for neuroimaging and MR angiography.

SAFETY AND BIOLOGICAL HAZARDS

As yet, there is no known biological risk from the magnetic field of an MRI unit. However, magnetic resonance imaging units require special consideration of the environment in which they are installed because of possible interactions between their extremely strong magnetic fields with ferromagnetic materials and electromagnetic devices. Included among devices that are affected by MRI units are cathode ray tubes, gamma cameras, cardiac pacemakers, and radio broadcasting and receiving equipment. Other equipment affected by magnetic fields includes computers (including the MRI computer itself), x-ray tubes, image intensification systems, computed tomography units, ultrasound units, electron microscopes, credit cards, analog watches, and any other devices that operate on electromagnetic principles. Safe operating distances for these devices depend on the strength of the MRI magnet and may range up to 500 feet for a 1.5 T magnet.

The MRI unit itself can be seriously affected by moving ferromagnetic devices, such as elevators and automobiles, and by strong electromagnetic devices, such as power transformers and radio broadcasting antennas. Although ferromagnetic sheets can be used to shield the MRI unit and the main resonance frequency can be adjusted slightly to avoid ranges conflicting with other equipment, these measures can compromise the imaging ability of the unit.

Safety Factors

Because magnetic fields change so dramatically with distance, it is easy for someone who is not knowledgeable about them to be misled on safety considerations. Accidents around MRI units occur when ferromagnetic materials such as oxygen tanks, IV poles, mop buckets, scissors, and personal items such as earrings and belt buckles enter the field. These items can become lethal projectiles. Magnetic media, such as computer and audio disks, and magnetized information strips on credit cards may be erased.

Other electronic devices, such as cardiac pacemakers and pocket pagers, and physiologic monitors, such as electrocardiographic monitors, may be damaged or turned off and will not work properly in a strong magnetic field. It is also possible that metal objects that have been surgically implanted, such as replacement hips, aneurysm clips and surgical staples, or foreign objects, such as buckshot or metallic debri in the eye, may be torqued during MRI examinations with catastrophic consequences. For example, torquing an aneurysm clip could open an artery and cause a fatal hemorrhage. Careful histories and, in some cases, fluoroscopic screening, are safety precautions that must be taken before MRI. Patients with histories of surgical implants or with employment histories in metal working must be interviewed with special care. The objects considered to contraindicate MRI examination are listed in Table 45-5.

A few steps closer to an MRI unit will increase the magnetic field attraction by the inverse cube

TABLE 45-5.	Objects That Contraindicate MRI Examination
Pacemakers	
Ferromagnetic cranial aneurysm clips	
Shrapnel or other metallic objects in vital locations	
Cochlear implants	

law. A distance of as little as one inch can make the difference between being able to hold onto an object and having it fly at incredible speed directly to the bore of the MRI unit. Remembering that an industrial electromagnet is capable of lifting an automobile or railroad car may help in understanding the power of an extremely strong magnetic field.

Within 10–20 feet of the magnet, wheelchairs and carts may begin to roll toward the MRI unit and within 5–10 feet, hairpins and pens may become projectiles. A cart may begin to roll from 20 feet away, but as it approaches the bore of the magnet the field may become strong enough to cause an oxygen tank or other object on the cart to become a projectile. It is important to emphasize to others that the magnetic field is operating at all times. Many persons assume that, as with most electromagnetic devices, the magnetic field is on only when the unit is in operation. The doors to the MRI scanning room should not only be locked, but padlocked during hours the unit is closed. This procedure prevents entry by persons with master passkeys during these hours.

Because of the cryogenically established superconductive conditions, superconductor magnets maintain their fields at all times and are therefore hazardous at all times. The extremely strong field must be treated with respect. The attractive force on an object as large as an oxygen tank makes it possible to fatally injure a patient or technologist if he or she is caught between the object and the MRI unit.

Biological Factors

The term used to describe the absorption of RF radiation is the **specific absorption rate (SAR)**. The SAR is indicated in units of watts per kilogram (W/kg). The United States Environmental Protec-

tion Agency (EPA) has concluded that adverse human health effects are associated with whole-body average SARs of 1–4 W/kg or greater. A primary concern is increased effects due to heating in geriatric and dehydrated patients. Consequently many agencies are considering RF radiation as a noncarcinogen but with uncertainty factors used in deriving exposure limits. The current FDA safe levels for exposure to RF during MR procedures are:

> The exposure to RF energy below the level of concern is an SAR of 0.4 W/kg or less averaged over the body; 8.0 W/kg or less spatial peak in any 1 g of tissue, and 3.2 W/kg or less averaged over the head, OR

> The exposure to RF energy that is insufficient to produce a core temperature increase of 1°C and localized heating to no greater than 38°C in the head, 39°C in the trunk, and 40°C in the extremities, except for patients with impaired system blood flow and/or perspiration (i.e., those with compromised thermoregulatory systems).

These conclusions are consistent with the recommendations of other agencies such as the United States National Council on Radiation Protection and Measurements (NCRP), International Radiation Protection Association (IRPA), the United States Food and Drug Administration (FDA), and the American National Standards Institute (ANSI). Although there have not been any published reports of harmful effects due to the use of MRI, the issue is under intense study and much additional information is expected in the years to come. In the United States, the FDA requires prominent posting of triangular warning signs at the 5 G (0.0005 T) line. There are two signs, one indicating a strong magnetic field, the other with markings and wording prohibiting pacemakers or loose metal objects.

Static magnetic fields appear to augment the T wave amplitude of the heart. This may occur when conductive fluids, such as blood, pass through the static magnetic field, thus generating low potentials that may affect the biopotentials of the heart. No arrhythmias or other heart rate alterations have yet been produced in laboratory animals or observed in patients undergoing MRI.

Intense gradient magnetic fields have been shown to induce electrical currents in body tissues such as nerve, muscle, skeletal, and heart. Light flashes due to physiological stimulation of the retina have also been observed. However, these field strengths are far above that used in MRI.

Radio frequency magnetic fields are known to produce thermal effects. Potential biological damage would depend on the ability of the specific biological system to metabolically absorb and distribute heat. Some effects, including ocular cataractogenesis due to thermal heating of the eye, have been recorded, although again at field levels well above those used in MRI.

Because of the lack of definitive data on the biological effects of MRI, pregnant women are seldom examined. However, when necessary, MRI studies are considered less hazardous to the fetus than computed tomography studies.

SUMMARY

Magnetic resonance imaging (MRI) uses magnetism and radio frequencies (RF) to create diagnostic sectional images of the body. The nucleus is spinning, thus creating a nuclear magnetic moment. This rotating charge acts as a current loop and produces a magnetic field. When a rotating nucleus is subjected to a magnetic field, it will begin to precess. MR imaging is accomplished through various measurements of this movement of the nuclear magnetic field.

The frequency of precession is called the Larmor frequency and is critical to MR imaging. Production of the nuclear magnetic resonance signal requires applying a Larmor frequency RF and then listening to the RF emissions from the protons. Digital imaging reconstruction techniques are then used to create sectional and three-dimensional images.

The primary parameters controlling the MRI process include proton spin density (PD, NEX or NSA, or ρ), repetition time (TR), echo time (TE), inversion time (TI), spin-lattice or longitudinal relaxation time (T_1), and spin-spin or transverse relaxation time (T_2). The parameters that are used vary depending on the pulse sequence used.

The localization of information for the MR image requires three electromagnetic coils to produce magnetic field gradients corresponding to the x, y, and z axes to be imaged. The RF that are detected from these gradient coils can then be analyzed to determine not only the type of atom they came from but also the atom's precise location within the imaging matrix.

The primary variable in the data collection procedure during MRI is the sequence of RF pulses that are used to cause the protons to precess. Partial saturation, spin-echo, inversion recovery, and gradient-echo are the major sequences, although most MRI is done with spin-echo pulse sequences. There are many modifications of spin-echo sequences, including multisection and multiecho sequences.

A typical MRI unit consists of a stationary magnet within which are fitted gradient and radio frequency (RF) coils. The stationary magnet must be extremely strong; current field strengths range from 0.06–3.0 T. A table for the patient and a large computer for image processing, display, and storage complete the system.

The primary image quality factor is often called brightness, which is actually the density of the MR image. The RF signal strength determines brightness, although it is also affected by field strength, section thickness, the MRI parameters (ρ, TI, TE, TR, T_1, T_2), motion, spatial resolution, S/N, and scan time. Image contrast is controlled by manipulating the MRI parameters to produce T_1 and T_2 weighted images. Chemical shift artifacts may occur at fat-water interfaces although chemical shift imaging may provide useful diagnostic information in the future. Paramagnetic contrast agents are used to enhance image contrast. As yet, there is no known biological risk from the magnetic field of an MRI unit. However, magnetic resonance imaging units require special restrictions to their access because of possible interactions between their extremely strong magnetic fields and ferromagnetic materials and electromagnetic devices. Accidents around MRI units occur when ferromagnetic materials such as oxygen tanks, IV poles, mop buckets, scissors, and personal items such as earrings and belt buckles enter the field. These items can become lethal projectiles.

The Food and Drug Administration suggests limiting whole or partial body exposure to 2.0 T for static magnetic fields, 3.0 T/sec for gradient fields, and a specific absorption rate (SAR) of 0.4 W/kg for RF fields.

REVIEW QUESTIONS

1. What is the source of the magnetic fields within the body that are used during MRI?

2. What is precession?

3. What is TI? TR? TE? T_1? T_2?

4. How do the gradient coils select an image section?

5. What is accomplished by an RF pulse during a pulse sequence?

6. What occurs at each step during a spin-echo pulse sequence?

7. How can MR image noise be reduced by improving the S/N?

8. How is MR image contrast increased? decreased?

9. Describe appropriate safety measures for protection of all persons who approach the MRI unit magnetic field.

REFERENCES AND RECOMMENDED READING

Andrew, E. R. (1982). Nuclear magnetic resonance imaging. In P. N. T. Wells (Ed.). *Scientific basis of medical imaging.* Edinburgh: Churchill Livingstone.

Atkinson, D. J. (1990). Pulse sequence design. In R. R. Edelman & J. R. Hesselink (Eds.). *Clinical magnetic resonance imaging.* Philadelphia: W. B. Saunders.

Axel, L. (1988). Chemical shift imaging. In D. D. Stark & W. G. Bradley (Eds.) *Magnetic resonance imaging.* St. Louis, MO: Elsevier/C. V. Mosby.

Ayton, V. T., Smith, M. A., & Bingham, J. B. (1989). Practical consideration for patient investigation using a high field magnetic resonance system. *Radiography Today, 55*(620), 12.

Barrafate, D. (1985). MRI: A technologist's perspective. The *Canadian Journal of Medical Radiation Technology, 16*(3), 73.

Barrafate, D., & Henkelman, M. (1985). MRI and surgical clips. *The Canadian Journal of Medical Radiation Technology, 16*(3), 101.

Bloch, F. (1946). Nuclear induction. *Physics Review, 70,* 460–474.

Bloch, F. (1998). The principle of nuclear induction. In *Nobel Lectures in Physics: 1901–1995.* New York: World Scientific Publishers.

Bloch, F., Hansen, W. W., & Packard, M. E. (1946). Nuclear induction. *Physics Review, 69,* 127.

Bushberg, J. T., Seibert, J. A., Leidholdt, E. M., & Boone, J. M. (2002). *The essential physics of medical imaging* (2nd ed.) Philadelphia: Lippincott Williams & Wilkins.

Bushong, S. C. (1996). *Magnetic resonance imaging: Physical and biological principles* (2nd ed.). St. Louis, MO: Elsevier/C. V. Mosby.

Bushong, S. C. (2004). *Radiologic science for technologists: Physics, biology, and protection* (8th ed.). St. Louis, MO: Elsevier/C. V. Mosby.

Curry, T. S., Dowdey, J. E., & Murry, R. C. (1990). *Christensen's introduction to the physics of diagnostic radiology* (4th ed.). Philadelphia: Lea and Febiger.

Damadian, R. (1971). Tumor detection by nuclear magnetic resonance. *Science, 171,* 1151–1153.

Damadian, R. 1981. *(NMR) in medicine.* Berlin: Springer-Verlag.

Damadian, R., Goldsmith, M., & Minkoff, L. (1977). NMR in cancer XVI: FONAR image of the live human body. *Physiological Chemistry and Physics, 9,* 97–100.

Damadian, R., Zaner, K., Hor, D., DiMaio, T., Minkoff, L., & Goldsmith, M. (1973). Nuclear magnetic resonance as a new tool in cancer research: Human tumors by NMR. *Annals of the New York Academy of Science, 222,* 1048–1076.

Davis, P. (1981). Potential hazards in NMR imaging: Heating effects of changing magnetic fields and RF fields on small metallic implants. *American Journal of Roentgenology, 137*, 857–860.

Edelman, R. R., & Hesselink, J. R. (1990). *Clinical magnetic resonance imaging.* Philadelphia: W. B. Saunders.

Elster, A. D. (1986). *Magnetic resonance imaging: A reference guide and atlas.* Philadelphia: J. B. Lippincott.

Fitzsimmons, J. R., & Mick, R. C. (1985). Image quality and magnetic field strength in NMR imaging. *Applied Radiology, 14*(2), 52.

Fodor, J., & Mallot, J. (1984). MRI: A new imaging modality. *Radiologic Technology, 56*(1), 17.

Forster, E. (1985). *Equipment for diagnostic radiography.* Lancaster, U.K.: MTP Press.

Friedman, B. R., Jones, J. P., Chaves-Munoz, G., Salmon, A. P., & Merritt, C. R. B. (1989). *Principles of MRI.* New York: McGraw-Hill.

Grey, M. L., & Coffey, C. W. (1987). Methods for evaluating image quality in magnetic resonance imaging. *Radiologic Technology, 58*(4), 339.

Heiken, J. P., & Brown, J. J. (Eds.). (1991). *Manual of clinical magnetic resonance imaging* (2nd ed.). New York: Raven.

Hendee, W. R., & Ritenour, R. (1993). *Medical imaging physics* (3rd ed.). St. Louis, MO: C. V. Mosby.

Hinshaw, W. S., Bottomley, P. A., & Holland, G. N. (1977). Radiographic thin-section image of the human wrist by nuclear magnetic resonance. *Nature, 270*(22/29), 722–723.

Kaut, C. (1992). *MRI workbook for technologists.* New York: Raven.

Lauterbur, P. C. (1973). Image formation by induced local interactions: Examples employing nuclear magnetic resonance. *Nature, 242*, 190–191.

Lipcamon, J. D., Chiu, L. C., Phillips, J. J., & Pottany, P. M. (1988). MRI of the upper abdomen using motion artifact suppression technique. *Radiologic Technology, 59*(5), 415.

Lufkin, R. B. (1990). *The MRI manual.* St. Louis, MO: Elsevier/C. V. Mosby.

Morgan, C. J., & Hendee, W. R. (1984). *Introduction to magnetic resonance imaging.* Denver: Multi-Media.

Nelson, T. R., Ritenour, E. R., Davis, K., & Pretorius, D. H. (1985a). MRI: The basic physical and clinical concepts Part 1. *Radiologic Technology, 56*(6), 410.

Nelson, T. R, Ritenour, E. R., Davis, K., & Pretorius, D. H. (1985b). MRI: The basic physical and clinical concepts Part 2. *Radiologic Technology, 57*(1), 26.

Nelson, T. R., Ritenour, E. R., Davis, K., Pretorius, D. H., & Hendrick, R. E. (1985c). MRI: The basic physical and clinical concepts Part 3. *Radiologic Technology, 57*(2), 142.

Olendorf, W., & Olendorf, W., Jr. (1991). *MRI primer.* New York: Raven.

Philips Medical Systems. (1984). *Principles of MR imaging* (Publication 1984–11). The Netherlands: Author.

Purcell, E. (1998). Research in nuclear magnetism. *Nobel lectures in physics: 1901–1995.* New York: World Scientific Publishers.

Purcell, E. M., Torrey, H. C., & Pound, R. V. (1946). Resonance absorption by nuclear magnetic moments in a solid. *Physics Review, 69*, 37–83.

Rollo, F. D., & Patton, J. A. (1981). Nuclear magnetic resonance imaging. Radiographic films and screen-film systems. In C. M. Coulam, J. J. Erickson, F. D. Rollo, & A. E. James (Eds.), *The physical basis of medical imaging.* New York: Appleton-Century-Crofts.

Russel, R., Dallas-Hultema, C., & Cohen, M. D. (1986). MRI techniques in children. *Radiologic Technology, 57*(5), 428.

Schellock, F. G., & Kanal, E. (1994). *Magnetic resonance bioeffects, safety, and patient management.* New York: Raven.

Seeram, E. (1985). *X-ray imaging equipment: An introduction.* Springfield, IL: Charles C Thomas.

Sigal, R. (1988). *Magnetic resonance imaging: Basis for interpretation.* Berlin: Springer-Verlag.

Smith, H., & Ranallo, F. N. (1989). *A non-mathematical approach to basic MRI.* Madison, WI: Medical Physics.

Sobol, W. T. (1994). Artifacts in magnetic resonance imaging. *Applied Radiology, 23*(8), 11–16.

Stark, D. D., & Bradley, W. (Eds.). (1988). *Magnetic resonance imaging.* St. Louis, MO: C. V. Mosby.

Westbrook, C. (1994). *Handbook of MRI technique.* Oxford: Blackwell Scientific.

Westbrook, C., & Kaut, C. (1993). *MRI in practice.* Oxford: Blackwell Scientific.

Wolbarst, A. B. (1993). *Physics of radiology.* Norwalk, CT: Appleton & Lange.

Wolfe, G., & Popp, C. (1984). *NMR: A primer for medical imaging.* Thorofare, NJ: Slack Book Division.

Woodward, P., & Freimarck, R. D. (1995). *MRI for technologists.* New York: McGraw-Hill.

Young, S. W. (1984). *Nuclear magnetic resonance imaging: Basic principles.* New York: Raven.

On a New Kind of Rays*

by W. C. Röntgen

(1) A discharge from a large induction coil is passed through a Hittorf's vacuum tube, or through a well-exhausted Crookes' or Lenard's tube. The tube is surrounded by a fairly close-fitting shield of black paper; it is then possible to see, in a completely darkened room, that paper covered on one side with barium platinocyanide lights up with brilliant fluorescence when brought into the neighbourhood of the tube, whether the painted side or the other be turned towards the tube. The fluorescence is still visible at two metres distance. It is easy to show that the origin of the fluorescence lies within the vacuum tube.

(2) It is seen, therefore, that some agent is capable of penetrating black cardboard which is quite opaque to ultra-violet light, sunlight, or arc-light. It is therefore of interest to investigate how far other bodies can be penetrated by the same agent. It is readily shown that all bodies possess this same transparency, but in very varying degrees. For example, paper is very transparent; the fluorescent screen will light up when placed behind a book of a thousand pages; printer's ink offers no marked resistance. Similarly the fluorescence shows behind two packs of cards; a single card does not visibly diminish the brilliancy of the light. So, again, a single thickness of tinfoil hardly casts a shadow on the screen; several have to be superposed to produce a marked effect. Thick blocks of wood are still transparent. Boards of pine two or three centimetres thick absorb only very little. A piece of sheet aluminium, 15 mm. thick, still allowed the x-rays (as I will call the rays, for the sake of brevity) to pass, but greatly reduced the fluorescence. Glass plates of similar thickness behave similarly; lead glass is, however, much more opaque than glass free from lead. Ebonite several centimetres thick is transparent. If the hand be held before the fluorescent screen, the shadow shows the bones darkly, with only faint outlines of the surrounding tissues.

Water and several other fluids are very transparent. Hydrogen is not markedly more permeable than air. Plates of copper, silver, lead, gold, and platinum also allow the rays to pass, but only when the metal is thin. Platinum .2 mm. thick allows some rays to pass; silver and copper are more transparent. Lead 1.5 mm. thick is practically opaque. If a square rod of wood 20 mm. in the side be painted on one face with white lead, it casts little shadow when it is so turned that the painted face is parallel to the x-rays, but a strong shadow if the rays have to pass through the painted side. The salts of the metals, either solid or in solution, behave generally as the metals themselves.

(3) The preceding experiments lead to the conclusion that the density of the bodies is the property whose variation mainly affects their permeability. At least no other property seems so marked in this connection. But that the density alone does not determine the transparency is shown by an experiment wherein plates of similar thickness of Iceland spar, glass, aluminium, and quartz were employed as screens. Then the Iceland spar showed itself much less transparent than the other bodies, though of approximately the same density. I have not remarked any strong fluorescence of Iceland spar compared with glass (see below, No. 4).

(4) Increasing thickness increases the hindrance offered to the rays by all bodies. A picture has been impressed on a photographic plate of a number of superposed layers of tinfoil, like steps, presenting thus a regularly increasing thickness. This is to be

*This article was reprinted from Nature, No. 1369, Vol. 53, January 23, 1896. By W. C. Röntgen. Translated by Arthur Stanton from the *Sitsungsberichte der Würsburger Physikmedic. Gesellschaft*, 1895.

submitted to photometric processes when a suitable instrument is available.

(5) Pieces of platinum, lead, zinc, and aluminium foil were so arranged as to produce the same weakening of the effect. The annexed table shows the relative thickness and density of the equivalent sheets of metal.

	Thickness	Relative Thickness	Density
platinum	.08 mm	1	21.5
lead	.050 "	3	11.3
zinc	.100 "	6	7.1
aluminum	3.500 "	200	2.6

From these values it is clear that in no case can we obtain the transparency of a body from the product of its density and thickness. The transparency increases much more rapidly than the product decreases.

(6) The fluorescence of barium platinocyanide is not the only noticeable action of the x-rays. It is to be observed that other bodies exhibit fluorescence, e.g. calcium sulphide, uranium glass, Iceland spar, rock-salt, etc.

Of special interest in this connection is the fact that photographic dry plates are sensitive to the x-rays. It is thus possible to exhibit the phenomena so as to exclude the danger of error. I have thus confirmed many observations originally made by eye observation with the fluorescent screen. Here the power of the x-rays to pass through wood or cardboard becomes useful. The photographic plate can be exposed to the action without removal of the shutter of the dark slide or other protecting case, so that the experiment need not be conducted in darkness. Manifestly, unexposed plates must not be left in their box near the vacuum tube.

It seems now questionable whether the impression on the plate is a direct effect of the x-rays, or a secondary result induced by the fluorescence of the material of the plate. Films can receive the impression as well as ordinary dry plates.

I have not been able to show experimentally that the x-rays give rise to any calorific effects. These,

however, may be assumed, for the phenomena of fluorescence show that the x-rays are capable of transformation. It is also certain that all the x-rays falling on a body do not leave it as such.

The retina of the eye is quite insensitive to these rays: the eye placed close to the apparatus sees nothing. It is clear from the experiments that this is not due to want of permeability on the part of the structures of the eye.

(7) After my experiments on the transparency of increasing thicknesses of different media, I proceeded to investigate whether the x-rays could be deflected by a prism. Investigations with water and carbon bisulphide on mica prisms of 30° showed no deviation either on the photographic or the fluorescent plate. For comparison, light rays were allowed to fall on the prism as the apparatus was set up for the experiment. They were deviated 10 mm. and 20 mm. respectively in the case of the two prisms.

With prisms of ebonite and aluminium, I have obtained images on the photographic plate, which point to a possible deviation. It is, however, uncertain, and at most would point to a refractive index 1.05. No deviation can be observed by means of the fluorescent screen. Investigations with the heavier metals have not as yet led to any result, because of their small transparency and the consequent enfeebling of the transmitted rays.

On account of the importance of the question it is desirable to try in other ways whether the x-rays are susceptible of refraction. Finely powdered bodies allow in thick layers but little of the incident light to pass through, in consequence of refraction and reflection. In the case of the x-rays, however, such layers of powder are for equal masses of substance equally transparent with the coherent solid itself. Hence we cannot conclude any regular reflection or refraction of the x-rays. The research was conducted by the aid of finely-powdered rock-salt, fine electrolytic silver powder, and zinc dust already many times employed in chemical work. In all these cases the result, whether by the fluorescent screen or the photographic method, indicated no difference in transparency between the powder and the coherent solid.

It is, hence, obvious that lenses cannot be looked upon as capable of concentrating the x-rays; in effect, both an ebonite and a glass lens of large size prove to be without action. The shadow photograph of a round rod is darker in the middle than at the edge; the image of a cylinder filled with a body more transparent than its walls exhibits the middle brighter than the edge.

(8) The preceding experiments, and others which I pass over, point to the rays being incapable of regular reflection. It is, however, well to detail an observation which at first sight seemed to lead to an opposite conclusion.

I exposed a plate, protected by a black paper sheath, to the x-rays, so that the glass side lay next to the vacuum tube. The sensitive film was partly covered with star-shaped pieces of platinum, lead, zinc, and aluminium. On the developed negative the star-shaped impression showed dark under platinum, lead, and more markedly, under zinc; the aluminium gave no image. It seems, therefore, that these three metals can reflect the x-rays; as, however, another explanation is possible, I repeated the experiment with this only difference, that a film of thin aluminium foil was interposed between the sensitive film and the metal stars. Such an aluminium plate is opaque to ultra-violet rays, but transparent to x-rays. In the result the images appeared as before, this pointing still to the existence of reflection at metal surfaces.

If one considers this observation in connection with others, namely, on the transparency of powders, and on the state of the surface not being effective in altering the passage of the x-rays through a body, it leads to the probable conclusion that regular reflection does not exist, but that bodies behave to the x-rays as turbid media to light.

Since I have obtained no evidence of refraction at the surface of different media, it seems probable that the x-rays move with the same velocity in all bodies, and in a medium which penetrates everything, and in which the molecules of bodies are embedded. The molecules obstruct the x-rays, the more effectively as the density of the body concerned is greater.

(9) It seemed possible that the geometrical arrangement of the molecules might affect the action of a body upon the x-rays, so that, for example, Iceland spar might exhibit different phenomena according to the relation of the surface of the plate to the axis of the crystal. Experiments with quartz and Iceland spar on this point lead to a negative result.

(10) It is known that Lenard, in his investigations on kathode rays, has shown that they belong to the ether, and can pass through all bodies. Concerning the x-rays the same may be said.

In his latest work, Lenard has investigated the absorption coefficients of various bodies for the kathode rays, including air at atmospheric pressure, which gives 4.10, 3.40, 3.10 for 1 cm., according to the degree of exhaustion of the gas in discharge tube. To judge from the nature of the discharge, I have worked at about the same pressure, but occasionally at greater or smaller pressures. I find, using a Weber's photometer, that the intensity of the fluorescent light varies nearly as the inverse square of the distance between screen and discharge tube. This result is obtained from three very consistent sets of observations at distances of 100 and 200 mm. Hence air absorbs the x-rays much less than the kathode rays. This result is in complete agreement with the previously described result, that the fluorescence of the screen can be still observed at 2 metres from the vacuum tube. In general, other bodies behave like air; they are more transparent for the x-rays than for the kathode rays.

(11) A further distinction, and a noteworthy one, results from the action of a magnet. I have not succeeded in observing any deviation of the x-rays even in very strong magnetic fields.

The deviation of kathode rays by the magnet is one of their peculiar characteristics; it has been observed by Hertz and Lenard, that several kinds of kathode rays exist, which differ by their power of exciting phosphorescence, their susceptibility of absorption, and their deviation by the magnet; but a notable deviation has been observed in all cases which have yet been investigated, and I think that such deviation affords a characteristic not to be set aside lightly.

(12) As the result of many researches, it appears that the place of most brilliant phosphorescence of the walls of the discharge-tube is the chief seat whence the x-rays originate and spread in all directions; that is, the x-rays proceed from the front where the kathode rays strike the glass. If one deviates the kathode rays within the tube by means of a magnet, it is seen that the x-rays proceed from a new point, *i.e.* again from the end of the kathode rays.

Also for this reason the x-rays, which are not deflected by a magnet, cannot be regarded as kathode rays which have passed through the glass, for that passage cannot, according to Lenard, be the cause of the different deflection of the rays. Hence I conclude that the x-rays are not identical with the kathode rays, but are produced from the kathode rays at the glass surface of the tube.

(13) The rays are generated not only in glass. I have obtained them in an apparatus closed by an aluminium plate 2 mm. thick. I purpose later to investigate the behaviour of other substances.

(14) The justification of the term "rays," applied to the phenomena, lies partly in the regular shadow pictures produced by the interposition of a more or less permeable body between the source and a photographic plate or fluorescent screen.

I have observed and photographed many such shadow pictures. Thus, I have an outline of part of a door covered with lead paint; the image was produced by placing the discharge-tube on one side of the door, and the sensitive plate on the other. I have also a shadow of the bones of the hand (Figure A–1), of a wire wound upon a bobbin, of a set of weights in a box, of a compass card and needle completely enclosed in a metal case (Figure A–2), of a piece of metal where the x-rays show the want of homogeneity, and of other things.

For the rectilinear propagation of the rays, I have a pin-hole photograph of the discharge apparatus covered with black paper. It is faint but unmistakable.

(15) I have sought for interference effects of the x-rays, but possibly, in consequence of their small intensity, without result.

(16) Researches to investigate whether electrostatic forces act on the x-rays are begun but not yet concluded.

(17) If one asks, what then are these x-rays; since they are not kathode rays, one might suppose, from their power of exciting fluorescence and chemical action, them to be due to ultra-violet light. In opposition to this view a weighty set of considera-

FIGURE A-1 Photograph of the bones in the fingers of a living human hand. The third finger has a ring upon it. *(Courtesy of the American College of Radiology)*

FIGURE A-2 Photograph of a compass card and needle completely enclosed in a metal case.

tions presents itself. If x-rays be indeed ultra-violet light, then that light must possess the following properties.

(a) It is not refracted in passing from air into water, carbon bisulphide, aluminium, rock-salt, glass or zinc.

(b) It is incapable of regular reflection at the surfaces of the above bodies.

(c) It cannot be polarised by any ordinary polarising media.

(d) The absorption by various bodies must depend chiefly on their density.

That is to say, these ultra-violet rays must behave quite differently from the visible, infrared, and hitherto known ultra-violet rays.

These things appear so unlikely that I have sought for another hypothesis.

A kind of relationship between the new rays and light rays appears to exist; at least the formation of shadows, fluorescence, and the production of chemical action point in this direction. Now it has been known for a long time, that besides the transverse vibrations which account for the phenomena of light, it is possible that longitudinal vibrations should exist in the ether, and, according to the view of some physicists, must exist. It is granted that their existence has not yet been made clear, and their properties are not experimentally demonstrated. Should not the new rays be ascribed to longitudinal waves in the ether?

I must confess that I have in the course of this research made myself more and more familiar with this thought, and venture to put the opinion forward, while I am quite conscious that the hypothesis advanced still requires a more solid foundation.

Agfa's Troubleshooting the Radiographic System: Symptoms and Possible Causes*

Low Density

A. Underexposure

1. Wrong Exposure Factors
   a. Too low kilovoltage
   b. Too low milliamperage
   c. Too short exposure
   d. Too great focal-film distance
2. Meters out of calibration
3. Timer out of calibration
4. Inaccurate setting of meters or timer
5. Drop in incoming line voltage
   a. Elevators, welders, furnaces, blowers, etc. on same circuit
   b. Insufficient size of power line or transformers
6. Photocell timer out of adjustment
7. Incorrect centering of patient to photocell
8. Central ray of X-ray tube not directed on film
   a. X-ray tube rotated in casing
9. Distance out of grid radius
10. Bucky timer inaccurate
11. One or more valve tubes burned out (Full wave rectifying machines)

B. Underdevelopment

1. Improper development
   a. Time too short
   b. Temperature too low (Hydroquinone inactive below 55 °F, or 13 °C)
   c. Combination of both
   d. Inaccurate thermometer
2. Exhausted developer
   a. Chemical activity used up
   b. Activity destroyed by contamination
3. Diluted developer
   a. Water overflowed from wash tank
   b. Insufficient chemical mixed originally due to tank actually larger than rating
   c. Improper additions
4. Incorrectly mixed developer
   a. Exact capacity of tank unknown
   b. Mixing ingredients in wrong sequence
   c. Omission of ingredients
   d. Unbalanced formula composition

High Density

A. Overexposure

1. Wrong exposure factors
   a. Too high kilovoltage
   b. Too high milliamperage
   c. Too long exposure
   d. Too short focal-film distance
2. Meters out of calibration
3. Timer out of calibration
4. Inaccurate setting of meters or timer
5. Surge in incoming line voltage
6. Photocell timer out of adjustment
7. Incorrect centering of patient to photocell

B. Improper development

1. Time too long
2. Temperature too high

* Reprinted with permission from Agfa Corporation, 10 South Academy Street, Greensville, NC 29601.

3. Combination of both
4. Inaccurate thermometer
5. Insufficient dilution of concentrated developer
6. Omission of bromide when mixing

C. Fog—see section on "FOG"

1. Light struck
2. Radiation
3. Chemical
4. Film deterioration

Low Contrast

A. Overpenetration from too high kilovoltage

1. Overmeasurement of part to be examined
2. Incorrect estimate of material or tissue density
3. Meters out of calibration
4. Meters inaccurately set
5. Surge in incoming line voltage
6. Undermeasurement of focal-film distance

B. Scattered radiation

1. Failure to use Bucky diaphragm
2. Failure to use stationary grid
3. Failure to use cutout diaphragm
4. Failure to use suitable cones
5. Failure to use lead backing cassette

C. Too short exposure

1. Timer out of calibration
2. Timer inaccurately set
3. Overload relay kicked out

D. Improper development

High Contrast

A. Underpenetration from too low kilovoltage

1. Undermeasurement of part to be examined
2. In parts of varying thickness, setting of kilovoltage for thinner sections

3. Meters out of calibration
4. Meters inaccurately set
5. Drop in incoming line voltage
   a. Elevators, welders, furnaces, etc. on same line
   b. Insufficient size of power line or transformer
6. Overmeasurement of focal-film distance

B. Too long exposure

1. Timer out of calibration
2. Timer inaccurately set

C. Improper development

Fog

A. Unsafe light

1. Light leaks into processing room
   a. Leaks through doors, windows, etc.
   b. Poorly designed labyrinth entrance
      1. Bright light at outer entrance
      2. Reflection from white uniforms of persons passing through
   c. Sparking of motors
      1. Ventilating fans
      2. Dryer fans
      3. Mixers-barium
      4. Light leaks in film carrying box
2. Safelights
   a. Bulb too bright
   b. Improper filter
      1. Not dense enough
      2. Cracked
      3. Bleached
      4. Shrunken
3. Luminous clock and watch faces
4. Lighting matches in darkroom
5. Where film is carried from machine to darkroom in containers, container may leak light

B. Radiation

1. Insufficient protection
   a. During delivery or transportation in laboratory or shop

b. Film storage bin

c. Loaded cassette racks—steel back should face toward source of radiation

d. Not enough protection for loading darkroom

2. Improper storage

a. Radium

b. Isotopes

c. X-ray machines

C. Chemical

1. Prolonged development (See item B under "HIGH DENSITY")

2. Developer contaminated

a. Foreign matter of any kind (Metals, etc.)

3. Contaminated chemicals

D. Deterioration of film

1. Age (Use oldest film first)

2. Storage conditions

a. Too high temperatures

1. Hot room

2. Cool room but near radiator or hot pipe

b. Too high humidity

1. Damp room

2. Moist air

3. Ammonia or other fumes present in darkroom or other work area

3. Delivery conditions

a. Moisture precipitation when cold box of film is opened in hot, humid room

b. Fresh boxes should be stored overnight at room temperature before opening

E. Excessive pressure on emulsions of unprocessed film

1. During storage

2. During manipulation in darkroom

F. Loaded cassettes stored near heat, sunlight or radiation

Stains on Radiographs

A. Yellow

1. Exhausted, oxidized developer

a. Old

b. Covers left off

c. Scum on developer surface

1. Oil from pipelines

2. Impure water used when mixing

3. Dust

2. Prolonged development

3. Insufficient rinsing

4. Exhausted fixing bath

B. Dichroic

1. Old, exhausted developer

a. Colloidal metallic silver

2. Nearly exhausted fixer

3. Developer containing small amounts of fixer or scum

4. Films partially fixed in weak fixer, exposed to light and refixed

5. Prolonged intermediate rinse in contaminated rinse water

Green tinted

A. Insufficient fixing or washing

Deposits on Radiographs

A. Metallic

1. Oxidized products from developer

2. Silver salts reacting with hydrogen sulfide in air to form silver sulfide

3. Silver loaded fixer

B. White or crystalline

1. Milky fixer

a. Hardener portion added too fast while mixing

b. Hardener portion added when too hot

   c. Excessive acidity
   d. Developer splashed into fixer
   e. Insufficient rinsing
  2. Prolonged washing

C. Grit

  1. Dirty water
  2. Dirt in dryer

Marks on Emulsion Surfaces

A. Runs

  1. Insufficient fixing
   a. Weakened fixer
   b. Unbalanced formula
   c. Exhausted ingredients
   d. Low acid content
    1. Deficient when fresh
    2. Diluted from rinse water
    3. Neutralized by developer because of insufficient or no rinsing
  2. Drying temperature too high
  3. Contact with hot viewing box

B. Blisters

  1. Formation of gas bubbles in gelatin
   a. Carbonate of developer reacting with acid of fixer
   b. Unbalanced processing temperatures
    1. Combination of hot fixer and cool developer
    2. Combination of cool fixer and hot developer
   c. Excessive acidity of fixer
   d. No agitation of film when first placed in fixer

C. Reticulation

  1. Non-uniform processing temperatures
   a. Developer (Hot)
   b. Fixer (Cool)
   c. Wash
  2. Weakened fixer with little hardening action

D. Frilling

  1. Weakened fixer with little hardening action
  2. Hot processing solutions
   a. Developer
   b. Fixer
   c. Wash

E. Drying marks from uneven drying of gelatin

  1. Excessive drying temperatures
  2. Extremely low humidity
  3. Puddies (Buckshot marks)
   a. Drops of water striking semi-dried emulsion surface
  4. Streaks
   a. Drops of water running down semi-dried emulsion surface
    1. Water splashes
    2. Drying air flow too rapid
    3. Insufficient or uneven squeeze last roller pair waterrack

F. White spots

  1. Screens pitted
  2. Grit or dust present on film or screens
  3. Chemical dust settling on film or screens (Particles of certain chemical dusts will also cause black spots)

G. Artifacts

  1. Crescents—rough handling
  2. Smudge marks—fingerprints or finger abrasions
  3. Bands in marginal areas usually due to screen mounting medium

Slow Drying

A. Waterlogged films

  1. Insufficient hardening in fixer
   a. Too short fixing period
   b. Weakened fixer from splashing

    c. Exhausted fixer

    d. Insufficient acidity (carry over dev. fixer)

  2. Wash water too warm

B. Incoming air too humid

C. Incoming air too cold

D. Air velocity too low

Streaks on Radiographs

A. Insufficient agitation while processing

B. Fog

C. Chemically active deposits (Dried chemicals)

D. Pressure fog

E. Scratches

  1. Careless handling

  2. Grit present in air, cassettes, or on illuminator

F. Exposure to white light before complete fixing

G. Uneven drying due to high temperature and low humidity

Lack of Detail or Fuzziness

A. Motion (Tube, film, subject)

  1. Inadequate immobilization

  2. Too long exposure

  3. Vibration of floor

  4. Slipping of subject on mount

  5. Stepping on and off operator's platform during exposure where control and tube are mounted on common mobile base

  6. Failure to arrest tube vibration after positioning before making exposure

B. Poor contact of intensifying screens

C. Improper distance relationship

  1. Object film distance too great

  2. Target film distance too short

D. Improper focal spot

  1. Too large

  2. Damaged (Cracked or pitted)

Static

A. Low humidity

B. Insulation

  1. Use of rubber gloves, shoes, finger cots, etc.

  2. Insulated flooring

C. Improper handling in:

  1. Removal from box

  2. Removal from interleaving paper

  3. Loading cassette

  4. Unloading cassette

  5. Loading hanger

  6. Films stacked before processing

Troubleshooting Guide-FUJI

IMAGE CONTRAST AND DENSITY

Contrast		
Problem	Possible Cause	Solutions
Image contrast consistently too low.	Contrast parameter set too low	Increase the GA. A 10% change in contrast equals .10 change in the GA. Change the GT (gradient type). This change affects other parameters such as GA, GS, and GC.
Image contrast consistently too high.	Contrast parameter set too high	Decrease the GA. A 10% change in contrast equals .10 change in the GA. Change the GT (gradient type). This change affects other parameters such as GA, GS, and GC.
Image contrast inconsistently too low in contrast.	Grid cut-off	Improper alignment of grid.

Contrast and Density		
Problem	Possible Cause	Solutions
Image contrast and density are too high or too low.	Improper selection of anatomical menu	Check to see that the image was processed under the correct menu name.
Image contrast and/or density increase or decrease day to day.	Film processing	Check the density (calibration) on the laser printer; adjust if needed. Check the chemicals for fatigue. Replenish or replace as needed.

Density		
Problem	Possible Cause	Solutions
Image is inconsistently dark and flat.	Improper exposure technique for EDR	Overlap of exposure when doing two on one exposures. Scatter radiation on the gap between split exposures. Blurred collimation edge. Improper split image pattern.
Image is white or unexposed.	Gross overexposure	Reduce the radiographic exposure. If the "S" number goes below <25 and the "L" value is greater than 2.0, image quality may be compromised.

(Courtesy of FUJIFILM Medical Systems USA, Inc.)

IMAGE QUALITY

Sharpness (Appearance of Unsharpness)		
Problem	Possible Cause	Solutions
Image looks unsharp in certain areas of interest.	Image contrast and/or density set too low	A higher contrast or higher density may improve the impression on sharpness. Try a slight increase in the GA or GS.
	RE too low	Increasing the RE increases sharpness. Note: Increasing the RE will increase the noise.
	RN too low	Higher frequency enhancement. Too much frequency enhancement will increase the graininess or artifacts.
	RT not adequate for this menu	The following RTs (U, T, P, and F) may increase the sharpness, especially in the low-density (bright) regions. RT of F will be the sharpest.

Graininess		
Problem	Possible Cause	Solutions
Overall image graininess for images in the same anatomical menu.	RE set too high	RE should be 0.0 to 1.0 for an enhanced image (too low of RE can seem like an unsharp image).
	RN set too high	Enhancement on a lower frequency.
	RT not adequate for this menu	RT's of Q, R, S may decrease graininess, especially in the low-density (bright) region.
	Contrast too high	Lower the GA to decrease the contrast. The impression of graininess may improve with lower contrast. A slight increase in the GS might be necessary.
	2K image data files "blown" up to life size images on larger cassette size studies	This occurs due to high levels of noise induced by the magnification process used to enlarge an image capture in a 2K $\times$ 2K format. An increase in exposure, compared to the original manufacturer's intentions may be required. Fuji HQ (4K $\times$ 4K) image capture is available to sites that require full resolution on all cassette sizes with no increase in exposure necessary.

Problem	Possible Cause	Solutions
Inconsistent grainy images	X-ray exposures too low	Increase X-ray exposure. As dose decreases X-ray noise (quantum noise increases). "S" numbers greater than 500-exhibit underexposure. Note: Even when a phototimer is used, resulting mAs may change depending on the type of cassette and detector (mostly due to backscatter characteristics from the cassette/detector). If the phototimer was optimized for conventional screen/film, it should be checked and adjusted when starting to use CR system.
	Wrong anatomical menu	Use the proper anatomical menu for the body part.
	Excessive scatter on image	Improper collimation. Only area of interest should be exposed; avoid, including extra anatomy. Use a grid on thickness over 10 cm.
	Grid cut-off	Improper alignment of grid.

Artifacts		
Problem	Possible Cause	Solutions
Artifacts appear on the border high-contrast anatomies and materials, such as bone and metal.	RE set too high	Strong enhancement may cause image processing artifact around high contrast edges.
White, irregular artifact appear on the image.	Mechanical damage to the phosphor	Check the surface of the IP, see if there is mechanical damage of the same shape.
White, grain-like artifacts appear on the image.	Phosphor damage or dust	Check the surface of the IP and see if any dust has adhered to it. If so, wipe it away using the proper cleaning technique.
		If there is no obvious dust, check the color of the IP surface. If the IP has a slight yellowish color, it means that moisture has damaged the protective layer and phosphor itself.
		Note: If liquid was left on the surface of the IP for a period of time, it might penetrate the phosphor. This usually happens if something other than anhydrous ethanol was used to clean the IP or if IP was put into the cassette before is was completely dried.

Artifacts Continued

Artifacts		
Problem	Possible Cause	Solutions
Appearance of double exposed images.	Double exposed	The auto density adjustment of CR images will produce a radiograph with normal appearing density and contrast if a previously used IP is accidentally re-exposed.
	Erasure systems malfunction	Contact the technical support hot line.

Improving Image Characteristics–KODAK

Use the following table to look up a general quality problem and find possible solutions.

Two tools are available for you to improve an image quality problem:

a. Changing contrast and brightness

b. Trained users can change user parameters

If you cannot correct the problem, contact the Kodak Technical Support Center (TSC) for further assistance.

Image Problem	Recommendations
Image is too light	• Decrease the brightness and then adjust the contrast if needed. If this causes clipping in the region of interest, switch to the raw image and adjust brightness and contrast on the raw image.
	• If images are consistently too light, contact your Kodak representative to increase the Density Shift in the system preferences for the body part, projection, and version.
Image is too dark	• Increase the brightness, and then adjust the contrast if needed. If this causes clipping in the region of interest, switch to the raw image and adjust brightness and contrast on the raw image.
	• If images are consistently too dark, contact your Kodak representative to decrease the Density Shift in the system preferences for the body part, projection, and version.
Image is too flat	• Increase the contrast, and adjust the brightness if needed.
	• If images are consistently too flat, contact your Kodak representative to increase the Contrast Factor in the system preferences for the body part and projection.
Image contrast is too high	• Decrease the brightness.
	• Change the tonescale type to Raw Data.
	• If image contrast is consistently too high, contact your Kodak representative to decrease the Contrast Factor in the system preferences for the body part, projection, and version.
Image is too grainy when no edge enhancement is applied (i.e., None is chosen for edge enhancement)	The image may be underexposed. Check the exposure index in the exam information.

(Used with permission of Eastman Kodak Company)

Image Problem	Recommendations

Image is too grainy with edge enhancement applied	• The image may be underexposed. Check the exposure index in the exam information.
	• Reduce the level of edge enhancement.
	• Change the tonescale to Raw Data tonescale type and adjust contrast and brightness. Remove edge enhancement by changing it to None.
	• If you are using Custom values to enhance a Chest exam:
	  – Lower the High Density Boost to reduce noise in the lung region.
	  – Decrease the Low Density Boost to reduce noise in the mediastinum or bony regions.
	• If the enhanced images are consistently too grainy, speak to your Kodak representative about specifying a lower USM boost factor in the system preferences for the body part, projection, and version.

No image	• Confirm an image was captured on the plate. You can check this by changing the tonescale type to Raw Data and setting the edge enhancement to None. • If the image was captured, adjust the contrast and brightness to produce an acceptable image.
Image is all white or all black	• Check the GAMMA correction level through the Calibration button on the Administrative menu. If the GAMMA is set to 0, the image will be black. If set to 5, the image will be white. • Confirm an image was captured on the plate. You can check this by changing the tonescale type to Raw Data and setting the edge enhancement to None. • Remove black surround.
Printed image has stripes running through it	• Check laser printer for errors; find out if problem is restricted to one QCW or for all prints produced on that particular printer. • Check clinical and diagnostic workstations to see if the same problems occurs when viewing the distributed image.
Image does not show enough detail	• If large edges are not clearly defined, increase the matrix size. • If small edges are not clearly defined, decrease the matrix size. • If the area missing detail is in a low density region, increase the low density boost. • If the area missing detail is in a high density region, increase the high density boost.

Answers to Case Studies

The Case of the Mysterious Mammals

Chapter 1, p. 18
Bats

The Case of the Unidentified Flying Object in the Skull

Chapter 5, p. 104
This patient was shot in the left temporal region by an arrow. The shaft was broken off prior to the time the radiograph was taken.

The Case of Lumpy

Chapter 15, p. 237
Theodore Bear

The Case of the Injured Animal

Chapter 16, p. 243
This is a rodent, a muskrat. The cause of death was a severed thoracic vertebral column, the result of being caught in a trap in the Ohio woods.

The Case of the White Snakes

Chapter 17, p. 254
The radiographer failed to observe that the high-voltage cables were within the primary beam field. Observe the sheath of grounding net inside the upper cable.

The Case of the Colon in the Spider's Web

Chapter 20, p. 302
This patient was unable to hold the barium within the colon and the sheet has become barium soaked. The wrinkled sheet is dense enough to make a distinct image under the patient.

The Case of the Line in the Stomach

Chapter 22, p. 330
The stomach is half filled with liquid barium. The line is an air-fluid level between the air and barium.

The Case of the Missing Lower Pelvis

Chapter 23, p. 341
This patient is quite obese and the large volume of soft tissue that has fallen down over the pelvis is demonstrated with an appropriate density. However, these technical factors produce much too much density for the pelvis. A second radiograph to demonstrate the pelvis, shown here, fails to demonstrate the abdomen. A case of "You can't have your cake and eat it too."

The Case of the Deep Sea Rodeo

Chapter 24, p. 354
A seahorse

The Case of the Animal with the Large Calcified Tumor-Like Mass

Chapter 28, p. 416
A chicken's egg about to be laid

The Case of the Last Dinner

Chapter 35, p. 515
There are no skeletal remains of the snake's last dinner on this image, but it's good practice to always examine your radiographs with careful attention to detail; the last dinner could have been demonstrated if it had been eaten more recently.

The Case of the Dripping Film

Chapter 38, p. 551
The horizontal lines are pi lines, so called because they are spaced apart by pi times the diameter of the first film processing roller. They are caused when developer precipitates onto the top rollers at the level of the chemistry when left in the tank overnight. When the first film is processed, the precipitate is deposited on the film emulsion each time the roller turns. The drip marks are most likely from developer solution that was splattered onto the film while it was being held vertically before processing.

The Case of the Ghostly Plants

Chapter 41, p. 597
A peony

The Case of the Mysterious Mammal

Chapter 44, p. 672
Loggerhead turtle *(Caretta, caretta)*

Epigraph Sources and Credits

Chapter 1 "Helping with the Math Homework" reprinted with permission of Louisiana State University Press from *In All This Rain* by John Stone. Copyright 1980 by John Stone.

Chapters 2, 3, 7, 8, 9, and 38 from Otto Glasser, *Dr. W. C. Röntgen*, 2nd edition, 1972. Courtesy of Charles C Thomas, Publisher, Springfield, Illinois.

Chapters 4 and 31 from *The Magic Mountain (Der Zauberberg)* by Thomas Mann, originally published by S. Fischer Verlag, Berlin, 1924; translated from the German by H. T. Lowe-Porter, New York: Alfred A. Knopf, 1965.

Chapter 5 by permission from "One More Time," copyright, Patricia Goedicke.

Chapters 6, 13, and 29 from W. D. Coolidge, "Experiences with the Roentgen-Ray Tube," *American Journal of Roentgenology*, 54, 6, 1945.

Chapter 10 by permission, copyright Celia Gilbert, "X-Ray" from *Queen of Darkness*, Viking Press, New York, NY, 1977.

Chapters 11, 28, 32, and 36 from E. C. Jerman, "An Analysis of the End-Result: The Radiograph," *Radiology*, 6, 59–62, 1926.

Chapter 12 from A. H. Compton in the preface to the first edition of *X-Rays and Electrons*, reprinted in *X-Rays in Theory and Experiment*, by A. H. Compton and H. K. Allison, 2nd edition, New York: Van Nostrand and Company, 1935.

Chapter 14 by Lawrence K. Russell, *Life*, March 12, 1896.

Chapter 15 lyrics from the song "X-Ray Vision" from the Capitol-EMI album *Mystery Ticket*, by Moon Martin, Pete Sinfield, and Terry Taylor, copyright 1982, Paper Music, Ltd.

Chapter 16 from William Carlos Williams, *The Autobiography of William Carlos Williams*, copyright 1951, William Carlos Williams. Reprinted by permission of New Directions Publishing Corporation.

Chapter 17 lyrics from the song "I'm Looking through You" from the Capitol-EMI Records, Inc. album, *Rubber Soul*, by John Lennon and Paul McCartney, Northern Songs, Ltd., copyright 1965, EMI Records, Inc.

Chapter 18 from Hollis E. Potter, "The Bucky Diaphragm Principle Applied to Roentgenography," *The American Journal of Roentgenology*, 7, 292–295, 1920.

Chapter 19 quoted from the Jerman Memorial Lecture given by Arthur W. Fuchs during the 1950 Annual Meeting of the American Society of X-Ray Technicians in Cincinnati, Ohio.

Chapter 20 reprinted by permission of Margaret Atwood, from *Selected Poems I*, published by Houghton Mifflin, U.S.A and *Selected Poems 1966–1984*, published by McClelland and Stewart, Canada, copyright 1968.

Chapter 21 reprinted by permission of the estate of Howard Moss from "In The X-Ray Room" from *New Selected Poems*, Antheneum Press, copyright MacMillan Publishing Company, 1985.

Chapter 22 as quoted in *From Immigrant to Inventor*, the autobiography of M. Pupin, in *Trail of the Invisible Light* by Otto Glasser as published by Charles C Thomas, Publisher, Springfield, Illinois, 1965.

Chapter 23 as quoted from *Pall Mall Gazette*, March, 1986 by Arthur W. Fuchs in "Radiography of 1896," Image 9: 4–17, 1960.

Chapter 24 by permission from Christopher C. Kuni, *Introduction to Computers and Digital Processing in Medical Imaging*, Chicago, Mosby-Year Book, Inc., 1988.

Chapter 25 from William Shakespeare Sonnet XXIV.

Chapter 26 from Oscar Wilde.

Chapter 27 from Gerhart S. Schwarz, *Unit-Step Radiography*, 1961. Courtesy of Charles C Thomas, Publisher, Springfield, Illinois.

Chapter 30 quoted from Merrill C. Sosman.

Chapter 33 William B. Hendee and Raymond P. Rossi in *Quality Assurance for Radiographic X-Ray Units and Associated Equipment*, Rockville, MD: U.S. Department of Health, Education, and Welfare, Public Health Service, Food and Drug Administration, Bureau of Radiological Health, HEW Publication FDA 79–8094, 1979.

Chapter 34 from Arthur W. Fuchs in the Preface to *Principles of Radiographic Exposure and Processing*, 1st edition, 1949. Charles C Thomas, Publisher, Springfield, Illinois.

Chapter 35 quoted from the Jerman Memorial Lecture given by John B. Cahoon, Jr. during the 1961 Annual Meeting of the American Society of X-Ray Technicians.

Chapter 37 from the text of the chapter.

Chapter 39 from William Shakespeare, *Hamlet*, III, iv, 18.

Chapter 40 Arthur W. Fuchs, "Edison and Roentgenology," *The American Journal of Roentgenology and Radium Therapy*, 57, (2), 145–156, 1947.

Chapter 41 from French patent 536464, June 3, 1921 by Andre-Edmund-Marie-Bocage, entitled "Method of, and Apparatus for, Radiography on a Moving Plate," as quoted by J. T. Littleton in *Tomography: Physical Principles and Clinical Applications*. Section 17: Golden's Diagnostic Radiology Series. Baltimore, MD: Williams & Wilkins, 1976.

Chapter 42 attributed to Hippocrates.

Chapter 43 from Margaret Hoing (The First Lady of Radiologic Technology) in *A History of the American Society of X-Ray Technicians*, Chicago: American Society of Radiologic Technologists, 1952.

Chapter 44 quoted from Allan Cormack, upon being informed that he and Godfrey Hounsfield were to share the 1979 Nobel Prize for Medicine for the invention of computed tomography.

Chapter 45 from Edward M. Purcell, "Research in Nuclear Magnetism," *Nobel Lectures: Physics 1901–1995*, New York: World Scientific Publishing, 1998.

Glossary

abscess An encapsulated infection.

absolute value The meaning of a number equal to the distance of that number from zero on the number line.

acceptance limits The range of images determined to be of good quality by a given individual or department.

acromegaly An overgrowth of the hands, feet, face, and jaw resulting from hypersecretion of growth hormones.

activator A chemical used in film developing in the fixer solution to maintain an acidic pH to enhance the functioning of the clearing agent.

active osteomyelitis Initial loss in bone tissue resulting from a bone infection.

activity Describes the quantity of radioactive material; expressed as the number of radioactive atoms that undergo decay per unit time.

actual focal spot The physical area of the focal track that is impacted.

added filtration Any filtration that occurs outside the tube and housing before the image receptor.

additive condition A disease that causes body tissues to thicken, increase in atomic number, or increase in density, requiring an increase in technical factors to achieve proper image receptor exposure.

adhesive A thin coating applied to the base material before it is coated with the emulsion to prevent bubbles or other distortion during processing or handling.

admittance The measure of resistance in an AC current when the expression 1/R is used.

aerophagia A psychological disorder resulting in abnormal swallowing of air.

afterglow Delayed phosphorescent emission; also called screen lag.

agitation Stirring up of the processing solutions.

air core transformer Arrangement of two coils of wire in proximity to facilitate induction.

air kerma The kinetic energy released per unit of mass air.

ALARA As low as reasonably achievable.

algebraic expression A mathematical sentence or term consisting of letters and/or numbers that are multiplied, divided, added, subtracted, or raised to a power.

aliasing Occurs when spatial frequency exceeds the Nyquist frequency and the incoming data are sampled less than twice per cycle.

alpha particle Contains two protons and two neutrons, is equivalent to a helium nucleus, and is emitted from the nuclei of heavy elements as they undergo radioactive decay; has a great mass and a positive charge.

alternating current (AC) Electrons move first in one direction and then reverse and move in the opposite direction.

ammeter A device used to measure current connected in a series; measured in amperes.

amp (A) The unit of current; also known as the ampere.

ampere (A) The unit of current; also known as the amp.

amplitude The intensity of the wave defined by its maximal height.

analog computer A machine that handles data composed of continuously varying electrical currents.

anatomically programmed radiography A computerized exposure control system; technique charts using existing exposure systems that are stored in the data memory banks.

annihilation reaction Matter being converted back into energy as a result of a positron combining with a negative electron, which creates two photons moving in opposite directions.

anode The positive side of the x-ray tube; serves as a target surface for high-voltage electrons from the filament, conducts the high voltage from the cathode back into the x-ray generator circuitry, and serves as the primary thermal conductor.

anode assembly Consists of the anode, stator, and rotor.

anode cooling chart Permits the calculation of the time necessary for the anode to cool enough for additional exposures to be taken.

anode heel effect Due to the geometry of the angled anode target, the radiation intensity is greater on the cathode side.

anorexia nervosa A psychological eating disorder resulting in extreme weight loss.

antihalation coating A substance applied to the back of a single-emulsion film designed to absorb light coming from the emulsion and preventing backscatter.

aortic aneurysm A large dilation of the aorta.

aperture diaphragm A flat sheet of metal, usually lead, with a hole cut in the center and attached to the x-ray port.

approximate entrance skin exposure An estimation of the dose of radiation related to a specific type of radiologic exam or procedure.

armature A coil of wire that acts as a conductor.

array detection Information received from an entire area at once.

artificial permanent magnet Manufactured from steel alloy called alnico, composed of aluminum, nickel, and cobalt.

ascites Fluid accumulation within the peritoneal cavity.

aseptic necrosis Death of tissue.

atelectasis Collapse of the lung.

atom The smallest particle of an element that still possesses the chemical properties of that element.

atomic mass number (A) The mass of an atom; used when precision is not necessary; is equal to the number of protons and neutrons in the nucleus of an atom.

atomic mass unit (amu) The mass of the particles of an atom.

atomic number The number of nuclear protons in an atom unique to each element; also known as the Z number.

atomic reactor A device that converts nuclear energy to electrical energy.

atrophy A wasting away of body tissue with diminished cell proliferation.

attenuation The reduction in the number of x-ray photons in the beam, and subsequent loss of energy, as the beam passes through matter.

automatic exposure control A device programmed to terminate the radiographic exposure time; also called automatic exposure device.

automatic exposure device A device programmed to terminate the radiographic exposure time; also called automatic exposure control.

autotransformer A transformer that automatically sets by adjustments.

average gradient The average slope of the D log E curve at the straight line portion of the curve.

backscatter radiation Photons that deflect back toward the source, traveling in the opposite direction of the incident photon.

band-pass filtering Amplifies or deletes all but a selected range or band of frequencies.

bandwidth The frequency response from the incoming signal.

base The base material that the film is made from; it is usually polyester, tough, stable, rigid, and uniformly lucent; it usually contains a blue tint.

base plus fog The density at no exposure; the density that is inherent in the film.

battery A device that converts chemical energy into electrical energy.

becquerel The SI unit for activity.

beta particle Identical to an electron, except it is emitted from the nuclei of radioactive materials; it is very light and negatively charged.

bias focusing Engagement of a small focal spot while a negative voltage that is applied to the focusing cup acts to reduce the size of the electron stream, creating a smaller focal spot.

binary machine language Language used by computers that operates with a two-symbol alphabet; 0 for off or 1 for on.

bit Binary digits.

blur The streaking or smearing that results in the loss of nearly all recorded detail of objects outside the focal plane.

bowel obstruction Abnormal accumulation of air and fluid resulting from a blockage in the bowel.

bremsstrahlung interaction An incident electron interacts with the force field of the nucleus, causing the incident electron to slow down, thus diverting the electron's course. The electron loses energy and changes direction. The energy lost is a bremsstrahlung photon, and the photon energy is half the difference between the entering and exiting kinetic energy of the electron.

brightness The concept of density as it is displayed on a soft-copy monitor for digitial images.

bronchiectasis Chronic dilation of the bronchi.

brush A device, attached to slip rings that allows the circuit to remain stationary while the armature rotates without breaking the electrical contact between them.

byte An 8-bit word.

calcified stones Calcium deposits in the form of stones that can be found in the gallbladder and kidneys.

calibrate To adjust a tool of measurement to zero.

caliper A device used to measure part thickness.

capacitor A device capable of accumulating and storing an electrical charge.

carcinoma Malignancy.

cardiomegaly Enlargement of the heart.

c-arm tube suspension system A type of radiography equipment that utilizes a c-shaped arm device to support the tube and the image receptor that allows the tube and image receptor to be rotated to new positions.

carriage The arm that supports the fluoroscopic equipment suspended over the table.

cathode The negative side of the x-ray tube; produces a thermionic cloud, conducts the high voltage to the gap between the cathode and anode, and focuses the electron stream as it heads for the anode.

cathode assembly Consists of the filament, focusing cup, and associated wiring.

cathode ray tube (CRT) imaging A type of imaging that requires a film that is sensitive to the light emitted by the CRT; also called video imaging.

caudad Longitudinal angulation in which the tube is angled toward the patient's feet.

central processing unit (CPU) The part of the computer that directs information to and from the various components that make up the computer system.

cephalad Longitudinal angulation in which the tube is angled toward the patient's head.

characteristic cascade The reaction of electrons dropping into the holes created during a characteristic interaction until there is only a hole in the outer shell.

characteristic curve A radiographic relationship between the amount of exposure and the resultant density on the film; also known as D log E curve, sensitometric curve, and Hurter and Driffield curve.

characteristic interaction The incident electron interacts with an inner shell electron, knocking out the inner shell electron and continuing in a slightly different direction, which creates a hole in the inner shell, making the shell unstable.

characteristic peak Occurs when K-shell emissions reach their effective energy range of 69 keV.

characteristic photon An x-ray photon created by the electron transfer from one shell to another.

chemical energy The form of energy released during a chemical reaction.

chemical fog The effect on a film when unexposed silver halides are reduced.

chemical precipitation A type of silver recovery system that uses chemicals to break down in the fixer and release electrons; the silver is heavy and falls to the bottom of the tank.

chronic osteomyelitis New bone growth at the site of a chronic bone infection.

circuit breaker A device constructed to interrupt a circuit before a dangerous temperature is reached.

circulation system A part of the automatic processing system designed to stabilize temperatures, agitate solutions, mix the chemistry, and filter the solutions.

cirrhosis Fibrotic changes in the liver causing the liver to enlarge and ascites to develop.

clearing agent The primary agent of the fixer.

clearing time Twice the time necessary for the milky appearance of the film to disappear.

closed-core transformer Arrangement of two coils of wire each filled with an iron core in proximity to facilitate induction that converges the inside and outside lines of force through the core.

coating The phase of the film production process in which the adhesive layer is applied to the base, then the emulsion and, finally, the supercoat.

coercivity The energy that caused reorientation of the magnetic dipoles.

coherent scatter An interaction between x-rays and matter characterized by interaction between a very low-energy x-ray photon and matter causing the electron to vibrate at the same frequency as the incident photon, which then produces a secondary photon with the same energy and wavelength as the incident photon but which travels in a different direction; also called classical scatter or unmodified scatter.

collimater pitch The pitch of a single detector within a MDCT array of image receptors.

collimator A set of lead shutters at right angles to one another which move in opposing pairs.

commutator ring A single ring that is divided in half, with each half connected to one end of the armature wire.

compensating filter Used to even out unequal densities.

compound A complex substance; two or more elements that are chemically united in a definite proportion.

compound filter The use of two or more materials to complement one another in their absorbing abilities; also known as K-edge filters.

compression band A piece of equipment used to restrain a patient or compress abdominal tissue.

Compton effect An interaction between x-rays and matter characterized by an incident x-ray photon interacting with a loosely bound outer-shell electron, resulting in removal of the electron from the shell, which then proceeds in a different direction as a scattered photon; also known as Compton scattering.

Compton electron The dislodged electron resulting from Compton scattering; also called a recoil electron.

Compton scattered photon The photon that exits the atom in a different direction as a result of Compton scattering.

Compton scattering An interaction between x-rays and matter characterized by an incident x-ray photon interacting with a loosely bound outer-shell electron, resulting in removal of the electron from the shell, which then proceeds in a different direction as a scattered photon; also known as Compton effect.

computed radiography (CR) A type of indirect digital radiography; the radiographer must move the detector between image acquisition and display.

computed tomography unit Specialized radiography equipment that allows the taking of sectional images.

concentration Law of electrostatics that states the greatest intensity of charge will be on the surface where the curvature is the sharpest.

conductance The measure of resistance in a DC current when the expression 1/R is used.

conduction band An area within the force field of an atom beyond the valence band.

conductor A material that allows electrons to flow freely.

cone A circular aperture diaphragm with metal extensions that flare or diverge with the upper diameter smaller than the bottom flared end.

cone cell Cells in the retina of the eye that are responsible for color vision.

congestive heart failure Increased venous congestion in the heart resulting from diminished cardiac output.

contact surgical radiography A type of imaging which uses nonscreen film in sterilized packages.

contrast One of the properties that comprise visibility of detail; the difference between adjacent densities.

contrast mask A tool to help focus on contrast in a selected area.

contrast media injection device Type of instrument that is used to inject contrast media into vessels for radiographic studies.

contrast perception The ability to visually distinguish differences in density or contrast.

conversion efficiency The ability of the phosphor to emit as much light per x-ray photon interaction as possible which is related to the screen speed.

convolution The process of modifying pixel values by a mathematical formula; also referred to as mask.

coulomb per kilogram A radiographically derived unit of the SI system, abbreviated as C/kg, formerly known as the roentgen.

criss-cross grid Two linear grids placed on top of one another so that the lead strips form a criss-cross pattern.

cross-hatched grid Two linear grids placed on top of one another so that the lead strips form a criss-cross pattern.

crossover effect Blurring of the image caused by light from one screen crossing into the light from another screen.

crossover network Part of the automatic processing transport system designed to bend and turn the film when it reaches the top of the transport rack and must be directed down to the next tank or section.

cryogen Cooling agent.

crystal production The part of the film manufacturing process that must be done in total darkness Silver nitrate and potassium bromide are combined in the presence of gelatin; the silver bromide precipitates out and the potassium nitrate can be washed away as a waste product.

curie (Ci) The unit of activity.

current The quantity or the number of electrons flowing.

cylinder A circular aperture diaphragm with metal extensions that have the same diameter at the top and bottom.

D log E curve A radiographic relationship between the amount of exposure and the resultant density on the film; also known as characteristic curve, sensitometric curve, and Hurter and Driffield curve.

D_{max} The maximum density the film is capable of recording.

data Collected facts.

deconvolution The process of returning the pixel values to their original level by a reverse process.

definition One of the geometric properties of image quality; the degree of geometric sharpness or accuracy of structural lines actually recorded in the image; also referred to as detail, recorded detail, sharpness, spatial resolution.

degenerative arthritis Inflammation of the joints resulting in destruction of adjoining joint tissue.

densitometer An instrument that provides a readout of the amount of blackening (density) on a film.

density One of the photographic properties that comprise visibility of detail; the degree of overall blackening of the film.

destructive condition A disease that causes body tissues to thin, decrease in atomic number, or decrease in density, requiring a decrease in technical factors to achieve proper image receptor exposure.

detail One of the geometric properties of image quality; the degree of geometric sharpness or accuracy of structural lines actually recorded in the image; also referred to as recorded detail, definition, sharpness, spatial resolution.

detail extremity radiography A type of imaging that uses fine-grain films with slow-speed screens.

deterministic effect Results of radiation exposure for which a threshold dose of radiation is assumed (e.g., cataracts, sterility).

developing The step in film processing; silver is deposited at the latent image sites and an image becomes visible.

diagnostic Methods used to determine the source or cause of a disease, disorder, or traumatic injury.

diamagnetic Materials weakly repelled by all magnetic fields (e.g., beryllium, bismuth, lead).

dielectric The insulation between two plates in a capacitor.

digital angiography Produces one image similar to the last fluoroscopy hold vascular image; also called spot imaging.

digital cineradiography Takes numerous exposures (frames) in a second of time.

digital computer A unit that processes data composed of discrete quantities of current.

digital mammography unit A dedicated breast imaging machine that utilizes a CR/DR image receptor system.

digital subtraction angiography Eliminates bone and soft tissue structures from an image so that only the contrast-filled vessels remain.

digital tomosynthesis Digital radiographic tomography.

diode A rectifying semiconductor made by sandwiching p-type crystal with an n-type to form a p-n junction.

direct acquisition A type of digital radiography in which the detector and reader are a permanent part of a table or wall unit; cassettes are not needed; converts incoming x-ray photons directly to an electronic signal.

direct current (DC) All electrons travel in the same direction.

direct digital radiography (DR) A type of digital radiography in which the detector and reader are a permanent part of a table or wall unit; cassettes are not needed.

direct square law A direct relationship is necessary to compensate for the changes in intensity and film density.

direct variation One quantity is a multiple of a second quantity.

distortion One of the geometric properties affecting radiographic image quality; a misrepresentation of the size and shape of the structures being examined.

distribution Law of electrostatics that states charges reside on the surfaces of conductors but are evenly distributed throughout nonconductors.

dose limit Radiation exposure limits that are pertinent to the protection of radiation workers.

dosimeter A mechanism that can measure amounts of radiation.

drive system Part of the automatic processing transport system designed as a series of mechanical devices to turn the numerous rollers in the processor from power supplied by a single motor.

dryer system The final stage of film processing that removes the excess water, cools and dries the film, and seals the film for viewing and storage.

drying The process of film developing in which hot air is forced over both sides of the film as it exits the processor.

dual focus A two-filament arrangement within the x-ray tube.

duplication film A type of film designed to provide an exact image of the original film.

duplitized Describes a film that is coated with emulsion of both sides.

dwell time The time allotted for the fixer in a silver recovery unit to sit to permit chemical reactions to occur.

dynamic range The concept of contrast as it is displayed on a soft-copy monitor for digital images; range of density/brightness of the display monitor light emission.

dynamometer Used to measure alternating current when electromagnets are used.

echo time (TE) The time between a 90-degree pulse and the echo during a spin-echo pulse sequence.

eddy current loss Result of currents opposing the cause which produced them.

edema Swelling.

edge enhancement Increase in contrast due to high-pass filtering; also known as sharpening.

edge spread function (ESF) Expression of the boundaries of an image.

effective dose The sum of the weighted equivalent doses for all irradiated tissues and organs; used to measure the radiation and organ system specific damage in man.

effective focal spot The area of the focal spot that is projected out of the tube toward the object being radiographed.

effective target angle In mammography, measured from the vertical central ray point.

electric current Electrons that are moving in predominantly the same direction.

electric field A force field; the result of the composite forces of the charges residing within an object.

electrical circuit A pathway that permits electrons to move in a complete circle from their source, through resisting electrical devices and back to the source.

electrical energy The result of movement of electrons; also known as electricity.

electricity The result of movement of electrons; also known as electrical energy.

electrification Describes the process of electron charges being added to or subtracted from an object.

electrolytic A type of silver recovery system that passes a current from a cathode to an anode through the fixer; the ionized silver is attracted to the negatively charged cathode.

electromagnet Temporary magnet produced by moving electric current.

electromagnetic energy A form of energy resulting from electric and magnetic disturbances in space.

electromagnetic radiation (EM) A form of energy that is the result of electric and magnetic disturbances in space.

electromagnetic relay A device used to protect the radiographer from electric shock by isolating control buttons on the x-ray console from the actual circuit in which high voltage is flowing; similar to a circuit breaker.

electromagnetic spectrum Describes the different forms of electromagnetic radiation.

electromotive force (emf) The force or strength of electron flow; also known as potential difference.

electron (e$^-$) Negatively charged subatomic particle of an atom.

electron binding energy (E$_b$) The amount of energy needed to remove the electron from the atom.

electron volt (eV) Measurement of the binding energy of an electron; the energy one electron will have when it is accelerated by an electrical potential of 1 volt.

electronic medical record All patient medical documentation stored in electronic formats.

electrostatic The study of the distribution of fixed charges, or electrons, that are at rest.

element A simple substance; it cannot be broken down into any simpler substances by ordinary means.

elongation Projection of an object, making it appear longer than it really is.

emaciation A generalized wasting of body tissue.

emphysema The overdistention of lung tissues by air.

empyema Pus in the thoracic cavity.

emulsion with crystals A gelatin in which photosensitive silver halide crystals are suspended. It is an extremely thin coating that acts as a neutral lucent suspension medium for the silver halide crystals to separate and allow chemicals to interact with them.

entrance roller Specially designed crossover network to begin the film traveling from the feed tray down into the developer section.

entrance skin exposure The area where the maximum exposure received by the patient lies.

envelope The entire cathode and anode assembly is housed within this glass or metal structure.

equation A statement that contains an equal sign.

equivalent equation Equations that have the same solutions.

excitation Process in which electrons in an atom are moved to a higher energy state without actually being removed from the atom.

exposure amplitude The total distance the tube travels during the tomographic exposure.

exposure maintenance formula A direct square law; mAs must increase when distance increases, and vice versa, in order to maintain image receptor exposure.

exposure switch A remote control device that permits current to flow through the circuit.

extended cycle A technique for processing radiographs whereby the speed of a standard film can be increased up to 35 percent and radiographic contrast increased measurably, by doubling the time the film is in the developer solution.

external beam evaluation The measurement of the quantity and quality of the external radiation beam.

extrafocal radiation Photons that were not produced at the focal spot; also called off-focus radiation.

farad (f) The unit of capacitance.

ferromagnetic Materials that are highly permeable and susceptible to induction (e.g., iron, cobalt, nickel).

fibrosarcoma Malignant tumor of the metaphysics of bone resulting in reduction of bone composition.

field survey instrument Portable device used to measure radiation in a given location.

15 percent rule An increase in kVp by 15 percent that causes a doubling in exposure and vice versa.

filament A small coil of thin thoriated tungsten wire.

filament circuit Supplies the filament of the x-ray tube with properly modified power.

film badge dosimeter Two pieces of film having different sensitivities to x-rays contained within a light, tight envelope; the film emulsion darkens in response to the radiation exposure received.

film processing system The equipment used to process radiographic film for viewing of the radiographic image

filter Any material designed to effectively absorb photons from the x-ray beam.

fixed A piece of equipment that remains in one place and is not movable.

fixing The process of removing undeveloped silver halides to make the image permanent for viewing.

flat field detector Descriptive term used for the plates used in both direct and indirect digital systems.

flat panel detector Descriptive term used for the plates used in both direct and indirect digital systems.

Fleming's hand rules A series of easily remembered aids to help with the relationship between electricity and magnetism.

flip angle Rotation of magnetization due to a Larmor frequency pulse.

flood replenishment A type of replenishing system used for low-volume systems; controlled by a timer that floods the developer and fixer tanks with replenisher at regular intervals.

floor suspension system A type of radiography unit that uses a tube support column mounted on the floor.

floor-to-ceiling suspension system A type of radiography unit that uses a pair of rails for longitudinal positioning.

fluorescence The ability of a material to emit light instantaneously in responses to excitation within 1 nanosecond.

fluoroscopic screen A specialized x-ray tube with an image receptor which can be viewed during an x-ray exposure.

fluoroscopic spot filming A type of imaging that is done with 70 mm roll film or 105 mm film chips that are sensitive to green light.

fluoroscopy A dynamic radiographic examination; involves active diagnosis during an examination.

flux density Determined by field strength and the arc in which the lines of flux are located.

flux gain A measurement of the increase in light photons due to the conversion efficiency of the output screen.

focal plane The section; also section level, layer height, object plane, depth of focus.

focal point The portion of the anode where the high-voltage electron stream will impact.

focal spot The portion of the anode where the high-voltage electron stream will impact.

focal track The portion of the anode where the high-voltage electron stream will impact. When discussing a rotating anode this describes the circular path that will be impacted by the electron beam.

focus The portion of the anode where the high-voltage electron stream will impact.

focused grid A grid created with the central grid strips parallel with the strips becoming more inclined as they move away from the central axis; the lines would intersect along a point in space called the line of convergence.

focusing cup A shallow depression in the cathode assembly designed to house the filament.

footboard A piece of equipment used with a tilting table that allows the patient to stand when the table is upright.

foreshortening Projection of an object, making it appear shorter than it really is.

fractional focal spot A very small focal spot; usually a fraction of a millimeter in size.

free induction decay (FID) The simplest form of loss of the MR signal due to protons becoming out of phase with one another.

frequency The number of waves that passes a particular point in a given time frame.

friction Electrification that occurs when one object is rubbed against another and, due to differences in the number of electrons available on each, electrons travel from one to the other.

fulcrum The pivot point around which the motions of the tube and the image receptor are centered.

full-wave rectification The conversion of the opposing half of the incoming electron flow to always move in the same direction, instead of discarding half the cycle.

fuse A device constructed to interrupt a circuit before a dangerous temperature is reached.

galvanometer Used to measure direct current when permanent magnets are used.

gamma A measure of the slope of the straight line portion of the D log E curve at the speed point.

gantry The movable frame of the CT unit.

gasses A light mixture that has neither shape nor volume.

gauss (G) The unit used for measuring magnetic flux density.

generator A device that converts mechanical energy to electrical energy using moving lines of flux in relationship to a conductor to induce current; also known as a dynamo.

genetic Describes the effects of radiation that appear in the descendants of the individual being irradiated.

gout A metabolic disease that can cause a reduction in bone composition.

gradient point The slope of any portion of the D log E curve.

gray (Gy) Unit of absorbed energy or dose; 1 joule of energy absorbed in each kilogram of absorbing material.

grid A device used to improve contrast of the radiographic image.

grid-biased A type of tube that quickly regulates the flow of electrons, producing x-ray photons.

grid-controlled A type of tube that quickly regulates the flow of electrons, producing x-ray photons.

grid cut-off The result of the primary beam being angled into the lead strips.

grid frequency The number of grid lines per inch or centimeter.

grid-pulsed A type of tube that quickly regulates the flow of electrons producing x-ray photons.

grid ratio The ratio of the height of the lead strips to the distance between the strips.

ground potential A neutral reference point for discussing charges; the earth is defined as zero.

gyromagnetic ratio The ratio of the magnetic moment to the moment of inertia.

halation An effect on a radiographic image caused when light that is reflected from the air interfaces on the back of the base material.

half-value layer (HVL) The amount of absorbing material that will reduce the intensity of the primary beam to one-half its original value.

half-wave rectification Suppressed rectification resulting from only half of the incoming alternating current being converted to pulsating direct current; called self-rectification.

handgrip A piece of equipment that allows the patient to grip when the table is being tilted for added support and reassurance.

hard copy Images that are visualized on film.

hardener A chemical used in film processing that controls the swelling of the gelatin to prevent scratches and abrasions to the emulsion during processing; in a fixer solution must function in an acidic environment.

hardware Computer equipment.

head unit Specialized radiography equipment used to conduct cranial studies.

heat The result of the motion of atoms and molecules; also known as thermal energy.

heat exchanger The part of the automatic processing system in which a thermostat is used to heat the developer which is then routed to a circulation coil to heat the fixer by conduction.

hemothorax The filling of the pleural cavity with blood.

high-pass filtering Amplifies or deletes all but the high frequencies.

histogram Generated by dividing a scanned area into pixels and determining the signal intensity for each pixel; can be calculated for specific anatomy and procedures.

hospital information system (HIS) The electronic database used in the hospital to store, generate, and retrieve information on patients.

housing cooling chart Permits the calculation of the time necessary for the housing to cool enough for additional exposures to be made.

Hurter and Driffield (H&D) curve A radiographic relationship between the amount of exposure and the resultant density on the film; also known as characteristic curve, sensitometric curve, and D log E curve.

hydrocephalus Dilatation of fluid-filled cerebral ventricles resulting in enlargement of the head.

hydroquinone A developing agent that slowly reduces silver and produces heavy density.

hydrothorax The filling of the pleural cavity with serous fluid.

hyperparathyroidism Oversecretion of the parathyroid hormone, causing calcium to leave bone and enter the bloodstream.

hysteresis loss Results from energy expended as the continually changing AC current magnetizes, demagnetizes, and remagnetizes the core material; also called lagging loss.

I^2R loss Results from the inherent resistance to current flow that is found in all conductors; power lost from resistance is proportional to the square of current; sometimes called copper loss.

identity An equation in which all numeric values substituted for the unknown will give a true statement.

image intensification tube Video camera and monitor used to view fluoroscopic images.

image receptor (film) The medium used to capture the radiographic image for recording.

imaging noise Background information that the imaging receptor receives.

incident electron The electrons from the thermionic cloud that arrive at the anode target.

incoming-line current The alternating current that is supplied to buildings; usually supplied in three-phase power cycle; also called the mains.

indirect acquisition The radiographer must move the detector between image acquisition and display; a two-part process involving a scintillator (which converts incoming x-ray photons to light) and a photodetector (which converts light to an electronic signal).

induction The process of electrical fields acting on one another without contact.

inductive reactance The ability of an alternating current to switch directions, causing the opposing potential difference to induce against the incoming supply of electrons; measured in ohms of resistance.

inherent filtration Results from the composition of the tube and housing.

insulator A material that inhibits electron flow.

integral dose The total amount of energy imparted to matter; the product of dose and the mass over which the energy is imparted.

intensification factor The most accurate factor that measures the speed or sensitivity of an intensifying screen; a measurement of the amplification of the image that occurs due to the screen's ability to convert x-ray photons to light.

intensifying screen Device used to amplify the incoming x-ray beam and reduce patient radiation dose.

inverse square law Law of electrostatics that states the force between two charges is directly proportional to the product of their magnitudes and inversely proportional to the square of the distance between them.

inverse variation When two quantities are multiplied, their product is a constant.

inversion time (TI) The time between a 180-degree pulse and a 90-degree inversion pulse in an inversion recovery pulse sequence.

ion An atom that has gained or lost an electron.

ionic solution Charged particles dissolved within a solution.

ionization The process of adding or removing an electron from an atom.

ionization chamber device An automatic exposure control device used to terminate the exposure after a desired exposure has been reached.

isotope Atoms that have the same number of protons in the nucleus but differ in the number of neutrons.

K-edge filter The use of two or more materials to complement one another in their absorbing abilities; also known as compound filters.

kerma Kinetic energy released in matter; the energy imparted directly to electrons per unit mass.

kilogram The standard unit of mass, abbreviated as kg.

kinetic energy The energy of motion.

K-shell absorption edge When the incident x-ray photons match the K-shell binding energy of the phosphor, there is an increase in characteristic production within the screen.

K-shell The orbital shell closest to the nucleus.

lambda The Greek letter that represents the measurement of a wavelength.

Larmor frequency In a static homogenous magnetic field, all protons in a nucleus of a given type element will rotate with exactly the same frequency.

laser film A type of film that is directly exposed by the laser used in the imaging camera.

latitude The range of exposures that will produce densities within the diagnostic range.

laws of electrostatics Rules relating how objects are electrified.

leakage radiation Any photons that escape from the housing except at the port.

like terms Terms (numbers) with identical literal factors (usually noted by a letter).

line spread function (LSF) Measurement of recorded detail, sharpness, and resolution; the ability of a film/screen system to accurately measure the boundaries of an image.

linear grid A grid with lead strips running in only one direction.

line-focus principle Used to reduce the effective area of the focal spot.

lines of flux The force fields that are created when magnetic dipoles orient to create a magnet; also called lines of force and magnetic field.

lines of force The force fields that are created when magnetic dipoles orient to create a magnet; also called lines of flux and magnetic field.

line pairs per millimeter (lp/mm) Measurement of recorded detail, sharpness, and resolution; the minimum size and space between objects that can be visualized on the final image.

low-pass filtering Amplifies or deletes all but the low frequencies.

luminescence The ability of a material to emit light in response to excitation.

M theory Electrons and quarks may not be particles, but instead may be extremely small loops of rapidly vibrating string-like matter.

Mach effect Each time the eye sees a change in density, there is a change in the intensity of the impulses sent to the brain.

magnet An object that exhibits a uniformly strong magnetic field.

magnetic dipole Groups of atoms with their net magnetic field moving in the same direction; also know as magnetic domains.

magnetic domain Groups of atoms with their net magnetic field moving in the same direction; also know as magnetic dipoles.

magnetic field The force fields that are created when magnetic dipoles orient to create a magnet; also called lines of flux and lines of force.

magnetic resonance The effect that occurs when an electromagnetic RF field that is alternating, or resonating, at the Larmor frequency is applied in addition to the static field, causing protons to alternate from parallel to antiparallel.

main circuit Supplies the x-ray tube with properly modified power.

mains The alternating current that is supplied to buildings; usually supplied in three-phase power cycle; also called the incoming-line current.

main switch The switch that generates the power to the x-ray tube.

mammography X-ray examination of the breast.

mammography unit Specialized radiography equipment for studies and imaging of the breast tissues.

mask The process of modifying pixel values by a mathematical formula; also referred to as convolution.

masking Indicates the frequencies that have been suppressed during the filtering process.

mass The quantity of matter contained in an object.

matrix A square series of boxes that gives form to the image.

mechanical energy The result of the action of machines or physical movement; can be potential or kinetic.

metallic conductor The most common pathway for the movement of electrical current (e.g., copper).

metallic replacement A fixer recovery unit in which the fixer acid breaks down the iron in a steel screen or in steel wool and displaces it with silver.

meter The standard unit of length, abbreviated as m.

milliamperage (mA) A measurement of x-ray tube current—the number of electrons crossing the tube from cathode to anode per second.

milliamperage-second (mAs) The product of tube current and exposure time.

milliampere-second timer A device used in falling load generators and some capacitor units to monitor the product of mA and time on the secondary side of the high-voltage step-up transformer.

minification gain Resulting from the same number of electrons that were produced at the large input screen being compressed into the area of the small output screen.

minimum reaction (or response) time The length of time necessary for the AEC to respond to the radiation and for the generator to terminate the exposure.

minimum response time The length of time necessary for the AEC to respond to the ionization and send a signal to terminate the exposure.

mixing The period of film production in which the shredded emulsion is melted at a precise temperature to properly sensitize the crystals.

mixture The combination of two or more substances.

mobile system A type of radiography equipment that can be brought to the patient anywhere the patient may be.

modulation transfer function (MTF) Measurement of recorded detail, sharpness, and resolution; measures the resolving ability of a film/screen combination.

molecule Two or more atoms chemically united; the smallest particle of a compound that still possesses the characteristics of the compound.

molybdenum In mammography, the anode is made of this element.

motor A device that is supplied with electrical current to produce mechanical motion.

movement Second law of electrostatics that states only negative charges move along solid conductors.

multiple myeloma A malignant tumor arising from plasma cells of bone marrow, causing a reduction in bone composition.

mutual induction The result of two coils being placed in close proximity with a varying current supplied to the first coil, which then induces a similar flow in the second coil.

natural magnet Created when iron oxide remains in the earth's magnetic field for ages, slowly orienting the magnetic dipoles in the same direction (e.g., lodestones).

negatron A negatively charged electron resulting from pair production.

neutron (n^0) Subatomic particle of an atom containing no charge.

nonmagnetic Materials not affected by magnetic fields and cannot be magnetized (e.g., wood, glass, rubber, plastic).

nu Greek letter used to denote the number of cycles per second.

nuclear energy The energy stored in the bond of the nucleus of an atom.

nuclear magnetic moment The rotating charge within a spinning nucleus which produces a magnetic field.

nucleon The protons and neutrons that make up the nucleus.

nucleus The small dense center of an atom; consists of protons and neutrons.

Nyquist criterion The sampling of the spatial resolution frequency signal twice from each cycle in digital systems.

occasionally exposed worker Workers whose duties may occasionally bring them into areas where radiation exposure may occur.

occupationally exposed worker Workers who have a significant potential for exposure to radiation in the course of their employment.

octet rule The number of electrons in the outermost shell never exceeds eight electrons.

off-focus radiation Photons that were not produced at the focal spot; also called extrafocal radiation.

ohm (Ω) The unit of resistance.

opacity The ability of a film to stop light.

open equation An equation that contains at least one unknown (variable).

open-core transformer Arrangement of two coils of wire each filled with an iron core in proximity to facilitate induction.

optical density numbers The numbers displayed by a densitometer.

optically stimulated luminescence (OSL) dosimeter Measures radiation that passes through a thin strip of aluminum oxide. A laser light simulates the aluminum oxide, which becomes luminescent in proportion to the amount of radiation exposure.

optimal kVp The maximum kVp level that will produce images with appropriate contrast that are consistently within acceptance limits.

orbital magnetic moment The motion of a charged particle creates a magnetic force field perpendicular to the motion.

orthochromatic A film that is not sensitive to the red spectrum.

osteitis deformans New bone growth resulting from an increase in bone cell activity.

osteoblastic metastases New bone growth resulting from the spread of cancer in bone.

osteochondroma A tumor in the bone and cartilage.

osteolytic metastases Destruction of bone due to malignancies that have spread to the bone.

osteomalacia A defect in bone mineralization, causing decreased composition.

osteoporosis A defect in bone production due to failure of osteoblasts to lay down bone matrix.

overhead suspension system A type of radiography unit that allows control of longitudinal and transverse positioning as well as vertical distance.

Paget's disease New bone growth resulting from an increase in bone cell activity.

pair production An interaction between x-rays and matter characterized by the conversion of the energy of an x-ray photon into matter in the form of two electrons.

panchromatic A film that is sensitive to all colors.

panoramic dental and facial unit Specialized radiography equipment for combined tomography of facial and dental structures.

pantomography A type of tomography that permits a slit scan of curved surfaces such as the face and head.

parallel circuit An electric circuit designed to send electrons through various resistance devices by giving each component its own branch.

parallel grid A grid created with the lead and interspace strips running parallel to one another; the lines will never intersect.

paramagnetic Materials that have a low permeability and weak attraction to magnetic fields (e.g., aluminum).

particulate radiation High-energy electrons, neutrons, and protons that produce ionization in matter by direct atomic collisions.

pass box A lightproof container set in the wall of the darkroom used to pass film through for processing.

pathology The medical science concerned with all aspects of disease, including the structural and functional changes caused by a disease process.

patient equivalent phantom A dummy or surrogate device that can be imaged that will mimic the thickness of an actual patient; used to control quality and acceptance levels of radiographic images.

penetrability The ability of the x-ray to pass through structures and tissues.

penetrometer A series of increasingly thick, uniform absorbers.

penumbra A geometric unsharpness around the periphery of the image.

period The time required to complete one cycle of the wave.

permeability The ease with which a material can be magnetized.

personnel monitoring device Instrument worn by health care workers who work regularly in radiation-exposed environments.

phenidone A chemical that quickly reduces silver, enhancing fine detail and subtle shades of gray, and works only in areas of light exposure.

phosphor layer A layer of material used in an intensifying screen that is capable of absorbing the energy of an incident x-ray photon and then emitting light photons.

phosphorescence The ability of a material to delay emission of light in response to excitation.

photodisintegration An interaction between x-rays and matter characterized by the interaction between a high-energy photon and the nucleus. The high-energy photon strikes the nucleus; the nucleus absorbs all the photons energy and then emits a nuclear fragment.

photoelectric absorption An interaction between x-rays and matter characterized by an incident electron with slightly greater energy than the binding energy of the electrons in the inner shells, ejecting an electron from the inner shell while being absorbed in the reaction, resulting in an ionized atom.

photoelectron An ionized atom with a missing inner-shell electron resulting from ejection of the electron due to photoelectric absorption.

photon A small bundle of energy. The specific amount of energy depends on frequency; also known as a quantum.

phototimer Often used to describe all automatic exposure controls; this type of AED is rarely used in modern radiography.

picture archiving and communication system (PACS) A computer system that can manage images in an electronic form.

pitch The extension or contraction of the helix; the ratio of the distance the table moves during one 360-degree tube rotation to the total beam collimation.

pixel Picture elements; individual matrix boxes.

pleural effusions The filling of the pleural cavity with blood or serous fluid.

pneumoconiosis The inhalation of dust particles, causing fibrotic scarring of the lungs.

pneumonectomy The removal of a lung.

pneumonia Inflammation of lung tissues, causing fluid to fill the alveolar spaces.

pneumonitis Inflammation of lung tissues, causing fluid to fill the alveolar spaces.

pneumothorax Free air in the pleural cavity that displaces lung tissue.

pocket dosimeter A personal use ionization chamber. When exposed to radiation, ionization occurs in the chamber, which neutralizes a positively charged electrode that will appear as movement of an exposure scale.

point spread function (PSF) Expression of the boundaries of an image; determined by a mathematical measurement of an image produced at a single point.

positive beam limitation device (PBL) An automatic collimator that adjusts to the size and placement of the cassette.

positron A positively charged electron resulting from pair production.

potential difference The force or strength of electron flow; also known as electromotive force (emf).

potential energy The energy an object has because of its position.

potentiometer A variable resistor that permits a variable contact to slide along a series circuit of resistance coils.

power loss formula Calculation that can provide an understanding of the changes in resistance to heat output.

precession Rotation of the axis of rotation within a nucleus when it encounters a magnetic field; causes a loss in momentum.

preservative A chemical used in film processing to help decrease the oxidation of the reducing agents when they are combined with air; also used in fixer solution to aid in removal of silver from the emulsion.

primary barrier A shielding structure that can be struck by the primary x-ray beam exiting the x-ray tube.

primary coil The coil first supplied with the current.

prime factor Factors related to x-ray emission that are under the direct control of the radiographer; milliamperage, kilovoltage, and distance.

program Operating instructions.

progressive scanning Increases resolution by scanning all 525 lines in order.

protective coat A layer of material used in an intensifying screen applied to the top of the phosphor layer to protect it from abrasions and stains; usually thick plastic.

protective device Items worn by the radiation worker to reduce exposure to radiation.

protective housing The entire cathode and anode assembly is housed within this metal structure.

proton (p^+) Positively charged subatomic particle of an atom.

proton (spin) density The quantity of resonating spins in a tissue.

proton spin density image The effect that is measured by the number of protons spinning in tissue volume.

pulmonary edema The filling of the interstitial lung tissues and alveoli with fluid.

pyramid problem Acceptable images depend on many factors. If any of those factors are off, it can cause a problem in various other factors, thus a pyramid affect of problems is the result.

quality assurance All activities that provide adequate confidence that a radiology service will render consistently high-quality images and services.

quality control The aspect of quality assurance that monitors technical equipment to maintain superior standards.

quality factor Radiation weighting factor, specific to specific types of radiation; accounts for the biological effectiveness of the specific radiation.

quantum A small bundle of energy. The specific amount of energy depends on frequency; also known as a photon.

quantum mottle A lack of sufficient incoming data to process an image; also known as quantum noise.

quantum noise A lack of sufficient incoming data to process an image; also known as quantum mottle.

quark Subnuclear structure that makes up protons and neutrons.

quenching Overheating of the superconducting magnet due to vaporization of gasses needed to maintain the environment for superconduction.

rad Term used to describe the measurement related to the absorbed dose of radiation; unit of absorbed energy or dose applicable to any material; 100 ergs of energy absorbed in 1 gram of absorbing material.

radiation Energy emitted and transferred through matter.

radiation fog The result of scattered photons striking the radiographic film and placing a density on the film that is unrelated to the patient's anatomy.

radiation worker An individual, who through occupational risk, has a certain likelihood of exposure to ionizing radiation in the course of his or her normal duties.

radiographic tube rating chart A guide regarding the most common technical factor combinations that can be used without overloading the tube.

radiology information system (RIS) A database of images and patient records specific to the imaging department.

ramping The process of bringing the superconducting magnet to the necessary temperature by using cryogens.

random-access memory (RAM) Temporary storage for programming and operating instructions during use that are constantly changing.

rate of precession The angular velocity of the nuclear magnetic field.

read-only memory (ROM) Basic operating instructions that never change.

reciprocity law The density on an x-ray film should remain unchanged as long as the intensity and duration of the x-ray exposure remains unchanged.

reciprocity law failure Failure to maintain consistent exposures when extremely short or long exposure times are used.

recoil electron The dislodged electron resulting from Compton scattering; also called a Compton electron.

recorded detail One of the geometric properties of image quality; the degree of geometric sharpness or accuracy of structural lines actually recorded in the image; also referred to as detail, definition, sharpness, spatial resolution.

rectification The process by which alternating current is changed to pulsating direct current.

reducing agent A chemical used in film developing that provides electrons to the silver ions attached to the sensitivity specks of the silver halide crystals.

reference axis target angle In mammography, measured from the center of the x-ray beam as in conventional radiography.

reference axis The angled central ray as used in mammography.

reflective layer A layer of material used in an intensifying screen to reflect light toward the film.

relative speed The most useful rating of intensifying screens; expressed with par-screens and film being arbitrarily assigned a relative speed number of 100 as a control point.

rem Term used to describe the measurement of the biologically equivalent dose.

repetition time (TR) The time interval between pulse sequences.

replenishment system Replaces chemicals that are depleted through the chemical reactions of processing, oxidation, and evaporation.

repulsion-attraction Law of electrostatics that states like charges repel and unlike charges attract.

resin A type of silver recovery system that uses acid to form resin ions. The silver is attracted to the resin; the resin is processed to remove the silver.

resistance The amount of opposition to the current in the circuit.

resolution The ability to accurately image an object; measured by the ability to see pairs of lines.

resolving power The ability to accurately image an object; measured by the ability to see pairs of lines.

restrainer A chemical used in film processing added to the developer to restrict the reducing action to those crystals with sensitivity speck gates.

retentivity The ability of a material to stay magnetized.

reversal The process of reducing the intensity of the latent image, producing less density.

rheostat A device constructed to interrupt a circuit before a dangerous temperature is reached.

rhodium In mammography, newer anodes are made from this substance.

ripening The period of film production during which silver halides are allowed to grow.

rod cell Cells in the retina of the eye that are sensitive to dim light.

roentgen (R) Term used to describe the measurement related to exposure; the unit of exposure in air; the quantity of x-rays or gamma rays required to produce a given amount of ionization in a unit mass of air.

rotating anode An anode assembly that turns during exposure.

rotor A hollow copper cylinder or cuff that is attached to the anode disk by a molybdenum shaft.

saturation current As kVp increases, a greater percentage of the thermionically emitted electrons are driven toward the anode.

scale of contrast The number of useful visible densities or shades of gray.

scanning Examining a particular area for information.

scattering The interaction of x-ray photons and matter that causes a change in direction of the photons.

sclerosis An increase in bone hardening resulting from a chronic inflammation of the bone.

screen lag Delayed phosphorescent emission; also called afterglow.

second The standard unit of time, abbreviated as s.

secondary barrier A shielding structure that can be struck by scattered and leakage radiation.

secondary coil The coil in which a current is inducted by the primary coil.

secondary radiation A characteristic photon created by the electron transfer from one shell to another but occurring outside the x-ray target.

section interval The distance between the fulcrum levels.

section thickness The width of the focal plane which is controlled by the exposure angle.

self-induction The ability of an alternating current to switch directions, causing an opposing potential difference to induce against the incoming supply of electrons; allows direct current to flow while at the same time hindering alternating current.

self-rectification Suppressed rectification resulting from only half of the incoming alternating current being converted to pulsating direct current; called half-wave rectification.

semiconductor A material that allows electrons to flow freely under certain conditions (conductor) or that inhibits electron flow under certain conditions (insulator).

sensitivity speck An impurity added to silver halide crystals (usually gold-silver sulfide) to act as an electrode that attracts free silver ions during latent image formation.

sensitometer An instrument designed to expose a reproducible uniform, optical step wedge onto a film.

sensitometric curve A radiographic relationship between the amount of exposure and the resultant density on the film; also known as characteristic curve, D log E curve, and Hurter and Driffield curve.

sensitometry The measurement of the characteristic responses of film to exposure and processing.

series circuit An electric circuit designed to send electrons through various resistance devices by linking them one after the other.

sharpening Increase in contrast due to high-pass filtering; also known as edge enhancement.

sharpness One of the geometric properties of image quality; the degree of geometric sharpness or accuracy of structural lines actually recorded in the image; also referred to as detail, definition, recorded detail, spatial resolution.

shell The energy level occupied by an electron determined by the distance from the nucleus.

shell-type transformer Arrangement of two coils of wire each filled with an iron core in proximity to facilitate induction.

shim coils Corrective magnetic coils.

shoulder supports A piece of equipment that keeps the patient from sliding off the table when the table is tilted head down.

sievert (Sv) The product of the absorbed dose in gray and the radiation weighting factor.

signal-to-noise ratio White noise or "snow."

silicon-controlled rectifier (SCR) A complex semiconductor useful for high-speed switching of the primary high-voltage x-ray circuit; also known as a thyristor.

silver bromide Type of silver halide crystal used to create x-ray films.

silver chloride Type of silver halide crystal used to create x-ray films.

silver iodide Type of silver halide crystal used to create x-ray films.

silver iodobromide Type of silver halide crystal used to create x-ray films.

simulator unit Specialized radiography equipment that allows verification of radiation therapy prior to actual treatment.

sine wave The type of curve produced by an AC generator.

single-phase power Power supply that allows the potential difference to drop to zero with every change in the direction of current flow.

slip ring A device with attached brushes that allows the circuit to remain stationary while the armature rotates without breaking the electrical contact between them.

slow scanning Increases resolution.

smoothing A type of low-pass filtering accomplished by averaging each pixel's value with that of adjacent pixels.

soft copy Images visualized on monitors, either flat panel technology or older cathode ray tubes.

software Programs used on a computer.

solar converter A device that converts solar photons to electrical energy.

solarization The process of reducing the intensity of the latent image, producing less density.

solenoid A coil consisting of a series of loops, which serve to increase the flux density.

solvent Chemicals used in developing film suspended in water.

somatic Describes the effects of radiation that appear in the individual who was irradiated.

space charge cloud The ejection of electrons from the surface of the wire due to increased heat, causing an electron cloud; also called thermionic emission.

space charge effect As more and more electrons build up in the area of the filament, their negative charges begin to oppose the emission of additional electrons.

spatial resolution One of the geometric properties of image quality; the degree of geometric sharpness or accuracy of structural lines actually recorded in the image; also referred to as detail, definition, sharpness, recoded detail. In digital images, it can be expressed in terms of three dimensions of the image.

specific absorption rate (SAR) The absorption of RF radiation.

spectral emission An indication of the precise wavelength of light emitted by the phosphor.

speed exposure point The log exposure that will produce the speed point for a given film.

speed point The point on the D log E curve where a density of ODD $1.0 + b + f$ is achieved.

spin magnetic moment The magnetic effect created by electrons spinning on their axes.

spin-lattice relaxation time (T_1) The time required for precessing spins to align with the constant external magnetic field to 63 percent of the maximum possible strength.

spin-spin relaxation time (T_2) The time required after precessing spins have aligned at an angle to the external magnetic field due to an RF pulse for them to lose 63 percent of their coherence due to interactions between the spins.

standby replenishment A type of flood replenishing system used for low-volume systems; controlled by a timer that floods the developer and fixer tanks with replenisher at regular intervals.

standby switch Shuts down a processing system after 2 minutes of inactivity; must be manually activated to bring the unit up for processing.

starter solution A solution of acetic acid and potassium bromide that is added to the replenisher solution when starting a fresh tank of developer.

static discharge The result of electrons jumping the gap between two objects, one negatively charged and one positively charged, resulting in the equalization of the charges of the two objects.

stationary anode An anode assembly that is immobile.

stator Induction-motor electromagnets that turn the anode.

step wedge A type of penetrometer that is wedge shaped and has different levels or steps.

step-down transformer A device used to decrease the voltage from the primary to the secondary coil.

step-up transformer A device used to increase the voltage from the primary to the secondary coil.

stochastic effects Results of radiation exposure for which no threshold dose of radiation exists (e.g., cancer, genetic effects).

straight line portion The useful range of densities on the D log E curve.

string theory The idea that matter behaves differently depending on the vibration on the string-like matter.

structural protective barriers Fixed x-ray facilities that are constructed of materials having effective x-ray attenuating properties and are of thickness sufficient to reduce exposures to desired levels.

subject contrast The degree of differential absorption resulting from the differing absorption characteristics of the tissues in the body.

subject density The impact the subject (patient) has on the resulting radiographic density.

subject detail The impact that the position of the structures of interest with the body has on the recorded detail.

subject distortion The impact that the position of the structures of interest within the body has on distortion.

substance A material that has a definite and constant composition.

superadditivity When two reducing agents are combined, forming a PQ developer, their reducing ability is the sum of their independent abilities.

supercoat A layer of hard, protective gelatin designed to prevent the soft emulsion underneath from being physically or chemically abused due to handling.

superconductor A material that allows electrons to flow freely.

surface coil An RF coil shaped to conform to the body part being imaged.

Système International d'Unités (SI units) An international system of units based on the metric system.

tailing If the silver recovery is not sufficient, a second process is undergone to process the solution after it has gone through the first unit.

target The portion of the anode where the high-voltage electron stream will impact.

target interaction The actions that take place when the electrons strike their target or focal spot.

targeting A magnification technique which permits an area of interest to be selected for reformatting.

temperature A measure of thermal energy.

temperature control system The part of the automatic processing unit that maintains all three solutions at compatible temperatures.

10-day rule The practice of waiting 10 days after a woman's menstrual flow to conduct a radiographic examination or study.

tesla (T) The unit used for measuring magnetic flux density.

therapeutic Methods used to treat and rehabilitate a disease, disorder, or traumatic injury.

thermal energy The result of the motion of atoms and molecules; also known as heat.

thermal noise Results from the increase of Brownian motion, which, in turn, increase body temperature.

thermionic emission The ejection of electrons from the surface of the wire due to increased heat, causing an electron cloud; also called the space charge cloud.

thermoluminescent dosimeter (TLD) Small chips of thermoluminescent material, usually lithium fluoride. When exposed to radiation, the chips enter a metastable state; when exposed to heat they give off visible light.

Thoreaus filter A type of compound filter consisting of tin, copper, and aluminum, in that order, typically used in radiation therapy.

three-phase 12-pulse A full-wave rectification produces a voltage ripple never dropping below 90–95 percent of the peak kilovoltage setting.

three-phase power Power supply generated as each wave peaks drops toward zero. The overall potential difference is boosted back to peak by the next phase wave; the sum of the phasing never drops to zero.

three-phase six-pulse A full-wave rectification produces a voltage ripple that produces six usable pulses per cycle.

threshold detection A visual phenomenon involving the perception of extremely small or faint details.

thyristor A complex semiconductor useful for high-speed switching of the primary high-voltage x-ray circuit; also known as a silicon-controlled rectifier (SCR).

tilting A piece of equipment that is movable and can be angled according to need.

timed replenishment A type of flood replenishing system used for low-volume systems; controlled by a timer that floods the developer and fixer tanks with replenisher at regular intervals.

timer Device used to end the exposure at an accurately measured preset time.

tomographic amplitude The total distance the tube travels; tomographic arc or tomographic angle.

tomography A radiographic technique that employs motion to show anatomical structures lying in a plane of tissue while blurring or eliminating the detail in images of structures above and below the plane of interest.

tomography unit Specialized radiography equipment that allow movement in an arc during exposure.

total brightness gain A measurement of the increase in image intensity achieved by an image intensification tube.

total filtration The sum of inherent and added filtration.

total repeat rate A figure that is calculated as a percentage of the total number of images produced during the period of the study.

transformer A device in which two coils are placed near one another without electrical connection. The number of turns in the coils differs, causing a change in current in the secondary coil; this serves to either increase or decrease the voltage.

transport racks Part of the automatic processing transport system consisting of three rollers designed to move film through a processing tank.

transport system Part of the automatic processing system designed to move a film through developer, fixer, wash, and dryer sections of the processor.

trough filter A type of compensating filter used to even out densities such as in the mediastinum.

tube rating chart Provides a guide regarding the most common technical factor combinations that can be used without overloading the tube.

tuberculosis Infection by mycobacteria, causing inflammation of the lungs.

tumor An abnormal new growth in tissue.

urologic unit Specialized radiography equipment that allow study of the urological and genital structures.

vacuum A space from which air has been removed.

valence The chemical combining characteristic of an element; determined by the number of electrons in the outermost shell.

valence energy band The outermost (sometimes the next-to-outermost) orbital shell.

visual acuity The ability of the eye to resolve detail.

volt (V) The unit of potential difference.

voltage (V) The unit of potential difference.

voltage ripple The net voltage produced during full-wave rectification.

voltmeter A device used to measure current connected in parallel; measures potential difference in volts.

volume replenishment Type of replenishment system used for high-volume systems; activates when films enter the processor.

voxel Three-dimensional volume correlating to each pixel.

washing The process of using water to remove as much of the fixer and developer solutions as possible.

wavelength The distance between two successive points on a wave.

Weber (Wb) SI unit used to measure magnetic flux.

wedge filter A type of compensating filter used to even out densities such as in the foot or lower extremities.

weight The force that an object exerts under the influence of gravity.

window A structure where the primary x-ray beams exits the envelope, which allows less absorption or scatter of photons.

window level The digital processing that produces changes in density/brightness.

window width The digital processing that produces changes in the range of density/brightness, which can be used to control contrast.

wiring The parts within the cathode assembly that connect the elements of the assembly together.

x-ray quality A measurement of the penetrating ability of the x-ray beam.

x-ray quantity A measure of the number of x-ray photons in the useful beam.

z number The number of nuclear protons in an atom, unique to each element; also known as the atomic number.

zero potential A neutral reference point for discussing charges. The earth is defined as zero; also known as ground potential.

zonography Narrow-angle tomography.

Index